Lippincott's Illustrated Reviews: Biochemistry

Fifth Edition

Lippincott's Illustrated Reviews: Biochemistry

Fifth Edition

Richard A. Harvey, PhD
Professor Emeritus
Department of Biochemistry
University of Medicine and Dentistry of New Jersey–
Robert Wood Johnson Medical School
Piscataway, New Jersey

Denise R. Ferrier, PhD
Professor
Department of Biochemistry and Molecular Biology
Drexel University College of Medicine
Philadelphia, Pennsylvania

Wolters Kluwer | Lippincott Williams & Wilkins
Health

Philadelphia · Baltimore · New York · London
Buenos Aires · Hong Kong · Sydney · Tokyo

Acquisitions Editor: Susan Rhyner
Product Manager: Jennifer Verbiar
Designer: Holly Reid McLaughlin

Printed in China

Library of Congress Cataloging-in-Publication Data

Harvey, Richard A., Ph. D.
  Biochemistry / Richard A. Harvey, Denise R. Ferrier ; computer graphics, Michael Cooper. -- 5th ed.
    p. cm.
  Rev. ed. of: Biochemistry / Pamela C. Champe, Richard A. Harvey, Denise R. Ferrier. 4th ed. c2008.
  Includes bibliographical references and index.
  ISBN 978-1-60831-412-6 (alk. paper)
  1. Biochemistry--Outlines, syllabi, etc. 2. Biochemistry--Examinations, questions, etc. 3. Clinical biochemistry--Outlines, syllabi, etc. 4. Clinical biochemistry--Examinations, questions, etc. I. Ferrier, Denise R. II. Title.
  QP514.2.C48 2010
  612'.015--dc22
2010008046

The publishers have made every effort to trace the copyright holders for borrowed material. If they have inadvertently overlooked any, they will be pleased to make the necessary arrangements at the first opportunity.

Contributing Authors (Chapter 26)

Susan K. Fried, PhD
Professor
Department of Medicine
Section of Endocrinology, Diabetes and Nutrition
Boston University School of Medicine
Boston, Massachusetts

Richard B. Horenstein, MD
Assistant Professor
Department of Medicine
Division of Endocrinology, Diabetes and Nutrition
University of Maryland Medical Center
Baltimore, Maryland

Computer Graphics:

Michael Cooper
Cooper Graphics
www.cooper247.com

This book is dedicated to the
memory of our dear friend and
colleague Pamela Champe,
whose commitment to her
students and love of biochemistry
made her the consummate
teacher and mentor.

Contents

Amino Acids

1

I. OVERVIEW

Proteins are the most abundant and functionally diverse molecules in living systems. Virtually every life process depends on this class of molecules. For example, enzymes and polypeptide hormones direct and regulate metabolism in the body, whereas contractile proteins in muscle permit movement. In bone, the protein collagen forms a framework for the deposition of calcium phosphate crystals, acting like the steel cables in reinforced concrete. In the bloodstream, proteins, such as hemoglobin and plasma albumin, shuttle molecules essential to life, whereas immunoglobulins fight infectious bacteria and viruses. In short, proteins display an incredible diversity of functions, yet all share the common structural feature of being linear polymers of amino acids. This chapter describes the properties of amino acids. Chapter 2 explores how these simple building blocks are joined to form proteins that have unique three-dimensional structures, making them capable of performing specific biologic functions.

II. STRUCTURE OF THE AMINO ACIDS

Although more than 300 different amino acids have been described in nature, only 20 are commonly found as constituents of mammalian proteins. [Note: These are the only amino acids that are coded for by DNA, the genetic material in the cell (see p. 395).] Each amino acid (except for proline, which has a secondary amino group) has a carboxyl group, a primary amino group, and a distinctive side chain ("R-group") bonded to the α-carbon atom (Figure 1.1A). At physiologic pH (approximately pH 7.4), the carboxyl group is dissociated, forming the negatively charged carboxylate ion ($-COO^-$), and the amino group is protonated ($-NH_3^+$). In proteins, almost all of these carboxyl and amino groups are combined through peptide linkage and, in general, are not available for chemical reaction except for hydrogen bond formation (Figure 1.1B). Thus, it is the nature of the side chains that ultimately dictates the role

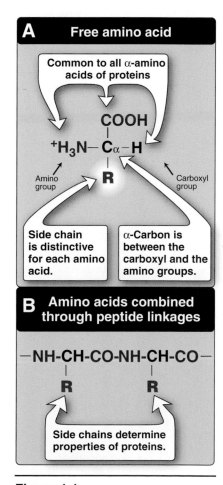

Figure 1.1
Structural features of amino acids (shown in their fully protonated form).

an amino acid plays in a protein. It is, therefore, useful to classify the amino acids according to the properties of their side chains, that is, whether they are nonpolar (have an even distribution of electrons) or polar (have an uneven distribution of electrons, such as acids and bases; Figures 1.2 and 1.3).

A. Amino acids with nonpolar side chains

Each of these amino acids has a nonpolar side chain that does not gain or lose protons or participate in hydrogen or ionic bonds (Figure 1.2). The side chains of these amino acids can be thought of as "oily" or lipid-like, a property that promotes hydrophobic interactions (see Figure 2.10, p. 19).

1. **Location of nonpolar amino acids in proteins:** In proteins found in aqueous solutions—a polar environment—the side chains of the nonpolar amino acids tend to cluster together in the interior of the protein (Figure 1.4). This phenomenon, known as the hydrophobic

NONPOLAR SIDE CHAINS

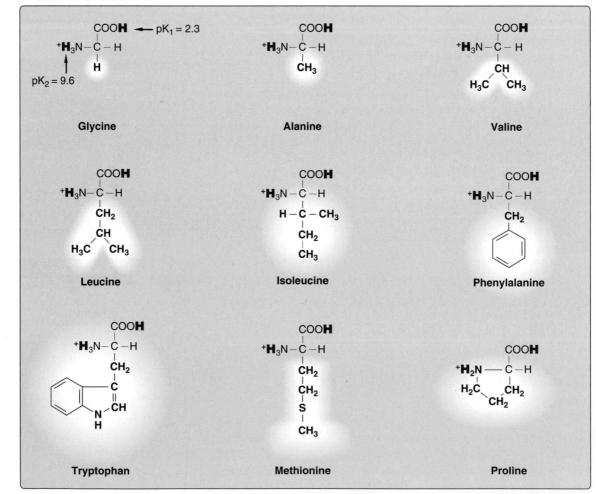

Figure 1.2
Classification of the 20 amino acids commonly found in proteins, according to the charge and polarity of their side chains at acidic pH is shown here and continues in Figure 1.3. Each amino acid is shown in its fully protonated form, with dissociable hydrogen ions represented in red print. The pK values for the α-carboxyl and α-amino groups of the nonpolar amino acids are similar to those shown for glycine. (Continued in Figure 1.3.)

UNCHARGED POLAR SIDE CHAINS

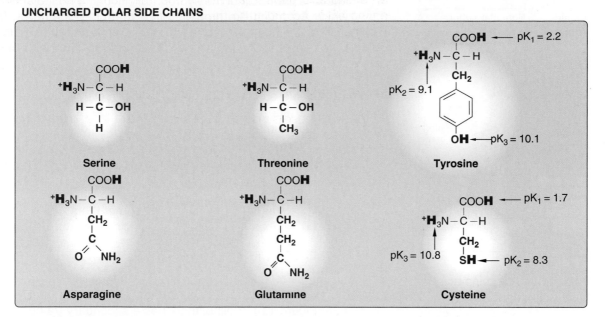

ACIDIC SIDE CHAINS

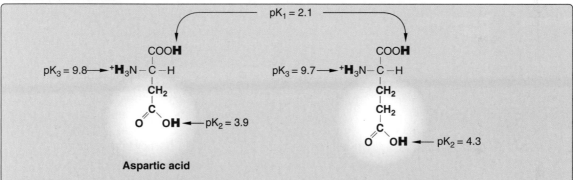

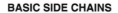

Aspartic acid

BASIC SIDE CHAINS

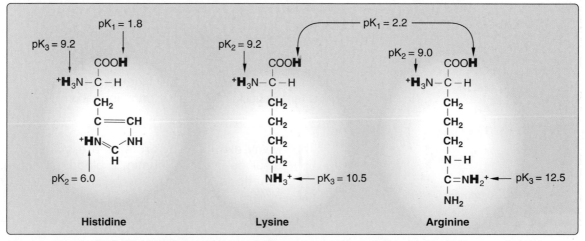

Figure 1.3

Classification of the 20 amino acids commonly found in proteins, according to the charge and polarity of their side chains at acidic pH (continued from Figure 1.2).

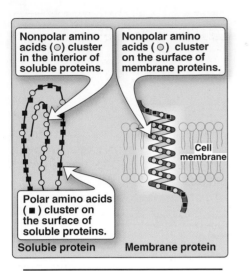

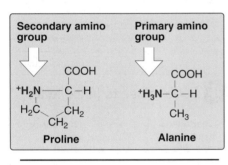

Figure 1.4
Location of nonpolar amino acids in soluble and membrane proteins.

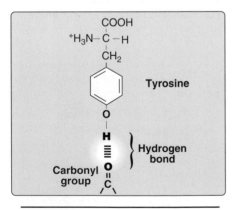

Figure 1.5
Comparison of the secondary amino group found in proline with the primary amino group found in other amino acids, such as alanine.

Figure 1.6
Hydrogen bond between the phenolic hydroxyl group of tyrosine and another molecule containing a carbonyl group.

effect, is the result of the hydrophobicity of the nonpolar R-groups, which act much like droplets of oil that coalesce in an aqueous environment. The nonpolar R-groups thus fill up the interior of the folded protein and help give it its three-dimensional shape. However, for proteins that are located in a hydrophobic environment, such as a membrane, the nonpolar R-groups are found on the outside surface of the protein, interacting with the lipid environment (see Figure 1.4). The importance of these hydrophobic interactions in stabilizing protein structure is discussed on p. 19.

> Sickle cell anemia, a sickling disease of red blood cells, results from the substitution of polar glutamate by nonpolar valine at the sixth position in the β subunit of hemoglobin (see p. 36).

2. **Proline:** Proline differs from other amino acids in that proline's side chain and α-amino N form a rigid, five-membered ring structure (Figure 1.5). Proline, then, has a secondary (rather than a primary) amino group. It is frequently referred to as an imino acid. The unique geometry of proline contributes to the formation of the fibrous structure of collagen (see p. 45), and often interrupts the α-helices found in globular proteins (see p. 26).

B. Amino acids with uncharged polar side chains

These amino acids have zero net charge at neutral pH, although the side chains of cysteine and tyrosine can lose a proton at an alkaline pH (see Figure 1.3). Serine, threonine, and tyrosine each contain a polar hydroxyl group that can participate in hydrogen bond formation (Figure 1.6). The side chains of asparagine and glutamine each contain a carbonyl group and an amide group, both of which can also participate in hydrogen bonds.

1. **Disulfide bond:** The side chain of cysteine contains a sulfhydryl group (–SH), which is an important component of the active site of many enzymes. In proteins, the –SH groups of two cysteines can become oxidized to form a dimer, cystine, which contains a covalent cross-link called a disulfide bond (–S–S–). (See p. 19 for a further discussion of disulfide bond formation.)

> Many extracellular proteins are stabilized by disulfide bonds. Albumin, a blood protein that functions as a transporter for a variety of molecules, is an example.

2. **Side chains as sites of attachment for other compounds:** The polar hydroxyl group of serine, threonine, and, rarely, tyrosine, can serve as a site of attachment for structures such as a phosphate group. In addition, the amide group of asparagine, as well as the hydroxyl group of serine or threonine, can serve as a site of attachment for oligosaccharide chains in glycoproteins (see p. 165).

C. Amino acids with acidic side chains

The amino acids aspartic and glutamic acid are proton donors. At physiologic pH, the side chains of these amino acids are fully ionized, containing a negatively charged carboxylate group (–COO⁻). They are, therefore, called aspartate or glutamate to emphasize that these amino acids are negatively charged at physiologic pH (see Figure 1.3).

D. Amino acids with basic side chains

The side chains of the basic amino acids accept protons (see Figure 1.3). At physiologic pH the side chains of lysine and arginine are fully ionized and positively charged. In contrast, histidine is weakly basic, and the free amino acid is largely uncharged at physiologic pH. However, when histidine is incorporated into a protein, its side chain can be either positively charged or neutral, depending on the ionic environment provided by the polypeptide chains of the protein. This is an important property of histidine that contributes to the role it plays in the functioning of proteins such as hemoglobin (see p. 31).

E. Abbreviations and symbols for commonly occurring amino acids

Each amino acid name has an associated three-letter abbreviation and a one-letter symbol (Figure 1.7). The one-letter codes are determined by the following rules:

1. **Unique first letter:** If only one amino acid begins with a particular letter, then that letter is used as its symbol. For example, I = isoleucine.

2. **Most commonly occurring amino acids have priority:** If more than one amino acid begins with a particular letter, the most common of these amino acids receives this letter as its symbol. For example, glycine is more common than glutamate, so G = glycine.

3. **Similar sounding names:** Some one-letter symbols sound like the amino acid they represent. For example, F = phenylalanine, or W = tryptophan ("twyptophan" as Elmer Fudd would say).

4. **Letter close to initial letter:** For the remaining amino acids, a one-letter symbol is assigned that is as close in the alphabet as possible to the initial letter of the amino acid, for example, K = lysine. Furthermore, B is assigned to Asx, signifying either aspartic acid or asparagine, Z is assigned to Glx, signifying either glutamic acid or glutamine, and X is assigned to an unidentified amino acid.

F. Optical properties of amino acids

The α-carbon of an amino acid is attached to four different chemical groups and is, therefore, a chiral or optically active carbon atom. Glycine is the exception because its α-carbon has two hydrogen substituents and, therefore, is optically inactive. Amino acids that have an asymmetric center at the α-carbon can exist in two forms, designated D and L, that are mirror images of each other (Figure 1.8). The two forms in each pair are termed stereoisomers, optical isomers, or enantiomers. All amino acids found in proteins are of the L-configuration. However, D-amino acids are found in some antibiotics and in plant and bacterial cell walls. (See p. 253 for a discussion of D-amino acid metabolism.)

---

1 **Unique first letter:**

Cysteine	=	Cys	=	**C**
Histidine	=	His	=	**H**
Isoleucine	=	Ile	=	**I**
Methionine	=	Met	=	**M**
Serine	=	Ser	=	**S**
Valine	=	Val	=	**V**

2 **Most commonly occurring amino acids have priority:**

Alanine	=	Ala	=	**A**
Glycine	=	Gly	=	**G**
Leucine	=	Leu	=	**L**
Proline	=	Pro	=	**P**
Threonine	=	Thr	=	**T**

3 **Similar sounding names:**

Arginine	=	Arg	=	**R** ("a**R**ginine")
Aspara**g**i**n**e	=	Asn	=	**N** (contains N)
Aspartate	=	Asp	=	**D** ("aspar**D**ic")
Glutamate	=	Glu	=	**E** ("glut**E**mate")
Glutami**n**e	=	Gln	=	**Q** ("**Q**-tamine")
Phenylalanine	=	Phe	=	**F** ("**F**enylalanine")
Tyrosine	=	Tyr	=	**Y** ("t**Y**rosine")
Trptophan	=	Trp	=	**W** (double ring in the molecule)

4 **Letter close to initial letter:**

Aspartate or asparagine	=	Asx =	**B** (near A)
Glutamate or glutamine	=	Glx =	**Z**
Lysine	=	Lys =	**K** (near L)
Undetermined amino acid	=		**X**

Figure 1.7
Abbreviations and symbols for the commonly occurring amino acids.

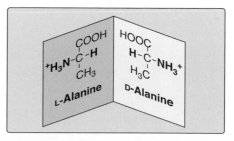

Figure 1.8
D and L forms of alanine are mirror images.

III. ACIDIC AND BASIC PROPERTIES OF AMINO ACIDS

Amino acids in aqueous solution contain weakly acidic α-carboxyl groups and weakly basic α-amino groups. In addition, each of the acidic and basic amino acids contains an ionizable group in its side chain. Thus, both free amino acids and some amino acids combined in peptide linkages can act as buffers. Recall that acids may be defined as proton donors and bases as proton acceptors. Acids (or bases) described as "weak" ionize to only a limited extent. The concentration of protons in aqueous solution is expressed as pH, where pH = log 1/[H^+] or $-\log$ [H^+]. The quantitative relationship between the pH of the solution and concentration of a weak acid (HA) and its conjugate base (A^-) is described by the Henderson-Hasselbalch equation.

A. Derivation of the equation

Consider the release of a proton by a weak acid represented by HA:

$$HA \quad \rightleftarrows \quad H^+ \quad + \quad A^-$$

weak   proton   salt form
acid   or conjugate base

The "salt" or conjugate base, A^-, is the ionized form of a weak acid. By definition, the dissociation constant of the acid, K_a, is

$$K_a = \frac{[H^+][A^-]}{[HA]}$$

[Note: The larger the K_a, the stronger the acid, because most of the HA has dissociated into H^+ and A^-. Conversely, the smaller the K_a, the less acid has dissociated and, therefore, the weaker the acid.] By solving for the [H^+] in the above equation, taking the logarithm of both sides of the equation, multiplying both sides of the equation by -1, and substituting pH = $-\log$ [H^+] and pK_a = $-\log K_a$, we obtain the Henderson-Hasselbalch equation:

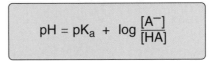

$$pH = pK_a + \log \frac{[A^-]}{[HA]}$$

B. Buffers

A buffer is a solution that resists change in pH following the addition of an acid or base. A buffer can be created by mixing a weak acid (HA) with its conjugate base (A^-). If an acid such as HCl is then added to such a solution, A^- can neutralize it, in the process being converted to HA. If a base is added, HA can neutralize it, in the process being converted to A^-. Maximum buffering capacity occurs at a pH equal to the pK_a, but a conjugate acid/base pair can still serve as an effective buffer when the pH of a solution is within approximately ± 1 pH unit of the pK_a. If the

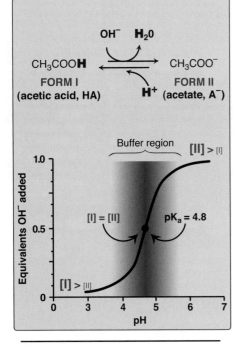

Figure 1.9
Titration curve of acetic acid.

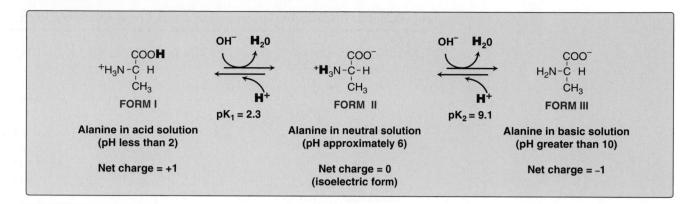

Figure 1.10
Ionic forms of alanine in acidic, neutral, and basic solutions.

amounts of HA and A⁻ are equal, the pH is equal to the pK_a. As shown in Figure 1.9, a solution containing acetic acid (HA = CH_3-COOH) and acetate (A⁻ = CH_3-COO^-) with a pK_a of 4.8 resists a change in pH from pH 3.8 to 5.8, with maximum buffering at pH 4.8. At pH values less than the pK_a, the protonated acid form (CH_3-COOH) is the predominant species. At pH values greater than the pK_a, the deprotonated base form (CH_3-COO^-) is the predominant species in solution.

C. Titration of an amino acid

1. **Dissociation of the carboxyl group:** The titration curve of an amino acid can be analyzed in the same way as described for acetic acid. Consider alanine, for example, which contains both an α-carboxyl and an α-amino group. At a low (acidic) pH, both of these groups are protonated (shown in Figure 1.10). As the pH of the solution is raised, the −COOH group of Form I can dissociate by donating a proton to the medium. The release of a proton results in the formation of the carboxylate group, −COO⁻. This structure is shown as Form II, which is the dipolar form of the molecule (see Figure 1.10). This form, also called a zwitterion, is the isoelectric form of alanine, that is, it has an overall (net) charge of zero.

2. **Application of the Henderson-Hasselbalch equation:** The dissociation constant of the carboxyl group of an amino acid is called K_1, rather than K_a, because the molecule contains a second titratable group. The Henderson-Hasselbalch equation can be used to analyze the dissociation of the carboxyl group of alanine in the same way as described for acetic acid:

$$K_1 = \frac{[H^+][II]}{[I]}$$

where I is the fully protonated form of alanine, and II is the isoelectric form of alanine (see Figure 1.10). This equation can be rearranged and converted to its logarithmic form to yield:

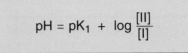

$$pH = pK_1 + \log \frac{[II]}{[I]}$$

3. Dissociation of the amino group: The second titratable group of alanine is the amino ($-NH_3^+$) group shown in Figure 1.10. This is a much weaker acid than the $-COOH$ group and, therefore, has a much smaller dissociation constant, K_2. [Note: Its pK_a is therefore larger.] Release of a proton from the protonated amino group of Form II results in the fully deprotonated form of alanine, Form III (see Figure 1.10).

4. pKs of alanine: The sequential dissociation of protons from the carboxyl and amino groups of alanine is summarized in Figure 1.10. Each titratable group has a pK_a that is numerically equal to the pH at which exactly one half of the protons have been removed from that group. The pK_a for the most acidic group ($-COOH$) is pK_1, whereas the pK_a for the next most acidic group ($-NH_3^+$) is pK_2.

5. Titration curve of alanine: By applying the Henderson-Hasselbalch equation to each dissociable acidic group, it is possible to calculate the complete titration curve of a weak acid. Figure 1.11 shows the change in pH that occurs during the addition of base to the fully protonated form of alanine (I) to produce the completely deprotonated form (III). Note the following:

a. Buffer pairs: The $-COOH/-COO^-$ pair can serve as a buffer in the pH region around pK_1, and the $-NH_3^+/-NH_2$ pair can buffer in the region around pK_2.

b. When pH = pK: When the pH is equal to pK_1 (2.3), equal amounts of Forms I and II of alanine exist in solution. When the pH is equal to pK_2 (9.1), equal amounts of Forms II and III are present in solution.

c. Isoelectric point: At neutral pH, alanine exists predominantly as the dipolar Form II in which the amino and carboxyl groups are ionized, but the net charge is zero. The isoelectric point (pI) is the pH at which an amino acid is electrically neutral, that is, in which the sum of the positive charges equals the sum of the negative charges. For an amino acid, such as alanine, that has only two dissociable hydrogens (one from the α-carboxyl and one from the α-amino group), the pI is the average of pK_1 and pK_2 (pI = [2.3 + 9.1]/2 = 5.7, see Figure 1.11). The pI is thus midway between pK_1 (2.3) and pK_2 (9.1). pI corresponds to the pH at which the Form II (with a net charge of zero) predominates, and at which there are also equal amounts of Forms I (net charge of +1) and III (net charge of −1).

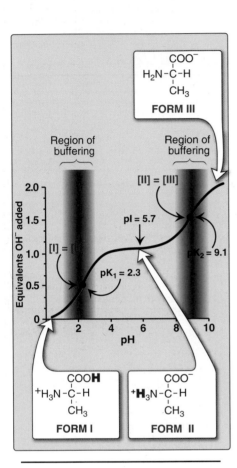

Figure 1.11
The titration curve of alanine.

> Separation of plasma proteins by charge typically is done at a pH above the pI of the major proteins, thus, the charge on the proteins is negative. In an electric field, the proteins will move toward the positive electrode at a rate determined by their net negative charge. Variations in the mobility pattern are suggestive of certain diseases.

6. Net charge of amino acids at neutral pH: At physiologic pH, amino acids have a negatively charged group ($-COO^-$) and a positively charged group ($-NH_3^+$), both attached to the α-carbon. [Note: Glutamate, aspartate, histidine, arginine, and lysine have additional potentially charged groups in their side chains.] Substances, such as amino acids, that can act either as an acid or a base are defined as amphoteric, and are referred to as ampholytes (amphoteric electrolytes).

D. Other applications of the Henderson-Hasselbalch equation

The Henderson-Hasselbalch equation can be used to calculate how the pH of a physiologic solution responds to changes in the concentration of a weak acid and/or its corresponding "salt" form. For example, in the bicarbonate buffer system, the Henderson-Hasselbalch equation predicts how shifts in the bicarbonate ion concentration, [HCO_3^-], and CO_2 influence pH (Figure 1.12A). The equation is also useful for calculating the abundance of ionic forms of acidic and basic drugs. For example, most drugs are either weak acids or weak bases (Figure 1.12B). Acidic drugs (HA) release a proton (H^+), causing a charged anion (A^-) to form.

$$HA \quad \rightleftarrows \quad H^+ + A^-$$

Weak bases (BH^+) can also release a H^+. However, the protonated form of basic drugs is usually charged, and the loss of a proton produces the uncharged base (B).

$$BH^+ \quad \rightleftarrows \quad B + H^+$$

A drug passes through membranes more readily if it is uncharged. Thus, for a weak acid such as aspirin, the uncharged HA can permeate through membranes and A^- cannot. For a weak base, such as morphine, the uncharged form, B, penetrates through the cell membrane and BH^+ does not. Therefore, the effective concentration of the permeable form of each drug at its absorption site is determined by the relative concentrations of the charged and uncharged forms. The ratio between the two forms is determined by the pH at the site of absorption, and by the strength of the weak acid or base, which is represented by the pK_a of the ionizable group. The Henderson-Hasselbalch equation is useful in determining how much drug is found on either side of a membrane that separates two compartments that differ in pH, for example, the stomach (pH 1.0–1.5) and blood plasma (pH 7.4).

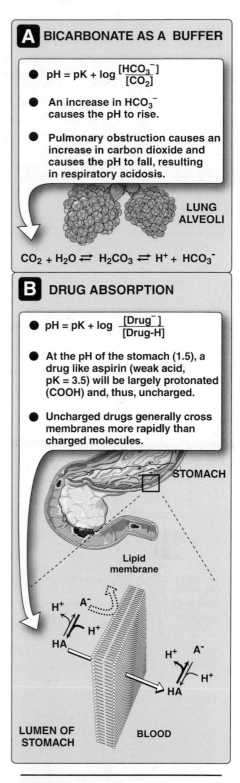

A BICARBONATE AS A BUFFER

- $pH = pK + \log \dfrac{[HCO_3^-]}{[CO_2]}$

- An increase in HCO_3^- causes the pH to rise.

- Pulmonary obstruction causes an increase in carbon dioxide and causes the pH to fall, resulting in respiratory acidosis.

LUNG ALVEOLI

$$CO_2 + H_2O \rightleftarrows H_2CO_3 \rightleftarrows H^+ + HCO_3^-$$

B DRUG ABSORPTION

- $pH = pK + \log \dfrac{[Drug^-]}{[Drug-H]}$

- At the pH of the stomach (1.5), a drug like aspirin (weak acid, pK = 3.5) will be largely protonated (COOH) and, thus, uncharged.

- Uncharged drugs generally cross membranes more rapidly than charged molecules.

STOMACH

Lipid membrane

H^+ A^-

H^+

HA

H^+ A^-

H^+

HA

LUMEN OF STOMACH

BLOOD

Figure 1.12
The Henderson-Hasselbalch equation is used to predict: A, changes in pH as the concentrations of HCO_3^- or CO_2 are altered; or B, the ionic forms of drugs.

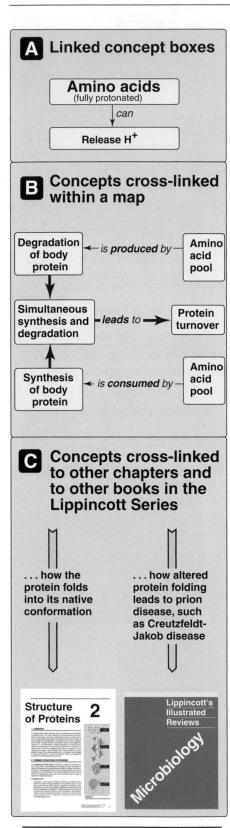

Figure 1.13
Symbols used in concept maps.

IV. CONCEPT MAPS

Students sometimes view biochemistry as a blur of facts or equations to be memorized, rather than a body of concepts to be understood. Details provided to enrich understanding of these concepts inadvertently turn into distractions. What seems to be missing is a road map—a guide that provides the student with an intuitive understanding of how various topics fit together to make sense. The authors have, therefore, created a series of biochemical concept maps to graphically illustrate relationships between ideas presented in a chapter, and to show how the information can be grouped or organized. A concept map is, thus, a tool for visualizing the connections between concepts. Material is represented in a hierarchic fashion, with the most inclusive, most general concepts at the top of the map, and the more specific, less general concepts arranged beneath. The concept maps ideally function as templates or guides for organizing information, so the student can readily find the best ways to integrate new information into knowledge they already possess.

A. How is a concept map constructed?

1. **Concept boxes and links:** Educators define concepts as "perceived regularities in events or objects." In our biochemical maps, concepts include abstractions (for example, free energy), processes (for example, oxidative phosphorylation), and compounds (for example, glucose 6-phosphate). These broadly defined concepts are prioritized with the central idea positioned at the top of the page. The concepts that follow from this central idea are then drawn in boxes (Figure 1.13A). The size of the type indicates the relative importance of each idea. Lines are drawn between concept boxes to show which are related. The label on the line defines the relationship between two concepts, so that it reads as a valid statement, that is, the connection creates meaning. The lines with arrowheads indicate in which direction the connection should be read (Figure 1.14).

2. **Cross-links:** Unlike linear flow charts or outlines, concept maps may contain cross-links that allow the reader to visualize complex relationships between ideas represented in different parts of the map (Figure 1.13B), or between the map and other chapters in this book or companion books in the series (Figure 1.13C). Cross-links can thus identify concepts that are central to more than one discipline, empowering students to be effective in clinical situations, and on the United States Medical Licensure Examination (USMLE) or other examinations, that bridge disciplinary boundaries. Students learn to visually perceive nonlinear relationships between facts, in contrast to cross-referencing within linear text.

V. CHAPTER SUMMARY

Each amino acid has an **α-carboxyl group** and a primary **α-amino group** (except for proline, which has a **secondary amino group**). At physiologic pH, the α-carboxyl group is dissociated, forming the negatively charged carboxylate ion ($-COO^-$), and the α-amino group is protonated ($-NH_3^+$). Each amino acid also contains one of 20 distinctive

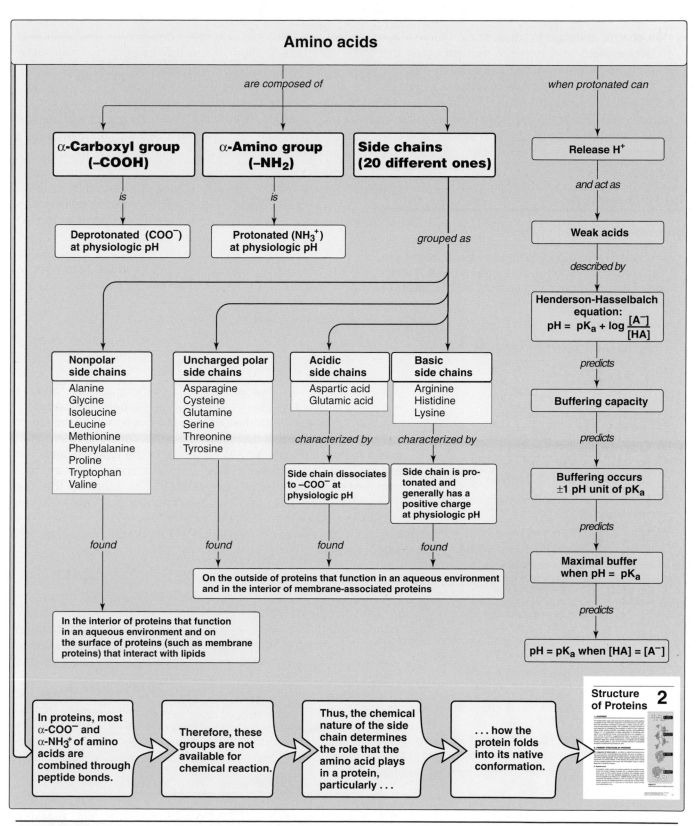

Figure 1.14
Key concept map for amino acids.

side chains attached to the α-carbon atom. The chemical nature of this side chain determines the function of an amino acid in a protein, and provides the basis for classification of the amino acids as **nonpolar**, **uncharged polar**, **acidic**, or **basic**. All free amino acids, plus charged amino acids in peptide chains, can serve as **buffers**. The quantitative relationship between the pH of a solution and the concentration of a weak acid (HA) and its conjugate base (A⁻) is described by the **Henderson-Hasselbalch equation**. Buffering occurs within ±1pH unit of the pK_a, and is maximal when pH = pK_a, at which [A⁻] = [HA]. The α-carbon of each amino acid (except glycine) is attached to four different chemical groups and is, therefore, a **chiral** or **optically active** carbon atom. Only the L-form of amino acids is found in proteins synthesized by the human body.

Study Questions

Choose the ONE correct answer.

1.1 The letters A through E designate certain regions on the titration curve for glycine (shown below). Which one of the following statements concerning this curve is correct?

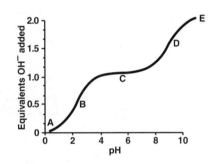

A. Point A represents the region where glycine is deprotonated.

B. Point B represents a region of minimal buffering.

C. Point C represents the region where the net charge on glycine is zero.

D. Point D represents the pK of glycine's carboxyl group.

E. Point E represents the pI for glycine.

Correct answer = C. C represents the isoelectric point or pI, and as such is midway between pK_1 and pK_2 for this monoamino monocarboxylic acid. Glycine is fully protonated at Point A. Point B represents a region of maximum buffering, as does Point D. Point E represents the region where glycine is fully deprotonated.

1.2 Which one of the following statements concerning the peptide shown below is correct?

Gly-Cys-Glu-Ser-Asp-Arg-Cys

A. The peptide contains glutamine.

B. The peptide contains a side chain with a secondary amino group.

C. The peptide contains a majority of amino acids with side chains that would be positively charged at pH 7.

D. The peptide is able to form an internal disulfide bond.

Correct answer = D. The two cysteine residues can, under oxidizing conditions, form a disulfide bond. Glutamine's 3-letter abbreviation is Gln. Proline (Pro) contains a secondary amino group. Only one (Arg) of the seven would have a positively charged side chain at pH 7.

1.3 Given that the pI for glycine is 6.1, to which electrode, positive or negative, will glycine move in an electric field at pH 2? Explain.

Correct answer = negative electrode. When the pH is less than the pI, the charge on glycine is positive because the α-amino group is fully protonated. (Recall that glycine has H as its R group).

Structure
of Proteins

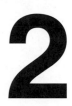

I. OVERVIEW

The 20 amino acids commonly found in proteins are joined together by peptide bonds. The linear sequence of the linked amino acids contains the information necessary to generate a protein molecule with a unique three-dimensional shape. The complexity of protein structure is best analyzed by considering the molecule in terms of four organizational levels, namely, primary, secondary, tertiary, and quaternary (Figure 2.1). An examination of these hierarchies of increasing complexity has revealed that certain structural elements are repeated in a wide variety of proteins, suggesting that there are general "rules" regarding the ways in which proteins achieve their native, functional form. These repeated structural elements range from simple combinations of α-helices and β–sheets forming small motifs, to the complex folding of polypeptide domains of multifunctional proteins (see p. 18).

II. PRIMARY STRUCTURE OF PROTEINS

The sequence of amino acids in a protein is called the primary structure of the protein. Understanding the primary structure of proteins is important because many genetic diseases result in proteins with abnormal amino acid sequences, which cause improper folding and loss or impairment of normal function. If the primary structures of the normal and the mutated proteins are known, this information may be used to diagnose or study the disease.

A. Peptide bond

In proteins, amino acids are joined covalently by peptide bonds, which are amide linkages between the α-carboxyl group of one amino acid and the α-amino group of another. For example, valine and alanine can form the dipeptide valylalanine through the formation of a peptide bond (Figure 2.2). Peptide bonds are not broken by conditions that denature proteins, such as heating or high concentrations of urea (see p. 20). Prolonged exposure to a strong acid or base at elevated temperatures is required to hydrolyze these bonds nonenzymatically.

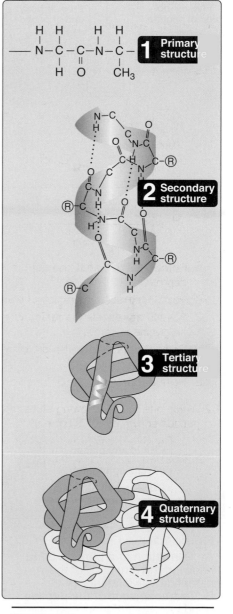

Figure 2.1
Four hierarchies of protein structure.

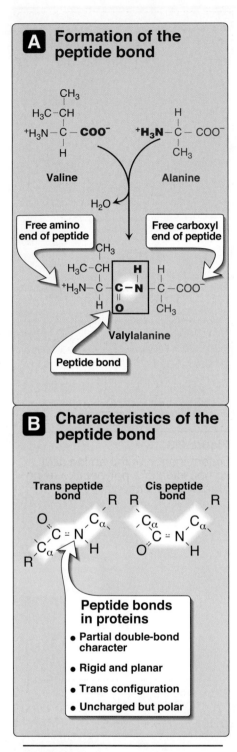

Figure 2.2
A. Formation of a peptide bond, showing the structure of the dipeptide valylalanine.
B. Characteristics of the peptide bond.

1. **Naming the peptide:** By convention, the free amino end (N-terminal) of the peptide chain is written to the left and the free carboxyl end (C-terminal) to the right. Therefore, all amino acid sequences are read from the N- to the C-terminal end of the peptide. For example, in Figure 2.2A, the order of the amino acids is "valine, alanine." Linkage of many amino acids through peptide bonds results in an unbranched chain called a polypeptide. Each component amino acid in a polypeptide is called a "residue" because it is the portion of the amino acid remaining after the atoms of water are lost in the formation of the peptide bond. When a polypeptide is named, all amino acid residues have their suffixes (-ine, -an, -ic, or -ate) changed to -yl, with the exception of the C-terminal amino acid. For example, a tripeptide composed of an N-terminal valine, a glycine, and a C-terminal leucine is called valylglycylleucine.

2. **Characteristics of the peptide bond:** The peptide bond has a partial double-bond character, that is, it is shorter than a single bond, and is rigid and planar (Figure 2.2B). This prevents free rotation around the bond between the carbonyl carbon and the nitrogen of the peptide bond. However, the bonds between the α-carbons and the α-amino or α-carboxyl groups can be freely rotated (although they are limited by the size and character of the R-groups). This allows the polypeptide chain to assume a variety of possible configurations. The peptide bond is generally a trans bond (instead of cis, see Figure 2.2B), in large part because of steric interference of the R-groups when in the cis position.

3. **Polarity of the peptide bond:** Like all amide linkages, the $-C=O$ and $-NH$ groups of the peptide bond are uncharged, and neither accept nor release protons over the pH range of 2–12. Thus, the charged groups present in polypeptides consist solely of the N-terminal (α-amino) group, the C-terminal (α-carboxyl) group, and any ionized groups present in the side chains of the constituent amino acids. The $-C=O$ and $-NH$ groups of the peptide bond are polar, and are involved in hydrogen bonds, for example, in α-helices and β-sheet structures, described on pp. 16–17.

B. Determination of the amino acid composition of a polypeptide

The first step in determining the primary structure of a polypeptide is to identify and quantitate its constituent amino acids. A purified sample of the polypeptide to be analyzed is first hydrolyzed by strong acid at 110°C for 24 hours. This treatment cleaves the peptide bonds and releases the individual amino acids, which can be separated by cation-exchange chromatography. In this technique, a mixture of amino acids is applied to a column that contains a resin to which a negatively charged group is tightly attached. [Note: If the attached group is positively charged, the column becomes an anion-exchange column.] The amino acids bind to the column with different affinities, depending on their charges, hydrophobicity, and other characteristics. Each amino acid is sequentially released from the chromatography column by eluting with solutions of increasing ionic strength and pH (Figure 2.3). The separated amino acids contained in the eluate from the column are quantitated by heating them with ninhydrin—a reagent that forms a purple compound with most amino acids, ammonia, and amines. The amount of each amino acid is determined spectrophotometrically by measuring the amount of light absorbed by the ninhydrin derivative. The analysis described above is performed using an amino acid analyzer—an automated machine whose components are depicted in Figure 2.3.

C. Sequencing of the peptide from its N-terminal end

Sequencing is a stepwise process of identifying the specific amino acid at each position in the peptide chain, beginning at the N-terminal end. Phenylisothiocyanate, known as Edman reagent, is used to label the amino-terminal residue under mildly alkaline conditions (Figure 2.4). The resulting phenylthiohydantoin (PTH) derivative introduces an instability in the N-terminal peptide bond that can be selectively hydrolyzed without cleaving the other peptide bonds. The identity of the amino acid derivative can then be determined. Edman reagent can be applied repeatedly to the shortened peptide obtained in each previous cycle.

D. Cleavage of the polypeptide into smaller fragments

Many polypeptides have a primary structure composed of more than 100 amino acids. Such molecules cannot be sequenced directly from end to end. However, these large molecules can be cleaved at specific sites, and the resulting fragments sequenced. By using more than one cleaving agent (enzymes and/or chemicals) on separate samples of the purified polypeptide, overlapping fragments can be generated that permit the proper ordering of the sequenced fragments, thus providing a complete amino acid sequence of the large polypeptide (Figure 2.5). Enzymes that hydrolyze peptide bonds are termed *peptidases* (*proteases*). [Note: *Exopeptidases* cut at the ends of proteins, and are divided into *aminopeptidases* and *carboxypeptidases*. *Carboxypeptidases* are used in determining the C-terminal amino acid. *Endopeptidases* cleave within a protein.]

E. Determination of a protein's primary structure by DNA sequencing

The sequence of nucleotides in a protein-coding region of the DNA specifies the amino acid sequence of a polypeptide. Therefore, if the nucleotide sequence can be determined, it is possible, from knowledge of the genetic code (see p. 431), to translate the sequence of nucleotides into the corresponding amino acid sequence of that

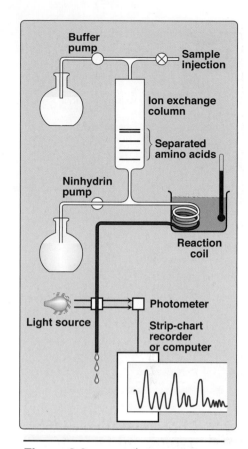

Figure 2.3
Determination of the amino acid composition of a polypeptide using an amino acid analyzer.

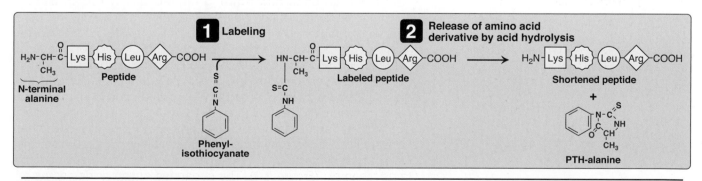

Figure 2.4
Determination of the amino-terminal residue of a polypeptide by Edman degradation.

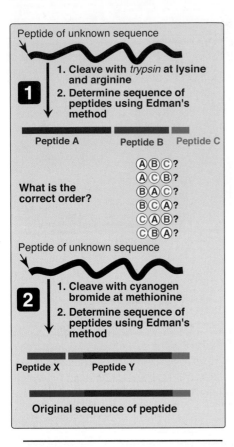

Figure 2.5
Overlapping of peptides produced by the action of *trypsin* and cyanogen bromide.

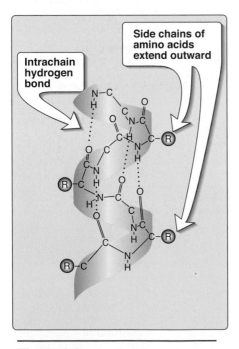

Figure 2.6
α-Helix showing peptide backbone.

polypeptide. This indirect process, although routinely used to obtain the amino acid sequences of proteins, has the limitations of not being able to predict the positions of disulfide bonds in the folded chain, and of not identifying any amino acids that are modified after their incorporation into the polypeptide (posttranslational modification, see p. 443). Therefore, direct protein sequencing is an extremely important tool for determining the true character of the primary sequence of many polypeptides.

III. SECONDARY STRUCTURE OF PROTEINS

The polypeptide backbone does not assume a random three-dimensional structure, but instead generally forms regular arrangements of amino acids that are located near to each other in the linear sequence. These arrangements are termed the secondary structure of the polypeptide. The α-helix, β-sheet, and β-bend (β-turn) are examples of secondary structures frequently encountered in proteins. [Note: The collagen α-chain helix, another example of secondary structure, is discussed on p. 45.]

A. α-Helix

Several different polypeptide helices are found in nature, but the α-helix is the most common. It is a spiral structure, consisting of a tightly packed, coiled polypeptide backbone core, with the side chains of the component amino acids extending outward from the central axis to avoid interfering sterically with each other (Figure 2.6). A very diverse group of proteins contains α-helices. For example, the keratins are a family of closely related, fibrous proteins whose structure is nearly entirely α-helical. They are a major component of tissues such as hair and skin, and their rigidity is determined by the number of disulfide bonds between the constituent polypeptide chains. In contrast to keratin, myoglobin, whose structure is also highly α-helical, is a globular, flexible molecule (see p. 26).

1. **Hydrogen bonds:** An α-helix is stabilized by extensive hydrogen bonding between the peptide-bond carbonyl oxygens and amide hydrogens that are part of the polypeptide backbone (see Figure 2.6). The hydrogen bonds extend up and are parallel to the spiral from the carbonyl oxygen of one peptide bond to the −NH− group of a peptide linkage four residues ahead in the polypeptide. This ensures that all but the first and last peptide bond components are linked to each other through intrachain hydrogen bonds. Hydrogen bonds are individually weak, but they collectively serve to stabilize the helix.

2. **Amino acids per turn:** Each turn of an α-helix contains 3.6 amino acids. Thus, amino acid residues spaced three or four residues apart in the primary sequence are spatially close together when folded in the α-helix.

3. **Amino acids that disrupt an α-helix:** Proline disrupts an α-helix because its secondary amino group is not geometrically compatible with the right-handed spiral of the α-helix. Instead, it inserts a kink in the chain, which interferes with the smooth, helical structure. Large numbers of charged amino acids (for example, gluta-

mate, aspartate, histidine, lysine, or arginine) also disrupt the helix by forming ionic bonds, or by electrostatically repelling each other. Finally, amino acids with bulky side chains, such as tryptophan, or amino acids, such as valine or isoleucine, that branch at the β-carbon (the first carbon in the R-group, next to the α-carbon) can interfere with formation of the α-helix if they are present in large numbers.

B. β-Sheet

The β-sheet is another form of secondary structure in which all of the peptide bond components are involved in hydrogen bonding (Figure 2.7A). The surfaces of β-sheets appear "pleated," and these structures are, therefore, often called "β-pleated sheets." When illustrations are made of protein structure, β-strands are often visualized as broad arrows (Figure 2.7B).

1. **Comparison of a β-sheet and an α-helix:** Unlike the α-helix, β-sheets are composed of two or more peptide chains (β-strands), or segments of polypeptide chains, which are almost fully extended. Note also that in β-sheets the hydrogen bonds are perpendicular to the polypeptide backbone (see Figure 2.7A).

2. **Parallel and antiparallel sheets:** A β-sheet can be formed from two or more separate polypeptide chains or segments of polypeptide chains that are arranged either antiparallel to each other (with the N-terminal and C-terminal ends of the β-strands alternating as shown in Figure 2.7B), or parallel to each other (with all the N-termini of the β-strands together as shown in Figure 2.7C). When the hydrogen bonds are formed between the polypeptide backbones of separate polypeptide chains, they are termed interchain bonds. A β-sheet can also be formed by a single polypeptide chain folding back on itself (see Figure 2.7C). In this case, the hydrogen bonds are intrachain bonds. In globular proteins, β-sheets always have a right-handed curl, or twist, when viewed along the polypeptide backbone. [Note: Twisted β-sheets often form the core of globular proteins.]

> The α-helix and β-sheet structures provide maximal hydrogen bonding for peptide bond components within the interior of polypeptides.

C. β-Bends (reverse turns, β-turns)

β-Bends reverse the direction of a polypeptide chain, helping it form a compact, globular shape. They are usually found on the surface of protein molecules, and often include charged residues. [Note: β-Bends were given this name because they often connect successive strands of antiparallel β-sheets.] β-Bends are generally composed of four amino acids, one of which may be proline—the amino acid that causes a "kink" in the polypeptide chain. Glycine, the amino acid with the smallest R-group, is also frequently found in β-bends. β-Bends are stabilized by the formation of hydrogen and ionic bonds.

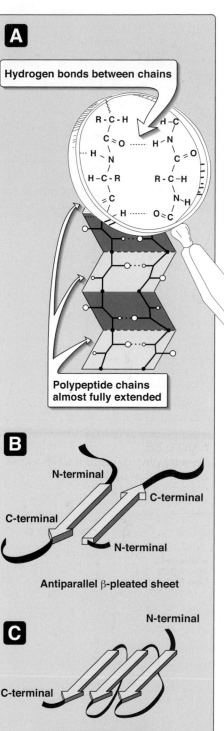

Figure 2.7
A. Structure of a β-sheet. B. An antiparallel β-sheet with the β-strands represented as broad arrows. C. A parallel β-sheet formed from a single polypeptide chain folding back on itself.

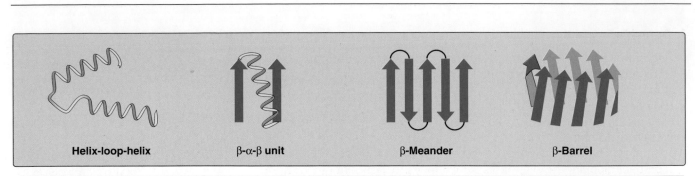

Figure 2.8
Some common structural motifs combining α-helices and/or β-sheets. The names describe their schematic appearance.

D. Nonrepetitive secondary structure

Approximately one half of an average globular protein is organized into repetitive structures, such as the α-helix and/or β-sheet. The remainder of the polypeptide chain is described as having a loop or coil conformation. These nonrepetitive secondary structures are not "random," but rather simply have a less regular structure than those described above. [Note: The term "random coil" refers to the disordered structure obtained when proteins are denatured (see p. 20).]

E. Supersecondary structures (motifs)

Globular proteins are constructed by combining secondary structural elements (α-helices, β-sheets, nonrepetitive sequences). These form primarily the core region—that is, the interior of the molecule. They are connected by loop regions (for example, β-bends) at the surface of the protein. Supersecondary structures are usually produced by packing side chains from adjacent secondary structural elements close to each other. Thus, for example, α-helices and β-sheets that are adjacent in the amino acid sequence are also usually (but not always) adjacent in the final, folded protein. Some of the more common motifs are illustrated in Figure 2.8.

Proteins that bind to DNA contain a limited number of motifs. The helix-loop-helix motif is an example found in a number of proteins that function as transcription factors (see p. 455).

IV. TERTIARY STRUCTURE OF GLOBULAR PROTEINS

The primary structure of a polypeptide chain determines its tertiary structure. "Tertiary" refers both to the folding of domains (the basic units of structure and function, see discussion below), and to the final arrangement of domains in the polypeptide. The structure of globular proteins in aqueous solution is compact, with a high-density (close packing) of the atoms in the core of the molecule. Hydrophobic side chains are buried in the interior, whereas hydrophilic groups are generally found on the surface of the molecule.

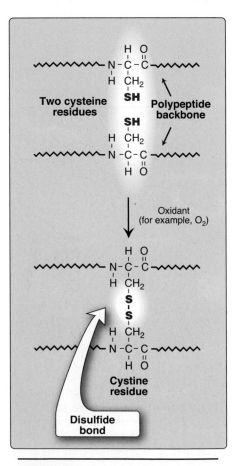

Figure 2.9
Formation of a disulfide bond by the oxidation of two cysteine residues, producing one cystine residue.

A. Domains

Domains are the fundamental functional and three-dimensional structural units of polypeptides. Polypeptide chains that are greater than 200 amino acids in length generally consist of two or more domains. The core of a domain is built from combinations of super-secondary structural elements (motifs). Folding of the peptide chain within a domain usually occurs independently of folding in other domains. Therefore, each domain has the characteristics of a small, compact globular protein that is structurally independent of the other domains in the polypeptide chain.

B. Interactions stabilizing tertiary structure

The unique three-dimensional structure of each polypeptide is determined by its amino acid sequence. Interactions between the amino acid side chains guide the folding of the polypeptide to form a compact structure. The following four types of interactions cooperate in stabilizing the tertiary structures of globular proteins.

1. **Disulfide bonds:** A disulfide bond is a covalent linkage formed from the sulfhydryl group (–SH) of each of two cysteine residues, to produce a cystine residue (Figure 2.9). The two cysteines may be separated from each other by many amino acids in the primary sequence of a polypeptide, or may even be located on two different polypeptide chains; the folding of the polypeptide chain(s) brings the cysteine residues into proximity, and permits covalent bonding of their side chains. A disulfide bond contributes to the stability of the three-dimensional shape of the protein molecule, and prevents it from becoming denatured in the extracellular environment. For example, many disulfide bonds are found in proteins such as immunoglobulins that are secreted by cells.

2. **Hydrophobic interactions:** Amino acids with nonpolar side chains tend to be located in the interior of the polypeptide molecule, where they associate with other hydrophobic amino acids (Figure 2.10). In contrast, amino acids with polar or charged side chains tend to be located on the surface of the molecule in contact with the polar solvent. [Note: Recall that proteins located in nonpolar (lipid) environments, such as a membrane, exhibit the reverse arrangement (see Figure 1.4, p. 4).] In each case, a segregation of R-groups occurs that is energetically most favorable.

3. **Hydrogen bonds:** Amino acid side chains containing oxygen- or nitrogen-bound hydrogen, such as in the alcohol groups of serine and threonine, can form hydrogen bonds with electron-rich atoms, such as the oxygen of a carboxyl group or carbonyl group of a peptide bond (Figure 2.11; see also Figure 1.6, p. 4). Formation of hydrogen bonds between polar groups on the surface of proteins and the aqueous solvent enhances the solubility of the protein.

4. **Ionic interactions:** Negatively charged groups, such as the carboxylate group (–COO⁻) in the side chain of aspartate or glutamate, can interact with positively charged groups, such as the amino group (–NH₃⁺) in the side chain of lysine (see Figure 2.11).

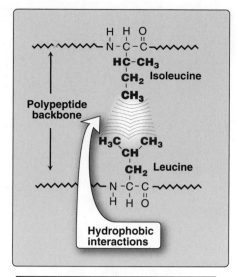

Figure 2.10
Hydrophobic interactions between amino acids with nonpolar side chains.

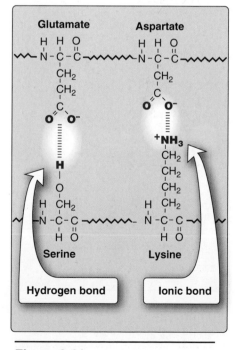

Figure 2.11
Interactions of side chains of amino acids through hydrogen bonds and ionic bonds (salt bridges).

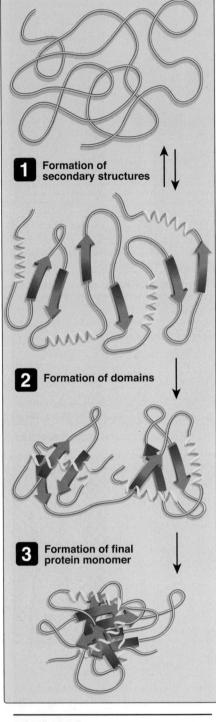

1 Formation of
secondary structures

2 Formation of domains

3 Formation of final
protein monomer

Figure 2.12
Steps in protein folding.

C. Protein folding

Interactions between the side chains of amino acids determine how a long polypeptide chain folds into the intricate three-dimensional shape of the functional protein. Protein folding, which occurs within the cell in seconds to minutes, employs a shortcut through the maze of all folding possibilities. As a peptide folds, its amino acid side chains are attracted and repulsed according to their chemical properties. For example, positively and negatively charged side chains attract each other. Conversely, similarly charged side chains repel each other. In addition, interactions involving hydrogen bonds, hydrophobic interactions, and disulfide bonds all exert an influence on the folding process. This process of trial and error tests many, but not all, possible configurations, seeking a compromise in which attractions outweigh repulsions. This results in a correctly folded protein with a low-energy state (Figure 2.12).

D. Denaturation of proteins

Protein denaturation results in the unfolding and disorganization of the protein's secondary and tertiary structures, which are not accompanied by hydrolysis of peptide bonds. Denaturing agents include heat, organic solvents, mechanical mixing, strong acids or bases, detergents, and ions of heavy metals such as lead and mercury. Denaturation may, under ideal conditions, be reversible, in which case the protein refolds into its original native structure when the denaturing agent is removed. However, most proteins, once denatured, remain permanently disordered. Denatured proteins are often insoluble and, therefore, precipitate from solution.

E. Role of chaperones in protein folding

It is generally accepted that the information needed for correct protein folding is contained in the primary structure of the polypeptide. Given that premise, it is difficult to explain why most proteins when denatured do not resume their native conformations under favorable environmental conditions. One answer to this problem is that a protein begins to fold in stages during its synthesis, rather than waiting for synthesis of the entire chain to be totally completed. This limits competing folding configurations made available by longer stretches of nascent peptide. In addition, a specialized group of proteins, named "chaperones," are required for the proper folding of many species of proteins. The chaperones—also known as "heat shock" proteins—interact with the polypeptide at various stages during the folding process. Some chaperones are important in keeping the protein unfolded until its synthesis is finished, or act as catalysts by increasing the rates of the final stages in the folding process. Others protect proteins as they fold so that their vulnerable, exposed regions do not become tangled in unproductive interactions.

V. QUATERNARY STRUCTURE OF PROTEINS

Many proteins consist of a single polypeptide chain, and are defined as monomeric proteins. However, others may consist of two or more polypeptide chains that may be structurally identical or totally unrelated. The arrangement of these polypeptide subunits is called the quaternary structure of the protein. Subunits are held together by noncovalent interactions (for example, hydrogen bonds, ionic bonds, and hydrophobic interactions). Subunits may either function independently of each other, or may work cooperatively, as in hemoglobin, in which the binding of oxygen to one subunit of the tetramer increases the affinity of the other subunits for oxygen (see p. 29).

> Isoforms are proteins that perform the same function but have different primary structures. They can arise from different genes or from tissue-specific processing of the product of a single gene. If the proteins function as enzymes, they are referred to as isozymes (see p. 65).

VI. PROTEIN MISFOLDING

Protein folding is a complex, trial-and-error process that can sometimes result in improperly folded molecules. These misfolded proteins are usually tagged and degraded within the cell (see p. 444). However, this quality control system is not perfect, and intracellular or extracellular aggregates of misfolded proteins can accumulate, particularly as individuals age. Deposits of these misfolded proteins are associated with a number of diseases.

A. Amyloid disease

Misfolding of proteins may occur spontaneously, or be caused by a mutation in a particular gene, which then produces an altered protein. In addition, some apparently normal proteins can, after abnormal proteolytic cleavage, take on a unique conformational state that leads to the formation of long, fibrillar protein assemblies consisting of β-pleated sheets. Accumulation of these insoluble, spontaneously aggregating proteins, called amyloids, has been implicated in many degenerative diseases—particularly in the age-related neurodegenerative disorder, Alzheimer disease. The dominant component of the amyloid plaque that accumulates in Alzheimer disease is amyloid β (Aβ), a peptide containing 40–42 amino acid residues. X-ray crystallography and infrared spectroscopy demonstrate a characteristic β-pleated sheet conformation in nonbranching fibrils. This peptide, when aggregated in a β-pleated sheet configuration, is neurotoxic, and is the central pathogenic event leading to the cognitive impairment characteristic of the disease. The Aβ that is deposited in the brain in Alzheimer disease is derived by proteolytic cleavages from the larger amyloid precursor protein—a single transmembrane protein expressed on the cell surface in the brain and other tissues (Figure 2.13). The Aβ peptides aggregate, generating the amyloid that is found in the brain parenchyma and around blood vessels. Most cases of Alzheimer disease are not genetically based, although at least 5–10% of cases are familial. A second biologic factor involved in the development of Alzheimer disease is the accumulation of neurofibrillary tangles inside neurons. A key component of these tangled fibers is an abnormal form of the tau (τ) protein, which in its healthy version helps in the assembly of the microtubular structure. The defective τ, however, appears to block the actions of its normal counterpart.

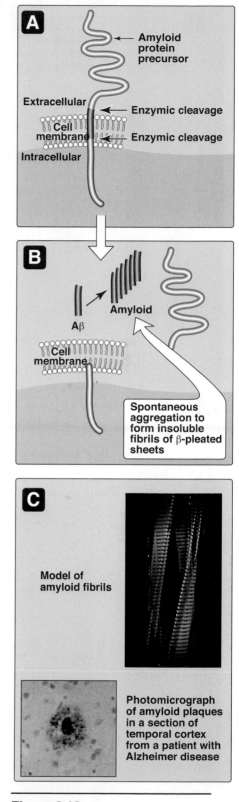

Figure 2.13
Formation of amyloid plaques found in Alzheimer disease.

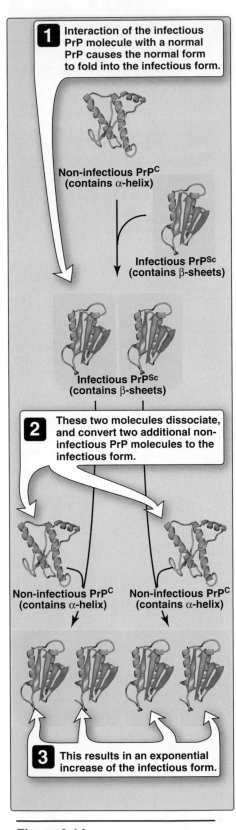

1 Interaction of the infectious PrP molecule with a normal PrP causes the normal form to fold into the infectious form.

Non-infectious PrP^C (contains α-helix)

Infectious PrP^{Sc} (contains β-sheets)

Infectious PrP^{Sc} (contains β-sheets)

2 These two molecules dissociate, and convert two additional non-infectious PrP molecules to the infectious form.

Non-infectious PrP^C (contains α-helix)   Non-infectious PrP^C (contains α-helix)

3 This results in an exponential increase of the infectious form.

Figure 2.14
One proposed mechanism for multiplication of infectious prion agents.

B. Prion disease

The prion protein (PrP) has been strongly implicated as the causative agent of transmissible spongiform encephalopathies (TSEs), including Creutzfeldt-Jakob disease in humans, scrapie in sheep, and bovine spongiform encephalopathy in cattle (popularly called "mad cow disease").[1] After an extensive series of purification procedures, scientists were astonished to find that the infectivity of the agent causing scrapie in sheep was associated with a single protein species that was not complexed with detectable nucleic acid. This infectious protein is designated PrP^{Sc} (Sc = scrapie). It is highly resistant to proteolytic degradation, and tends to form insoluble aggregates of fibrils, similar to the amyloid found in some other diseases of the brain. A noninfectious form of PrP^C (C = cellular), encoded by the same gene as the infectious agent, is present in normal mammalian brains on the surface of neurons and glial cells. Thus, PrP^C is a host protein. No primary structure differences or alternate posttranslational modifications have been found between the normal and the infectious forms of the protein. The key to becoming infectious apparently lies in changes in the three-dimensional conformation of PrP^C. It has been observed that a number of α-helices present in noninfectious PrP^C are replaced by β-sheets in the infectious form (Figure 2.14). It is presumably this conformational difference that confers relative resistance to proteolytic degradation of infectious prions, and permits them to be distinguished from the normal PrP^C in infected tissue. The infective agent is thus an altered version of a normal protein, which acts as a "template" for converting the normal protein to the pathogenic conformation. The TSEs are invariably fatal, and no treatment is currently available that can alter this outcome.

VII. CHAPTER SUMMARY

Central to understanding protein structure is the concept of the **native conformation** (Figure 2.15), which is the functional, fully-folded protein structure (for example, an active enzyme or structural protein). The unique three-dimensional structure of the native conformation is determined by its **primary structure**, that is, its amino acid sequence. Interactions between the amino acid side chains guide the folding of the polypeptide chain to form **secondary**, **tertiary**, and (sometimes) **quaternary** structures, which cooperate in stabilizing the native conformation of the protein. In addition, a specialized group of proteins named "**chaperones**" is required for the proper folding of many species of proteins. **Protein denaturation** results in the unfolding and disorganization of the protein's structure, which are not accompanied by hydrolysis of peptide bonds. Denaturation may be reversible or, more commonly, irreversible. Disease can occur when an apparently normal protein assumes a conformation that is cytotoxic, as in the case of Alzheimer disease and the **transmissible spongiform encephalopathies (TSEs)**, including **Creutzfeldt-Jakob disease**. In **Alzheimer disease,** normal proteins, after abnormal chemical processing, take on a unique conformational state that leads to the formation of neurotoxic **amyloid protein** assemblies consisting of β-pleated sheets. In TSEs, the infective agent is an altered version of a normal **prion protein** that acts as a "template" for converting normal protein to the pathogenic conformation.

INFO LINK [1]See Chapter 31 in *Lippincott's Illustrated Reviews: Microbiology* for a more detailed discussion of prions.

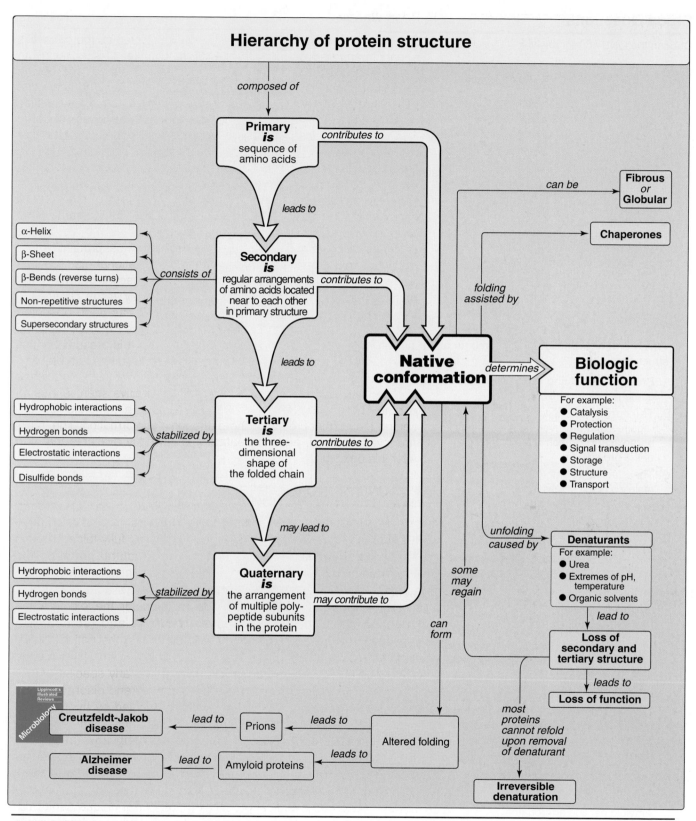

Figure 2.15
Key concept map for protein structure.

Study Questions

Choose the ONE correct answer.

2.1 A peptide bond:

A. has a partial double-bond character.

B. is ionized at physiologic pH.

C. is cleaved by agents that denature proteins, such as organic solvents and high concentrations of urea.

D. is stable to heating in strong acids.

E. occurs most commonly in the cis configuration.

Correct answer = A. The peptide bond has a partial double-bond character. Unlike its components—the α-amino and α-carboxyl groups—the −NH and −C=O of the peptide bond do not accept or give off protons. The peptide bond is not cleaved by organic solvents or urea, but is labile to strong acids. It is usually in the trans configuration.

2.2 Which one of the following statements is correct?

A. The α-helix can be composed of more than one polypeptide chain.

B. β-Sheets exist only in the antiparallel form.

C. β-Bends often contain proline.

D. Domains are a type of secondary structure.

E. The α-helix is stabilized primarily by ionic interactions between the side chains of amino acids.

Correct answer = C. β-Bends often contain proline, which provides a kink. The α-helix differs from the β-sheet in that it always involves the coiling of a single polypeptide chain. The β-sheet occurs in both parallel and antiparallel forms. Domains are elements of tertiary structure. The α-helix is stabilized primarily by hydrogen bonds between the −C=O and −NH− groups of peptide bonds.

2.3 Which one of the following statements about protein structure is correct?

A. Proteins consisting of one polypeptide can have quaternary structure.

B. The formation of a disulfide bond in a protein requires that the two participating cysteine residues be adjacent to each other in the primary sequence of the protein.

C. The stability of quaternary structure in proteins is mainly a result of covalent bonds among the subunits.

D. The denaturation of proteins always leads to irreversible loss of secondary and tertiary structure.

E. The information required for the correct folding of a protein is contained in the specific sequence of amino acids along the polypeptide chain.

Correct answer = E. The correct folding of a protein is guided by specific interactions between the side chains of the amino acid residues of a polypeptide chain. The two cysteine residues that react to form the disulfide bond may be a great distance apart in the primary structure (or on separate polypeptides), but are brought into close proximity by the three-dimensional folding of the polypeptide chain. Denaturation may either be reversible or irreversible. Quaternary structure requires more than one polypeptide chain. These chains associate through noncovalent interactions.

2.4 An 80-year-old man presented with impairment of higher intellectual function and alterations in mood and behavior. His family reported progressive disorientation and memory loss over the last 6 months. There is no family history of dementia. The patient was tentatively diagnosed with Alzheimer disease. Which one of the following best describes the disease?

A. It is associated with β-amyloid—an abnormal protein with an altered amino acid sequence.

B. It results from accumulation of denatured proteins that have random conformations.

C. It is associated with the accumulation of amyloid precursor protein.

D. It is associated with the deposition of neurotoxic amyloid peptide aggregates.

E. It is an environmentally produced disease not influenced by the genetics of the individual.

F. It is caused by the infectious form of a host-cell protein.

Correct answer = D. Alzheimer disease is associated with long, fibrillar protein assemblies consisting of β-pleated sheets found in the brain and elsewhere. The disease is associated with abnormal processing of a normal protein. The accumulated altered protein occurs in a β-pleated sheet configuration that is neurotoxic. The Aβ amyloid that is deposited in the brain in Alzheimer disease is derived by proteolytic cleavages from the larger amyloid precursor protein—a single transmembrane protein expressed on the cell surface in the brain and other tissues. Most cases of Alzheimer disease are sporadic, although at least 5–10% of cases are familial. Prion diseases, such as Creutzfeldt-Jakob, are caused by the infectious form (PrP^{Sc}) of a host-cell protein (PrP^{C}).

Globular Proteins

3

I. OVERVIEW

The previous chapter described the types of secondary and tertiary structures that are the bricks-and-mortar of protein architecture. By arranging these fundamental structural elements in different combinations, widely diverse proteins can be constructed that are capable of various specialized functions. This chapter examines the relationship between structure and function for the clinically important globular hemeproteins. Fibrous structural proteins are discussed in Chapter 4.

II. GLOBULAR HEMEPROTEINS

Hemeproteins are a group of specialized proteins that contain heme as a tightly bound prosthetic group. (See p. 54 for a discussion of prosthetic groups.) The role of the heme group is dictated by the environment created by the three-dimensional structure of the protein. For example, the heme group of a cytochrome functions as an electron carrier that is alternately oxidized and reduced (see p. 76). In contrast, the heme group of the enzyme *catalase* is part of the active site of the enzyme that catalyzes the breakdown of hydrogen peroxide (see p. 148). In hemoglobin and myoglobin, the two most abundant hemeproteins in humans, the heme group serves to reversibly bind oxygen.

A. Structure of heme

Heme is a complex of protoporphyrin IX and ferrous iron (Fe^{2+}) (Figure 3.1). The iron is held in the center of the heme molecule by bonds to the four nitrogens of the porphyrin ring. The heme Fe^{2+} can form two additional bonds, one on each side of the planar porphyrin ring. In myoglobin and hemoglobin, one of these positions is coordinated to the side chain of a histidine residue of the globin molecule, whereas the other position is available to bind oxygen (Figure 3.2). (See p. 278 for a discussion of the synthesis and degradation of heme.)

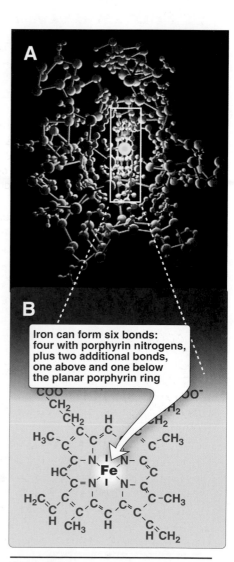

Figure 3.1
A. Hemeprotein (cytochrome c).
B. Structure of heme.

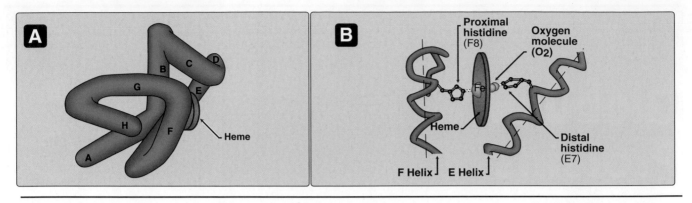

Figure 3.2
A. Model of myoglobin showing helices A to H. B. Schematic diagram of the oxygen-binding site of myoglobin.

B. Structure and function of myoglobin

Myoglobin, a hemeprotein present in heart and skeletal muscle, functions both as a reservoir for oxygen, and as an oxygen carrier that increases the rate of transport of oxygen within the muscle cell. Myoglobin consists of a single polypeptide chain that is structurally similar to the individual subunit polypeptide chains of the hemoglobin molecule. This homology makes myoglobin a useful model for interpreting some of the more complex properties of hemoglobin.

1. **α-Helical content:** Myoglobin is a compact molecule, with approximately 80% of its polypeptide chain folded into eight stretches of α-helix. These α-helical regions, labeled A to H in Figure 3.2A, are terminated either by the presence of proline, whose five-membered ring cannot be accommodated in an α-helix (see p. 16), or by β-bends and loops stabilized by hydrogen bonds and ionic bonds (see p. 17).

2. **Location of polar and nonpolar amino acid residues:** The interior of the myoglobin molecule is composed almost entirely of nonpolar amino acids. They are packed closely together, forming a structure stabilized by hydrophobic interactions between these clustered residues (see p. 19). In contrast, charged amino acids are located almost exclusively on the surface of the molecule, where they can form hydrogen bonds, both with each other and with water.

3. **Binding of the heme group:** The heme group of myoglobin sits in a crevice in the molecule, which is lined with nonpolar amino acids. Notable exceptions are two histidine residues (Figure 3.2B). One, the proximal histidine (F8), binds directly to the iron of heme. The second, or distal histidine (E7), does not directly interact with the heme group, but helps stabilize the binding of oxygen to the ferrous iron. The protein, or globin, portion of myoglobin thus creates a special microenvironment for the heme that permits the reversible binding of one oxygen molecule (oxygenation). The simultaneous loss of electrons by the ferrous iron (oxidation) occurs only rarely.

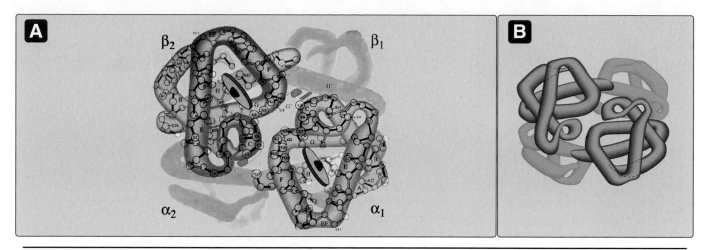

Figure 3.3
A. Structure of hemoglobin showing the polypeptide backbone. B. Simplified drawing showing the helices.

C. Structure and function of hemoglobin

Hemoglobin is found exclusively in red blood cells (RBCs), where its main function is to transport oxygen (O_2) from the lungs to the capillaries of the tissues. Hemoglobin A, the major hemoglobin in adults, is composed of four polypeptide chains—two α chains and two β chains—held together by noncovalent interactions (Figure 3.3). Each subunit has stretches of α-helical structure, and a heme-binding pocket similar to that described for myoglobin. However, the tetrameric hemoglobin molecule is structurally and functionally more complex than myoglobin. For example, hemoglobin can transport H^+ and CO_2 from the tissues to the lungs, and can carry four molecules of O_2 from the lungs to the cells of the body. Furthermore, the oxygen-binding properties of hemoglobin are regulated by interaction with allosteric effectors (see p. 29).

> Obtaining O_2 from the atmosphere solely by diffusion greatly limits the size of organisms. Circulatory systems overcome this, but transport molecules such as hemoglobin are also required because O_2 is only slightly soluble in aqueous solutions such as blood.

1. **Quaternary structure of hemoglobin:** The hemoglobin tetramer can be envisioned as being composed of two identical dimers, $(\alpha\beta)_1$ and $(\alpha\beta)_2$, in which the numbers refer to dimers one and two. The two polypeptide chains within each dimer are held tightly together, primarily by hydrophobic interactions (Figure 3.4). [Note: In this instance, hydrophobic amino acid residues are localized not only in the interior of the molecule, but also in a region on the surface of each subunit. Interchain hydrophobic interactions form strong associations between α-subunits and β-subunits in the

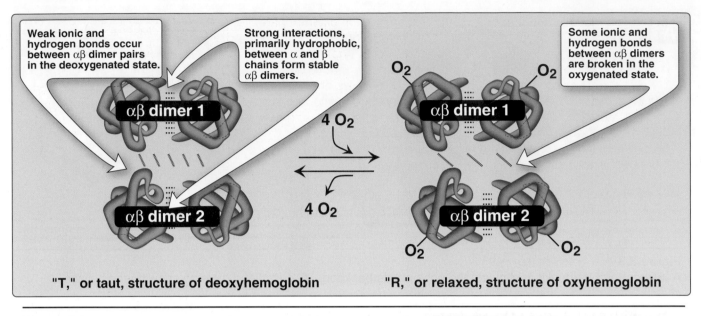

Weak ionic and hydrogen bonds occur between αβ dimer pairs in the deoxygenated state.

Strong interactions, primarily hydrophobic, between α and β chains form stable αβ dimers.

Some ionic and hydrogen bonds between αβ dimers are broken in the oxygenated state.

αβ dimer 1

αβ dimer 2

4 O₂

4 O₂

O_2 O_2

αβ dimer 1

αβ dimer 2

O_2 O_2

"T," or taut, structure of deoxyhemoglobin

"R," or relaxed, structure of oxyhemoglobin

Figure 3.4
Schematic diagram showing structural changes resulting from oxygenation and deoxygenation of hemoglobin.

dimers.] Ionic and hydrogen bonds also occur between the members of the dimer. In contrast, the two dimers are able to move with respect to each other, being held together primarily by polar bonds. The weaker interactions between these mobile dimers result in the two dimers occupying different relative positions in deoxyhemoglobin as compared with oxyhemoglobin (see Figure 3.4). [Note: The binding of O_2 to the heme iron pulls the iron into the plane of the heme. Because the iron is also linked to the proximal histidine (F8), there is movement of the globin chains that alters the interface between the αβ dimers.]

a. **T form:** The deoxy form of hemoglobin is called the "T," or taut (tense) form. In the T form, the two αβ dimers interact through a network of ionic bonds and hydrogen bonds that constrain the movement of the polypeptide chains. The T form is the low-oxygen-affinity form of hemoglobin.

b. **R form:** The binding of oxygen to hemoglobin causes the rupture of some of the ionic bonds and hydrogen bonds between the αβ dimers. This leads to a structure called the "R," or relaxed form, in which the polypeptide chains have more freedom of movement (see Figure 3.4). The R form is the high-oxygen-affinity form of hemoglobin.

D. Binding of oxygen to myoglobin and hemoglobin

Myoglobin can bind only one molecule of oxygen, because it contains only one heme group. In contrast, hemoglobin can bind four oxygen molecules—one at each of its four heme groups. The degree of saturation (Y) of these oxygen-binding sites on all myoglobin or hemoglobin molecules can vary between zero (all sites are empty) and 100% (all sites are full, Figure 3.5).

1. **Oxygen dissociation curve:** A plot of Y measured at different partial pressures of oxygen (pO_2) is called the oxygen dissociation curve. The curves for myoglobin and hemoglobin show important differences (see Figure 3.5). This graph illustrates that myoglobin has a higher oxygen affinity at all pO_2 values than does hemoglobin. The partial pressure of oxygen needed to achieve half-saturation of the binding sites (P_{50}) is approximately 1 mm Hg for myoglobin and 26 mm Hg for hemoglobin. The higher the oxygen affinity (that is, the more tightly oxygen binds), the lower the P_{50}. [Note: pO_2 may also be represented as PO_2.]

a. **Myoglobin (Mb):** The oxygen dissociation curve for myoglobin has a hyperbolic shape (see Figure 3.5). This reflects the fact that myoglobin reversibly binds a single molecule of oxygen. Thus, oxygenated (MbO_2) and deoxygenated (Mb) myoglobin exist in a simple equilibrium:

$$Mb + O_2 \rightleftarrows MbO_2$$

The equilibrium is shifted to the right or to the left as oxygen is added to or removed from the system. [Note: Myoglobin is designed to bind oxygen released by hemoglobin at the low pO_2 found in muscle. Myoglobin, in turn, releases oxygen within the muscle cell in response to oxygen demand.]

b. **Hemoglobin (Hb):** The oxygen dissociation curve for hemoglobin is sigmoidal in shape (see Figure 3.5), indicating that the subunits cooperate in binding oxygen. Cooperative binding of oxygen by the four subunits of hemoglobin means that the binding of an oxygen molecule at one heme group increases the oxygen affinity of the remaining heme groups in the same hemoglobin molecule (Figure 3.6). This effect is referred to as heme-heme interaction (see below). Although it is more difficult for the first oxygen molecule to bind to hemoglobin, the subsequent binding of oxygen occurs with high affinity, as shown by the steep upward curve in the region near 20–30 mm Hg (see Figure 3.5).

E. Allosteric effects

The ability of hemoglobin to reversibly bind oxygen is affected by the pO_2 (through heme-heme interactions as described above), the pH of the environment, the partial pressure of carbon dioxide, pCO_2, and the availability of 2,3-bisphosphoglycerate. These are collectively called allosteric ("other site") effectors, because their interaction at one site on the hemoglobin molecule affects the binding of oxygen to heme groups at other locations on the molecule. [Note: The binding of oxygen to myoglobin is not influenced by allosteric effectors.]

1. **Heme-heme interactions:** The sigmoidal oxygen dissociation curve reflects specific structural changes that are initiated at one heme group and transmitted to other heme groups in the hemoglobin tetramer. The net effect is that the affinity of hemoglobin for the last oxygen bound is approximately 300 times greater than its affinity for the first oxygen bound.

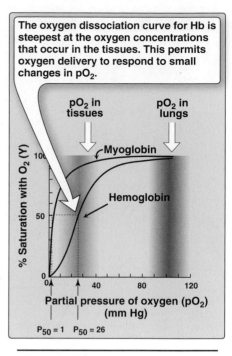

Figure 3.5
Oxygen dissociation curves for myoglobin and hemoglobin (Hb).

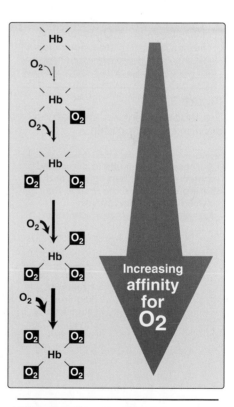

Figure 3.6
Hemoglobin (Hb) binds oxygen with increasing affinity.

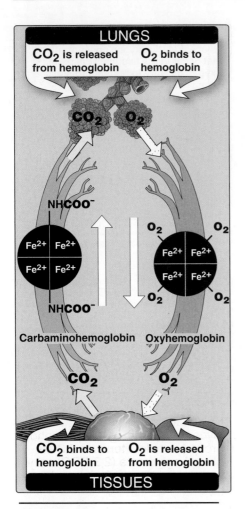

Figure 3.7
Transport of oxygen and carbon dioxide by hemoglobin.

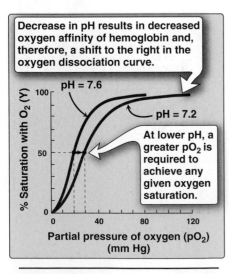

Figure 3.8
Effect of pH on the oxygen affinity of hemoglobin. Protons are allosteric effectors of hemoglobin.

a. Loading and unloading oxygen: The cooperative binding of oxygen allows hemoglobin to deliver more oxygen to the tissues in response to relatively small changes in the partial pressure of oxygen. This can be seen in Figure 3.5, which indicates pO_2 in the alveoli of the lung and the capillaries of the tissues. For example, in the lung, the concentration of oxygen is high and hemoglobin becomes virtually saturated (or "loaded") with oxygen. In contrast, in the peripheral tissues, oxyhemoglobin releases (or "unloads") much of its oxygen for use in the oxidative metabolism of the tissues (Figure 3.7).

b. Significance of the sigmoidal oxygen dissociation curve: The steep slope of the oxygen dissociation curve over the range of oxygen concentrations that occur between the lungs and the tissues permits hemoglobin to carry and deliver oxygen efficiently from sites of high to sites of low pO_2. A molecule with a hyperbolic oxygen dissociation curve, such as myoglobin, could not achieve the same degree of oxygen release within this range of partial pressures of oxygen. Instead, it would have maximum affinity for oxygen throughout this oxygen pressure range and, therefore, would deliver no oxygen to the tissues.

2. **Bohr effect:** The release of oxygen from hemoglobin is enhanced when the pH is lowered or when the hemoglobin is in the presence of an increased pCO_2. Both result in a decreased oxygen affinity of hemoglobin and, therefore, a shift to the right in the oxygen dissociation curve (Figure 3.8), and both, then, stabilize the T state. This change in oxygen binding is called the Bohr effect. Conversely, raising the pH or lowering the concentration of CO_2 results in a greater affinity for oxygen, a shift to the left in the oxygen dissociation curve, and stabilization of the R state.

   a. **Source of the protons that lower the pH:** The concentration of both CO_2 and H^+ in the capillaries of metabolically active tissues is higher than that observed in alveolar capillaries of the lungs, where CO_2 is released into the expired air. [Note: Organic acids, such as lactic acid, are produced during anaerobic metabolism in rapidly contracting muscle (see p. 103).] In the tissues, CO_2 is converted by *carbonic anhydrase* to carbonic acid:

$$CO_2 + H_2O \quad \rightleftarrows \quad H_2CO_3$$

which spontaneously loses a proton, becoming bicarbonate (the major blood buffer):

$$H_2CO_3 \quad \rightleftarrows \quad HCO_3^- + H^+$$

The H^+ produced by this pair of reactions contributes to the lowering of pH. This differential pH gradient (lungs having a higher pH, tissues a lower pH) favors the unloading of oxygen in the peripheral tissues, and the loading of oxygen in the lung. Thus, the oxygen affinity of the hemoglobin molecule responds to small shifts in pH between the lungs and oxygen-consuming tissues, making hemoglobin a more efficient transporter of oxygen.

b. Mechanism of the Bohr effect: The Bohr effect reflects the fact that the deoxy form of hemoglobin has a greater affinity for protons than does oxyhemoglobin. This effect is caused by ionizable groups, such as specific histidine side chains that have higher pK_as in deoxyhemoglobin than in oxyhemoglobin. Therefore, an increase in the concentration of protons (resulting in a decrease in pH) causes these groups to become protonated (charged) and able to form ionic bonds (also called salt bridges). These bonds preferentially stabilize the deoxy form of hemoglobin, producing a decrease in oxygen affinity.

The Bohr effect can be represented schematically as:

$$HbO_2 + H^+ \rightleftarrows HbH + O_2$$

oxyhemoglobin   deoxyhemoglobin

where an increase in protons (or a lower pO_2) shifts the equilibrium to the right (favoring deoxyhemoglobin), whereas an increase in pO_2 (or a decrease in protons) shifts the equilibrium to the left.

3. Effect of 2,3-bisphosphoglycerate on oxygen affinity: 2,3-Bisphosphoglycerate (2,3-BPG) is an important regulator of the binding of oxygen to hemoglobin. It is the most abundant organic phosphate in the RBC, where its concentration is approximately that of hemoglobin. 2,3-BPG is synthesized from an intermediate of the glycolytic pathway (Figure 3.9; see p. 101 for a discussion of 2,3-BPG synthesis in glycolysis).

a. Binding of 2,3-BPG to deoxyhemoglobin: 2,3-BPG decreases the oxygen affinity of hemoglobin by binding to deoxyhemoglobin but not to oxyhemoglobin. This preferential binding stabilizes the taut conformation of deoxyhemoglobin. The effect of binding 2,3-BPG can be represented schematically as:

$$HbO_2 + 2,3\text{-}BPG \rightleftarrows Hb\text{–}2,3\text{-}BPG + O_2$$

oxyhemoglobin   deoxyhemoglobin

b. Binding site of 2,3-BPG: One molecule of 2,3-BPG binds to a pocket, formed by the two β-globin chains, in the center of the deoxyhemoglobin tetramer (Figure 3.10). This pocket contains several positively charged amino acids that form ionic bonds with the negatively charged phosphate groups of 2,3-BPG. [Note: A mutation of one of these residues can result in hemoglobin variants with abnormally high oxygen affinity.] 2,3-BPG is expelled on oxygenation of the hemoglobin.

c. Shift of the oxygen dissociation curve: Hemoglobin from which 2,3-BPG has been removed has a high affinity for oxygen. However, as seen in the RBC, the presence of 2,3-BPG significantly reduces the affinity of hemoglobin for oxygen, shifting the oxygen dissociation curve to the right (Figure 3.11). This reduced affinity enables hemoglobin to release oxygen efficiently at the partial pressures found in the tissues.

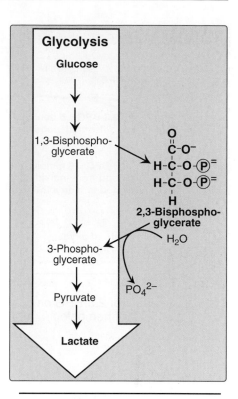

Figure 3.9
Synthesis of 2,3-bisphospho-glycerate. [Note: Ⓟ is a phosphoryl group.] In older literature 2,3-bis-phosphoglycerate (2,3-BPG) may be referred to as 2,3-diphospho-glycerate (2,3-DPG).

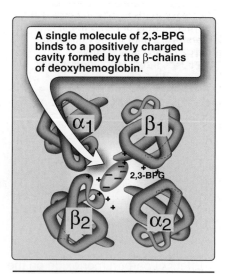

A single molecule of 2,3-BPG binds to a positively charged cavity formed by the β-chains of deoxyhemoglobin.

Figure 3.10
Binding of 2,3-BPG by deoxy-hemoglobin.

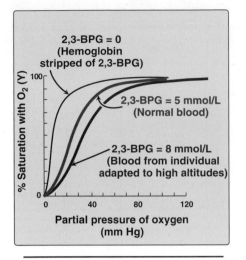

Figure 3.11
Allosteric effect of 2,3-BPG on the oxygen affinity of hemoglobin.

d. Response of 2,3-BPG levels to chronic hypoxia or anemia: The concentration of 2,3-BPG in the RBC increases in response to chronic hypoxia, such as that observed in chronic obstructive pulmonary disease (COPD) like emphysema, or at high altitudes, where circulating hemoglobin may have difficulty receiving sufficient oxygen. Intracellular levels of 2,3-BPG are also elevated in chronic anemia, in which fewer than normal RBCs are available to supply the body's oxygen needs. Elevated 2,3-BPG levels lower the oxygen affinity of hemoglobin, permitting greater unloading of oxygen in the capillaries of the tissues (see Figure 3.11).

e. Role of 2,3-BPG in transfused blood: 2,3-BPG is essential for the normal oxygen transport function of hemoglobin. However, storing blood in the currently available media results in a decrease in 2,3-PBG. Stored blood displays an abnormally high oxygen affinity, and fails to unload its bound oxygen properly in the tissues. Hemoglobin deficient in 2,3-BPG thus acts as an oxygen "trap" rather than as an oxygen transport system. Transfused RBCs are able to restore their depleted supplies of 2,3-BPG in 6–24 hours. However, severely ill patients may be compromised if transfused with large quantities of such 2,3-BPG–"stripped" blood. [Note: The maximum storage time for red cells has been doubled (21 to 42 days, with median time of 15 days) by changes in H^+, phosphate and hexose sugar concentration, and by the addition of adenine (see p. 291). Although the content of 2,3-BPG was not greatly affected by these changes, ATP production was increased and improved RBC survival.]

4. Binding of CO_2: Most of the CO_2 produced in metabolism is hydrated and transported as bicarbonate ion (see p. 9). However, some CO_2 is carried as carbamate bound to the N-terminal amino groups of hemoglobin (forming carbaminohemoglobin, see Figure 3.7), which can be represented schematically as follows:

$$Hb-NH_2 + CO_2 \rightleftarrows Hb-NH-COO^- + H^+$$

The binding of CO_2 stabilizes the T (taut) or deoxy form of hemoglobin, resulting in a decrease in its affinity for oxygen (see p. 28) and a right shift in the oxygen dissociation. In the lungs, CO_2 dissociates from the hemoglobin, and is released in the breath.

5. Binding of CO: Carbon monoxide (CO) binds tightly (but reversibly) to the hemoglobin iron, forming carbon monoxyhemoglobin (or carboxyhemoglobin). When CO binds to one or more of the four heme sites, hemoglobin shifts to the relaxed conformation, causing the remaining heme sites to bind oxygen with high affinity. This shifts the oxygen dissociation curve to the left, and changes the normal sigmoidal shape toward a hyperbola. As a result, the affected hemoglobin is unable to release oxygen to the tissues (Figure 3.12). [Note: The affinity of hemoglobin for CO is 220 times greater than for oxygen. Consequently, even minute concentrations of CO in the environment can produce toxic concentrations of carbon monoxyhemoglobin in the blood. For exam-

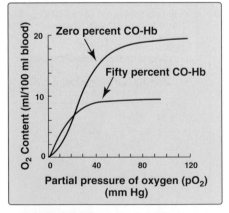

Figure 3.12
Effect of carbon monoxide on the oxygen affinity of hemoglobin. CO-Hb = carbon monoxy-hemoglobin.

ple, increased levels of CO are found in the blood of tobacco smokers. Carbon monoxide toxicity appears to result from a combination of tissue hypoxia and direct CO-mediated damage at the cellular level.] Carbon monoxide poisoning is treated with 100% oxygen at high pressure (hyperbaric oxygen therapy), which facilitates the dissociation of CO from the hemoglobin. [Note: CO inhibits Complex IV of the electron transport chain (see p. 76).] In addition to O_2, CO_2, and CO, nitric oxide gas (NO) also is carried by hemoglobin. NO is a potent vasodilator (see p. 151). It can be taken up (salvaged) or released from RBCs, thus modulating NO availability and influencing vessel diameter.

F. Minor hemoglobins

It is important to remember that human hemoglobin A (Hb A) is just one member of a functionally and structurally related family of proteins, the hemoglobins (Figure 3.13). Each of these oxygen-carrying proteins is a tetramer, composed of two α-globin polypeptides and two β-globin (or β-globin-like) polypeptides. Certain hemoglobins, such as Hb F, are normally synthesized only during fetal development, whereas others, such as Hb A_2, are synthesized in the adult, although at low levels compared with Hb A. Hb A can also become modified by the covalent addition of a hexose. For example, addition of glucose forms the glucosylated hemoglobin derivative, Hb A_{1c}.

1. **Fetal hemoglobin (Hb F):** Hb F is a tetramer consisting of two α chains identical to those found in Hb A, plus two γ chains ($\alpha_2\gamma_2$, see Figure 3.13). The γ chains are members of the β-globin gene family (see p. 35).

    a. **Hb F synthesis during development:** In the first month after conception, embryonic hemoglobins such as Hb Gower 1, composed of two α-like zeta (ζ) chains and two β-like epsilon (ε) chains ($\zeta_2\varepsilon_2$), are synthesized by the embryonic yolk sac. In the fifth week of gestation, the site of globin synthesis shifts, first to the liver and then to the marrow, and the primary product is Hb F. Hb F is the major hemoglobin found in the fetus and newborn, accounting for about 60% of the total hemoglobin in the erythrocytes during the last months of fetal life (Figure 3.14). Hb A synthesis starts in the bone marrow at about the eighth month of pregnancy and gradually replaces Hb F. (Figure 3.14 shows the relative production of each type of hemoglobin chain during fetal and postnatal life.) [Note: Hb F represents less than 1% of the Hb in most adults, and is concentrated in RBCs known as F-cells.]

    b. **Binding of 2,3-BPG to Hb F:** Under physiologic conditions, Hb F has a higher affinity for oxygen than does Hb A, as a result of Hb F binding only weakly to 2,3-BPG. [Note: The γ-globin chains of Hb F lack some of the positively charged amino acids that are responsible for binding 2,3-BPG in the β-globin chains.] Because 2,3-BPG serves to reduce the affinity of hemoglobin for oxygen, the weaker interaction between 2,3-BPG and Hb F results in a higher oxygen affinity for Hb F relative to Hb A. In contrast, if both Hb A and Hb F are stripped of their 2,3-BPG, they then have a similar affinity for oxygen.

Form	Chain composition	Fraction of total hemoglobin
HbA	$\alpha_2\beta_2$	90%
HbF	$\alpha_2\gamma_2$	<2%
HbA$_2$	$\alpha_2\delta_2$	2–5%
HbA$_{1c}$	$\alpha_2\beta_2$-glucose	3–9%

Figure 3.13
Normal adult human hemoglobins. [Note: The α-chains in these hemoglobins are identical.]

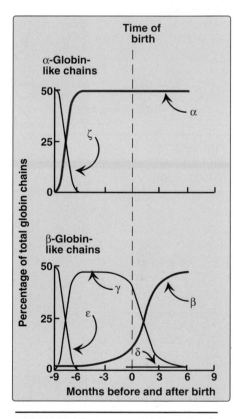

Figure 3.14
Developmental changes in hemoglobin.

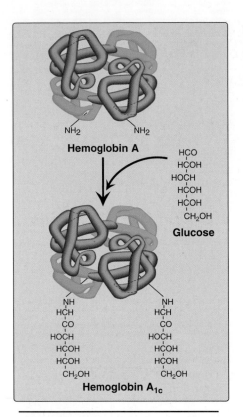

Figure 3.15
Nonenzymic addition of glucose to hemoglobin.

The higher oxygen affinity of Hb F facilitates the transfer of oxygen from the maternal circulation across the placenta to the RBCs of the fetus.

2. **Hemoglobin A$_2$ (Hb A$_2$):** Hb A$_2$ is a minor component of normal adult hemoglobin, first appearing shortly before birth and, ultimately, constituting about 2% of the total hemoglobin. It is composed of two α-globin chains and two δ-globin chains ($\alpha_2\delta_2$, see Figure 3.13).

3. **Hemoglobin A$_{1c}$ (HbA$_{1c}$):** Under physiologic conditions, Hb A is slowly and nonenzymically glycosylated, the extent of glycosylation being dependent on the plasma concentration of a particular hexose. The most abundant form of glycosylated hemoglobin is Hb A$_{1c}$. It has glucose residues attached predominantly to the NH$_2$ groups of the N-terminal valines of the β-globin chains (Figure 3.15). Increased amounts of Hb A$_{1c}$ are found in RBCs of patients with diabetes mellitus, because their Hb A has contact with higher glucose concentrations during the 120-day lifetime of these cells. (See p. 340 for a discussion of the use of this phenomenon in assessing average blood glucose levels in persons with diabetes.)

III. ORGANIZATION OF THE GLOBIN GENES

To understand diseases resulting from genetic alterations in the structure or synthesis of hemoglobins, it is necessary to grasp how the hemoglobin genes, which direct the synthesis of the different globin chains, are structurally organized into gene families and also how they are expressed.

A. α-Gene family

The genes coding for the α-globin-like and β-globin-like subunits of the hemoglobin chains occur in two separate gene clusters (or families) located on two different chromosomes (Figure 3.16). The α-gene cluster on chromosome 16 contains two genes for the α-globin chains. It also contains the ζ gene that is expressed early in development as a component of embryonic hemoblobin. [Note: Globin gene famillies also contain globin-like genes that are not expressed (that is, their genetic information is not used to produce globin chains). These are called pseudogenes.]

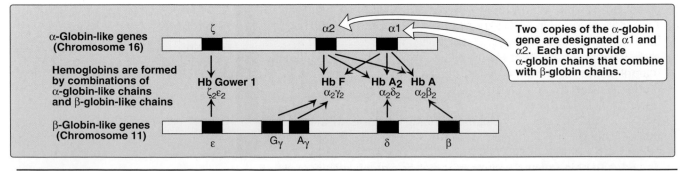

Figure 3.16
Organization of the globin gene families.

B. β-Gene family

A single gene for the β-globin chain is located on chromosome 11 (see Figure 3.16). There are an additional four β-globin-like genes: the ε gene (which, like the ζ gene, is expressed early in embryonic development), two γ genes (G_γ and A_γ that are expressed in Hb F), and the δ gene that codes for the globin chain found in the minor adult hemoglobin Hb A_2.

C. Steps in globin chain synthesis

Expression of a globin gene begins in the nucleus of red cell precursors, where the DNA sequence encoding the gene is transcribed. The RNA produced by transcription is actually a precursor of the messenger RNA (mRNA) that is used as a template for the synthesis of a globin chain. Before it can serve this function, two noncoding stretches of RNA (introns) must be removed from the mRNA precursor sequence, and the remaining three fragments (exons) joined in a linear manner. The resulting mature mRNA enters the cytosol, where its genetic information is translated, producing a globin chain. (A summary of this process is shown in Figure 3.17. A more detailed description of protein synthesis is presented in Chapter 31, p. 431.)

IV. HEMOGLOBINOPATHIES

Hemoglobinopathies have traditionally been defined as a family of genetic disorders caused by production of a structurally abnormal hemoglobin molecule, synthesis of insufficient quantities of normal hemoglobin, or, rarely, both. Sickle cell anemia (Hb S), hemoglobin C disease (Hb C), hemoglobin SC disease (Hb S + Hb C), and the thalassemia syndromes are representative hemoglobinopathies that can have severe clinical consequences. The first three conditions result from production of hemoglobin with an altered amino acid sequence (qualitative hemoglobinopathy), whereas the thalassemias are caused by decreased production of normal hemoglobin (quantitative hemoglobinopathy).

A. Sickle cell anemia (hemoglobin S disease)

Sickle cell anemia, the most common of the red cell sickling diseases, is a genetic disorder of the blood caused by a single nucleotide alteration (a point mutation) in the gene for β-globin. It is the most common inherited blood disorder in the United States, affecting 80,000 Americans. It occurs primarily in the African-American population, affecting one of 500 newborn African-American infants in the United States. Sickle cell anemia is a homozygous, recessive disorder. It occurs in individuals who have inherited two mutant genes (one from each parent) that code for synthesis of the β chains of the globin molecules. [Note: The mutant β-globin chain is designated β^S, and the resulting hemoglobin, $\alpha_2\beta^S_2$, is referred to as Hb S.] An infant does not begin showing symptoms of the disease until sufficient Hb F has been replaced by Hb S so that sickling can occur (see below). Sickle cell anemia is characterized by lifelong episodes of pain ("crises"), chronic hemolytic anemia with associated hyperbilirubinemia (see p. 284), and increased susceptibility to infections, usually beginning in early childhood. [Note: The lifetime of an

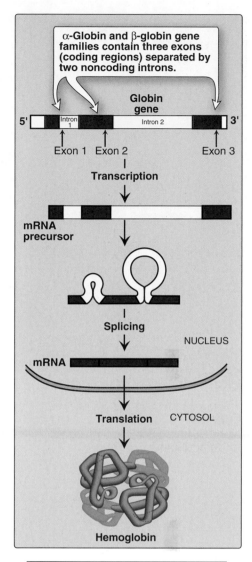

α-Globin and β-globin gene families contain three exons (coding regions) separated by two noncoding introns.

Figure 3.17
Synthesis of globin chains.

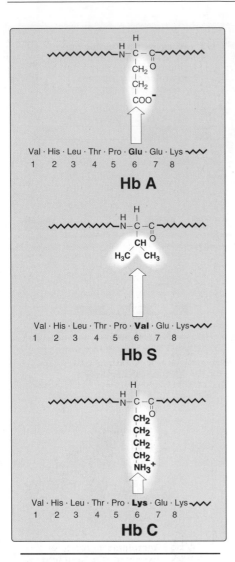

Figure 3.18
Amino acid substitutions in Hb S and Hb C.

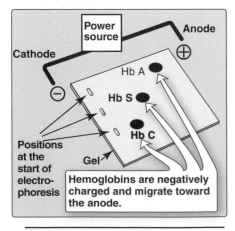

Figure 3.19
Diagram of hemoglobins A, S, and C after electrophoresis.

erythrocyte in sickle cell anemia is less than 20 days, compared with 120 days for normal RBCs; hence, the anemia.] Other symptoms include acute chest syndrome, stroke, splenic and renal dysfunction, and bone changes due to marrow hyperplasia. Heterozygotes, representing 1 in 12 African-Americans, have one normal and one sickle cell gene. The blood cells of such heterozygotes contain both Hb S and Hb A. These individuals have sickle cell trait. They usually do not show clinical symptoms and can have a normal life span.

1. **Amino acid substitution in Hb S β chains:** A molecule of Hb S contains two normal α-globin chains and two mutant β-globin chains (β^S), in which glutamate at position six has been replaced with valine (Figure 3.18). Therefore, during electrophoresis at alkaline pH, Hb S migrates more slowly toward the anode (positive electrode) than does Hb A (Figure 3.19). This altered mobility of Hb S is a result of the absence of the negatively charged glutamate residues in the two β chains, thus rendering Hb S less negative than Hb A. [Note: Electrophoresis of hemoglobin obtained from lysed RBCs is routinely used in the diagnosis of sickle cell trait and sickle cell disease.]

2. **Sickling and tissue anoxia:** The replacement of the charged glutamate with the nonpolar valine forms a protrusion on the β-globin that fits into a complementary site on the β chain of another hemoglobin molecule in the cell (Figure 3.20). At low oxygen tension, deoxyhemoglobin S polymerizes inside the RBC, forming a network of fibrous polymers that stiffen and distort the cell, producing rigid, misshapen erythrocytes. Such sickled cells frequently block the flow of blood in the narrow capillaries. This interruption in the supply of oxygen leads to localized anoxia (oxygen deprivation) in the tissue, causing pain and eventually death (infarction) of cells in the vicinity of the blockage. The anoxia also leads to an increase in deoxygenated Hb S. [Note: The mean diameter of RBCs is 7.5 μm, whereas that of the microvasculature is 3–4 μm. Instead of squeezing through the microvasculature like Hb A–containing RBCs, sickled cells have a decreased ability to deform and an increased tendency to adhere to vessel walls, and so have difficulty moving through small vessels.]

3. **Variables that increase sickling:** The extent of sickling and, therefore, the severity of disease is enhanced by any variable that increases the proportion of Hb S in the deoxy state (that is, reduces the affinity of Hb S for oxygen). These variables include decreased oxygen tension as a result of high altitudes or flying in a nonpressurized plane, increased pCO$_2$, decreased pH, dehydration, and an increased concentration of 2,3-BPG in erythrocytes.

4. **Treatment:** Therapy involves adequate hydration, analgesics, aggressive antibiotic therapy if infection is present, and transfusions in patients at high risk for fatal occlusion of blood vessels. Intermittent transfusions with packed red cells reduce the risk of stroke, but the benefits must be weighed against the complications of transfusion, which include iron overload (hemosiderosis), bloodborne infections, and immunologic complications. Hydroxyurea, an antitumor drug, is therapeutically useful because it increases circulating levels of Hb F, which decreases RBC sickling. This leads to decreased frequency of painful crises and reduces mortality.

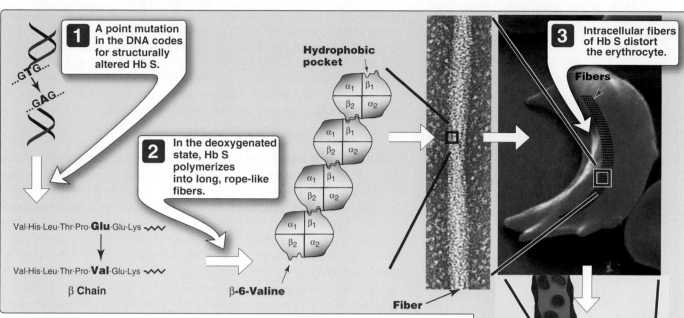

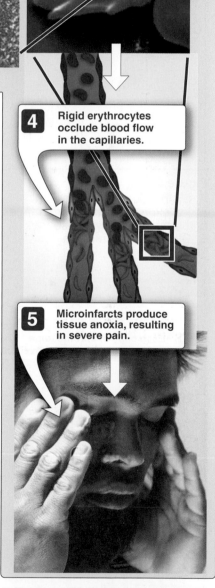

Figure 3.20
Molecular and cellular events leading to sickle cell crisis.

5. Possible selective advantage of the heterozygous state: The high frequency of the β^S mutation among black Africans, despite its damaging effects in the homozygous state, suggests that a selective advantage exists for heterozygous individuals. For example, heterozygotes for the sickle cell gene are less susceptible to malaria, caused by the parasite <u>Plasmodium</u> <u>falciparum</u>. This organism spends an obligatory part of its life cycle in the RBC. One theory is that because these cells in individuals heterozygous for Hb S, like those in homozygotes, have a shorter life span than normal, the parasite cannot complete the intracellular stage of its development. This fact may provide a selective advantage to heterozygotes living in regions where malaria is a major cause of death. Figure 3.21 illustrates that in Africa, the geographic distribution of sickle cell anemia is similar to that of malaria. The morbidity and mortality associated with sickle cell anemia has led to its inclusion in newborn screening panels to allow prophylactic antibiotic therapy to begin soon after the birth of an affected child.

B. Hemoglobin C disease

Like Hb S, Hb C is a hemoglobin variant that has a single amino acid substitution in the sixth position of the β-globin chain (see Figure 3.18). In this case, however, a lysine is substituted for the glutamate (as compared with a valine substitution in Hb S). [Note: This substitution causes Hb C to move more slowly toward the anode than Hb A or Hb S does (see Figure 3.19).] Patients homozygous for hemoglobin C generally have a relatively mild, chronic hemolytic anemia. These patients do not suffer from infarctive crises, and no specific therapy is required.

C. Hemoglobin SC disease

Hemoglobin SC disease is another of the red cell sickling diseases. In this disease, some β-globin chains have the sickle cell mutation, whereas other β-globin chains carry the mutation found in Hb C disease. [Note: Patients with Hb SC disease are doubly hetero-

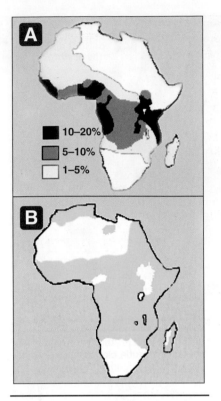

Figure 3.21
A. Distribution of sickle cell in Africa expressed as a percentage of the population with disease.
B. Distribution of malaria in Africa.

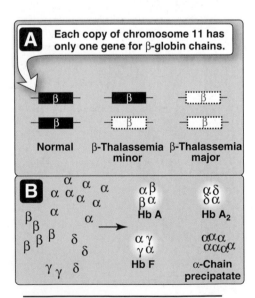

Figure 3.22
A. β-Globin gene mutations in the β-thalassemias. B. Hemoglobin tetramers formed in ß-thalassemias.

zygous (compound heterozygote) because both of their β-globin genes are abnormal, although different from each other.] Hemoglobin levels tend to be higher in Hb SC disease than in sickle cell anemia, and may even be at the low end of the normal range. The clinical course of adults with Hb SC anemia differs from that of sickle cell anemia in that symptoms such as painful crises are less frequent and less severe; however, there is significant clinical variability.

D. Methemoglobinemias

Oxidation of the heme component of hemoglobin to the ferric (Fe^{3+}) state forms methemoglobin, which cannot bind oxygen. This oxidation may be caused by the action of certain drugs, such as nitrates, or endogenous products, such as reactive oxygen intermediates (see p. 148). The oxidation may also result from inherited defects, for example, certain mutations in the α- or β-globin chain promote the formation of methemoglobin (Hb M). Furthermore, a deficiency of *NADH-cytochrome b_5 reductase* (also called *NADH-methemoglobin reductase*), the enzyme responsible for the conversion of methemoglobin (Fe^{3+}) to hemoglobin (Fe^{2+}), leads to the accumulation of methemoglobin. [Note: The erythrocytes of newborns have approximately half the capacity of those of adults to reduce methemoglobin. They are therefore particularly susceptible to the effects of methemoglobin-producing compounds.] The methemoglobinemias are characterized by "chocolate cyanosis" (a brownish-blue coloration of the skin and mucous membranes) and chocolate-colored blood, as a result of the dark-colored methemoglobin. Symptoms are related to the degree of tissue hypoxia, and include anxiety, headache, and dyspnea. In rare cases, coma and death can occur. Treatment is with methylene blue, which is oxidized as Fe^{+3} is reduced.

E. Thalassemias

The thalassemias are hereditary hemolytic diseases in which an imbalance occurs in the synthesis of globin chains. As a group, they are the most common single gene disorders in humans. Normally, synthesis of the α- and β-globin chains is coordinated, so that each α-globin chain has a β-globin chain partner. This leads to the formation of $\alpha_2\beta_2$ (Hb A). In the thalassemias, the synthesis of either the α- or the β-globin chain is defective. A thalassemia can be caused by a variety of mutations, including entire gene deletions, or substitutions or deletions of one to many nucleotides in the DNA. [Note: Each thalassemia can be classified as either a disorder in which no globin chains are produced (α°- or β°-thalassemia), or one in which some chains are synthesized, but at a reduced level (α+- or β+-thalassemia).]

1. **β-Thalassemias:** In these disorders, synthesis of β-globin chains is decreased or absent, typically as a result of point mutations that affect the production of functional mRNA; however, α-globin chain synthesis is normal. α-Globin chains cannot form stable tetramers and, therefore, precipitate, causing the premature death of cells initially destined to become mature RBCs. Increase in $\alpha_2\gamma_2$ (Hb F) and $\alpha_2\delta_2$ (Hb A_2) also occurs. There are only two copies of the β-globin gene in each cell (one on each chromosome 11). Therefore, individuals with β-globin gene defects have either β-thalassemia trait (β-thalassemia minor) if they have only one defective β-globin gene, or β-thalassemia major (Cooley anemia)

if both genes are defective (Figure 3.22). Because the β-globin gene is not expressed until late in fetal gestation, the physical manifestations of β-thalassemias appear only several months after birth. Those individuals with β-thalassemia minor make some β chains, and usually do not require specific treatment. However, those infants born with β-thalassemia major are seemingly healthy at birth, but become severely anemic, usually during the first or second year of life due to ineffective erythropoiesis. Skeletal changes as a result of extramedullary hematopoiesis also are seen. These patients require regular transfusions of blood. [Note: Although this treatment is lifesaving, the cumulative effect of the transfusions is iron overload (a syndrome known as hemosiderosis). Use of iron chelation therapy has improved morbidity and mortality.] The increasing use of bone marrow replacement therapy has been a boon to these patients.

2. **α-Thalassemias:** These are defects in which the synthesis of α-globin chains is decreased or absent, typically as a result of deletional mutations. Because each individual's genome contains four copies of the α-globin gene (two on each chromosome 16), there are several levels of α-globin chain deficiencies (Figure 3.23). If one of the four genes is defective, the individual is termed a silent carrier of α-thalassemia, because no physical manifestations of the disease occur. If two α-globin genes are defective, the individual is designated as having α-thalassemia trait. If three α-globin genes are defective, the individual has Hb H (β_4) disease—a mildly to moderately severe hemolytic anemia. If all four α-globin genes are defective, Hb Bart (γ_4) disease with hydrops fetalis and fetal death results, because α-globin chains are required for the synthesis of Hb F. [Note: Hemoglobinopathies that result in increased O_2 affinity typically are characterized by increased production of RBCs, whereas those that result in decreased O_2 affinity are characterized by anemia.]

V. CHAPTER SUMMARY

Hemoglobin A, the major hemoglobin in adults, is composed of four polypeptide chains (two α chains and two β chains, $\alpha_2\beta_2$) held together by noncovalent interactions (Figure 3.24). The subunits occupy different relative positions in deoxyhemoglobin compared with oxyhemoglobin. The **deoxy form** of hemoglobin is called the "**T**," or **taut (tense) form**. It has a constrained structure that limits the movement of the polypeptide chains. The T form is the **low-oxygen-affinity form** of hemoglobin. The binding of oxygen to hemoglobin causes rupture of some of the ionic and hydrogen bonds. This leads to a structure called the "**R**," or **relaxed form**, in which the polypeptide chains have more freedom of movement. The R form is the **high-oxygen-affinity form** of hemoglobin. The **oxygen dissociation curve** for hemoglobin is **sigmoidal** in shape (in contrast to that of **myoglobin**, which is **hyperbolic**), indicating that the subunits cooperate in binding oxygen. **Cooperative binding** of oxygen by the four subunits of hemoglobin means that the binding of an oxygen molecule at one heme group increases the oxygen affinity of the remaining heme groups in the same hemoglobin molecule. Hemoglobin's **ability to bind**

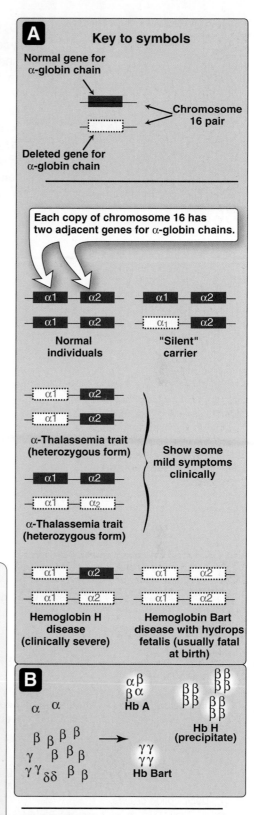

Figure 3.23
A. α-Globin gene deletions in the α-thalassemias. B. Hemoglobin tetramers formed in α-thalassemias.

oxygen reversibly is affected by the pO_2 (through heme-heme interactions), the **pH** of the environment, the pCO_2, and the availability of **2,3-bisphosphoglycerate (2,3-BPG)**. For example, the release of O_2 from Hb is enhanced when the pH is lowered or the pCO_2 is increased (the **Bohr effect**), such as in **exercising muscle**, and the oxygen dissociation curve of Hb is shifted to the right. To cope long-term with the effects of **chronic hypoxia** or **anemia**, the concentration of **2,3-BPG** in **RBCs** increases. **2,3-BPG** binds to the Hb and decreases its oxygen affinity, and it, therefore, also shifts the oxygen-dissociation curve to the right. **Carbon monoxide (CO)** binds tightly (but reversibly) to the hemoglobin iron, forming **carbon monoxyhemoglobin (Hb CO)**. **Hemoglobinopathies** are disorders caused either by production of a **structurally abnormal hemoglobin** molecule, synthesis of **insufficient quantities** of normal hemoglobin subunits, or, rarely, both (Figure 3.25). The sickling diseases **sickle cell anemia** (Hb S disease) and **hemoglobin SC disease**, as well as **hemoglobin C disease** and the **thalassemia syndromes** are representative hemoglobinopathies that can have severe clinical consequences.

Study Questions

Choose the ONE correct answer.

3.1 Which one of the following statements concerning the hemoglobins is correct?

A. Fetal blood has a higher affinity for oxygen than does adult blood because Hb F has a decreased affinity for 2,3-BPG.

B. Purified Hb F (stripped of 2,3-BPG) has a higher affinity for oxygen than does purified Hb A.

C. The globin chain composition of Hb F is $\alpha_2\delta_2$.

D. Hb A_{1c} differs from Hb A by a single, genetically determined amino acid substitution.

E. Hb A_2 appears early in fetal life.

Correct answer = A. Because 2,3-BPG reduces the affinity of hemoglobin for oxygen, the weaker interaction between 2,3-BPG and Hb F results in a higher oxygen affinity for Hb F relative to Hb A. In contrast, if both Hb A and Hb F are stripped of 2,3-BPG, they have a similar affinity for oxygen. Hb F consists of $\alpha_2\gamma_2$. Hb A_{1c} is a glycosylated form of Hb A, formed nonenzymatically in red cells. Hb A_2 is a minor component of normal adult hemoglobin, first appearing shortly before birth and rising to adult levels (about 2% of the total hemoglobin) by 6 months of age.

3.2 Which one of the following statements concerning the ability of acidosis to precipitate a crisis in sickle cell anemia is correct?

A. Acidosis decreases the solubility of Hb S.

B. Acidosis increases the affinity of hemoglobin for oxygen.

C. Acidosis favors the conversion of hemoglobin from the taut to the relaxed conformation.

D. Acidosis shifts the oxygen dissociation curve to the left.

E. Acidosis decreases the ability of 2,3-BPG to bind to hemoglobin.

Correct answer = A. Hb S is significantly less soluble in the deoxygenated form, compared with oxyhemoglobin S. A decrease in pH (acidosis) causes the oxygen dissociation curve to shift to the right, indicating a decreased affinity for oxygen. This favors the formation of the deoxy, or taut, form of hemoglobin, and can precipitate a sickle cell crisis. The binding of 2,3-BPG is increased, because it binds only to the deoxy form of hemoglobins.

3.3 Which one of the following statements concerning the binding of oxygen by hemoglobin is correct?

A. The Bohr effect results in a lower affinity for oxygen at higher pH values.

B. Carbon dioxide increases the oxygen affinity of hemoglobin by binding to the C-terminal groups of the polypeptide chains.

C. The oxygen affinity of hemoglobin increases as the percentage saturation increases.

D. The hemoglobin tetramer binds four molecules of 2,3-BPG.

E. Oxyhemoglobin and deoxyhemoglobin have the same affinity for protons (H^+).

Correct answer = C. The binding of oxygen at one heme group increases the oxygen affinity of the remaining heme groups in the same molecule. Carbon dioxide decreases oxygen affinity because it lowers the pH; moreover, binding of carbon dioxide to the N-termini stabilizes the taut, deoxy form. Hemoglobin binds one molecule of 2,3-BPG. Deoxyhemoglobin has a greater affinity for protons and, therefore, is a weaker acid.

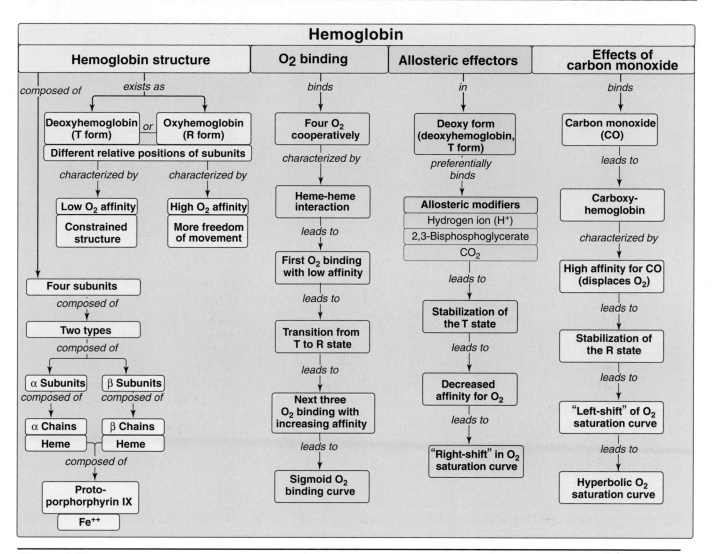

Figure 3.24
Key concept map for hemoglobin structure and function.

Study Questions (continued)

3.4 β-Lysine 82 in hemoglobin A is important for the binding of 2,3-BPG. In Hb Helsinki, this amino acid has been replaced by methionine. Which of the following should be true concerning Hb Helsinki?

A. It should be stabilized in the T, rather than the R, form.

B. It should have increased O_2 affinity and, consequently, decreased delivery of O_2 to tissues.

C. Its O_2 dissociation curve should be shifted to the right relative to Hb A.

D. It results in anemia.

Correct answer is B. Substitution of lysine by methionine decreases the ability of negatively charged phosphate groups in 2,3-BPG to bind the β subunits of hemoglobin. Because 2,3BPG decreases the O_2 affinity of hemoglobin, a reduction in 2,3-BPG should result in increased O_2 affinity and decreased delivery of O_2 to tissues. The R form is the high-oxygen-affinity form of hemoglobin. Increased O_2 affinity (decreased delivery) results in a left shift in the O_2 dissociation curve. Decreased O_2 delivery is compensated for by increased RBC production.

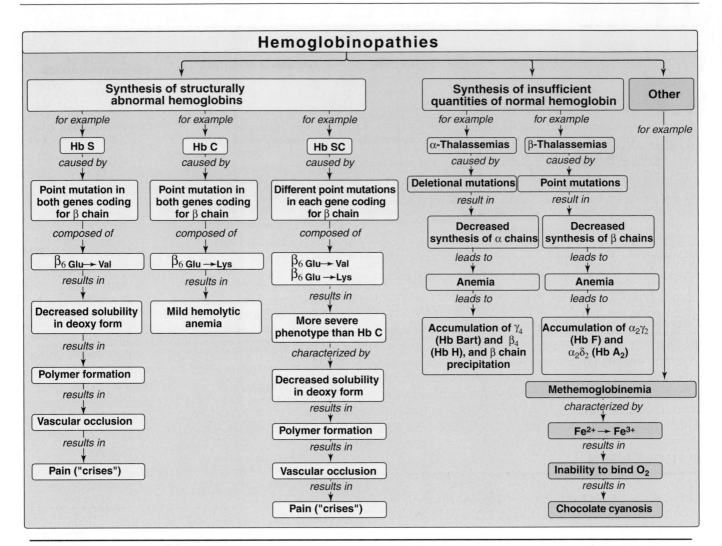

Figure 3.25
Key concept map for hemoglobinopathies.

Study Questions (continued)

3.5 A 67-year-old man presented to the emergency department with a 1 week history of angina and shortness of breath. He complained that his face and extremities had a "blue color." His medical history included chronic stable angina treated with isosorbide dinitrate and nitroglycerin. Blood obtained for analysis was chocolate-colored. Which one of the following is the most likely diagnosis?

A. Sickle cell anemia

B. Carboxyhemoglobinemia

C. Methemoglobinemia.

D. β-Thalassemia

E. Hemoglobin SC disease

Correct answer = C. Oxidation of the heme component of hemoglobin to the ferric (Fe^{3+}) state forms methemoglobin. This may be caused by the action of certain drugs, such as nitrates. The methemoglobinemias are characterized by chocolate cyanosis (a brownish-blue coloration of the skin and mucous membranes), and chocolate-colored blood as a result of the dark-colored methemoglobin. Symptoms are related to tissue hypoxia, and include anxiety, headache, dyspnea. In rare cases, coma and death can occur.

Fibrous Proteins

4

I. OVERVIEW

Collagen and elastin are examples of common, well-characterized fibrous proteins of the extracellular matrix that serve structural functions in the body. For example, collagen and elastin are found as components of skin, connective tissue, blood vessel walls, and sclera and cornea of the eye. Each fibrous protein exhibits special mechanical properties, resulting from its unique structure, which are obtained by combining specific amino acids into regular, secondary structural elements. This is in contrast to globular proteins, whose shapes are the result of complex interactions between secondary, tertiary, and, sometimes, quaternary structural elements.

II. COLLAGEN

Collagen is the most abundant protein in the human body. A typical collagen molecule is a long, rigid structure in which three polypeptides (referred to as "α chains") are wound around one another in a rope-like triple helix (Figure 4.1). Although these molecules are found throughout the body, their types and organization are dictated by the structural role collagen plays in a particular organ. In some tissues, collagen may be dispersed as a gel that gives support to the structure, as in the extracellular matrix or the vitreous humor of the eye. In other tissues, collagen may be bundled in tight, parallel fibers that provide great strength, as in tendons. In the cornea of the eye, collagen is stacked so as to transmit light with a minimum of scattering. Collagen of bone occurs as fibers arranged at an angle to each other so as to resist mechanical shear from any direction.

A. Types of collagen

The collagen superfamily of proteins includes more than 25 collagen types, as well as additional proteins that have collagen-like domains. The three polypeptide α chains are held together by hydrogen bonds between the chains. Variations in the amino acid sequence of the α chains result in structural components that are about the same size (approximately 1,000 amino acids long), but with slightly different properties. These α chains are combined to form the various types of collagen found in the tissues. For example, the most common collagen, type I, contains two chains called α1 and one chain called α2 ($\alpha1_2\alpha2$), whereas type II collagen contains three α1 chains ($\alpha1_3$). The

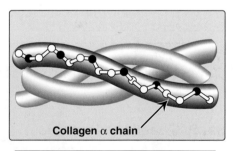

Collagen α chain

Figure 4.1
Triple-stranded helix of collagen.

TYPE	TISSUE DISTRIBUTION
	Fibril-forming
I	Skin, bone, tendon, blood vessels, cornea
II	Cartilage, intervertebral disk, vitreous body
III	Blood vessels, fetal skin
	Network-forming
IV	Basement membrane
VII	Beneath stratified squamous epithelia
	Fibril-associated
IX	Cartilage
XII	Tendon, ligaments, some other tissues

Figure 4.2
The most abundant types of collagen.

collagens can be organized into three groups, based on their location and functions in the body (Figure 4.2).

1. **Fibril-forming collagens:** Types I, II, and III are the fibrillar collagens, and have the rope-like structure described above for a typical collagen molecule. In the electron microscope, these linear polymers of fibrils have characteristic banding patterns, reflecting the regular staggered packing of the individual collagen molecules in the fibril (Figure 4.3). Type I collagen fibers are found in supporting elements of high tensile strength (for example, tendon and cornea), whereas fibers formed from type II collagen molecules are restricted to cartilaginous structures. The fibers derived from type III collagen are prevalent in more distensible tissues, such as blood vessels.

2. **Network-forming collagens:** Types IV and VII form a three-dimensional mesh, rather than distinct fibrils (Figure 4.4). For example, type IV molecules assemble into a sheet or meshwork that constitutes a major part of basement membranes.

> Basement membranes are thin, sheet-like structures that provide mechanical support for adjacent cells, and function as a semipermeable filtration barrier to macromolecules in organs such as the kidney and the lung.

3. **Fibril-associated collagens:** Types IX and XII bind to the surface of collagen fibrils, linking these fibrils to one another and to other components in the extracellular matrix (see Figure 4.2).

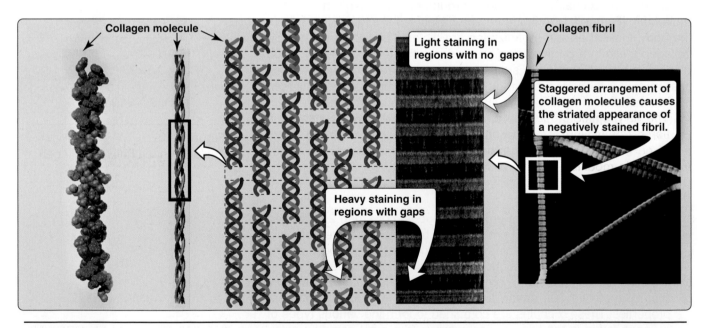

Figure 4.3
Collagen fibrils at right have a characteristic banding pattern, reflecting the regularly staggered packing of the individual collagen molecules in the fibril.

B. Structure of collagen

1. **Amino acid sequence:** Collagen is rich in proline and glycine, both of which are important in the formation of the triple-stranded helix. Proline facilitates the formation of the helical conformation of each α chain because its ring structure causes "kinks" in the peptide chain. [Note: The presence of proline dictates that the helical conformation of the α chain cannot be an α helix.] Glycine, the smallest amino acid, is found in every third position of the polypeptide chain. It fits into the restricted spaces where the three chains of the helix come together. The glycine residues are part of a repeating sequence, –Gly–X–Y–, where X is frequently proline and Y is often hydroxyproline (but can be hydroxylysine, Figure 4.5). Thus, most of the α chain can be regarded as a polytripeptide whose sequence can be represented as $(-Gly-Pro-Hyp-)_{333}$.

2. **Triple-helical structure:** Unlike most globular proteins that are folded into compact structures, collagen, a fibrous protein, has an elongated, triple-helical structure that places many of its amino acid side chains on the surface of the triple-helical molecule. [Note: This allows bond formation between the exposed R-groups of neighboring collagen monomers, resulting in their aggregation into long fibers.]

3. **Hydroxyproline and hydroxylysine:** Collagen contains hydroxyproline (hyp) and hydroxylysine (hyl), which are not present in most other proteins. These residues result from the hydroxylation of some of the proline and lysine residues after their incorporation into polypeptide chains (Figure 4.6). The hydroxylation is, thus, an example of posttranslational modification (see p. 443). Hydroxyproline is important in stabilizing the triple-helical structure of collagen because it maximizes interchain hydrogen bond formation.

4. **Glycosylation:** The hydroxyl group of the hydroxylysine residues of collagen may be enzymatically glycosylated. Most commonly, glucose and galactose are sequentially attached to the polypeptide chain prior to triple-helix formation (Figure 4.7).

C. Biosynthesis of collagen

The polypeptide precursors of the collagen molecule are formed in fibroblasts (or in the related osteoblasts of bone and chondroblasts of cartilage), and are secreted into the extracellular matrix. After enzymic modification, the mature collagen monomers aggregate and become cross-linked to form collagen fibers.

1. **Formation of pro-α chains:** Collagen is one of many proteins that normally function outside of cells. Like most proteins produced for export, the newly synthesized polypeptide precursors of α chains (prepro-α chains) contain a special amino acid sequence at their N-terminal ends. This sequence acts as a signal that, in the absence of additional signals, targets the polypeptide being synthesized for secretion from the cell. The signal sequence facilitates the binding of ribosomes to the rough endoplasmic reticulum (RER), and directs the passage of the prepro-α chain into the lumen of the RER. The signal sequence is rapidly cleaved in the RER to yield a precursor of collagen called a pro-α chain (see Figure 4.7).

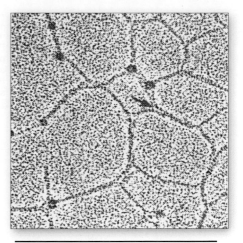

Figure 4.4
Electron micrograph of a polygonal network formed by association of collagen type IV monomers.

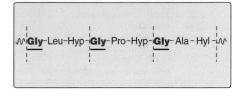

Figure 4.5
Amino acid sequence of a portion of the α1 chain of collagen. [Note: Hyp is hydroxyproline and Hyl is hydroxylysine.]

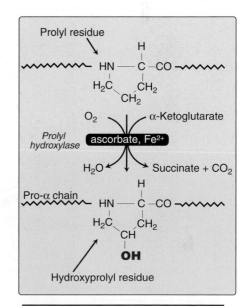

Figure 4.6
Hydroxylation of prolyl residues of pro-α chains of collagen by *prolyl hydroxylase*.

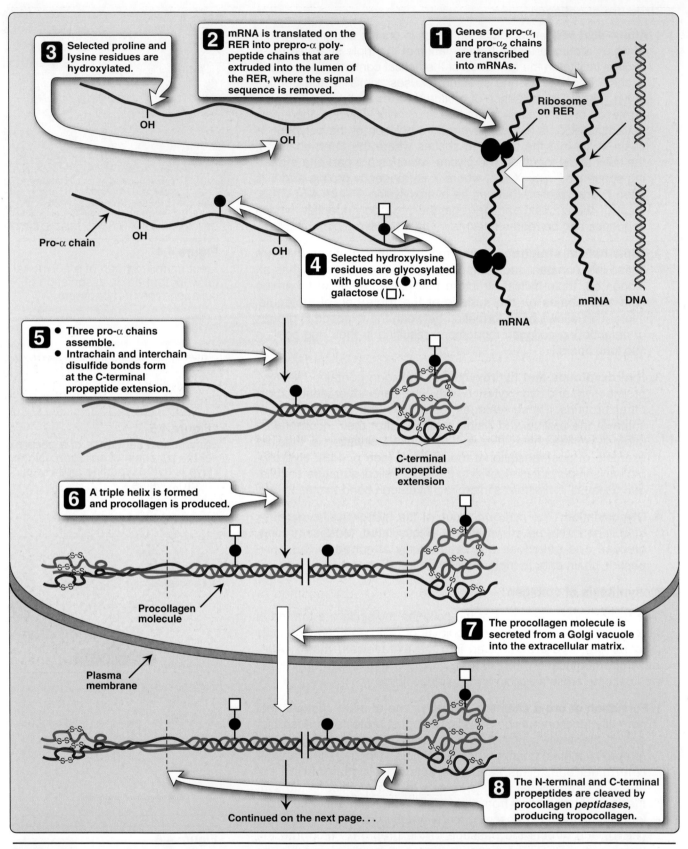

Figure 4.7
Synthesis of collagen. RER = rough endoplasmic reticulum. (*Continued on the next page*)

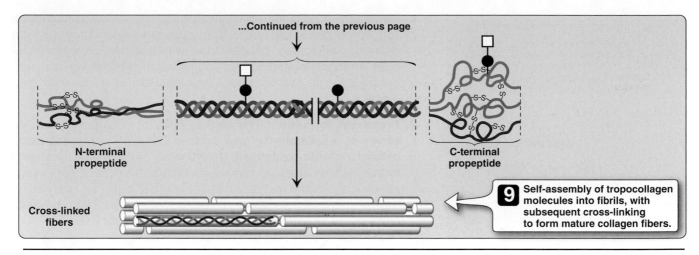

...Continued from the previous page

N-terminal
propeptide

C-terminal
propeptide

Cross-linked
fibers

9 Self-assembly of tropocollagen
molecules into fibrils, with
subsequent cross-linking
to form mature collagen fibers.

Figure 4.7
Synthesis of collagen. (*Continued from the previous page*)

2. **Hydroxylation:** The pro-α chains are processed by a number of
   enzymic steps within the lumen of the RER while the polypeptides
   are still being synthesized (see Figure 4.7). Proline and lysine
   residues found in the Y-position of the –Gly–X–Y– sequence can
   be hydroxylated to form hydroxyproline and hydroxylysine
   residues. These hydroxylation reactions require molecular oxygen,
   Fe^{2+}, and the reducing agent vitamin C (ascorbic acid, see p. 377),
   without which the hydroxylating enzymes, *prolyl hydroxylase* and
   lysyl hydroxylase, are unable to function (see Figure 4.6). In the case
   of ascorbic acid deficiency (and, therefore, a lack of prolyl and lysyl
   hydroxylation), interchain H-bond formation is impaired, as is formation of a stable triple helix. Additionally, collagen fibrils cannot be
   cross-linked (see below), greatly decreasing the tensile strength of
   the assembled fiber. The resulting deficiency disease is known as
   scurvy. Patients with ascorbic acid deficiency also often show
   bruises on the limbs as a result of subcutaneous extravasation of
   blood due to capillary fragility (Figure 4.8).

3. **Glycosylation:** Some hydroxylysine residues are modified by
   glycosylation with glucose or glucosyl-galactose (see Figure 4.7).

4. **Assembly and secretion:** After hydroxylation and glycosylation,
   pro-α chains form procollagen, a precursor of collagen that has a
   central region of triple helix flanked by the nonhelical amino- and
   carboxyl-terminal extensions called propeptides (see Figure 4.7).
   The formation of procollagen begins with formation of interchain
   disulfide bonds between the C-terminal extensions of the pro-α
   chains. This brings the three α chains into an alignment favorable
   for helix formation. The procollagen molecules move through the
   Golgi apparatus, where they are packaged in secretory vesicles.
   The vesicles fuse with the cell membrane, causing the release of
   procollagen molecules into the extracellular space.

5. **Extracellular cleavage of procollagen molecules:** After their
   release, the procollagen molecules are cleaved by *N*- and *C-pro-
   collagen peptidases,* which remove the terminal propeptides,
   releasing triple-helical tropocollagen molecules.

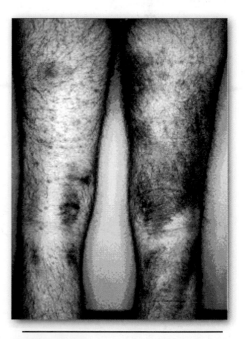

Figure 4.8
The legs of a 46-year-old man
with scurvy.

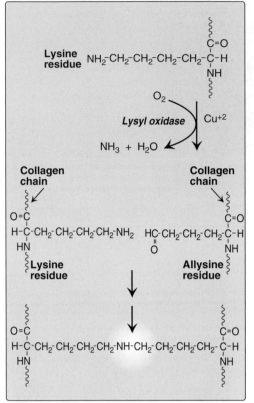

Figure 4.9
Formation of cross-links in collagen.

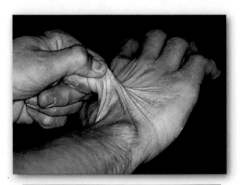

Figure 4.10
Stretchy skin of Ehlers-Danlos syndrome.

6. **Formation of collagen fibrils:** Individual tropocollagen molecules spontaneously associate to form collagen fibrils. They form an ordered, overlapping, parallel array, with adjacent collagen molecules arranged in a staggered pattern, each overlapping its neighbor by a length approximately three-quarters of a molecule (see Figure 4.7).

7. **Cross-link formation:** The fibrillar array of collagen molecules serves as a substrate for *lysyl oxidase*. This Cu^{2+}-containing extracellular enzyme oxidatively deaminates some of the lysyl and hydroxylysyl residues in collagen. The reactive aldehydes that result (allysine and hydroxyallysine) can condense with lysyl or hydroxylysyl residues in neighboring collagen molecules to form covalent cross-links and, thus, mature collagen fibers (Figure 4.9).

> *Lysyl oxidase* is one of several copper-containing enzymes. Others include *cytochrome oxidase* (see p. 76), *dopamine hydroxylase* (see p. 286), *superoxide dismutase* (see p.148) and *tyrosinase* (see p. 273). Disruption in copper homeostasis causes copper deficiency (X-linked Menkes disease) or overload (Wilson disease).

D. Degradation of collagen

Normal collagens are highly stable molecules, having half-lives as long as several years. However, connective tissue is dynamic and is constantly being remodeled, often in response to growth or injury of the tissue. Breakdown of collagen fibers is dependent on the proteolytic action of *collagenases*, which are part of a large family of matrix *metalloproteinases*. For type I collagen, the cleavage site is specific, generating three-quarter and one-quarter length fragments. These fragments are further degraded by other matrix *proteinases* to their constituent amino acids.

E. Collagen diseases: Collagenopathies

Defects in any one of the many steps in collagen fiber synthesis can result in a genetic disease involving an inability of collagen to form fibers properly and, thus, provide tissues with the needed tensile strength normally provided by collagen. More than 1,000 mutations have been identified in 22 genes coding for 12 of the collagen types. The following are examples of diseases that are the result of defective collagen synthesis.

1. **Ehlers-Danlos syndrome (EDS):** This disorder is a heterogeneous group of generalized connective tissue disorders that result from inheritable defects in the metabolism of fibrillar collagen molecules. EDS can result from a deficiency of collagen-processing enzymes (for example, *lysyl hydroxylase* or *procollagen peptidase*), or from mutations in the amino acid sequences of collagen types I, III, or V. The most clinically important mutations are found in the gene for type III collagen. Collagen containing mutant chains is not secreted, and is either degraded or accumulated to high levels in intracellular compartments. Because collagen type III is an important component of the arteries, potentially lethal vascular problems

occur. [Note: Although collagen type III is only a minor component of the collagen fibrils in the skin, patients with EDS also show, for unknown reasons, defects in collagen type I fibrils. This results in fragile, stretchy skin and loose joints (Figure 4.10).]

2. **Osteogenesis imperfecta (OI):** This disease, known as brittle bone syndrome, is also a heterogeneous group of inherited disorders distinguished by bones that easily bend and fracture (Figure 4.11). Retarded wound healing and a rotated and twisted spine leading to a "humped-back" (kyphotic) appearance are common features of the disease. Type I OI is called osteogenesis imperfecta tarda. The disease is the consequence of decreased production of $\alpha 1$ and $\alpha 2$ chains. It presents in early infancy with fractures secondary to minor trauma, and may be suspected if prenatal ultrasound detects bowing or fractures of long bones. Type II OI is called osteogenesis imperfecta congenita, and is the most severe. Patients die of pulmonary hypoplasia in utero or during the neonatal period. Most patients with severe OI have mutations in the gene for either the pro-$\alpha 1$ or pro-$\alpha 2$ chains of type I collagen. The most common mutations cause the replacement of glycine residues (in –Gly–X–Y–) by amino acids with bulky side chains. The resultant structurally abnormal pro-α chains prevent the formation of the required triple-helical conformation.

III. ELASTIN

In contrast to collagen, which forms fibers that are tough and have high tensile strength, elastin is a connective tissue protein with rubber-like properties. Elastic fibers composed of elastin and glycoprotein microfibrils are found in the lungs, the walls of large arteries, and elastic ligaments. They can be stretched to several times their normal length, but recoil to their original shape when the stretching force is relaxed.

A. Structure of elastin

Elastin is an insoluble protein polymer synthesized from a precursor, tropoelastin, which is a linear polypeptide composed of about 700 amino acids that are primarily small and nonpolar (for example, glycine, alanine, and valine). Elastin is also rich in proline and lysine, but contains only a little hydroxyproline and hydroxylysine. Tropoelastin is secreted by the cell into the extracellular space. There it interacts with specific glycoprotein microfibrils, such as fibrillin, which function as a scaffold onto which tropoelastin is deposited. Some of the lysyl side chains of the tropoelastin polypeptides are oxidatively deaminated by *lysyl oxidase*, forming allysine residues. Three of the allysyl side chains plus one unaltered lysyl side chain from the same or neighboring polypeptides form a desmosine cross-link (Figure 4.12). This produces elastin—an extensively interconnected, rubbery network that can stretch and bend in any direction when stressed, giving connective tissue elasticity (Figure 4.13). Mutations in the fibrillin-1 protein are responsible for Marfan syndrome—a connective tissue disorder characterized by impaired structural integrity in the skeleton, the eye, and the cardiovascular system. With this disease, abnormal fibrillin protein is incorporated into microfibrils along with normal fibrillin, inhibiting the formation of functional microfibrils. [Note: Patients with OI, EDS, or Marfan syndrome may have blue sclera due to tissue thinning that allows underlying pigment to show through.]

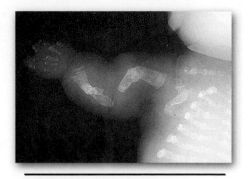

Figure 4.11
Lethal form (type II) of osteogenesis imperfecta in which the fractures appear in utero, as revealed by this radiograph of a stillborn fetus.

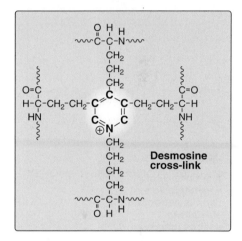

Figure 4.12
Desmosine cross-link in elastin.

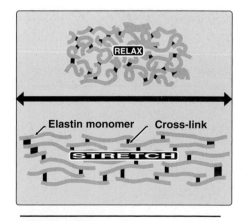

Figure 4.13
Elastin fibers in relaxed and stretched conformations.

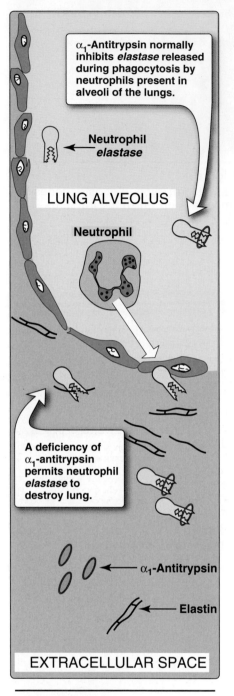

α₁-Antitrypsin normally inhibits *elastase* released during phagocytosis by neutrophils present in alveoli of the lungs.

Neutrophil *elastase*

LUNG ALVEOLUS

Neutrophil

A deficiency of α₁-antitrypsin permits neutrophil *elastase* to destroy lung.

α₁-Antitrypsin

Elastin

EXTRACELLULAR SPACE

Figure 4.14
Destruction of alveolar tissue by *elastase* released from neutrophils activated as part of the immune response to airborne pathogens.

B. Role of α₁-antitrypsin in elastin degradation

1. **α₁-Antitrypsin:** Blood and other body fluids contain a protein, α₁-antitrypsin (α₁-AT, A1AT, currently also called α₁-antiproteinase), that inhibits a number of proteolytic enzymes (also called *proteases* or *proteinases*) that hydrolyze and destroy proteins. [Note: The inhibitor was originally named α₁-antitrypsin because it inhibits the activity of *trypsin* (a proteolytic enzyme synthesized as trypsinogen by the pancreas, see p. 248.] α₁-AT comprises more than 90% of the α₁-globulin fraction of normal plasma. α₁-AT has the important physiologic role of inhibiting neutrophil *elastase*—a powerful *protease* that is released into the extracellular space, and degrades elastin of alveolar walls, as well as other structural proteins in a variety of tissues (Figure 4.14). Most of the α₁-AT found in plasma is synthesized and secreted by the liver. The remainder is synthesized by several tissues, including monocytes and alveolar macrophages, which may be important in the prevention of local tissue injury by *elastase*.

2. **Role of α₁-AT in the lungs:** In the normal lung, the alveoli are chronically exposed to low levels of neutrophil *elastase* released from activated and degenerating neutrophils. This proteolytic activity can destroy the elastin in alveolar walls if unopposed by the action of α₁-AT, the most important inhibitor of neutrophil *elastase* (see Figure 4.14). Because lung tissue cannot regenerate, emphysema results from the destruction of the connective tissue of alveolar walls.

3. **Emphysema resulting from α₁-AT deficiency:** In the United States, approximately 2–5% of patients with emphysema are predisposed to the disease by inherited defects in α₁-AT. A number of different mutations in the gene for α₁-AT are known to cause a deficiency of this protein, but one single purine base mutation (GAG → AAG, resulting in the substitution of lysine for glutamic acid at position 342 of the protein) is clinically the most widespread. The polymerization of the mutated protein in the endoplasmic reticulum of hepatocytes causes decreased secretion of α₁-AT by the liver. The accumulated polymer may result in cirrhosis (scarring of the liver). In the United States, the α₁-AT mutation is most common in Caucasians of Northern European ancestry. An individual must inherit two abnormal α₁-AT alleles to be at risk for the development of emphysema. In a heterozygote, with one normal and one defective gene, the levels of α₁-AT are sufficient to protect the alveoli from damage. [Note: A specific α₁-AT methionine is required for the binding of the inhibitor to its target *proteases*. Smoking causes the oxidation and subsequent inactivation of that methionine residue, thereby rendering the inhibitor powerless to neutralize *elastase*. Smokers with α₁-AT deficiency, therefore, have a considerably elevated rate of lung destruction and a poorer survival rate than nonsmokers with the deficiency.] The deficiency of *elastase* inhibitor can be reversed by augmentation therapy—weekly intravenous administration of α₁-AT. The α₁-AT diffuses from the blood into the lung, where it reaches therapeutic levels in the fluid surrounding the lung epithelial cells.

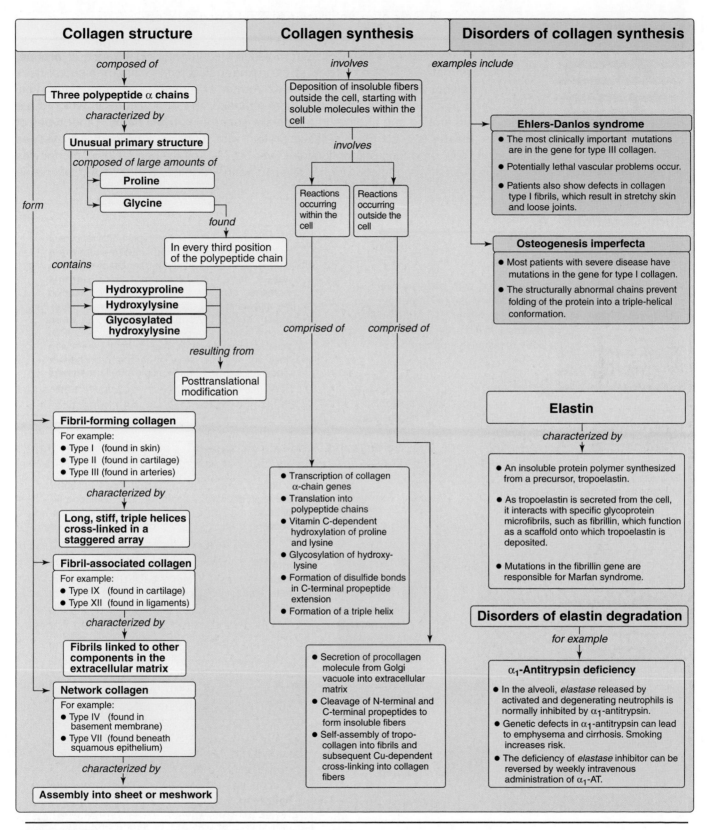

Figure 4.15
Key concept map for the fibrous proteins, collagen and elastin.

IV. CHAPTER SUMMARY

Collagen and elastin are fibrous proteins (Figure 4.15). Collagen molecules contain an abundance of **proline**, **lysine**, and **glycine**, the latter occurring at every third position in the primary structure. Collagen also contains **hydroxyproline**, **hydroxylysine**, and **glycosylated hydroxylysine**, each formed by posttranslational modification. Collagen molecules typically form **fibrils** containing a long, stiff, triple-stranded helical structure, in which three collagen polypeptide chains are wound around one another in a rope-like superhelix (**triple helix**). Other types of collagen form mesh-like networks. **Elastin** is a connective tissue protein with rubber-like properties in tissues such as the lung. **α1-Antitrypsin** (α_1-AT), produced primarily by the liver but also by tissues such as monocytes and alveolar macrophages, prevents elastin degradation in the alveolar walls. A deficiency of α_1-AT can cause **emphysema** and, in some cases, cirrhosis of the liver.

Study Questions

Choose the ONE best answer.

4.1 A 30-year-old woman presented with progressive shortness of breath. She denied the use of cigarettes. A family history revealed that her sister had suffered from unexplained lung disease. Which one of the following etiologies most likely explains this patient's pulmonary symptoms?

A. Deficiency of proline hydroxylase

B. Deficiency of α_1-antitrypsin

C. Deficiency in dietary vitamin C

D Decreased elastase activity

E. Increased collagenase activity

> Correct answer = B. α_1-Antitrypsin deficiency is a genetic disorder that can cause pulmonary emphysema even in the absence of cigarette use. A deficiency of α_1-antitrypsin permits increased elastase activity to destroy elastin in the alveolar walls, even in nonsmokers. α_1-Antitrypsin deficiency should be suspected when chronic obstructive pulmonary disease (COPD) develops in a patient younger than 45 years who does not have a history of chronic bronchitis or tobacco use, or when multiple family members develop obstructive lung disease at an early age. Choices A, C, and E refer to collagen, not elastin.

4.2 A seven-month-old child "fell over" while crawling, and now presents with a swollen leg. At age 1 month, the infant had multiple fractures in various states of healing (right clavicle, right humerus, right radius). At age 7 months, the infant has a fracture of a bowed femur, secondary to minor trauma (see x-ray at right). The bones are thin, have few trabecula, and have thin cortices. A careful family history ruled out nonaccidental trauma (child abuse) as a cause of the bone fractures. The child is most likely to have a defect in:

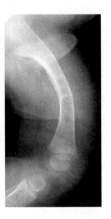

A. type I collagen.

B. type III collagen.

C. type IV collagen.

D. elastin.

E. fibrillin.

> Correct answer = A. The child most likely has osteogenesis imperfecta. Most cases arise from a defect in the genes encoding type I collagen. Bones in affected patients are thin, osteoporotic, often bowed with a thin cortex and deficient trabeculae, and extremely prone to fracture. This patient is affected with type I, osteogenesis imperfecta tarda. The disease presents in early infancy with fractures secondary to minor trauma. The disease may be suspected on prenatal ultrasound through detection of bowing or fractures of long bones. Type II, osteogenesis imperfecta congenita, is more severe, and patients die of pulmonary hypoplasia <u>in utero</u> or during the neonatal period. Defects in type III collagen are the most common cause of Ehlers-Danlos syndrome, characterized by lethal vascular problems and stretchy skin. Type IV collagen forms networks, not fibrils.

4.3 What is the differential basis of the liver and lung pathology seen in α_1-AT deficiency?

> With α_1-AT deficiency, the liver cirrhosis that can result is due to polymerization and retention of α_1-AT in the liver, its site of synthesis. The lung pathology is due to this retention-based deficiency in α_1-AT (a serin protease inhibitor or serpin) such that elastase (a serine protease) is unopposed.

Enzymes

5

I. OVERVIEW

Virtually all reactions in the body are mediated by enzymes, which are protein catalysts that increase the rate of reactions without being changed in the overall process. Among the many biologic reactions that are energetically possible, enzymes selectively channel reactants (called substrates) into useful pathways. Enzymes thus direct all metabolic events. This chapter examines the nature of these catalytic molecules and their mechanism of action.

II. NOMENCLATURE

Each enzyme is assigned two names. The first is its short, recommended name, convenient for everyday use. The second is the more complete systematic name, which is used when an enzyme must be identified without ambiguity.

A. Recommended name

Most commonly used enzyme names have the suffix "-ase" attached to the substrate of the reaction (for example, glucosidase and urease), or to a description of the action performed (for example, lactate dehydrogenase and adenylyl cyclase). [Note: Some enzymes retain their original trivial names, which give no hint of the associated enzymic reaction, for example, trypsin and pepsin.]

B. Systematic name

In the systematic naming system, enzymes are divided into six major classes (Figure 5.1), each with numerous subgroups. For a given enzyme, the suffix -ase is attached to a fairly complete description of the chemical reaction catalyzed, including the names of all the substrates; for example, lactate:NAD⁺ oxidoreductase. [Note: Each enzyme is also assigned a classification number.] The systematic names are unambiguous and informative, but are frequently too cumbersome to be of general use.

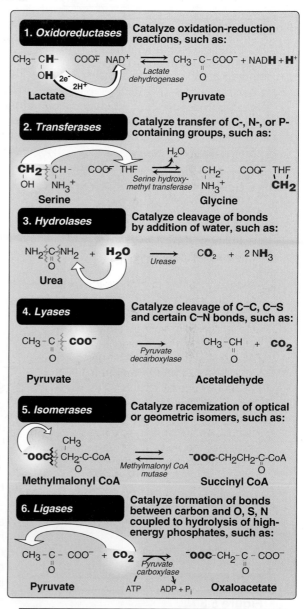

Figure 5.1
The six major classes of enzymes with examples. THF = tetrahydrofolate.

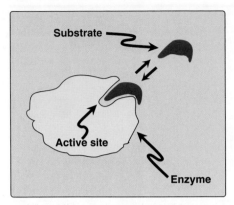

Figure 5.2
Schematic representation of an enzyme with one active site binding a substrate molecule.

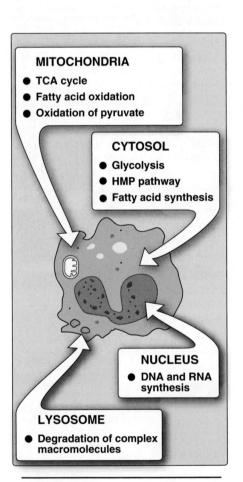

Figure 5.3
The intracellular location of some important biochemical pathways.

Potentially confusing enzyme nomenclature: *synthetase* (requires ATP), *synthase* (no ATP required); *phosphatase* (uses water to remove phosphoryl group), *phosphorylase* (uses P_i to break a bond and generate a phosphorylated product); *dehydrogenase* (NAD^+/FAD is electron acceptor in redox reaction), *oxidase* (O_2 is acceptor but oxygen atoms are not incorporated into substrate), *oxygenase* (one or both oxygens atoms are incorporated).

III. PROPERTIES OF ENZYMES

Enzymes are protein catalysts that increase the velocity of a chemical reaction, and are not consumed during the reaction. [Note: Some RNAs can act like enzymes, usually catalyzing the cleavage and synthesis of phosphodiester bonds. RNAs with catalytic activity are called ribozymes (see p. 439), and are much less commonly encountered than protein catalysts.]

A. Active sites

Enzyme molecules contain a special pocket or cleft called the active site. The active site contains amino acid side chains that participate in substrate binding and catalysis (Figure 5.2). The substrate binds the enzyme, forming an enzyme–substrate (ES) complex. Binding is thought to cause a conformational change in the enzyme (induced fit) that allows catalysis. ES is converted to an enzyme–product (EP) complex that subsequently dissociates to enzyme and product.

B. Catalytic efficiency

Enzyme-catalyzed reactions are highly efficient, proceeding from 10^3–10^8 times faster than uncatalyzed reactions. The number of molecules of substrate converted to product per enzyme molecule per second is called the turnover number, or k_{cat} and typically is 10^2–$10^4 s^{-1}$.

C. Specificity

Enzymes are highly specific, interacting with one or a few substrates and catalyzing only one type of chemical reaction. [Note: The set of enzymes made in a cell determines which metabolic pathways occur in that cell.]

D. Holoenzymes

Some enzymes require molecules other than proteins for enzymic activity. The term holoenzyme refers to the active enzyme with its nonprotein component, whereas the enzyme without its nonprotein moiety is termed an apoenzyme and is inactive. If the nonprotein moiety is a metal ion such as Zn^{2+} or Fe^{2+}, it is called a cofactor. If it is a small organic molecule, it is termed a coenzyme. Coenzymes that only transiently associate with the enzyme are called cosubstrates. Cosubstrates dissociate from the enzyme in an altered state (NAD^+ is an example, see p. 101). If the coenzyme is permanently associated with the enzyme and returned to its original form, it is called a prosthetic group (FAD is an example, see p. 110). Coenzymes frequently are derived from vitamins. For example, NAD^+ contains niacin and FAD contains riboflavin (see Chapter 28).

E. Regulation

Enzyme activity can be regulated, that is, increased or decreased, so that the rate of product formation responds to cellular need.

F. Location within the cell

Many enzymes are localized in specific organelles within the cell (Figure 5.3). Such compartmentalization serves to isolate the reaction substrate or product from other competing reactions. This provides a favorable environment for the reaction, and organizes the thousands of enzymes present in the cell into purposeful pathways.

IV. HOW ENZYMES WORK

The mechanism of enzyme action can be viewed from two different perspectives. The first treats catalysis in terms of energy changes that occur during the reaction, that is, enzymes provide an alternate, energetically favorable reaction pathway different from the uncatalyzed reaction. The second perspective describes how the active site chemically facilitates catalysis.

A. Energy changes occurring during the reaction

Virtually all chemical reactions have an energy barrier separating the reactants and the products. This barrier, called the free energy of activation, is the energy difference between that of the reactants and a high-energy intermediate that occurs during the formation of product. For example, Figure 5.4 shows the changes in energy during the conversion of a molecule of reactant A to product B as it proceeds through the transition state (high-energy intermediate), T*:

$$A \rightleftarrows T^* \rightleftarrows B$$

1. **Free energy of activation:** The peak of energy in Figure 5.4 is the difference in free energy between the reactant and T*, where the high-energy intermediate is formed during the conversion of reactant to product. Because of the high free energy of activation, the rates of uncatalyzed chemical reactions are often slow.

2. **Rate of reaction:** For molecules to react, they must contain sufficient energy to overcome the energy barrier of the transition state. In the absence of an enzyme, only a small proportion of a population of molecules may possess enough energy to achieve the transition state between reactant and product. The rate of reaction is determined by the number of such energized molecules. In general, the lower the free energy of activation, the more molecules have sufficient energy to pass through the transition state, and, thus, the faster the rate of the reaction.

3. **Alternate reaction pathway:** An enzyme allows a reaction to proceed rapidly under conditions prevailing in the cell by providing an alternate reaction pathway with a lower free energy of activation (Figure 5.4). The enzyme does not change the free energies of the reactants or products and, therefore, does not change the equilibrium of the reaction (see p. 71). It does, however, accelerate the rate with which equilibrium is reached.

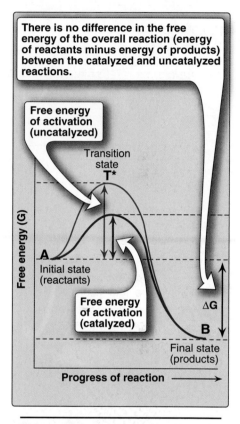

Figure 5.4
Effect of an enzyme on the activation energy of a reaction.

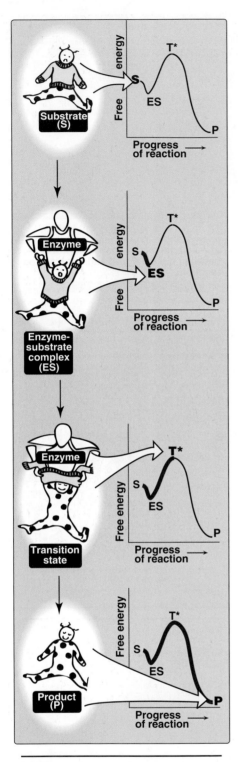

Figure 5.5
Schematic representation of energy changes accompanying formation of an enzyme–substrate complex and subsequent formation of a transition state.

B. Chemistry of the active site

The active site is not a passive receptacle for binding the substrate, but rather is a complex molecular machine employing a diversity of chemical mechanisms to facilitate the conversion of substrate to product. A number of factors are responsible for the catalytic efficiency of enzymes, including the following:

1. **Transition-state stabilization:** The active site often acts as a flexible molecular template that binds the substrate and initiates its conversion to the transition state, a structure in which the bonds are not like those in the substrate or the product (see T* at the top of the curve in Figure 5.4). By stabilizing the transition state, the enzyme greatly increases the concentration of the reactive intermediate that can be converted to product and, thus, accelerates the reaction.

2. **Other mechanisms:** The active site can provide catalytic groups that enhance the probability that the transition state is formed. In some enzymes, these groups can participate in general acid-base catalysis in which amino acid residues provide or accept protons. In other enzymes, catalysis may involve the transient formation of a covalent ES complex. [Note: The mechanism of action of *chymotrypsin*, an enzyme of protein digestion in the intestine, includes general base, general acid, and covalent catalysis. A histidine at the active site of the enzyme gains (general base) and loses (general acid) protons, mediated by the pK of histidine in proteins being close to physiologic pH. Serine at the active site forms a covalent link with the substrate.]

3. **Visualization of the transition state:** The enzyme-catalyzed conversion of substrate to product can be visualized as being similar to removing a sweater from an uncooperative infant (Figure 5.5). The process has a high energy of activation because the only reasonable strategy for removing the garment (short of ripping it off) requires that the random flailing of the baby results in both arms being fully extended over the head—an unlikely posture. However, we can envision a parent acting as an enzyme, first coming in contact with the baby (forming ES), then guiding the baby's arms into an extended, vertical position, analogous to the ES transition state. This posture (conformation) of the baby facilitates the removal of the sweater, forming the disrobed baby, which here represents product. [Note: The substrate bound to the enzyme (ES) is at a slightly lower energy than unbound substrate (S) and explains the small "dip" in the curve at ES.]

V. FACTORS AFFECTING REACTION VELOCITY

Enzymes can be isolated from cells, and their properties studied in a test tube (that is, <u>in vitro</u>). Different enzymes show different responses to changes in substrate concentration, temperature, and pH. This section describes factors that influence the reaction velocity of enzymes. Enzymic responses to these factors give us valuable clues as to how enzymes function in living cells (that is, <u>in vivo</u>).

A. Substrate concentration

1. **Maximal velocity:** The rate or velocity of a reaction (v) is the number of substrate molecules converted to product per unit time; velocity is usually expressed as µmol of product formed per minute. The rate of an enzyme-catalyzed reaction increases with substrate concentration until a maximal velocity (V_{max}) is reached (Figure 5.6). The leveling off of the reaction rate at high substrate concentrations reflects the saturation with substrate of all available binding sites on the enzyme molecules present.

2. **Hyperbolic shape of the enzyme kinetics curve:** Most enzymes show Michaelis-Menten kinetics (see p. 58), in which the plot of initial reaction velocity (v_o) against substrate concentration ([S]), is hyperbolic (similar in shape to that of the oxygen-dissociation curve of myoglobin, see p. 29). In contrast, allosteric enzymes do not follow Michaelis-Menton kinetics and show a sigmoidal curve (see p. 62) that is similar in shape to the oxygen dissociation curve of hemoglobin (see p. 29).

B. Temperature

1. **Increase of velocity with temperature:** The reaction velocity increases with temperature until a peak velocity is reached (Figure 5.7). This increase is the result of the increased number of molecules having sufficient energy to pass over the energy barrier and form the products of the reaction.

2. **Decrease of velocity with higher temperature:** Further elevation of the temperature results in a decrease in reaction velocity as a result of temperature-induced denaturation of the enzyme (see Figure 5.7).

> The optimum temperature for most human enzymes is between 35 and 40°C. Human enzymes start to denature at temperatures above 40°C, but thermophilic bacteria found in the hot springs have optimum temperatures of 70°C.

C. pH

1. **Effect of pH on the ionization of the active site:** The concentration of H+ affects reaction velocity in several ways. First, the catalytic process usually requires that the enzyme and substrate have specific chemical groups in either an ionized or un-ionized state in order to interact. For example, catalytic activity may require that an amino group of the enzyme be in the protonated form ($-NH_3^+$). At alkaline pH, this group is deprotonated, and the rate of the reaction, therefore, declines.

2. **Effect of pH on enzyme denaturation:** Extremes of pH can also lead to denaturation of the enzyme, because the structure of the catalytically active protein molecule depends on the ionic character of the amino acid side chains.

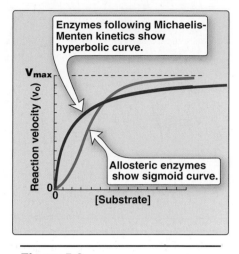

Figure 5.6
Effect of substrate concentration on reaction velocity.

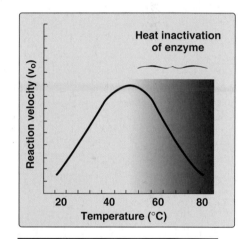

Figure 5.7
Effect of temperature on an enzyme-catalyzed reaction.

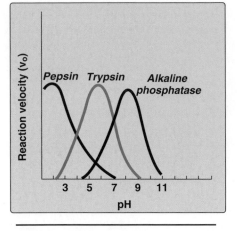

Figure 5.8
Effect of pH on enzyme-catalyzed reactions.

3. **The pH optimum varies for different enzymes:** The pH at which maximal enzyme activity is achieved is different for different enzymes, and often reflects the [H⁺] at which the enzyme functions in the body. For example, *pepsin*, a digestive enzyme in the stomach, is maximally active at pH 2, whereas other enzymes, designed to work at neutral pH, are denatured by such an acidic environment (Figure 5.8).

VI. MICHAELIS-MENTEN EQUATION

A. Reaction model

Leonor Michaelis and Maude Menten proposed a simple model that accounts for most of the features of enzyme-catalyzed reactions. In this model, the enzyme reversibly combines with its substrate to form an ES complex that subsequently yields product, regenerating the free enzyme. The model, involving one substrate molecule, is represented below:

$$E + S \underset{k_{-1}}{\overset{k_1}{\rightleftharpoons}} ES \overset{k_2}{\longrightarrow} E + P$$

where   S is the substrate
              E is the enzyme
              ES is the enzyme–substrate complex
              P is the product
              k_1, k_{-1}, and k_2 are rate constants

B. Michaelis-Menten equation

The Michaelis-Menten equation describes how reaction velocity varies with substrate concentration:

$$v_o = \frac{V_{max}[S]}{K_m + [S]}$$

where v_o = initial reaction velocity
              V_{max} = maximal velocity
              K_m = Michaelis constant = $(k_{-1} + k_2)/k_1$
              [S] = substrate concentration

The following assumptions are made in deriving the Michaelis-Menten rate equation:

1. **Relative concentrations of E and S:** The concentration of substrate ([S]) is much greater than the concentration of enzyme ([E]), so that the percentage of total substrate bound by the enzyme at any one time is small.

2. **Steady-state assumption:** [ES] does not change with time (the steady-state assumption), that is, the rate of formation of ES is equal to that of the breakdown of ES (to E + S and to E + P). In general, an intermediate in a series of reactions is said to be in steadystate when its rate of synthesis is equal to its rate of degradation.

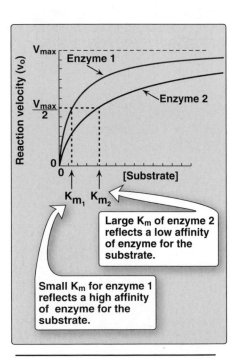

Figure 5.9
Effect of substrate concentration on reaction velocities for two enzymes: enzyme 1 with a small K_m, and enzyme 2 with a large K_m.

3. Initial velocity: Initial reaction velocities (v_o) are used in the analysis of enzyme reactions. This means that the rate of the reaction is measured as soon as enzyme and substrate are mixed. At that time, the concentration of product is very small and, therefore, the rate of the back reaction from P to S can be ignored.

C. Important conclusions about Michaelis-Menten kinetics

1. Characteristics of K_m: K_m—the Michaelis constant—is characteristic of an enzyme and its particular substrate, and reflects the affinity of the enzyme for that substrate. K_m is numerically equal to the substrate concentration at which the reaction velocity is equal to $\frac{1}{2}V_{max}$. K_m does not vary with the concentration of enzyme.

    a. Small K_m: A numerically small (low) K_m reflects a high affinity of the enzyme for substrate, because a low concentration of substrate is needed to half-saturate the enzyme—that is, to reach a velocity that is $\frac{1}{2}V_{max}$ (Figure 5.9).

    b. Large K_m: A numerically large (high) K_m reflects a low affinity of enzyme for substrate because a high concentration of substrate is needed to half-saturate the enzyme.

2. Relationship of velocity to enzyme concentration: The rate of the reaction is directly proportional to the enzyme concentration at all substrate concentrations. For example, if the enzyme concentration is halved, the initial rate of the reaction (v_o), as well as that of V_{max}, are reduced to half that of the original.

3. Order of reaction: When [S] is much less than K_m, the velocity of the reaction is approximately proportional to the substrate concentration (Figure 5.10). The rate of reaction is then said to be first order with respect to substrate. When [S] is much greater than K_m, the velocity is constant and equal to V_{max}. The rate of reaction is then independent of substrate concentration, and is said to be zero order with respect to substrate concentration (see Figure 5.10).

D. Lineweaver-Burk plot

When v_o is plotted against [S], it is not always possible to determine when V_{max} has been achieved, because of the gradual upward slope of the hyperbolic curve at high substrate concentrations. However, if $1/v_o$ is plotted versus $1/[S]$, a straight line is obtained (Figure 5.11). This plot, the Lineweaver-Burk plot (also called a double-reciprocal plot) can be used to calculate K_m and V_{max}, as well as to determine the mechanism of action of enzyme inhibitors.

1. The equation describing the Lineweaver-Burk plot is:

$$\frac{1}{v_o} = \frac{K_m}{V_{max}\,[S]} + \frac{1}{V_{max}}$$

where the intercept on the x-axis is equal to $-1/K_m$, and the intercept on the y-axis is equal to $1/V_{max}$.

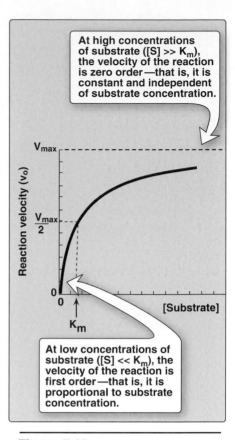

Figure 5.10
Effect of substrate concentration on reaction velocity for an enzyme-catalyzed reaction.

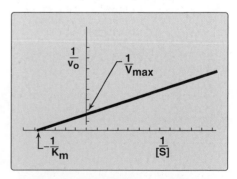

Figure 5.11
Lineweaver-Burk plot.

VII. INHIBITION OF ENZYME ACTIVITY

Any substance that can diminish the velocity of an enzyme-catalyzed reaction is called an inhibitor. In general, irreversible inhibitors bind to enzymes through covalent bonds. Reversible inhibitors typically bind to enzymes through noncovalent bonds, thus dilution of the enzyme–inhibitor complex results in dissociation of the reversibly bound inhibitor, and recovery of enzyme activity. The two most commonly encountered types of reversible inhibition are competitive and noncompetitive.

A. Competitive inhibition

This type of inhibition occurs when the inhibitor binds reversibly to the same site that the substrate would normally occupy and, therefore, competes with the substrate for that site.

1. **Effect on V_{max}:** The effect of a competitive inhibitor is reversed by increasing [S]. At a sufficiently high substrate concentration, the reaction velocity reaches the V_{max} observed in the absence of inhibitor (Figure 5.12).

2. **Effect on K_m:** A competitive inhibitor increases the apparent K_m for a given substrate. This means that, in the presence of a competitive inhibitor, more substrate is needed to achieve $\frac{1}{2}V_{max}$.

3. **Effect on the Lineweaver-Burk plot:** Competitive inhibition shows a characteristic Lineweaver-Burk plot in which the plots of the inhibited and uninhibited reactions intersect on the y-axis at $1/V_{max}$ (V_{max} is unchanged). The inhibited and uninhibited reactions show different x-axis intercepts, indicating that the apparent K_m is increased in the presence of the competitive inhibitor because $-1/K_m$ moves closer to zero from a negative value (see Figure 5.12).

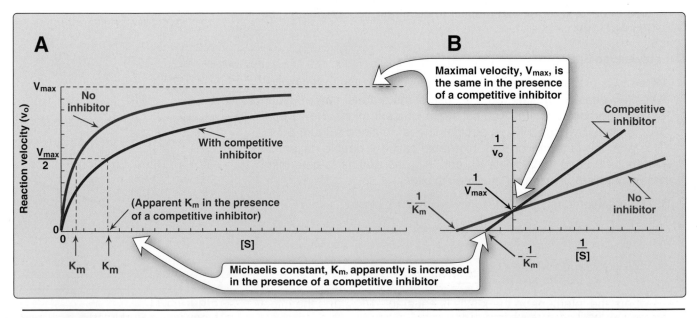

Figure 5.12
A. Effect of a competitive inhibitor on the reaction velocity (v_o) versus substrate ([S]) plot. B. Lineweaver-Burk plot of competitive inhibition of an enzyme.

4. Statin drugs as examples of competitive inhibitors: This group of antihyperlipidemic agents competitively inhibits the first committed step in cholesterol synthesis. This reaction is catalyzed by *hydroxymethylglutaryl–CoA reductase* (*HMG-CoA reductase*), see p. 220). Statin drugs, such as atorvastatin (Lipitor) and pravastatin (Pravachol),[1] are structural analogs of the natural substrate for this enzyme, and compete effectively to inhibit *HMG-CoA reductase*. By doing so, they inhibit de novo cholesterol synthesis, thereby lowering plasma cholesterol levels (Figure 5.13).

B. Noncompetitive inhibition

This type of inhibition is recognized by its characteristic effect on V_{max} (Figure 5.14). Noncompetitive inhibition occurs when the inhibitor and substrate bind at different sites on the enzyme. The noncompetitive inhibitor can bind either free enzyme or the ES complex, thereby preventing the reaction from occurring (Figure 5.15).

1. Effect on V_{max}: Noncompetitive inhibition cannot be overcome by increasing the concentration of substrate. Thus, noncompetitive inhibitors decrease the apparent V_{max} of the reaction.

2. Effect on K_m: Noncompetitive inhibitors do not interfere with the binding of substrate to enzyme. Thus, the enzyme shows the same K_m in the presence or absence of the noncompetitive inhibitor.

3. Effect on Lineweaver-Burk plot: Noncompetitive inhibition is readily differentiated from competitive inhibition by plotting $1/v_o$ versus $1/[S]$ and noting that the apparent V_{max} decreases in the presence of a noncompetitive inhibitor, whereas K_m is unchanged (see Figure 5.14).

4. Examples of noncompetitive inhibitors: Some inhibitors act by forming covalent bonds with specific groups of enzymes. For

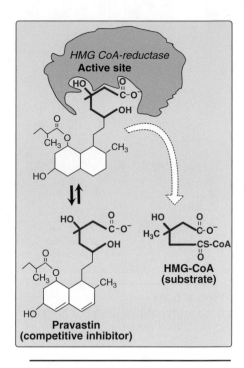

Figure 5.13
Pravastatin competes with HMG-CoA for the active site of *HMG-CoA reductase*.

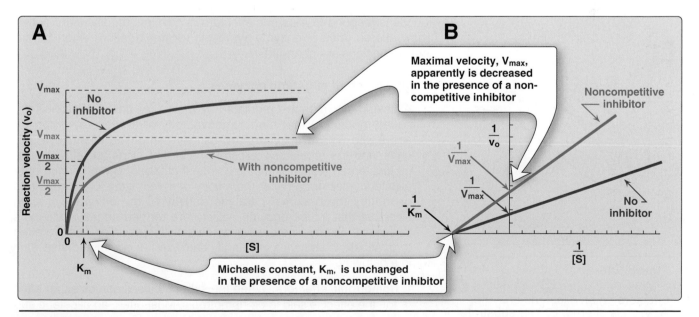

Figure 5.14
A. Effect of a noncompetitive inhibitor on the reaction velocity (v_o) versus substrate ([S]) plot. B. Lineweaver-Burk plot of noncompetitive inhibition of an enzyme.

[1]See Chapter 21 in *Lippincott's Illustrated Reviews: Pharmacolog* for a more detailed discussion of the drugs used to treat hyperlipidemia.

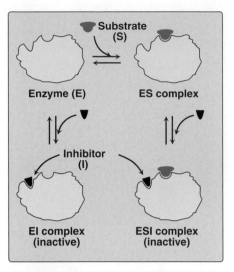

Figure 5.15
A noncompetitive inhibitor binding to both free enzyme and enzyme–substrate (ES) complex.

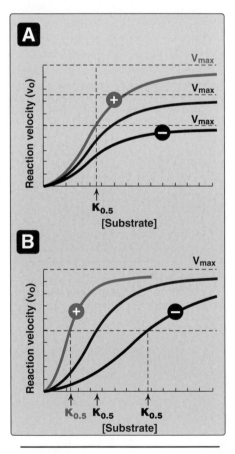

Figure 5.16
Effects of negative or positive ⊕ effectors on an allosteric enzyme. A. V_{max} is altered. B. The substrate concentration that gives half-maximal velocity ($K_{0.5}$) is altered.

example, lead forms covalent bonds with the sulfhydryl side chains of cysteine in proteins. The binding of the heavy metal shows non-competitive inhibition. *Ferrochelatase*, an enzyme that catalyzes the insertion of Fe^{2+} into protoporphyrin (a precursor of heme, see p. 279), is an example of an enzyme sensitive to inhibition by lead. Other examples of noncompetitive inhibition are certain insecticides, whose neurotoxic effects are a result of their covalent binding at the catalytic site of the enzyme *acetylcholinesterase* (an enzyme that cleaves the neurotransmitter, acetylcholine). [Note: Even though covalent bonds are formed, if active enzyme can be recovered, the inhibition is reversible.]

C. Enzyme inhibitors as drugs

At least half of the ten most commonly dispensed drugs in the United States act as enzyme inhibitors. For example, the widely prescribed β-lactam antibiotics, such as penicillin and amoxicillin,[2] act by inhibiting enzymes involved in bacterial cell wall synthesis. Drugs may also act by inhibiting extracellular reactions. This is illustrated by *angiotensin-converting enzyme* (ACE) inhibitors. They lower blood pressure by blocking the enzyme that cleaves angiotensin I to form the potent vasoconstrictor, angiotensin II.[3] These drugs, which include captopril, enalapril, and lisinopril, cause vasodilation and a resultant reduction in blood pressure.

VIII. REGULATION OF ENZYME ACTIVITY

The regulation of the reaction velocity of enzymes is essential if an organism is to coordinate its numerous metabolic processes. The rates of most enzymes are responsive to changes in substrate concentration, because the intracellular level of many substrates is in the range of the K_m. Thus, an increase in substrate concentration prompts an increase in reaction rate, which tends to return the concentration of substrate toward normal. In addition, some enzymes with specialized regulatory functions respond to allosteric effectors or covalent modification, or they show altered rates of enzyme synthesis (or degradation) when physiologic conditions are changed.

A. Regulation of allosteric enzymes

Allosteric enzymes are regulated by molecules called effectors (also called modifiers) that bind noncovalently at a site other than the active site. These enzymes are usually composed of multiple subunits, and the regulatory (allosteric) site that binds the effector may be located on a subunit that is not itself catalytic. The presence of an allosteric effector can alter the affinity of the enzyme for its substrate, or modify the maximal catalytic activity of the enzyme, or both. Effectors that inhibit enzyme activity are termed negative effectors, whereas those that increase enzyme activity are called positive effectors. Allosteric enzymes frequently catalyze the committed step early in a pathway.

1. Homotropic effectors: When the substrate itself serves as an effector, the effect is said to be homotropic. Most often, an allosteric substrate functions as a positive effector. In such a case, the presence of a substrate molecule at one site on the enzyme enhances the catalytic properties of the other substrate-binding sites—that is, their binding sites exhibit cooperativity. These enzymes show a sigmoidal curve when reaction velocity (v_o) is plotted against substrate concentration ([S]), Figure 5.16). This contrasts with the hyperbolic curve characteristic of enzymes following Michaelis-Menten kinetics, as previously discussed. [Note: The concept of cooperativity of substrate binding is analogous to the binding of oxygen to hemoglobin.] Positive and negative effectors of allosteric enzymes can affect either the V_{max}, the $K_{0.5}$, or both (see Figure 5.16).

2. **Heterotropic effectors:** The effector may be different from the substrate, in which case the effect is said to be heterotropic. For example, consider the feedback inhibition shown in Figure 5.17. The enzyme that converts D to E has an allosteric site that binds the endproduct, G. If the concentration of G increases (for example, because it is not used as rapidly as it is synthesized), the first irreversible step unique to the pathway is typically inhibited. Feedback inhibition provides the cell with appropriate amounts of a product it needs by regulating the flow of substrate molecules through the pathway that synthesizes that product. Heterotropic effectors are commonly encountered, for example, the glycolytic enzyme *phosphofructokinase-1* is allosterically inhibited by citrate, which is not a substrate for the enzyme (see p. 99).

B. Regulation of enzymes by covalent modification

Many enzymes may be regulated by covalent modification, most frequently by the addition or removal of phosphate groups from specific serine, threonine, or tyrosine residues of the enzyme. Protein phosphorylation is recognized as one of the primary ways in which cellular processes are regulated.

1. **Phosphorylation and dephosphorylation:** Phosphorylation reactions are catalyzed by a family of enzymes called *protein kinases* that use adenosine triphosphate (ATP) as a phosphate donor. Phosphate groups are cleaved from phosphorylated enzymes by the action of *phosphoprotein phosphatases* (Figure 5.18).

2. **Response of enzyme to phosphorylation:** Depending on the specific enzyme, the phosphorylated form may be more or less active than the unphosphorylated enzyme. For example, phosphorylation of *glycogen phosphorylase* (an enzyme that degrades glycogen) increases activity, whereas the addition of phosphate to *glycogen synthase* (an enzyme that synthesizes glycogen) decreases activity (see p. 132).

C. Induction and repression of enzyme synthesis

The regulatory mechanisms described above modify the activity of existing enzyme molecules. However, cells can also regulate the amount of enzyme present by altering the rate of enzyme degradation or, more typically, the rate of enzyme synthesis. The increase (induction) or decrease (repression) of enzyme synthesis leads to an alteration in the total population of active sites. Enzymes subject to regulation of synthesis are often those that are needed at only one

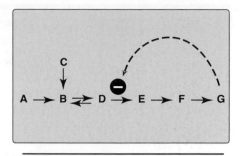

Figure 5.17
Feedback inhibition of a metabolic pathway.

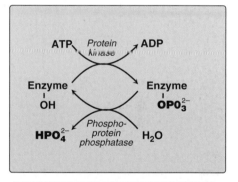

Figure 5.18
Covalent modification by the addition and removal of phosphate groups.

REGULATOR EVENT	TYPICAL EFFECTOR	RESULTS	TIME REQUIRED FOR CHANGE
Substrate inhibition	Substrate	Change in velocity (v_o)	Immediate
Product inhibition	Reaction product	Change in V_{max} and/or K_m	Immediate
Allosteric control	Pathway end product	Change in V_{max} and/or $K_{0.5}$	Immediate
Covalent modification	Another enzyme	Change in V_{max} and/or K_m	Immediate to minutes
Synthesis or degradation of enzyme	Hormone or metabolite	Change in the amount of enzyme	Hours to days

Figure 5.19
Mechanisms for regulating enzyme activity. [Note: Inhibition by pathway end product is also referred to as feedback inhibition.]

stage of development or under selected physiologic conditions. For example, elevated levels of insulin as a result of high blood glucose levels cause an increase in the synthesis of key enzymes involved in glucose metabolism (see p. 105). In contrast, enzymes that are in constant use are usually not regulated by altering the rate of enzyme synthesis. Alterations in enzyme levels as a result of induction or repression of protein synthesis are slow (hours to days), compared with allosterically or covalently regulated changes in enzyme activity, which occur in seconds to minutes. Figure 5.19 summarizes the common ways that enzyme activity is regulated.

IX. ENZYMES IN CLINICAL DIAGNOSIS

Plasma enzymes can be classified into two major groups. First, a relatively small group of enzymes are actively secreted into the blood by certain cell types. For example, the liver secretes zymogens (inactive precursors) of the enzymes involved in blood coagulation. Second, a large number of enzyme species are released from cells during normal cell turnover. These enzymes almost always function intracellularly, and have no physiologic use in the plasma. In healthy individuals, the levels of these enzymes are fairly constant, and represent a steady state in which the rate of release from damaged cells into the plasma is balanced by an equal rate of removal of the enzyme protein from the plasma. Increased plasma levels of these enzyme may indicate tissue damage (Figure 5.20).

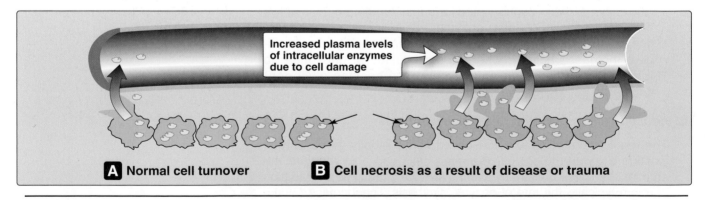

Increased plasma levels of intracellular enzymes due to cell damage

A Normal cell turnover   **B** Cell necrosis as a result of disease or trauma

Figure 5.20
Release of enzymes from normal and diseased or traumatized cells.

Plasma is the fluid, noncellular part of blood. Laboratory assays of enzyme activity most often use serum, which is obtained by centrifugation of whole blood after it has been allowed to coagulate. Plasma is a physiologic fluid, whereas serum is prepared in the laboratory.

A. Alteration of plasma enzyme levels in disease states

Many diseases that cause tissue damage result in an increased release of intracellular enzymes into the plasma. The activities of many of these enzymes are routinely determined for diagnostic purposes in diseases of the heart, liver, skeletal muscle, and other tissues. The level of specific enzyme activity in the plasma frequently correlates with the extent of tissue damage. Thus, determining the degree of elevation of a particular enzyme activity in the plasma is often useful in evaluating the prognosis for the patient.

B. Plasma enzymes as diagnostic tools

Some enzymes show relatively high activity in only one or a few tissues. The presence of increased levels of these enzymes in plasma thus reflects damage to the corresponding tissue. For example, the enzyme *alanine aminotransferase* (*ALT*, see p. 251) is abundant in the liver. The appearance of elevated levels of *ALT* in plasma signals possible damage to hepatic tissue. [Note: Measurement of *ALT* is part of the liver function test panel.] Increases in plasma levels of enzymes with a wide tissue distribution provide a less specific indication of the site of cellular injury and limits their diagnostic value.

C. Isoenzymes and diseases of the heart

Most isoenzymes (also called isozymes) are enzymes that catalyze the same reaction. However, they do not necessarily have the same physical properties because of genetically determined differences in amino acid sequence. For this reason, isoenzymes may contain different numbers of charged amino acids and may, therefore, be separated from each other by electrophoresis (Figure 5.21). Different organs frequently contain characteristic proportions of different isoenzymes. The pattern of isoenzymes found in the plasma may, therefore, serve as a means of identifying the site of tissue damage. For example, the plasma levels of *creatine kinase* (*CK*) are commonly determined in the diagnosis of myocardial infarction. They are particularly useful when the electrocardiogram is difficult to interpret, such as when there have been previous episodes of heart disease.

1. **Quaternary structure of isoenzymes:** Many isoenzymes contain different subunits in various combinations. For example, *creatine kinase* (*CK*) occurs as three isoenzymes. Each isoenzyme is a dimer composed of two polypeptides (called B and M subunits) associated in one of three combinations: *CK1* = BB, *CK2* = MB, and *CK3* = MM. Each *CK* isoenzyme shows a characteristic electrophoretic mobility (see Figure 5.21). [Note: Virtually all *CK* in the brain is the BB isoform, whereas in skeletal muscle it is MM. In cardiac muscle, about one-third is MB with the rest as MM.]

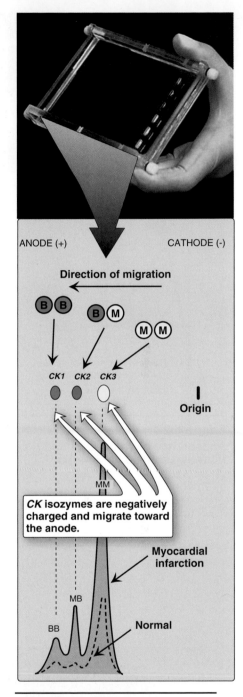

Figure 5.21
Subunit structure, electrophoretic mobility, and enzyme activity of *creatine kinase* (*CK*) isoenzymes.

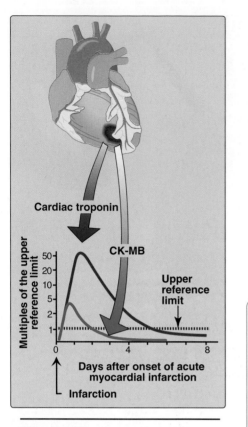

Figure 5.22
Appearance of *creatine kinase* (*CK*) and cardiac troponin in plasma after a myocardial infarction.

2. Diagnosis of myocardial infarction: Measurement of blood levels of proteins with cardiac specificity is used in the diagnosis of myocardial infarction (MI) because myocardial muscle is the only tissue that contains more than 5% of the total *CK* activity as the *CK2* (MB) isoenzyme. Appearance of this hybrid isoenzyme in plasma is virtually specific for infarction of the myocardium. Following an acute MI, this isoenzyme appears approximately 4–8 hours following onset of chest pain, reaches a peak of activity at approximately 24 hours, and returns to baseline after 48–72 hours (Figure 5.22). Troponin T and troponin I are regulatory proteins involved in myocardial contractility. They are released into the plasma in response to cardiac damage. Cardiac troponin I (cTnI) is highly sensitive and specific for damage to cardiac tissue. cTnI appears in plasma within 4–6 hours after an MI, peaks in 8–28 hours, and remains elevated for 3–10 days. Elevated serum troponins then, are more predictive of adverse outcomes in unstable angina or myocardial infarction than the conventional assay of *CK2*.

X. CHAPTER SUMMARY

Enzymes are **protein catalysts** that increase the velocity of a chemical reaction by lowering the energy of the transition state (Figure 5.23). Enzymes are not consumed during the reaction they catalyze. Enzyme molecules contain a special pocket or cleft called the **active site**. The active site contains amino acid side chains that participate in substrate binding and catalysis. The active site binds the substrate, forming an **enzyme–substrate (ES) complex**. Binding is thought to cause a conformational change in the enzyme (induced fit) that allows catalysis. ES is converted to enzyme-product (EP), which subsequently dissociates to enzyme and product. An enzyme allows a reaction to proceed rapidly under conditions prevailing in the cell by providing an **alternate reaction pathway** with a **lower free energy of activation**. The enzyme does not change the free energies of the reactants or products and, therefore, does not change the equilibrium of the reaction. Most enzymes show **Michaelis-Menten kinetics**, and a plot of the **initial reaction velocity (v_o)** against **substrate concentration ([S])** has a **hyperbolic** shape similar to the oxygen dissociation curve of myoglobin. Any substance that can diminish the velocity of such enzyme-catalyzed reactions is called an inhibitor. The two most commonly encountered types of reversible inhibition are **competitive** (which **increases** the **apparent K_m**) and **noncompetitive** (which **decreases** the **apparent V_{max}**). In contrast, the **multisubunit allosteric enzymes** frequently show a **sigmoidal curve** similar in shape to the oxygen dissociation curve of hemoglobin. They typically catalyze the **committed step (often the rate-limiting or slowest step)** of a pathway. Allosteric enzymes are regulated by molecules called **effectors** (also **modifiers**) that bind noncovalently at a site other than the active site. Effectors can be either **positive** (accelerate the enzyme-catalyzed reaction) or **negative** (slow down the reaction). An allosteric effector can alter the affinity of the enzyme for its substrate, or modify the maximal catalytic activity of the enzyme, or both. Enzymes can also be regulated by covalent modification, and by changes in the rate of synthesis or degradation. Enzymes have diagnostic and therapeutic value in medicine.

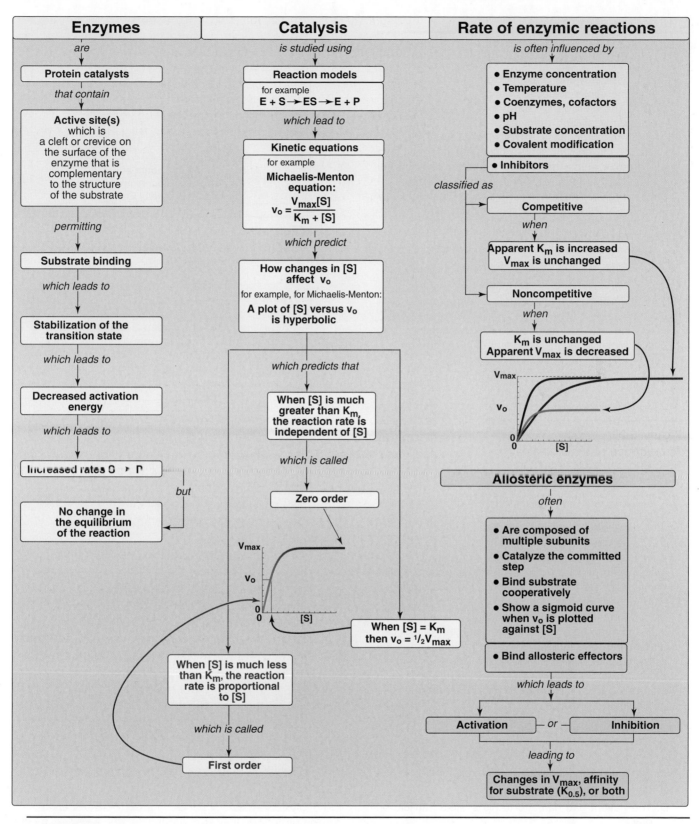

Figure 5.23
Key concept map for the enzymes. S = substrate, [S] = substrate concentration, P = product, E = enzyme, v_o = initial velocity, V_{max} = maximal velocity, K_m = Michaelis constant, $K_{0.5}$ = substrate concentration which gives half maximal velocity.

Study Questions

Choose the ONE correct answer.

5.1 In cases of ethylene glycol poisoning and its characteristic metabolic acidosis, treatment involves correction of the acidosis, removal of any remaining ethylene glycol, and administration of an inhibitor of alcohol dehydrogenase (ADH, alcohol:NAD$^+$ oxidoreductase), the enzyme that oxidizes ethylene glycol to the organic acids that cause the acidosis. Ethanol (grain alcohol) frequently is the inhibitor given to treat ethylene glycol poisoning; it works by competitively inhibiting ADH. As a competitive inhibitor, ethanol:

A. increases apparent K_m without affecting V_{max}.

B. decreases apparent K_m without affecting V_{max}.

C. increases apparent V_{max} without affecting K_m.

D. decreases apparent V_{max} without affecting K_m.

E. decreases both apparent V_{max} and apparent K_m.

5.2 ADH requires NAD$^+$ for catalytic activity. In the reaction catalyzed by ADH, an alcohol is oxidized to an aldehyde as NAD$^+$ is reduced to NADH and dissociates from the enzyme. The NAD$^+$ is functioning as a (an):

A. apoenzyme.

B. coenzyme-cosubstrate.

C. coenzyme-prosthetic group.

D. cofactor.

E. heterotropic effector.

5.3 A 70-year-old man was admitted to the emergency room with a 12-hour history of chest pain. Serum creatine kinase (CK) activity was measured at admission (day 1) and once daily (Figure 5.24). On day 2 after admission, he experienced cardiac arrhythmia, which was terminated by three cycles of electric cardioconversion, the latter two at maximum energy. [Note: Cardioconversion is performed by placing two paddles, 12 cm in diameter, in firm contact with the chest wall and applying a short electric voltage.] Normal cardiac rhythm was reestablished. He had no recurrence of arrhythmia over the next several days. His chest pain subsided and he was released on day 10. Which one of the following is most consistent with the data presented?

A. The patient had a myocardial infarction 48 to 64 hours prior to admission.

B. The patient had a myocardial infarction on day 2.

C. The patient had angina prior to admission.

D. The patient had damage to his skeletal muscle on day 2.

E. The data do not permit any conclusion concerning myocardial infarction prior to, or after, admission to the hospital.

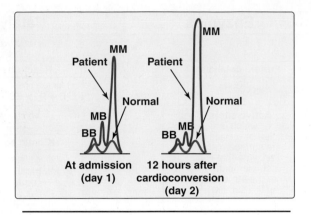

Figure 5.24
Serum *creatine kinase* levels.

Correct answer = A. In the presence of a competitive inhibitor, an enzyme appears to have a lower affinity for substrate, but as the substrate level is increased, the observed velocity approaches V_{max}. (See panel B of Figures 5.12 and 5.14 to compare effects of competitive and noncompetitive inhibitors.)

Correct answer = B. Coenzymes-cosubstrates are small organic molecules that associate transiently with an enzyme and leave the enzyme in a changed form. Coenzyme-prosthetic groups are small organic molecules that associate permanently with an enzyme and are returned to their original form on the enzyme. Cofactors are metal ions. Heterotropic effectors are not substrates.

Correct answer = D. The CK isoenzyme pattern at admission showed elevated MB isozyme, indicating that the patient had experienced a myocardial infarction in the previous 12–24 hours. [Note: 48–64 hours after an infarction, the MB isozyme would have returned to normal values.] On day 2, 12 hours after the cardioconversions, the MB isozyme had decreased, indicating no further damage to the heart. However, the patient showed an increased MM isozyme after cardioconversion. This suggests damage to muscle, probably a result of the convulsive muscle contractions caused by repeated cardioconversion. Angina is typically the result of transient spasms in the vasculature of the heart, and would not be expected to lead to tissue death that results in elevation in serum creatine kinase.

Bioenergetics and Oxidative Phosphorylation

6

I. OVERVIEW

Bioenergetics describes the transfer and utilization of energy in biologic systems. It makes use of a few basic ideas from the field of thermodynamics, particularly the concept of free energy. Changes in free energy (ΔG) provide a measure of the energetic feasibility of a chemical reaction and can, therefore, allow prediction of whether a reaction or process can take place. Bioenergetics concerns only the initial and final energy states of reaction components, not the mechanism or how much time is needed for the chemical change to take place. In short, bioenergetics predicts if a process is possible, whereas kinetics measures how fast the reaction occurs (see p. 54).

II. FREE ENERGY

The direction and extent to which a chemical reaction proceeds is determined by the degree to which two factors change during the reaction. These are enthalpy (ΔH, a measure of the change in heat content of the reactants and products) and entropy (ΔS, a measure of the change in randomness or disorder of reactants and products, Figure 6.1). Neither of these thermodynamic quantities by itself is sufficient to determine whether a chemical reaction will proceed spontaneously in the direction it is written. However, when combined mathematically (see Figure 6.1), enthalpy and entropy can be used to define a third quantity, free energy (G), which predicts the direction in which a reaction will spontaneously proceed.

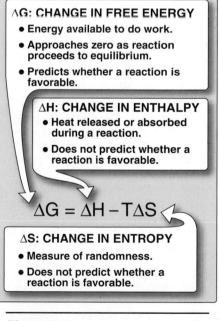

ΔG: CHANGE IN FREE ENERGY
- Energy available to do work.
- Approaches zero as reaction proceeds to equilibrium.
- Predicts whether a reaction is favorable.

ΔH: CHANGE IN ENTHALPY
- Heat released or absorbed during a reaction.
- Does not predict whether a reaction is favorable.

$$\Delta G = \Delta H - T\Delta S$$

ΔS: CHANGE IN ENTROPY
- Measure of randomness.
- Does not predict whether a reaction is favorable.

Figure 6.1
Relationship between changes in free energy (G), enthalpy (H), and entropy (S). T is the absolute temperature in degrees Kelvin ($^\circ K$): $^\circ K = {}^\circ C + 273$.

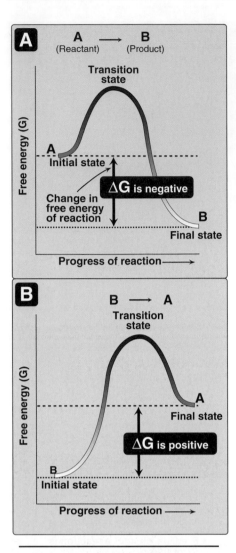

Figure 6.2
Change in free energy (ΔG) during a reaction. A. The product has a lower free energy (G) than the reactant. B. The product has a higher free energy than the reactant.

III. FREE ENERGY CHANGE

The change in free energy is represented in two ways, ΔG and ΔG°. The first, ΔG (without the superscript "o"), represents the change in free energy and, thus, the direction of a reaction at any specified concentration of products and reactants. ΔG, then, is a variable. This contrasts with the standard free energy change, ΔG° (with the superscript "o"), which is the energy change when reactants and products are at a concentration of 1 mol/L. [Note: The concentration of protons is assumed to be 10^{-7} mol/L, that is, pH = 7.] Although ΔG° represents energy changes at these nonphysiologic concentrations of reactants and products, it is nonetheless useful in comparing the energy changes of different reactions. Furthermore, ΔG° can readily be determined from measurement of the equilibrium constant (see p. 72). This section outlines the uses of ΔG; ΔG° is described on p. 71.

A. Sign of ΔG predicts the direction of a reaction

The change in free energy, ΔG, can be used to predict the direction of a reaction at constant temperature and pressure. Consider the reaction:

$$A \rightleftarrows B$$

1. **Negative ΔG:** If ΔG is a negative number, there is a net loss of energy, and the reaction goes spontaneously as written—that is, A is converted into B (Figure 6.2A). The reaction is said to be exergonic.

2. **Positive ΔG:** If ΔG is a positive number, there is a net gain of energy, and the reaction does not go spontaneously from B to A (see Figure 6.2B). Energy must be added to the system to make the reaction go from B to A, and the reaction is said to be endergonic.

3. **ΔG is zero:** If $\Delta G = 0$, the reactants are in equilibrium. [Note: When a reaction is proceeding spontaneously—that is, free energy is being lost—then the reaction continues until ΔG reaches zero and equilibrium is established.]

B. ΔG of the forward and back reactions

The free energy of the forward reaction (A $\rightarrow$ B) is equal in magnitude but opposite in sign to that of the back reaction (B $\rightarrow$ A). For example, if ΔG of the forward reaction is –5 kcal/mol, then that of the back reaction is +5 kcal/mol. [Note: ΔG can also be expressed in kilojoules per mole or kJ/mol (1 kcal = 4.2 kJ).]

C. ΔG depends on the concentration of reactants and products

The ΔG of the reaction A $\rightarrow$ B depends on the concentration of the reactant and product. At constant temperature and pressure, the following relationship can be derived:

$$\Delta G = \Delta G^\circ + RT \ln \frac{[B]}{[A]}$$

where ΔG° is the standard free energy change (see below)

R is the gas constant (1.987 cal/mol · degree)

T is the absolute temperature ($^\circ K$)

[A] and [B] are the actual concentrations of the reactant and product

ln represents the natural logarithm

A reaction with a positive ΔG° can proceed in the forward direction (have a negative overall ΔG) if the ratio of products to reactants ([B]/[A]) is sufficiently small (that is, the ratio of reactants to products is large). For example, consider the reaction:

$$\text{Glucose 6-phosphate} \rightleftarrows \text{fructose 6-phosphate}$$

Figure 6.3A shows reaction conditions in which the concentration of reactant, glucose 6-phosphate, is high compared with the concentration of product, fructose 6-phosphate. This means that the ratio of the product to reactant is small, and RT ln([fructose 6-phosphate]/[glucose 6-phosphate]) is large and negative, causing ΔG to be negative despite ΔG° being positive. Thus, the reaction can proceed in the forward direction.

D. Standard free energy change, ΔG°

The standard free energy change, ΔG°, is so called because it is equal to the free energy change, ΔG, under standard conditions—that is, when reactants and products are at 1 mol/L concentrations (see Figure 6.3B). Under these conditions, the natural logarithm of the ratio of products to reactants is zero (ln1 = 0) and, therefore, the equation shown at the top of this page becomes:

$$\Delta G = \Delta G^\circ + 0$$

1. **ΔG° is predictive only under standard conditions:** Under standard conditions, ΔG° can be used to predict the direction a reaction proceeds because, under these conditions, ΔG° is equal to ΔG. However, ΔG° cannot predict the direction of a reaction under physiologic conditions, because it is composed solely of constants (R, T, and K_{eq}) and is, therefore, not altered by changes in product or substrate concentrations.

2. **Relationship between ΔG° and K_{eq}:** In a reaction A→B, a point of equilibrium is reached at which no further net chemical change takes place—that is, when A is being converted to B as fast as B is being converted to A. In this state, the ratio of [B] to [A] is constant, regardless of the actual concentrations of the two compounds:

$$K_{eq} = \frac{[B]_{eq}}{[A]_{eq}}$$

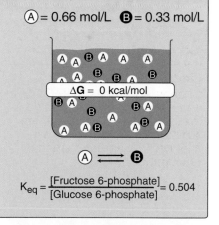

A Nonequilibrium conditions

Ⓐ = 0.9 mol/L   Ⓑ = 0.09 mol/L

ΔG = -0.96 kcal/mol

Ⓐ $\rightleftharpoons$ Ⓑ
Glucose 6-P   Fructose 6-P

B Standard conditions

Ⓐ = 1 mol/L   Ⓑ = 1 mol/L

$\Delta G = \Delta G^\circ$ = +0.4 kcal/mol

Ⓐ $\rightleftharpoons$ Ⓑ

C Equilibrium conditions

Ⓐ = 0.66 mol/L   Ⓑ = 0.33 mol/L

ΔG = 0 kcal/mol

Ⓐ $\rightleftharpoons$ Ⓑ

$$K_{eq} = \frac{[\text{Fructose 6-phosphate}]}{[\text{Glucose 6-phosphate}]} = 0.504$$

Figure 6.3
ΔG of a reaction depends on the concentration of reactant (A) and product (B). For the conversion of glucose 6-P to fructose 6-P, ΔG is negative when the ratio of reactant (A) to product (B) is large (top, panel A); is positive under standard conditions (middle, panel B); and is zero at equilibrium (bottom, panel C).

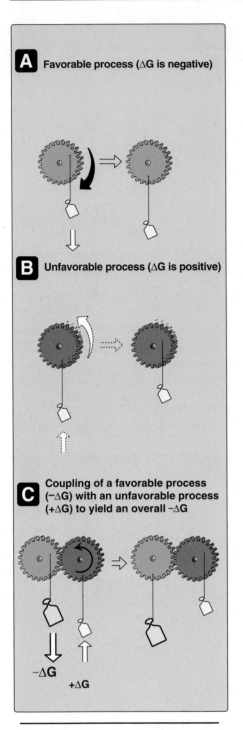

Figure 6.4
Mechanical model of coupling of favorable and unfavorable processes.

where K_{eq} is the equilibrium constant, and $[A]_{eq}$ and $[B]_{eq}$ are the concentrations of A and B at equilibrium. If the reaction A $\rightleftarrows$ B is allowed to go to equilibrium at constant temperature and pressure, then at equilibrium the overall free energy change (ΔG) is zero. Therefore,

$$\Delta G = 0 = \Delta G^{o} + RT \ln \frac{[B]_{eq}}{[A]_{eq}}$$

where the actual concentrations of A and B are equal to the equilibrium concentrations of reactant and product $[A]_{eq}$ and $[B]_{eq}$, and their ratio as shown above is equal to the K_{eq}. Thus,

$$\Delta G^{o} = -RT \ln K_{eq}$$

This equation allows some simple predictions:

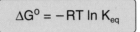

If $K_{eq} = 1$, then $\Delta G^{o} = 0$ A $\rightleftharpoons$ B

If $K_{eq} > 1$, then $\Delta G^{o} < 0$ A $\longrightarrow$ B

If $K_{eq} < 1$, then $\Delta G^{o} > 0$ A $\longleftarrow$ B

3. **ΔG^{o} of two consecutive reactions are additive:** The standard free energy changes (ΔG^{o}) are additive in any sequence of consecutive reactions, as are the free energy changes (ΔG). For example:

Glucose + ATP $\rightarrow$ glucose 6-P + ADP	$\Delta G^{o} = -4{,}000$ cal/mol
Glucose 6-P $\rightarrow$ fructose 6-P	$\Delta G^{o} = +400$ cal/mol
Glucose + ATP $\rightarrow$ fructose 6-P + ADP	$\Delta G^{o} = -3{,}600$ cal/mol

4. **ΔGs of a pathway are additive:** This additive property of free energy changes is very important in biochemical pathways through which substrates must pass in a particular direction (for example, A $\rightarrow$ B $\rightarrow$ C $\rightarrow$ D $\rightarrow$ ...). As long as the sum of the ΔGs of the individual reactions is negative, the pathway can potentially proceed as written, even if some of the individual reactions of the pathway have a positive ΔG. The actual rate of the reactions does, of course, depend on the lowering of activation energies by the enzymes that catalyze the reactions (see p. 55).

IV. ATP AS AN ENERGY CARRIER

Reactions or processes that have a large positive ΔG, such as moving ions against a concentration gradient across a cell membrane, are made possible by coupling the endergonic movement of ions with a second, spontaneous process with a large negative ΔG, such as the exergonic hydrolysis of adenosine triphosphate (ATP). [Note: In the absence of enzymes, ATP is a stable molecule because its hydrolysis has a high activation energy.] Figure 6.4 shows a mechanical model of energy coupling. A gear with an attached weight spontaneously turns in the direction that achieves the lowest energy state, in this case the weight seeks its lowest position (see Figure 6.4A). The reverse motion (see Figure 6.4B) is energetically unfavored and does not occur spontaneously. Figure 6.4C shows that the energetically favored movement of one gear can be used to turn a second gear in a direction that it would not move spontaneously. The simplest example of energy coupling in biologic reactions occurs when the energy-requiring and the energy-yielding reactions share a common intermediate.

A. Reactions are coupled through common intermediates

Two chemical reactions have a common intermediate when they occur sequentially so that the product of the first reaction is a substrate for the second. For example, given the reactions

$$A + B \rightarrow C + D$$

$$D + X \rightarrow Y + Z$$

D is the common intermediate and can serve as a carrier of chemical energy between the two reactions. Many coupled reactions use ATP to generate a common intermediate. These reactions may involve the transfer of a phosphate group from ATP to another molecule. Other reactions involve the transfer of phosphate from an energy-rich intermediate to adenosine diphosphate (ADP), forming ATP.

B. Energy carried by ATP

ATP consists of a molecule of adenosine (adenine + ribose) to which three phosphate groups are attached (Figure 6.5). If one phosphate is removed, ADP is produced; if two phosphates are removed, adenosine monophosphate (AMP) results. The standard free energy of hydrolysis of ATP, ΔG°, is approximately -7.3 kcal/mol for each of the two terminal phosphate groups. Because of this large negative ΔG°, ATP is called a high-energy phosphate compound.

V. ELECTRON TRANSPORT CHAIN

Energy-rich molecules, such as glucose, are metabolized by a series of oxidation reactions ultimately yielding CO_2 and water (Figure 6.6). The metabolic intermediates of these reactions donate electrons to specific coenzymes—nicotinamide adenine dinucleotide (NAD^+) and flavin adenine dinucleotide (FAD)—to form the energy-rich reduced coenzymes, NADH and $FADH_2$. These reduced coenzymes can, in turn, each donate a pair of electrons to a specialized set of electron carriers, collectively called the electron transport chain, described in this section. As electrons are passed down the electron transport chain, they lose much of their free energy. Part of this energy can be captured and stored by the production of ATP from ADP and inorganic phosphate (P_i). This process is called oxidative phosphorylation and is described on p. 77. The remainder of the free energy not trapped as ATP is used to drive ancillary reactions such as Ca^{2+} transport into mitochondria, and to generate heat.

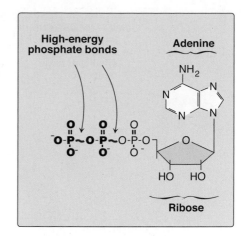

Figure 6.5
Adenosine triphosphate.

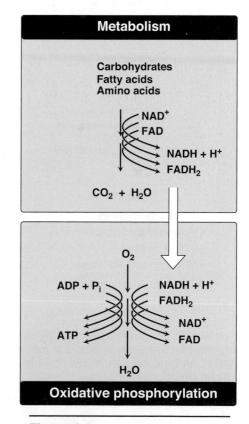

Figure 6.6
The metabolic breakdown of energy-yielding molecules.

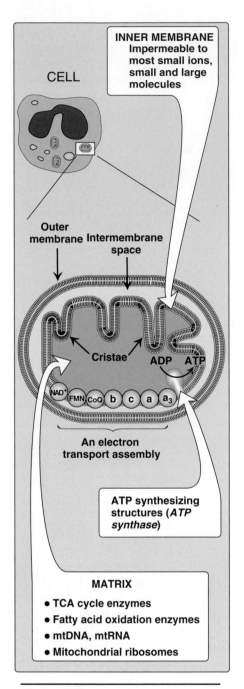

Figure 6.7
Structure of a mitochondrion showing schematic representation of the electron transport chain and ATP synthesizing structures on the inner membrane.
mtDNA = mitochondrial DNA; mtRNA = mitochondrial RNA. [Note: In contrast to the inner membrane, the outer membrane is highly permeable and the milieu of the intermembrane space is like that of the cytosol.]

A. Mitochondrion

The electron transport chain is present in the inner mitochondrial membrane and is the final common pathway by which electrons derived from different fuels of the body flow to oxygen. Electron transport and ATP synthesis by oxidative phosphorylation proceed continuously in all tissues that contain mitochondria.

1. **Membranes of the mitochondrion:** The components of the electron transport chain are located in the inner membrane. Although the outer membrane contains special pores, making it freely permeable to most ions and small molecules, the inner mitochondrial membrane is a specialized structure that is impermeable to most small ions, including H^+, Na^+, and K^+, and small molecules such as ATP, ADP, pyruvate, and other metabolites important to mitochondrial function (Figure 6.7). Specialized carriers or transport systems are required to move ions or molecules across this membrane. The inner mitochondrial membrane is unusually rich in protein, half of which is directly involved in electron transport and oxidative phosphorylation. The inner mitochondrial membrane is highly convoluted. The convolutions, called cristae, serve to greatly increase the surface area of the membrane.

2. **Matrix of the mitochondrion:** This gel-like solution in the interior of mitochondria is 50% protein. These molecules include the enzymes responsible for the oxidation of pyruvate, amino acids, fatty acids (by β-oxidation), and those of the tricarboxylic acid (TCA) cycle. The synthesis of glucose, urea, and heme occur partially in the matrix of mitochondria. In addition, the matrix contains NAD^+ and FAD (the oxidized forms of the two coenzymes that are required as hydrogen acceptors) and ADP and P_i, which are used to produce ATP. [Note: The matrix also contains mitochondrial RNA and DNA (mtRNA and mtDNA) and mitochondrial ribosomes.]

B. Organization of the electron transport chain

The inner mitochondrial membrane can be disrupted into five separate protein complexes, called Complexes I, II, III, IV, and V. Complexes I–IV each contain part of the electron transport chain (Figure 6.8). Each complex accepts or donates electrons to relatively mobile electron carriers, such as coenzyme Q and cytochrome c. Each carrier in the electron transport chain can receive electrons from an electron donor, and can subsequently donate electrons to the next carrier in the chain. The electrons ultimately combine with oxygen and protons to form water. This requirement for oxygen makes the electron transport process the respiratory chain, which accounts for the greatest portion of the body's use of oxygen. Complex V is a protein complex that contains a domain (F_o) that spans the inner mitochondrial membrane, and a domain (F_1) that appears as a sphere that protrudes into the mitochondrial matrix (see p. 78). Complex V catalyzes ATP synthesis and so is referred to as *ATP synthase*.

C. Reactions of the electron transport chain

With the exception of coenzyme Q, all members of this chain are proteins. These may function as enzymes as is the case with the

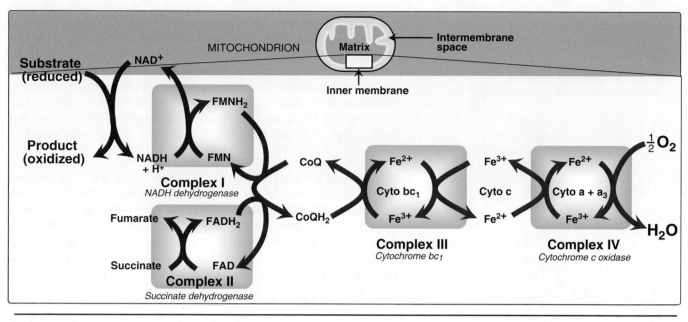

Figure 6.8
Electron transport chain. [Note: NADH, produced from a variety of oxidative (catabolic) processes, is the substrate for Complex I. Succinate, an intermediate of the TCA cycle, is the substrate for Complex II.]

dehydrogenases, may contain iron as part of an iron–sulfur center, may be coordinated with a porphyrin ring as in the cytochromes, or may contain copper as does the cytochrome a + a$_3$ complex.

1. **Formation of NADH:** NAD$^+$ is reduced to NADH by *dehydrogenases* that remove two hydrogen atoms from their substrate. (For examples of these reactions, see the discussion of the *dehydrogenases* found in the TCA cycle, p. 112.) Both electrons but only one proton (that is, a hydride ion, :H$^-$) are transferred to the NAD$^+$, forming NADH plus a free proton, H$^+$.

2. **NADH dehydrogenase:** The free proton plus the hydride ion carried by NADH are next transferred to *NADH dehydrogenase*, a protein complex (Complex I) embedded in the inner mitochondrial membrane. Complex I has a tightly bound molecule of flavin mononucleotide (FMN, a coenzyme structurally related to FAD, see Figure 28.15, p. 380) that accepts the two hydrogen atoms (2e$^-$+2H$^+$), becoming FMNH$_2$. *NADH dehydrogenase* also contains iron atoms paired with sulfur atoms to make iron–sulfur centers (Figure 6.9). These are necessary for the transfer of the hydrogen atoms to the next member of the chain, coenzyme Q (ubiquinone).

3. **Coenzyme Q:** Coenzyme Q (CoQ) is a quinone derivative with a long, hydrophobic isoprenoid tail. It is also called ubiquinone because it is ubiquitous in biologic systems. CoQ is a mobile carrier and can accept hydrogen atoms both from FMNH$_2$, produced on *NADH dehydrogenase* (Complex I), and from FADH$_2$, produced on *succinate dehydrogenase* (Complex II), *glycerophosphate dehydrogenase* (see p. 79), and *acyl CoA dehydrogenase* (see p. 192). CoQ transfers electrons to Complex III. CoQ, then, links the flavoproteins to the cytochromes.

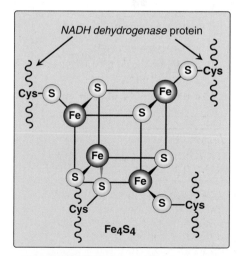

Figure 6.9
Iron-sulfur center of Complex I. [Note: Complexes II and III also contain iron-sulfur centers.

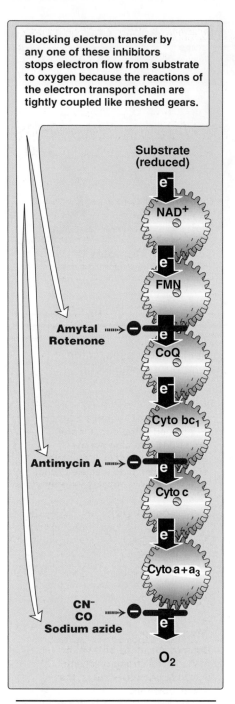

Figure 6.10
Site-specific inhibitors of electron transport shown using a mechanical model for the coupling of oxidation-reduction reactions. [Note: Figure illustrates normal direction of electron flow.]

4. **Cytochromes:** The remaining members of the electron transport chain are cytochromes. Each contains a heme group (a porphyrin ring plus iron). Unlike the heme groups of hemoglobin, the cytochrome iron is reversibly converted from its ferric (Fe^{3+}) to its ferrous (Fe^{2+}) form as a normal part of its function as a reversible carrier of electrons. Electrons are passed along the chain from CoQ to cytochromes bc_1 (Complex III), c, and a + a_3 (Complex IV, see Figure 6.8). [Note: Cytochrome c is associated with the outer face of the inner membrane and, like CoQ, is a mobile carrier of electrons.]

5. **Cytochrome a + a_3:** This cytochrome complex is the only electron carrier in which the heme iron has an available coordination site that can react directly with O_2, and so also is called *cytochrome oxidase*. At this site, the transported electrons, O_2, and free protons are brought together, and O_2 is reduced to water (see Figure 6.8). *Cytochrome oxidase* contains copper atoms that are required for this complex reaction to occur.

6. **Site-specific inhibitors:** Site-specific inhibitors of electron transport have been identified and are illustrated in Figure 6.10. These compounds prevent the passage of electrons by binding to a component of the chain, blocking the oxidation/reduction reaction. Therefore, all electron carriers before the block are fully reduced, whereas those located after the block are oxidized. [Note: Inhibition of electron transport inhibits ATP synthesis because these processes are tightly coupled.]

> Incomplete reduction of oxygen to water produces reactive oxygen species (ROS), such as superoxide ($O_2 \cdot^-$), hydrogen peroxide (H_2O_2) and hydroxyl radicals (OH$\cdot$). ROS damage DNA and proteins, and cause lipid peroxidation. Enzymes such as *superoxide dismutase (SOD)*, *catalase*, and *glutathione peroxidase* are cellular defenses against ROS.

D. Release of free energy during electron transport

Free energy is released as electrons are transferred along the electron transport chain from an electron donor (reducing agent or reductant) to an electron acceptor (oxidizing agent or oxidant). The electrons can be transferred as hydride ions (:H^-) to NAD^+, as hydrogen atoms ($\cdot$H) to FMN, coenzyme Q, and FAD, or as electrons (e^-) to cytochromes.

1. **Redox pairs:** Oxidation (loss of electrons) of one compound is always accompanied by reduction (gain of electrons) of a second substance. For example, Figure 6.11 shows the oxidation of NADH to NAD^+ accompanied by the reduction of FMN to $FMNH_2$. Such oxidation-reduction reactions can be written as the sum of two separate half-reactions, one an oxidation reaction and the other a reduction reaction (see Figure 6.11). NAD^+ and NADH form a redox pair, as do FMN and $FMNH_2$. Redox pairs differ in their tendency to lose electrons. This tendency is a characteristic of a particular redox pair, and can be quantitatively specified by a constant, E_o (the standard reduction potential), with units in volts.

2. Standard reduction potential (E_o): The E_o of various redox pairs can be ordered from the most negative E_o to the most positive. The more negative the E_o of a redox pair, the greater the tendency of the reductant member of that pair to lose electrons. The more positive the E_o, the greater the tendency of the oxidant member of that pair to accept electrons. Therefore, electrons flow from the pair with the more negative E_o to that with the more positive E_o. The E_o values for some members of the electron transport chain are shown in Figure 6.12. [Note: The components of the electron transport chain are arranged in order of increasingly positive E_0 values.]

3. ΔG^o is related to ΔE_o: The change in free energy is related directly to the magnitude of the change in E_o:

$$\Delta G^o = - n F \Delta E_o$$

n = number of electrons transferred (1 for a cytochrome, 2 for NADH, $FADH_2$, and coenzyme Q)

F = Faraday constant (23.1 kcal/volt · mol)

ΔE_o = E_o of the electron-accepting pair minus the E_o of the electron-donating pair

ΔG^o = change in the standard free energy

4. ΔG^o of ATP: The standard free energy for the phosphorylation of ADP to ATP is +7.3 kcal/mol. The transport of a pair of electrons from NADH to oxygen via the electron transport chain produces 52.58 kcal. Therefore, more than sufficient energy is available to produce three ATP from three ADP and three P_i (3 x 7.3 = 21.9 kcal/mol), sometimes expressed as a P:O ratio (ATP made per O atom reduced) of 3:1. The remaining calories are used for ancillary reactions or released as heat. [Note: P:O for $FADH_2$ is 2:1 because Complex I is bypassed.]

VI. OXIDATIVE PHOSPHORYLATION

The transfer of electrons down the electron transport chain is energetically favored because NADH is a strong electron donor and molecular oxygen is an avid electron acceptor. However, the flow of electrons from NADH to oxygen does not directly result in ATP synthesis.

A. Chemiosmotic hypothesis

The chemiosmotic hypothesis (also known as the Mitchell hypothesis) explains how the free energy generated by the transport of electrons by the electron transport chain is used to produce ATP from ADP + P_i.

1. Proton pump: Electron transport is coupled to the phosphorylation of ADP by the transport ("pumping") of protons (H^+) across the inner mitochondrial membrane from the matrix to the intermembrane space at Complexes I, III, and IV. This process creates an electrical gradient (with more positive charges on the outside of the membrane than on the inside) and a pH gradient (the outside of the membrane is at a lower pH than the inside, Figure 6.13). The energy generated by this proton gradient is sufficient to drive ATP

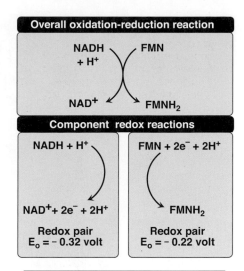

Figure 6.11
Oxidation of NADH by FMN, separated into two component redox pairs.

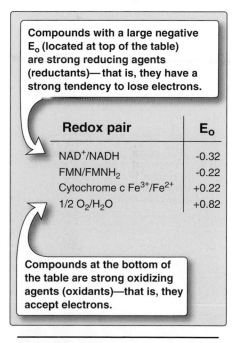

Figure 6.12
Standard reduction potentials of some reactions.

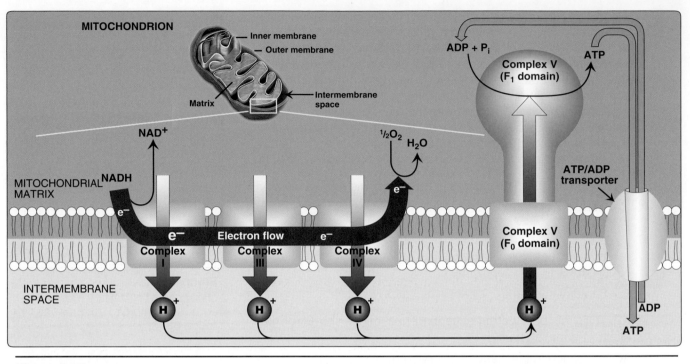

Figure 6.13
Electron transport chain shown coupled to the transport of protons. [Note: Protons are not pumped at Complex II.]

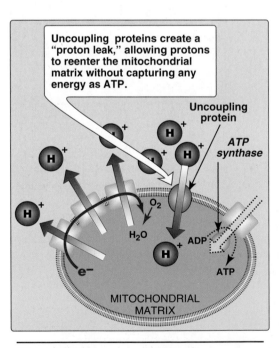

Figure 6.14
Transport of H⁺ across the mitochondrial membrane by 2,4-dinitrophenol.

synthesis. Thus, the proton gradient serves as the common intermediate that couples oxidation to phosphorylation.

2. **ATP synthase:** The enzyme complex *ATP synthase* (Complex V, see Figure 6.13) synthesizes ATP using the energy of the proton gradient generated by the electron transport chain. [Note: It is also called *F₁/F₀ ATPase* because the isolated enzyme can catalyze the hydrolysis of ATP to ADP and P_i.] The chemiosmotic hypothesis proposes that after protons have been pumped to the cytosolic side of the inner mitochondrial membrane, they reenter the matrix by passing through a channel in the membrane-spanning domain (F_o) of Complex V, driving rotation of F_o and, at the same time, dissipating the pH and electrical gradients. F_o rotation causes conformational changes in the extra-membranous F_1 domain that allow it to bind ADP + P_i, phosphorylate ADP to ATP, and release ATP.

a. **Oligomycin:** This drug binds to the F_o (hence the letter o) domain of *ATP synthase,* closing the H⁺ channel, preventing reentry of protons into the mitochondrial matrix, and thus preventing phosphorylation of ADP to ATP. Because the pH and electrical gradients cannot be dissipated in the presence of this drug, electron transport stops because of the difficulty of pumping any more protons against the steep gradients. This dependency of cellular respiration on the ability to phosphorylate ADP to ATP is known as respiratory control, and is the consequence of the tight coupling of these processes. Electron transport and phosphorylation are, therefore, again shown to be tightly coupled processes. Inhibition of one process inhibits the other. [Note: Respiratory control also results from decreased availability of ADP or P_i.]

b. Uncoupling proteins (UCP): UCPs occur in the inner mitochondrial membrane of mammals, including humans. These carrier proteins create a "proton leak," that is, they allow protons to re-enter the mitochondrial matrix without energy being captured as ATP (Figure 6.14). The energy is released as heat, and the process is called nonshivering thermogenesis. UCP1, also called thermogenin, is responsible for the heat production in the brown adipocytes of mammals. UCP1 is activated by fatty acids. Brown fat, unlike the more abundant white fat, uses almost 90% of its respiratory energy for thermogenesis in response to cold in the neonate, and during arousal in hibernating animals. However, humans appear to have little brown fat (except in the newborn), and UCP1 does not appear to play a major role in energy balance. [Note: Other uncoupling proteins (UCP2, UCP3) have been found in humans, but their significance remains unclear.]

c. Synthetic uncouplers: Electron transport and phosphorylation can also be uncoupled by compounds that increase the permeability of the inner mitochondrial membrane to protons. The classic example is 2,4-dinitrophenol, a lipophilic proton carrier that readily diffuses through the mitochondrial membrane. This uncoupler causes electron transport to proceed at a rapid rate without establishing a proton gradient, much as do the UCPs (see Figure 6.14). Again, energy is released as heat rather than being used to synthesize ATP. In high doses, aspirin and other salicylates uncouple oxidative phosphorylation. This explains the fever that accompanies toxic overdoses of these drugs.

B. Membrane transport systems

The inner mitochondrial membrane is impermeable to most charged or hydrophilic substances. However, it contains numerous transport proteins that permit passage of specific molecules from the cytosol (or more correctly, the intermembrane space) to the mitochondrial matrix.

1. ATP-ADP transport: The inner mitochondrial membrane requires specialized carriers to transport ADP and P_i from the cytosol (where ATP is used and converted to ADP in many energy-requiring reactions) into mitochondria, where ATP can be resynthesized. An adenine nucleotide carrier imports one molecule of ADP from the cytosol into mitochondria, while exporting one ATP from the matrix back into the cytosol (see Figure 6.13). [Note: A phosphate carrier is responsible for transporting P_i from the cytosol into mitochondria.]

2. Transport of reducing equivalents: The inner mitochondrial membrane lacks an NADH transporter, and NADH produced in the cytosol cannot directly enter the mitochondrial matrix. However, two electrons of NADH (also called reducing equivalents) are transported from the cytosol into the matrix using substrate shuttles. In the glycerophosphate shuttle (Figure 6.15A), two electrons are transferred from NADH to dihydroxyacetone phosphate by cytosolic *glycerophosphate dehydrogenase*. The glycerol 3-phosphate produced is oxidized by the mitochondrial isozyme as FAD is

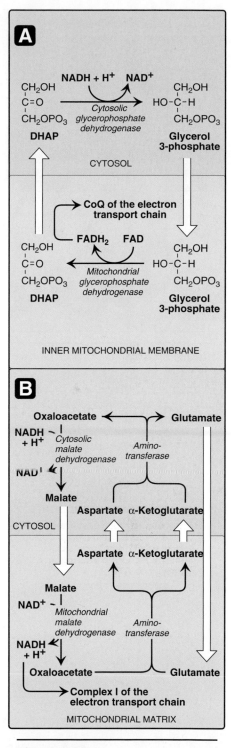

Figure 6.15
Substrate shuttles for the transport of electrons across the inner mitochondrial membrane. A. Glycerol 3-phosphate shuttle. B. Malate-aspartate shuttle. DHAP = dihydroxyacetone phosphate.

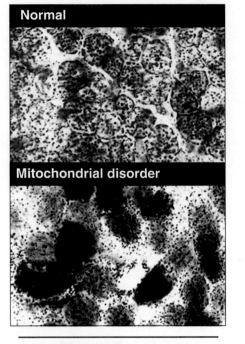

Figure 6.16
Muscle fibers from a patient with a mitochondrial myopathy show abnormal mitochondrial proliferation when stained for *succinate dehydrogenase*, an enzyme of Complex II.

reduced to $FADH_2$. CoQ of the electron transport chain oxidizes $FADH_2$. The glycerophosphate shuttle, therefore, results in the synthesis of two ATPs for each cytosolic NADH oxidized. This contrasts with the malate-aspartate shuttle (Figure 6.15B), which produces NADH (rather than $FADH_2$) in the mitochondrial matrix and, therefore, yields three ATPs for each cytosolic NADH oxidized by *malate dehydrogenase* as oxaloacetate is reduced to malate. A transport protein carries malate into the matrix.

C. Inherited defects in oxidative phosphorylation

Thirteen of the approximately 120 polypeptides required for oxidative phosphorylation are coded for by mtDNA and synthesized in mitochondria, whereas the remaining mitochondrial proteins are synthesized in the cytosol and transported into mitochondria. Defects in oxidative phosphorylation are more likely a result of alterations in mtDNA, which has a mutation rate about ten times greater than that of nuclear DNA. Tissues with the greatest ATP requirement (for example, central nervous system, skeletal and heart muscle, kidney, and liver) are most affected by defects in oxidative phosphorylation. Mutations in mtDNA are responsible for several diseases, including some cases of mitochondrial myopathies (Figure 6.16), and Leber hereditary optic neuropathy, a disease in which bilateral loss of central vision occurs as a result of neuroretinal degeneration, including damage to the optic nerve. The mtDNA is maternally inherited because mitochondria from the sperm cell do not enter the fertilized egg.

D. Mitochondria and apoptosis

The process of apoptosis or programmed cell death may be initiated through the intrinsic (mitochondrial-mediated) pathway by the formation of pores in the outer mitochondrial membrane. These pores allow cytochrome c to leave the intermembrane space and enter the cytosol. Once in the cytosol, cytochrome c, in association with proapoptotic factors, activates a family of proteolytic enzymes (the *caspases*), causing cleavage of key proteins and resulting in the morphologic and biochemical changes characteristic of apoptosis.

VII. CHAPTER SUMMARY

The change in **free energy** (ΔG) occurring during a reaction predicts the direction in which that reaction will spontaneously proceed. If ΔG is **negative** (that is, the product has a lower free energy than the substrate), the **reaction goes spontaneously**. If ΔG is **positive**, the reaction **does not go spontaneously**. If $\Delta G = 0$, the reactions are in **equilibrium**. The ΔG of the forward reaction (A → B) is equal in magnitude but opposite in sign to that of the back reaction (B → A). The ΔGs are **additive** in any sequence of consecutive reactions, as are the standard free energy changes ($\Delta G°$s). Therefore, reactions or processes that have a large, positive ΔG are made possible by **coupling** with cleavage of **adenosine triphosphate** (**ATP**), which has a large, negative ΔG. The reduced coenzymes **NADH** and **$FADH_2$** each donate a pair of electrons to a specialized set of electron carriers, consisting of **FMN**,

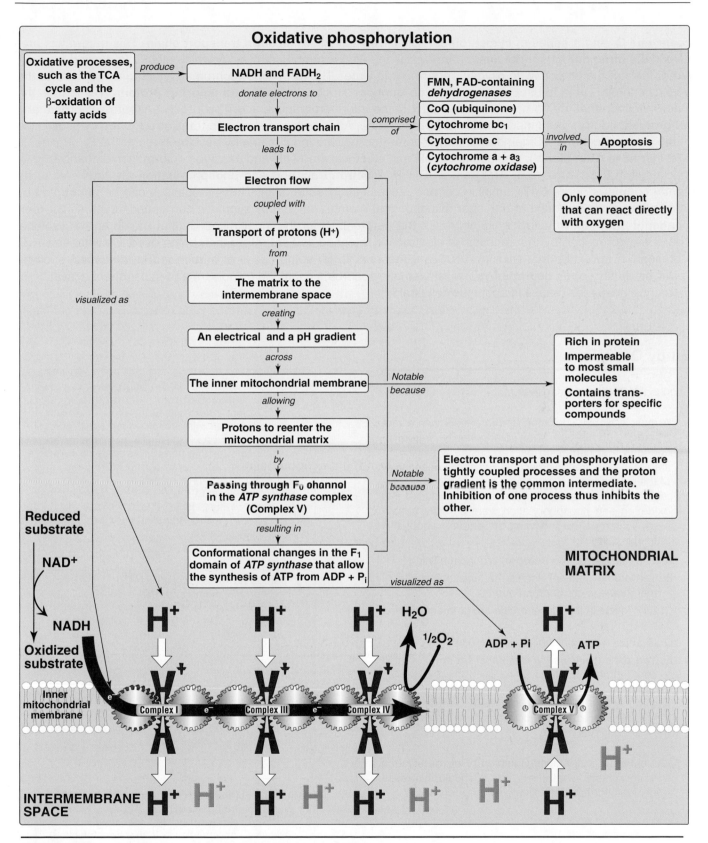

Figure 6.17

Summary of key concepts for oxidative phosphorylation. [Note: Electron flow and ATP synthesis are envisioned as sets of interlocking gears to emphasize the idea of coupling.]

coenzyme Q, and a series of **cytochromes**, collectively called the **electron transport chain**. This pathway is present in the **inner mitochondrial membrane**, and is the final common pathway by which electrons derived from different fuels of the body flow to oxygen, reducing it to water. The terminal cytochrome, cytochrome oxidase, is the only cytochrome able to bind oxygen. **Electron transport** is coupled to the **transport of protons** (H$^+$) across the inner mitochondrial membrane from the matrix to the intermembrane space. This process creates **electrical** and **pH gradients** across the inner mitochondrial membrane. After protons have been transferred to the cytosolic side of the inner mitochondrial membrane, they reenter the mitochondrial matrix by passing through the F_o channel in **ATP synthase (Complex V)**, dissipating the pH and electrical gradients and causing conformational changes in F_1 that result in the synthesis of ATP from ADP + P_i. **Electron transport** and **phosphorylation** are thus said to be **tightly coupled** (Figure 6.17). Inhibition of one process inhibits the other. These processes can be **uncoupled** by **uncoupling proteins** found in the inner mitochondrial membrane, and by synthetic compounds such as **2,4-dinitrophenol** and **aspirin**, all of which increase the permeability of the inner mitochondrial membrane to protons. The energy produced by the transport of electrons is released as **heat** rather than being used to synthesize ATP. Mutations in **mitochondrial DNA (mtDNA)** are responsible for some cases of **mitochondrial diseases**, such as **Leber hereditary optic neuropathy**. The release of cytochrome c into the cytoplasm and subsequent activation of proteolytic caspases results in apoptotic cell death.

Study Questions

Choose the ONE correct answer.

6.1 A muscle biopsy specimen from a patient with a rare disorder, Luft disease, showed abnormally large mitochondria that contained packed cristae when examined in the electron microscope. Basal ATPase activity of the mitochondria was seven times greater than normal. From these and other data it was concluded that oxidation and phosphorylation were partially uncoupled. Which of the following statements about this patient is correct?

A. The rate of electron transport is abnormally low.

B. The proton gradient across the inner mitochondrial membrane is greater than normal.

C. ATP levels in the mitochondria are greater than normal.

D. Cyanide would not inhibit electron flow.

E. The patient shows hypermetabolism and elevated core temperature.

6.2 Explain why and how the malate-aspartate shuttle moves NADH reducing equivalents from the cytosol to the mitochondrial matrix.

6.3 CO binds to and inhibits Complex IV of the electron transport chain. What effect, if any, should this respiratory inhibitor have on oxidative phosphorylation?

Correct answer = E. When phosphorylation is partially uncoupled from electron flow, one would expect a decrease in the proton gradient across the inner mitochondrial membrane and, hence, impaired ATP synthesis. In an attempt to compensate for this defect in energy capture, metabolism and electron flow to oxygen is increased. This hypermetabolism will be accompanied by elevated body temperature because the energy in fuels is largely wasted, appearing as heat. The electron transport chain will still be inhibited by cyanide.

There is no transporter for NADH in the inner mitochondrial membrane. However, NADH can be oxidized to NAD$^+$ by the cytoplasmic isozyme of malate dehydrogenase as oxaloacetate is reduced to malate. The malate is transported across the inner membrane, and the mitochondrial isozyme of malate dehydrogenase oxidizes it to oxaloacetate as mitochondrial NAD$^+$ is reduced to NADH. This NADH can be oxidized by Complex I of the electron transport chain, generating three ATP through the coupled processes of respiration and oxidative phosphorylation.

Inhibition of the electron transport chain by respiratory inhibitors such as CO results in an inability to maintain the proton gradient. Oxidative phosphorylation is therefore inhibited, as are ancillary reactions, because they also require the proton gradient.

Introduction to Carbohydrates

7

I. OVERVIEW

Carbohydrates are the most abundant organic molecules in nature. They have a wide range of functions, including providing a significant fraction of the dietary calories for most organisms, acting as a storage form of energy in the body, and serving as cell membrane components that mediate some forms of intercellular communication. Carbohydrates also serve as a structural component of many organisms, including the cell walls of bacteria, the exoskeleton of many insects, and the fibrous cellulose of plants. The empiric formula for many of the simpler carbohydrates is $(CH_2O)_n$, hence the name "hydrate of carbon."

II. CLASSIFICATION AND STRUCTURE OF CARBOHYDRATES

Monosaccharides (simple sugars) can be classified according to the number of carbon atoms they contain. Examples of some monosaccharides commonly found in humans are listed in Figure 7.1. Carbohydrates with an aldehyde as their most oxidized functional group are called aldoses, whereas those with a keto as their most oxidized functional group are called ketoses (Figure 7.2). For example, glyceraldehyde is an aldose, whereas dihydroxyacetone is a ketose. Carbohydrates that have a free carbonyl group have the suffix –ose. [Note: Ketoses (with some exceptions, for example, fructose) have an additional two letters in their suffix: –ulose, for example, xylulose.] Monosaccharides can be linked by glycosidic bonds to create larger structures (Figure 7.3). Disaccharides contain two monosaccharide units, oligosaccharides contain from three to about ten monosaccharide units, whereas polysaccharides contain more than ten monosaccharide units, and can be hundreds of sugar units in length.

A. Isomers and epimers

Compounds that have the same chemical formula but have different structures are called isomers. For example, fructose, glucose, mannose, and galactose are all isomers of each other, having the same chemical formula, $C_6H_{12}O_6$. Carbohydrate isomers that differ in configuration around only one specific carbon atom (with the exception of the carbonyl carbon, see "anomers" below) are defined as epimers of each other. For example, glucose and galactose are C-4

Generic names	Examples
3 Carbons: trioses	Glyceraldehyde
4 Carbons: tetroses	Erythrose
5 Carbons: pentoses	Ribose
6 Carbons: hexoses	Glucose
7 Carbons: heptoses	Sedoheptulose
9 Carbons: nonoses	Nouraminic acid

Figure 7.1
Examples of monosaccharides found in humans, classified according to the number of carbons they contain.

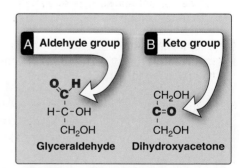

Figure 7.2
Examples of an aldose (A) and a ketose (B) sugar.

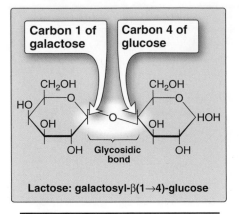

Figure 7.3
A glycosidic bond between two hexoses producing a disaccharide.

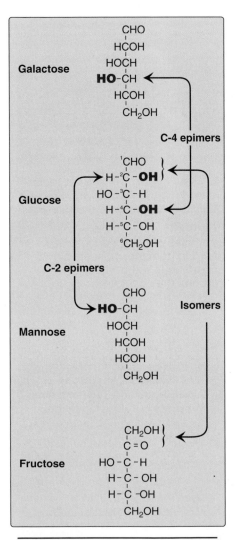

Figure 7.4
C-2 and C-4 epimers and an isomer of glucose.

epimers—their structures differ only in the position of the –OH group at carbon 4. [Note: The carbons in sugars are numbered beginning at the end that contains the carbonyl carbon—that is, the aldehyde or keto group (Figure 7.4).] Glucose and mannose are C-2 epimers. However, galactose and mannose are NOT epimers—they differ in the position of –OH groups at two carbons (2 and 4) and are, therefore, defined only as isomers (see Figure 7.4).

B. Enantiomers

A special type of isomerism is found in the pairs of structures that are mirror images of each other. These mirror images are called enantiomers, and the two members of the pair are designated as a D- and an L-sugar (Figure 7.5). The vast majority of the sugars in humans are D-sugars. In the D isomeric form, the –OH group on the asymmetric carbon (a carbon linked to four different atoms or groups) farthest from the carbonyl carbon is on the right, whereas in the L-isomer it is on the left. Enzymes known as *racemases* are able to interconvert D- and L-isomers.

C. Cyclization of monosaccharides

Less than 1% of each of the monosaccharides with five or more carbons exists in the open-chain (acyclic) form. Rather, they are predominantly found in a ring (cyclic) form, in which the aldehyde (or keto) group has reacted with an alcohol group on the same sugar, making the carbonyl carbon (carbon 1 for an aldose or carbon 2 for a ketose) asymmetric. [Note: Pyranose refers to a six-membered ring consisting of five carbons and one oxygen, for example, glucopyranose (Figure 7.6), whereas furanose denotes a five-membered ring with four carbons and one oxygen.]

1. **Anomeric carbon:** Cyclization creates an anomeric carbon (the former carbonyl carbon), generating the α and β configurations of the sugar, for example, α-D-glucopyranose and β-D-glucopryanose (see Figure 7.6). These two sugars are both glucose but are anomers of each other. [Note: In the α configuration, the OH on the anomeric C projects to the same side as the ring in a modified Fischer projection formula (Figure 7.6A), and is trans to the CH₂OH group in a Haworth projection formula (Figure 7.6B). Because the α and β forms are not mirror images, they are referred to as diastereomers.] Enzymes are able to distinguish between these two structures and use one or the other preferentially. For example, glycogen is synthesized from α-D-glucopyranose, whereas cellulose is synthesized from β-D-glucopyranose. The cyclic α and β anomers of a sugar in solution are in equilibrium with each other, and can be spontaneously interconverted (a process called mutarotation, see Figure 7.6).

2. **Reducing sugars:** If the hydroxyl group on the anomeric carbon of a cyclized sugar is not linked to another compound by a glycosidic bond, the ring can open. The sugar can act as a reducing agent, and is termed a reducing sugar. Such sugars can react with chromogenic agents (for example, Benedict's reagent or Fehling's solution) causing the reagent to be reduced and colored, with the aldehyde group of the acyclic sugar becoming oxidized. [Note:

Only the state of the oxygen in the aldehyde group determines if the sugar is reducing or nonreducing.]

A colorimetric test can detect a reducing sugar in urine. A positive result is indicative of an underlying pathology because sugars are not normally present in urine, and can be followed up by more specific tests to identify the reducing sugar.

D. Joining of monosaccharides

Monosaccharides can be joined to form disaccharides, oligosaccharides, and polysaccharides. Important disaccharides include lactose (galactose + glucose), sucrose (glucose + fructose), and maltose (glucose + glucose). Important polysaccharides include branched glycogen (from animal sources) and starch (plant sources) and unbranched cellulose (plant sources); each is a polymer of glucose. The bonds that link sugars are called glycosidic bonds. These are formed by enzymes known as *glycosyltransferases* that use nucleotide sugars such as UDP-glucose as substrates.

1. **Naming glycosidic bonds:** Glycosidic bonds between sugars are named according to the numbers of the connected carbons, and with regard to the position of the anomeric hydroxyl group of the sugar involved in the bond. If this anomeric hydroxyl is in the α configuration, the linkage is an α-bond. If it is in the β configuration, the linkage is a β-bond. Lactose, for example, is synthesized by forming a glycosidic bond between carbon 1 of β-galactose and carbon 4 of glucose. The linkage is, therefore, a $\beta(1\rightarrow4)$ glycosidic bond (see Figure 7.3). [Note: Because the anomeric end of the glucose residue is not involved in the glycosidic linkage it (and, therefore, lactose) remains a reducing sugar.]

E. Complex carbohydrates

Carbohydrates can be attached by glycosidic bonds to non-carbohydrate structures, including purine and pyrimidine bases (found in

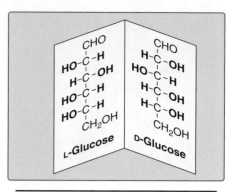

Figure 7.5
Enantiomers (mirror images) of glucose.

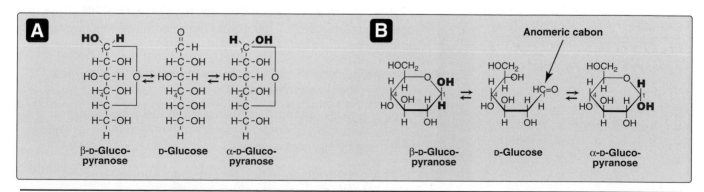

Figure 7.6
A The interconversion (mutarotation) of the α and β anomeric forms of glucose shown as modified Fischer projection formulas. B. The interconversion shown as Haworth projection formulas. Carbon 1 is the anomeric carbon. [Note: Glucose is a reducing sugar.]

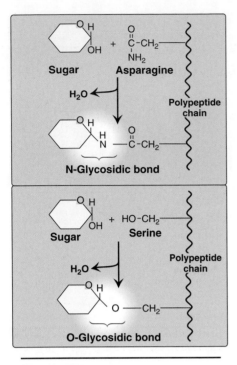

Figure 7.7
Glycosides: examples of N- and O-glycosidic bonds.

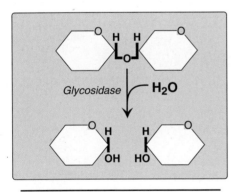

Figure 7.8
Hydrolysis of a glycosidic bond.

nucleic acids), aromatic rings (such as those found in steroids and bilirubin), proteins (found in glycoproteins and proteoglycans), and lipids (found in glycolipids).

1. **N- and O-glycosides:** If the group on the non-carbohydrate molecule to which the sugar is attached is an $-NH_2$ group, the structure is an N-glycoside and the bond is called an N-glycosidic link. If the group is an $-OH$, the structure is an O-glycoside, and the bond is an O-glycosidic link (Figure 7.7). [Note: All sugar–sugar glycosidic bonds are O-type linkages.]

III. DIGESTION OF DIETARY CARBOHYDRATES

The principal sites of dietary carbohydrate digestion are the mouth and intestinal lumen. This digestion is rapid and is catalyzed by enzymes known as *glycoside hydrolases* (*glycosidases*) that hydrolyze glycosidic bonds. Because there is little monosaccharide present in diets of mixed animal and plant origin, the enzymes are primarily *endoglycosidases* that hydrolyze polysaccharides and oliosaccharides, and *disacchari-dases* that hydrolyse tri- and disaccharides into their reducing sugar components (Figure 7.8). *Glycosidases* are usually specific for the structure and configuration of the glycosyl residue to be removed, as well as for the type of bond to be broken. The final products of carbohy-drate digestion are the monosaccharides, glucose, galactose and fruc-tose, which are absorbed by cells of the small intestine.

A. Digestion of carbohydrates begins in the mouth

The major dietary polysaccharides are of plant (starch, composed of amylose and amylopectin) and animal (glycogen) origin. During mas-tication, salivary α-*amylase* acts briefly on dietary starch and glyco-gen, hydrolyzing random $\alpha(1{\rightarrow}4)$ bonds. [Note: There are both $\alpha(1{\rightarrow}4)$- and $\beta(1{\rightarrow}4)$-*endoglucosidases* in nature, but humans do not produce the latter. Therefore, we are unable to digest cellulose—a carbohydrate of plant origin containing $\beta(1{\rightarrow}4)$ glycosidic bonds between glucose residues.] Because branched amylopectin and glycogen also contain $\alpha(1{\rightarrow}6)$ bonds, which α-*amylase* cannot hydrolyze, the digest resulting from its action contains a mixture of short, branched and unbranched oligosaccharides kown as dextrins (Figure 7.9) [Note: Disaccharides are also present as they, too, are resistant to *amylase*.] Carbohydrate digestion halts temporarily in the stomach, because the high acidity inactivates salivary α-*amylase*.

B. Further digestion of carbohydrates by pancreatic enzymes occurs in the small intestine

When the acidic stomach contents reach the small intestine, they are neutralized by bicarbonate secreted by the pancreas, and pan-creatic α-*amylase* continues the process of starch digestion.

C. Final carbohydrate digestion by enzymes synthesized by the intestinal mucosal cells

The final digestive processes occur primarily at the mucosal lining of the upper jejunum, and include the action of several *disacchari-*

dases (Figure 7.10). For example, *isomaltase* cleaves the α(1→6) bond in isomaltose and *maltase* cleaves maltose and maltotriose, each producing glucose, *sucrase* cleaves sucrose producing glucose and fructose, and *lactase* (*β-galactosidase*) cleaves lactose producing galactose and glucose. Trehalose, an α(1→1) disaccharide of glucose found in mushrooms and other fungi, is cleaved by *trehalase*. These enzymes are secreted through, and remain associated with, the luminal side of the brush border membranes of the intestinal mucosal cells. [Note: The substrates for *isomaltase* are broader than its name suggests, as it hydrolyzes the majority of maltose.]

> *Sucrase* and *isomaltase* are enzymic activities of a single protein which is cleaved into two functional subunits that remain associated in the cell membrane, forming the *sucrase-isomaltase* complex. *Maltase* forms a similar complex with an *exoglucosidase* (*glucoamylase*) that cleaves α(1→4) glycosidic bonds in dextrins.

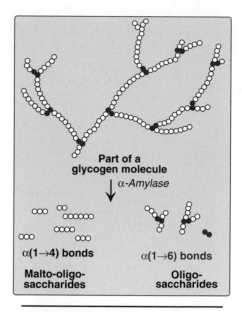

Figure 7.9
Degradation of dietary glycogen by salivary or pancreatic α-*amylase*.

D. Absorption of monosaccharides by intestinal mucosal cells

The duodenum and upper jejunum absorb the bulk of the dietary sugars. However, different sugars have different mechanisms of absorption. For example, galactose and glucose are transported into the mucosal cells by an active, energy-requiring process that requires a concurrent uptake of sodium ions; the transport protein is the sodium-dependent glucose cotransporter 1 (SGLT-1). Fructose uptake requires a sodium-independent monosaccharide transporter (GLUT-5) for its absorption. All three monosaccharides are transported from the intestinal mucosal cell into the portal circulation by yet another transporter, GLUT-2. (See p. 97 for a discussion of these transporters.)

E. Abnormal degradation of disaccharides

The overall process of carbohydrate digestion and absorption is so efficient in healthy individuals that ordinarily all digestible dietary carbohydrate is absorbed by the time the ingested material reaches the lower jejunum. However, because it is monosaccharides that are absorbed, any defect in a specific *disaccharidase* activity of the intestinal mucosa causes the passage of undigested carbohydrate into the large intestine. As a consequence of the presence of this osmotically active material, water is drawn from the mucosa into the large intestine, causing osmotic diarrhea. This is reinforced by the bacterial fermentation of the remaining carbohydrate to two- and three-carbon compounds (which are also osmotically active) plus large volumes of CO_2 and H_2 gas, causing abdominal cramps, diarrhea, and flatulence.

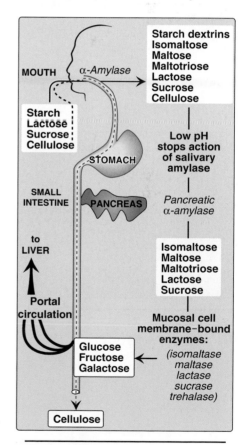

Figure 7.10
Digestion of carbohydrates. [Note: Indigestible cellulose enters the colon and is excreted.]

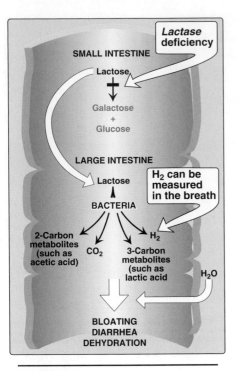

Figure 7.11
Abnormal lactose metabolism.

1. **Digestive enzyme deficiencies:** Genetic deficiencies of the individual *disaccharidases* result in disaccharide intolerance. Alterations in disaccharide degradation can also be caused by a variety of intestinal diseases, malnutrition, or drugs that injure the mucosa of the small intestine. For example, brush border enzymes are rapidly lost in normal individuals with severe diarrhea, causing a temporary, acquired enzyme deficiency. Thus, patients suffering or recovering from such a disorder cannot drink or eat significant amounts of dairy products or sucrose without exacerbating the diarrhea.

2. **Lactose intolerance:** More than three quarters of the world's adults are lactose intolerant (Figure 7.11). This is particularly manifested in certain populations. For example, up to 90% of adults of African or Asian descent are *lactase*-deficient and, therefore, are less able to metabolize lactose than individuals of Northern European origin. The age-dependent loss of *lactase* activity represents a reduction in the amount of enzyme rather than a modified inactive enzyme. It is thought to be caused by small variations in the DNA sequence of a region on chromosome 2 that controls expression of the gene for *lactase*, also on chromosome 2. Treatment for this disorder is to reduce consumption of milk while eating yogurts and cheeses, as well as green vegetables such as broccoli, to ensure adequate calcium intake; to use *lactase*-treated products; or to take *lactase* in pill form prior to eating. [Note: Because the loss of *lactase* is the norm for most of the world's adults, use of the term "adult hypolactasia" for lactose intolerance is becoming more common.]

3. **Sucrase-isomaltase complex deficiency:** This deficiency results in an intolerance of ingested sucrose. The disorder is found in about 10% of the Inuit people of Greenland and Canada, whereas 2% of North Americans are heterozygous for the deficiency. Treatment includes the dietary restriction of sucrose, and enzyme replacement therapy.

4. **Diagnosis:** Identification of a specific enzyme deficiency can be obtained by performing oral tolerance tests with the individual disaccharides. Measurement of hydrogen gas in the breath is a reliable test for determining the amount of ingested carbohydrate not absorbed by the body, but which is metabolized instead by the intestinal flora (see Figure 7.11).

IV. CHAPTER SUMMARY

Monosaccharides (simple sugars, Figure 7.12) containing an aldehyde group are called **aldoses** and those with a keto group are called **ketoses. Disaccharides**, **oligosaccharides**, and **polysaccharides** consist of monosaccharides linked by **glycosidic bonds**. Compounds with the same chemical formula are called **isomers**. If two monosaccharide isomers differ in configuration around one specific carbon atom (with the exception of the carbonyl carbon), they are defined as **epimers** of each other. If a pair of sugars are mirror images (**enantiomers**), the two members of the pair are designated as **D-** and **L-sugars**. When a

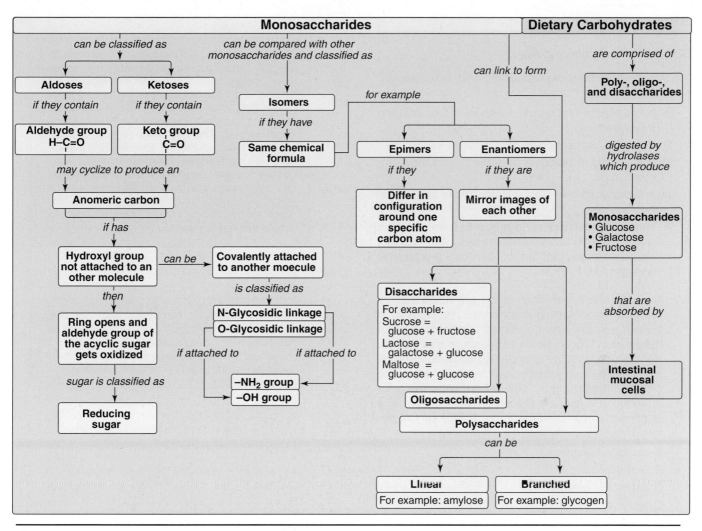

Figure 7.12
Key concept map for structure of monosaccharides.

sugar cyclizes, an **anomeric carbon** is created from the aldehyde group of an aldose or keto group of a ketose. This carbon can have two configurations, α or β. If the aldehyde group on an acyclic sugar gets oxidized as a chromogenic agent gets reduced, that sugar is a **reducing sugar**. A sugar with its anomeric carbon linked to another structure is called a **glycosyl residue**. Sugars can be attached either to an –NH$_2$ or an –OH group, producing **N-** and **O-glycosides**. **Salivary α-amylase** acts on **dietary polysaccharides** (glycogen, amylose, amylopectin), producing **oligosaccharides**. **Pancreatic α-amylase** continues the process of polysaccharide digestion. The final digestive processes occur at the **mucosal lining** of the **small intestine**. Several **disaccharidases** [for example, **lactase (β-galactosidase)**, **sucrase**, **maltase**, and **isomaltase**] produce monosaccharides (glucose, galactose, and fructose). These enzymes are secreted by and remain associated with the luminal side of the **brush border membranes** of **intestinal mucosal cells**. Absorption of the monosaccharides requires specific transporters. If carbohydrate degradation is deficient (as a result of heredity, intestinal disease, malnutrition, or drugs that injure the mucosa of the small intestine), undigested carbohydrate will pass into the large intestine, where it can cause **osmotic diarrhea**. Bacterial fermentation of the compounds produces large volumes of CO$_2$ and H$_2$ gas, causing abdominal cramps, diarrhea, and flatulence. **Lactose intolerance**, caused by a lack of **lactase**, is by far the most common of these deficiencies.

Study Question

Choose the ONE correct answer.

7.1 Which of the following statements best describes glucose?

    A. It is a ketose and usually exists as a furanose ring in solution.

    B. It is a C-4 epimer of galactose.

    C. It is utilized in biological systems only in the L-isomeric form.

    D. It is produced from dietary starch by the action of α-amylase.

    E. Homopolysaccharides of glucose, formed by the action of glycosyltransferases, are always branched molecules that contain only β-glycosidic linkages.

Correct answer = B. Glucose and galactose differ only in configuration around carbon 4, and so are C-4 epimers that are interconvertible by the action of an epimerase. Glucose is an aldose sugar that typically exists as a pyranose ring in solution; fructose, however, is a ketose with a furanose ring. The D-isomeric form of carbohydrates is most typically the form found in biologic systems, in contrast to amino acids. Salivary amylase does not produce monosaccharides. Homopolysaccharides of glucose include branched glycogen in which the glycosidic linkages are the α form, as well as unbranched cellulose that has β linkages.

7.2 A young black man entered his physician's office complaining of bloating and diarrhea. His eyes were sunken and the physician noted additional signs of dehydration. The patient's temperature was normal. He explained that the episode had occurred following a birthday party at which he had participated in an ice cream eating contest. The patient reported prior episodes of a similar nature following ingestion of a significant amount of dairy products. This clinical picture is most probably due to a deficiency in:

    A. salivary α-amylase.

    B. isomaltase.

    C. pancreatic α-amylase.

    D. sucrase.

    E. lactase.

Correct answer = E. The physical symptoms suggest a deficiency in an enzyme responsible for carbohydrate degradation. The symptoms observed following the ingestion of dairy products suggest that the patient is deficient in lactase.

7.3 Routine examination of the urine of an asymptomatic pediatric patient showed a positive reaction with Clinitest (a copper reduction method of detecting reducing sugars), but a negative reaction with the glucose oxidase test. Which one of the following sugars is least likely to be present (assuming a single elevated saccharide)?

    A. Lactose

    B. Fructose

    C. Sucrose

    D. Xylulose

    E. Galactose

Correct answer = C. Clinitest is a nonspecific test that produces a change in color if urine is positive for reducing substances, including reducing sugars (glucose, fructose, galactose, xylulose, lactose), amino acids, ascorbic acid, and certain drugs and drug metabolites. Because sucrose is not a reducing sugar, it is not detected by Clinitest. Glucose oxidase method will not detect increased levels of galactose or other sugars in urine. It is therefore important that a copper reduction method be used as a screening test. In those instances when the copper method is positive and the glucose oxidase method is negative, glucosuria is ruled out.

7.4 α-Glucosidase inhibitors such as acarbose and miglitol taken with meals are used in the treatment of diabetes. Explain. What effect should these drugs have on the digestion of lactose?

α-Glucosidase inhibitors slow the production of glucose from dietary carbohydrates, thereby reducing the post-prandial rise in blood glucose and facilitating better blood glucose control in diabetics. These drugs have no effect on lactose digestion because the disaccharide lactose contains a β-glycosidic bond, not an α.

Glycolysis

8

I. INTRODUCTION TO METABOLISM

In Chapter 5, individual enzymic reactions were analyzed in an effort to explain the mechanisms of catalysis. However, in cells, these reactions rarely occur in isolation, but rather are organized into multistep sequences called pathways, such as that of glycolysis (Figure 8.1). In a pathway, the product of one reaction serves as the substrate of the subsequent reaction. Different pathways can also intersect, forming an integrated and purposeful network of chemical reactions. These are collectively called metabolism, which is the sum of all the chemical changes occurring in a cell, a tissue, or the body. Most pathways can be classified as either catabolic (degradative) or anabolic (synthetic). Catabolic reactions break down complex molecules, such as proteins, polysaccharides, and lipids, to a few simple molecules, for example, CO_2, NH_3 (ammonia), and water. Anabolic pathways form complex end products from simple precursors, for example, the synthesis of the polysaccharide, glycogen, from glucose. [Note: Pathways that regenerate a component are called cycles.] In the following chapters, this text focuses on the central metabolic pathways that are involved in synthesizing and degrading carbohydrates, lipids, and amino acids.

A. Metabolic map

It is convenient to investigate metabolism by examining its component pathways. Each pathway is composed of multienzyme sequences, and each enzyme, in turn, may exhibit important catalytic or regulatory features. To provide the reader with the "big picture," a metabolic map containing the important central pathways of energy metabolism is presented in Figure 8.2. This map is useful in tracing connections between pathways, visualizing the purposeful "movement" of metabolic intermediates, and picturing the effect on the flow of intermediates if a pathway is blocked, for example, by a drug or an inherited deficiency of an enzyme. Throughout the next three units of this book, each pathway under discussion will be repeatedly featured as part of the major metabolic map shown in Figure 8.2.

B. Catabolic pathways

Catabolic reactions serve to capture chemical energy in the form of adenosine triphosphate (ATP) from the degradation of energy-rich fuel molecules. Catabolism also allows molecules in the diet (or nutrient molecules stored in cells) to be converted into building blocks needed for the synthesis of complex molecules. Energy generation by degradation of complex molecules occurs in three stages as shown in Figure 8.3. [Note: Catabolic pathways are typically oxidative, and require coenzymes such as NAD^+.]

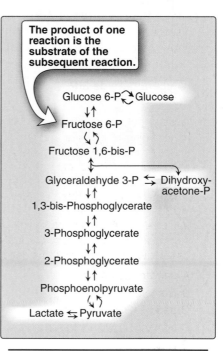

Figure 8.1
Glycolysis, an example of a metabolic pathway.

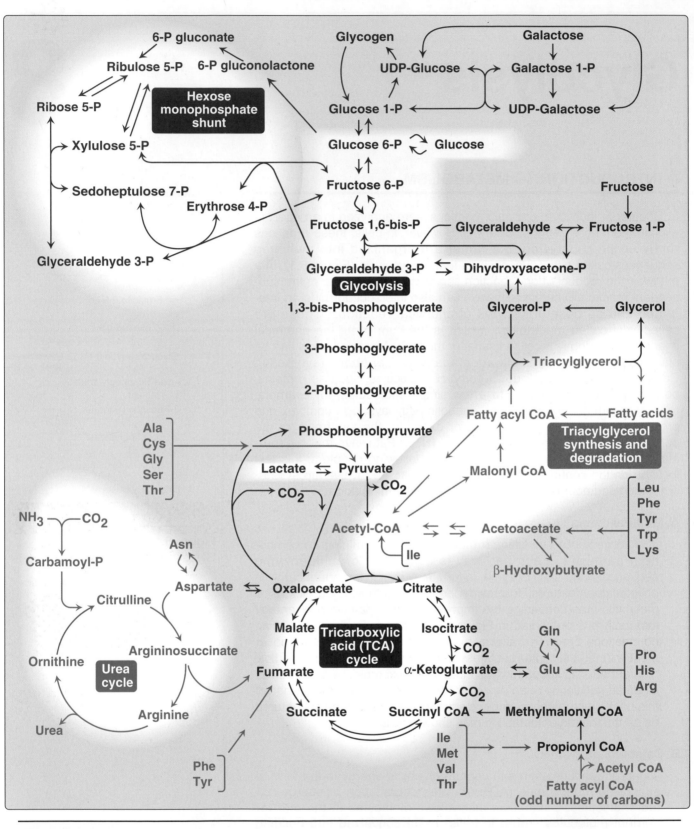

Figure 8.2
Important reactions of intermediary metabolism. Several important pathways to be discussed in later chapters are highlighted. Curved reaction arrows (⤸) indicate forward and reverse reactions that are catalyzed by different enzymes. The straight arrows (⇌) indicate forward and reverse reactions that are catalyzed by the same enzyme. **Blue text** = intermediates of carbohydrate metabolism; **brown text** = intermediates of lipid metabolism; **green text** = intermediates of protein metabolism.

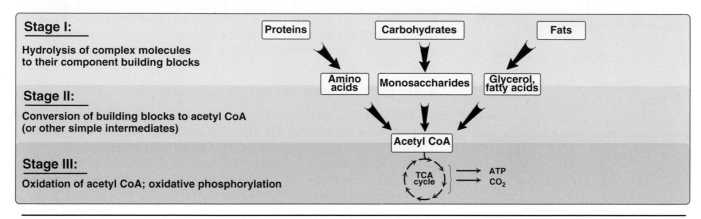

Figure 8.3
Three stages of catabolism.

1. **Hydrolysis of complex molecules:** In the first stage, complex molecules are broken down into their component building blocks. For example, proteins are degraded to amino acids, polysaccharides to monosaccharides, and fats (triacylglycerols) to free fatty acids and glycerol.

2. **Conversion of building blocks to simple intermediates:** In the second stage, these diverse building blocks are further degraded to acetyl coenzyme A (CoA) and a few other, simple molecules. Some energy is captured as ATP, but the amount is small compared with the energy produced during the third stage of catabolism.

3. **Oxidation of acetyl CoA:** The tricarboxylic acid (TCA) cycle (see p. 109) is the final common pathway in the oxidation of fuel molecules that produce acetyl CoA. Oxidation of acetyl CoA generates large amounts of ATP via oxidative phosphorylation as electrons flow from NADH and $FADH_2$ to oxygen (see p. 73).

C. Anabolic pathways

Anabolic reactions combine small molecules, such as amino acids, to form complex molecules, such as proteins (Figure 8.4). Anabolic reactions require energy (are endergonic), which is generally provided by the breakdown of ATP to adenosine diphosphate (ADP) and inorganic phosphate (P_i). Anabolic reactions often involve chemical reductions in which the reducing power is most frequently provided by the electron donor NADPH (see p. 147). Note that catabolism is a convergent process—that is, a wide variety of molecules are transformed into a few common end products. By contrast, anabolism is a divergent process in which a few biosynthetic precursors form a wide variety of polymeric or complex products.

II. REGULATION OF METABOLISM

The pathways of metabolism must be coordinated so that the production of energy or the synthesis of end products meets the needs of the cell. Furthermore, individual cells do not function in isolation but, rather, are part of a community of interacting tissues. Thus, a sophisticated communication system has evolved to coordinate the functions of the

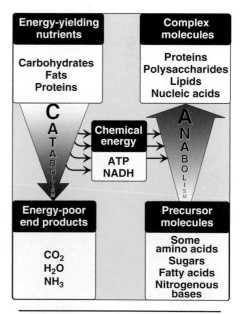

Figure 8.4
Comparison of catabolic and anabolic pathways.

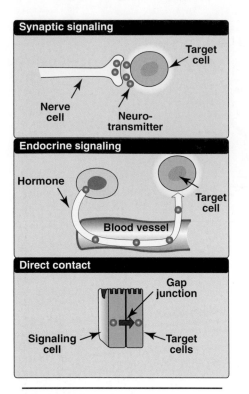

Figure 8.5
Some commonly used mechanisms for transmission of regulatory signals between cells.

body. Regulatory signals that inform an individual cell of the metabolic state of the body as a whole include hormones, neurotransmitters, and the availability of nutrients. These, in turn, influence signals generated within the cell (Figure 8.5).

A. Signals from within the cell (intracellular)

The rate of a metabolic pathway can respond to regulatory signals that arise from within the cell. For example, the rate of a pathway may be influenced by the availability of substrates, product inhibition, or alterations in the levels of allosteric activators or inhibitors. These intracellular signals typically elicit rapid responses, and are important for the moment-to-moment regulation of metabolism.

B. Communication between cells (intercellular)

The ability to respond to extracellular signals is essential for the survival and development of all organisms. Signaling between cells provides for long-range integration of metabolism, and usually results in a response that is slower than is seen with signals that originate within the cell. Communication between cells can be mediated, for example, by surface-to-surface contact and, in some tissues, by formation of gap junctions, allowing direct communication between the cytoplasms of adjacent cells. However, for energy metabolism, the most important route of communication is chemical signaling between cells by bloodborne hormones or by neurotransmitters.

C. Second messenger systems

Hormones or neurotransmitters can be thought of as signals, and their receptors as signal detectors. Each component serves as a link in the communication between extracellular events and chemical changes within the cell. Many receptors signal their recognition of a bound ligand by initiating a series of reactions that ultimately result in a specific intracellular response. "Second messenger" molecules—so named because they intervene between the original messenger (the neurotransmitter or hormone) and the ultimate effect on the cell—are part of the cascade of events that translates hormone or neurotransmitter binding into a cellular response. Two of the most widely recognized second messenger systems are the calcium/phosphatidylinositol system (see p. 205), and the *adenylyl cyclase* system, which is particularly important in regulating the pathways of intermediary metabolism.

D. Adenylyl cyclase

The recognition of a chemical signal by some membrane receptors, such as the β- and $α_2$-adrenergic receptors, triggers either an increase or a decrease in the activity of *adenylyl cyclase* (*adenylate cyclase*). This is a membrane-bound enzyme that converts ATP to 3',5'-adenosine monophosphate (also called cyclic AMP or cAMP). The chemical signals are most often hormones or neurotransmitters, each of which binds to a unique type of membrane receptor. Therefore, tissues that respond to more than one chemical signal must have several different receptors, each of which can be linked to *adenylyl cyclase*. These receptors, known as G protein-coupled receptors (GPCR), are characterized by an extracellular ligand-binding region, seven transmembrane helices, and an intracellular domain that interacts with G proteins (Figure 8.6).

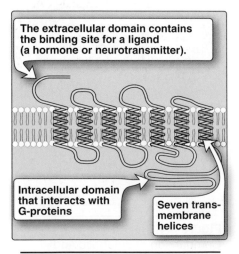

The extracellular domain contains the binding site for a ligand (a hormone or neurotransmitter).

Intracellular domain that interacts with G-proteins

Seven transmembrane helices

Figure 8.6
Structure of a typical G protein-coupled receptor (GPCR) of the plasma membrane.

1. **GTP-dependent regulatory proteins:** The effect of the activated, occupied GPCR on second messenger formation is not direct but, rather, is mediated by specialized trimeric proteins (α, β, γ subunits) of the cell membrane. These proteins, referred to as G proteins because they bind guanosine nucleotides (GTP and GDP), form a link in the chain of communication between the receptor and *adenylyl cyclase*. In the inactive form of a G protein, the α-subunit is bound to GDP (Figure 8.7). Binding of ligand causes a conformational change in the receptor, triggering replacement of this GDP with GTP. The GTP-bound form of the α subunit dissociates from the βγ subunits and moves to *adenylyl cyclase*, which is thereby activated. Many molecules of active Gα protein are formed by one activated receptor. [Note: The ability of a hormone or neurotransmitter to stimulate or inhibit *adenylyl cyclase* depends on the type of Gα protein that is linked to the receptor. One family of G proteins, designated G_s, stimulates *adenylyl cyclase*; another family, designated G_i, inhibits the enzyme (not shown in Figure 8.7).] The actions of the Gα–GTP complex are short-lived because Gα has an inherent *GTPase* activity, resulting in the rapid hydrolysis of GTP to GDP. This causes inactivation of the Gα, its dissociation from *adenylyl cyclase* and reassociation with the βγ dimer.

> Toxins from <u>Vibrio</u> <u>cholerae</u> (cholera) and <u>Bordetella</u> <u>pertussis</u> (whooping cough) cause inappropriate activation of *adenylyl cyclase* through covalent modification (ADP-ribosylation) of different G proteins. With cholera, the *GTPase* activity of $Gα_s$ is inhibited. With whooping cough, $Gα_i$ is inactivated.

2. **Protein kinases:** The next key link in the cAMP second messenger system is the activation by cAMP of a family of enzymes called cAMP-independent *protein kinases*, for example, *protein kinase A* (Figure 8.8). Cyclic AMP activates *protein kinase A* by binding to its two regulatory subunits, causing the release of active catalytic subunits. The active subunits catalyze the transfer of phosphate from ATP to specific serine or threonine residues of protein substrates. The phosphorylated proteins may act directly on the cell's ion channels, or, if enzymes, may become activated or inhibited. *Protein kinase A* can also phosphorylate proteins that bind to DNA, causing changes in gene expression. [Note: Several types of *protein kinases* are not cAMP-dependent, for example, *protein kinase C* described on p. 205.]

3. **Dephosphorylation of proteins:** The phosphate groups added to proteins by *protein kinases* are removed by *protein phosphatases*—enzymes that hydrolytically cleave phosphate esters (see Figure 8.8). This ensures that changes in protein activity induced by phosphorylation are not permanent.

4. **Hydrolysis of cAMP:** cAMP is rapidly hydrolyzed to 5'-AMP by *cAMP phosphodiesterase*, one of a family of enzymes that cleave the cyclic 3',5'-phosphodiester bond. 5'-AMP is not an intracellular signaling molecule. Thus, the effects of neurotransmitter- or hormone-mediated

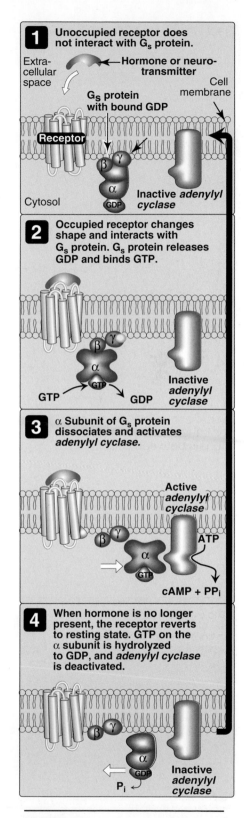

1 Unoccupied receptor does not interact with G_s protein.

Extracellular space — Hormone or neurotransmitter

G_s protein with bound GDP

Cell membrane

Receptor

Cytosol   Inactive *adenylyl cyclase*

2 Occupied receptor changes shape and interacts with G_s protein. G_s protein releases GDP and binds GTP.

GTP   GDP   Inactive *adenylyl cyclase*

3 α Subunit of G_s protein dissociates and activates *adenylyl cyclase*.

Active *adenylyl cyclase*

ATP

cAMP + PP$_i$

4 When hormone is no longer present, the receptor reverts to resting state. GTP on the α subunit is hydrolyzed to GDP, and *adenylyl cyclase* is deactivated.

P$_i$ Inactive *adenylyl cyclase*

Figure 8.7
The recognition of chemical signals by certain membrane receptors triggers an increase (or, less often, a decrease) in the activity of *adenylyl cyclase*.

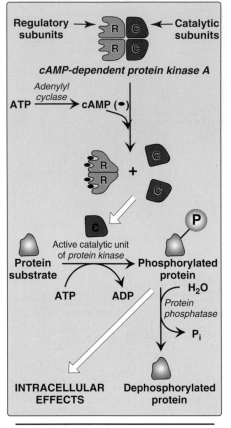

Figure 8.8
Actions of cAMP.

increases of cAMP are rapidly terminated if the extracellular signal is removed. [Note: *Phosphodiesterase* is inhibited by methylxanthine derivatives, such as theophylline and caffeine.[1]]

III. OVERVIEW OF GLYCOLYSIS

The glycolytic pathway is employed by all tissues for the breakdown of glucose to provide energy (in the form of ATP) and intermediates for other metabolic pathways. Glycolysis is at the hub of carbohydrate metabolism because virtually all sugars—whether arising from the diet or from catabolic reactions in the body—can ultimately be converted to glucose (Figure 8.9A). Pyruvate is the end product of glycolysis in cells with mitochondria and an adequate supply of oxygen. This series of ten reactions is called aerobic glycolysis because oxygen is required to reoxidize the NADH formed during the oxidation of glyceraldehyde 3-phosphate (Figure 8.9B). Aerobic glycolysis sets the stage for the oxidative decarboxylation of pyruvate to acetyl CoA, a major fuel of the TCA (or citric acid) cycle. Alternatively, pyruvate is reduced to lactate as NADH is oxidized to NAD⁺ (Figure 8.9C). This conversion of glucose to lactate is called anaerobic glycolysis because it can occur without the participation of oxygen. Anaerobic glycolysis allows the production of ATP in tissues that lack mitochondria (for example, red blood cells) or in cells deprived of sufficient oxygen.

IV. TRANSPORT OF GLUCOSE INTO CELLS

Glucose cannot diffuse directly into cells, but enters by one of two transport mechanisms: a Na⁺-independent, facilitated diffusion transport system or a Na⁺-monosaccharide cotransporter system.

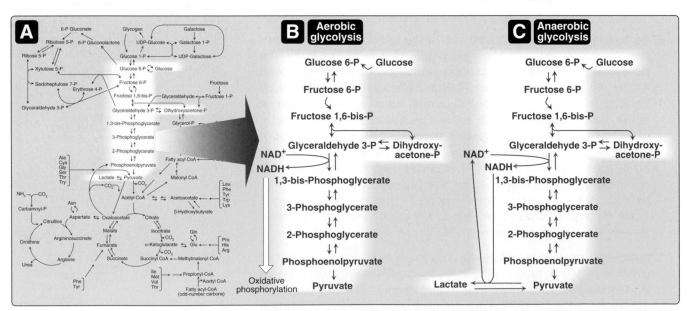

Figure 8.9
A. Glycolysis shown as one of the essential pathways of energy metabolism. B. Reactions of aerobic glycolysis. C. Reactions of anaerobic glycolysis.

 [1]See Chapter 10 in *Lippincott's Illustrated Reviews: Pharmacology* for a discussion of the use of methylxanthine derivatives as drugs.

A. Na⁺-independent facilitated diffusion transport

This system is mediated by a family of 14 glucose transporters in cell membranes. They are designated GLUT-1 to GLUT-14 (glucose transporter isoforms 1–14). These transporters exist in the membrane in two conformational states (Figure 8.10). Extracellular glucose binds to the transporter, which then alters its conformation, transporting glucose across the cell membrane.

1. **Tissue specificity of GLUT gene expression:** The glucose transporters display a tissue-specific pattern of expression. For example, GLUT-3 is the primary glucose transporter in neurons. GLUT-1 is abundant in erythrocytes and blood brain barrier, but is low in adult muscle, whereas GLUT-4 is abundant in adipose tissue and skeletal muscle. [Note: The number of GLUT-4 transporters active in these tissues is increased by insulin. (See p. 311 for a discussion of insulin and glucose transport.)] The other GLUT isoforms also have tissue-specific distributions.

2. **Specialized functions of GLUT isoforms:** In facilitated diffusion, glucose movement follows a concentration gradient, that is, from a high glucose concentration to a lower one. For example, GLUT-1, GLUT-3, and GLUT-4 are primarily involved in glucose uptake from the blood. In contrast, GLUT-2, which is found in the liver and kidney, can either transport glucose into these cells when blood glucose levels are high, or transport glucose from these cells when blood glucose levels are low (for example, during fasting). [Note: GLUT-2 is also found in pancreatic β cells.] GLUT-5 is unusual in that it is the primary transporter for fructose (instead of glucose) in the small intestine and the testes.

B. Na⁺-monosaccharide cotransporter system

This is an energy-requiring process that transports glucose "against" a concentration gradient—that is, from low glucose concentrations outside the cell to higher concentrations within the cell. This system is a carrier-mediated process in which the movement of glucose is coupled to the concentration gradient of Na⁺, which is transported into the cell at the same time. The carrier is a sodium-dependent–glucose transporter or SGLT. This type of transport occurs in the epithelial cells of the intestine (see p. 87), renal tubules, and choroid plexus. [Note: The choroid plexus, part of the blood brain barrier, also contains GLUT-1.]

V. REACTIONS OF GLYCOLYSIS

The conversion of glucose to pyruvate occurs in two stages (Figure 8.11). The first five reactions of glycolysis correspond to an energy investment phase in which the phosphorylated forms of intermediates are synthesized at the expense of ATP. The subsequent reactions of glycolysis constitute an energy generation phase in which a net of two molecules of ATP are formed by substrate-level phosphorylation (see p. 102) per glucose molecule metabolized.

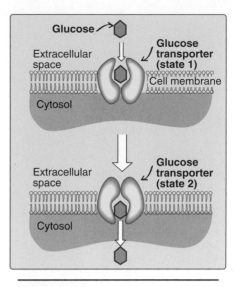

Figure 8.10
Schematic representation of the facilitated transport of glucose through a cell membrane. [Note: GLUT proteins contain 12 transmembrane helices.]

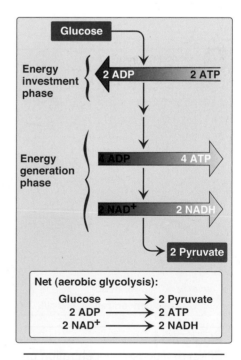

Figure 8.11
Two phases of aerobic glycolysis.

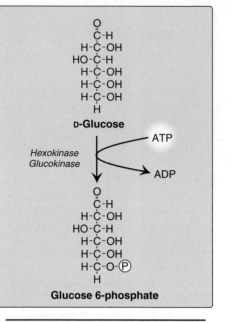

Figure 8.12
Energy investment phase:
phosphorylation of glucose.

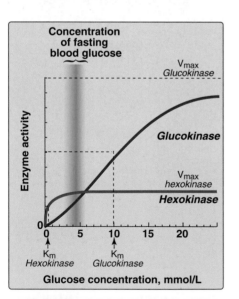

Figure 8.13
Effect of glucose concentration on
the rate of phosphorylation
catalyzed by *hexokinase* and
glucokinase.

A. Phosphorylation of glucose

Phosphorylated sugar molecules do not readily penetrate cell membranes, because there are no specific transmembrane carriers for these compounds, and because they are too polar to diffuse through the lipid core of membranes. The irreversible phosphorylation of glucose (Figure 8.12), therefore, effectively traps the sugar as cytosolic glucose 6-phosphate, thus committing it to further metabolism in the cell. Mammals have several isozymes of the enzyme *hexokinase* that catalyze the phosphorylation of glucose to glucose 6-phosphate.

1. **Hexokinase:** In most tissues, the phosphorylation of glucose is catalyzed by *hexokinase*, one of three regulatory enzymes of glycolysis (see also *phosphofructokinase* and *pyruvate kinase*). *Hexokinase* has broad substrate specificity and is able to phosphorylate several hexoses in addition to glucose. *Hexokinase* is inhibited by the reaction product, glucose 6-phosphate, which accumulates when further metabolism of this hexose phosphate is reduced. *Hexokinase* has a low K_m (and, therefore, a high affinity, see p. 59) for glucose. This permits the efficient phosphorylation and subsequent metabolism of glucose even when tissue concentrations of glucose are low (Figure 8.13). *Hexokinase*, however, has a low V_{max} for glucose and, therefore, cannot sequester (trap) cellular phosphate in the form of phosphorylated hexoses, or phosphorylate more sugars than the cell can use.

2. **Glucokinase:** In liver parenchymal cells and β cells of the pancreas, *glucokinase* (also called *hexokinase D*, or *type IV*) is the predominant enzyme responsible for the phosphorylation of glucose. In β cells, *glucokinase* functions as the glucose sensor, determining the threshold for insulin secretion (see p. 310). In the liver, the enzyme facilitates glucose phosphorylation during hyperglycemia. [Note: *Hexokinase* also serves as a glucose sensor in neurons of the hypothalamus, playing a key role in the adrenergic response to hypoglycemia (see p. 315.] Despite the popular but misleading name *glucokinase*, the sugar specificity of the enzyme is similar to that of other *hexokinase* isozymes.

   a. **Kinetics:** *Glucokinase* differs from *hexokinase* in several important properties. For example, it has a much higher K_m, requiring a higher glucose concentration for half-saturation (see Figure 8.13). Thus, *glucokinase* functions only when the intracellular concentration of glucose in the hepatocyte is elevated, such as during the brief period following consumption of a carbohydrate-rich meal, when high levels of glucose are delivered to the liver via the portal vein. *Glucokinase* has a high V_{max}, allowing the liver to effectively remove the flood of glucose delivered by the portal blood. This prevents large amounts of glucose from entering the systemic circulation following a carbohydrate-rich meal, and thus minimizes hyperglycemia during the absorptive period. [Note: GLUT-2 insures that blood glucose equilibrates rapidly across the membrane of the hepatocyte.]

   b. **Regulation by fructose 6-phosphate and glucose:** *Glucokinase* activity is not directly inhibited by glucose 6-phosphate as are the other *hexokinases*, but rather is indirectly inhibited by fructose 6-phosphate (which is in equilibrium with glucose 6-phosphate, a product of *glucokinase*), and is indirectly stimulated by glucose (a substrate of *glucokinase*) via the following mechanism. Glucokinase regulatory protein (GKRP) in the liver regulates the activity of *glucokinase* through reversible binding. In the presence of fructose 6-phosphate, *glucokinase* is translocated into the nucleus and binds tightly to the regulatory protein, thus rendering the enzyme inactive (Figure 8.14). When glucose levels in the blood (and also in the hepatocyte, as a result of GLUT-2) increase, *glucokinase* is released from the regulatory protein, and the enzyme re-enters the cytosol where it phosphorylates glucose to glucose 6-phosphate. [Note: Fructose 1-phosphate inhibits formation of the *glucokinase*-GKRP complex.]

> *Glucokinase* functions as a glucose sensor in the maintenance of blood glucose homeostasis. Mutations that decrease the activity of *glucokinase* are the cause of a rare form of diabetes, maturity onset diabetes of the young type 2 (MODY 2).

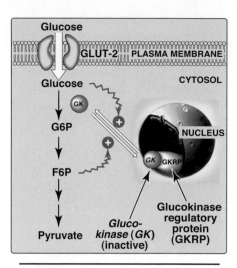

Figure 8.14
Regulation of *glucokinase* activity by glucokinase regulatory protein.

B. Isomerization of glucose 6-phosphate

The isomerization of glucose 6-phosphate to fructose 6-phosphate is catalyzed by *phosphoglucose isomerase* (Figure 8.15). The reaction is readily reversible and is not a rate-limiting or regulated step.

C. Phosphorylation of fructose 6-phosphate

The irreversible phosphorylation reaction catalyzed by *phosphofructokinase-1* (*PFK-1*) is the most important control point and the rate-limiting and committed step of glycolysis (Figure 8.16). *PFK-1* is controlled by the available concentrations of the substrates ATP and fructose 6-phosphate, and by regulatory substances described below.

1. **Regulation by energy levels within the cell:** *PFK-1* is inhibited allosterically by elevated levels of ATP, which act as an "energy-rich" signal indicating an abundance of high-energy compounds. Elevated levels of citrate, an intermediate in the TCA cycle (see p. 109), also inhibit *PFK-1*. Conversely, *PFK-1* is activated allosterically by high concentrations of AMP, which signal that the cell's energy stores are depleted. [Note: Citrate inhibition favors the use of glucose for glycogen synthesis, see p.125.]

2. **Regulation by fructose 2,6-bisphosphate:** Fructose 2,6-bisphosphate is the most potent activator of *PFK-1* (see Figure 8.16), and is able to activate the enzyme even when ATP levels are high. Fructose 2,6-bisphosphate is formed by *phosphofructokinase-2* (*PFK-2*), an enzyme different than *PFK-1*. *PFK-2* is a bifunctional protein that has both the *kinase* activity that produces fructose 2,6-bisphosphate and a *phosphatase* activity that dephosphorylates fructose 2,6-bisphosphate back to fructose 6-phosphate. In liver, the *kinase* domain is active if dephosphorylated and is inactive if phosphorylated (Figure 8.17). [Note: Fructose 2,6-bisphos-

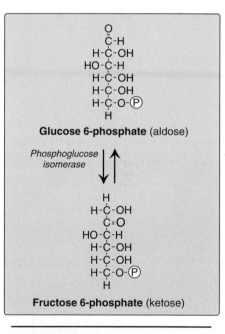

Figure 8.15
Aldose-ketose isomerization of glucose 6-phosphate to fructose 6-phosphate.

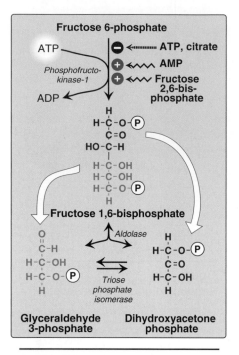

Figure 8.16
Energy investment phase (continued):
Conversion of fructose 6-phosphate
to triose phosphates.

phate is an inhibitor of *fructose 1,6-bisphosphatase*, an enzyme of gluconeogenesis (see p. 120 for a discussion of the regulation of gluconeogenesis). The reciprocal actions of fructose 2,6-bisphosphate on glycolysis (activation) and gluconeogenesis (inhibition) ensure that both pathways are not fully active at the same time, preventing a futile cycle in which glucose would be converted to pyruvate followed by resynthesis of glucose from pyruvate.]

a. **During the well-fed state:** Decreased levels of glucagon and elevated levels of insulin, such as occur following a carbohydrate-rich meal, cause an increase in fructose 2,6-bisphosphate and, thus, in the rate of glycolysis in the liver (see Figure 8.17). Fructose 2,6-bisphosphate, therefore, acts as an intracellular signal, indicating that glucose is abundant.

b. **During starvation:** Elevated levels of glucagon and low levels of insulin, such as occur during fasting (see p. 327), decrease the intracellular concentration of hepatic fructose 2,6-bisphosphate. This results in a decrease in the overall rate of glycolysis and an increase in gluconeogenesis.

D. Cleavage of fructose 1,6-bisphosphate

Aldolase cleaves fructose 1,6-bisphosphate to dihydroxyacetone phosphate and glyceraldehyde 3-phosphate (see Figure 8.16). The reaction is reversible and not regulated. [Note: *Aldolase B*, the isoform in the liver and kidney, also cleaves fructose 1-phosphate, and functions in the metabolism of dietary fructose (see p. 138).]

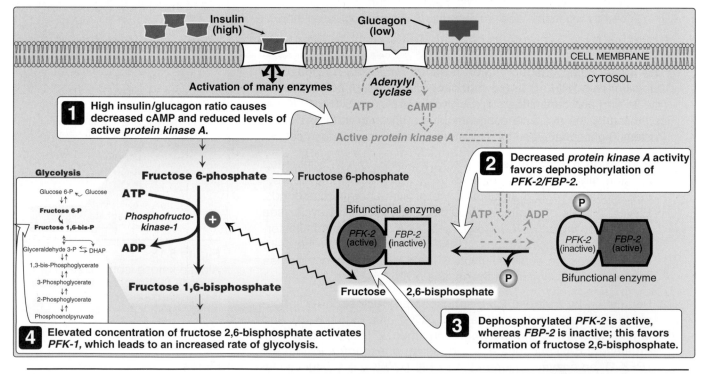

Figure 8.17
Effect of elevated insulin concentration on the intracellular concentration of fructose 2,6-bisphosphate in liver.
PFK-2 = phosphofructokinase-2; FBP-2 = fructose bisphosphatase-2.

E. Isomerization of dihydroxyacetone phosphate

Triose phosphate isomerase interconverts dihydroxyacetone phosphate and glyceraldehyde 3-phosphate (see Figure 8.16). Dihydroxyacetone phosphate must be isomerized to glyceraldehyde 3-phosphate for further metabolism by the glycolytic pathway. This isomerization results in the net production of two molecules of glyceraldehyde 3-phosphate from the cleavage products of fructose 1,6-bisphosphate.

F. Oxidation of glyceraldehyde 3-phosphate

The conversion of glyceraldehyde 3-phosphate to 1,3-bisphosphoglycerate by *glyceraldehyde 3-phosphate dehydrogenase* is the first oxidation-reduction reaction of glycolysis (Figure 8.18). [Note: Because there is only a limited amount of NAD^+ in the cell, the NADH formed by this reaction must be reoxidized to NAD^+ for glycolysis to continue. Two major mechanisms for oxidizing NADH are: 1) the NADH-linked conversion of pyruvate to lactate (anaerobic, see p. 96), and 2) oxidation of NADH via the respiratory chain (aerobic, see p. 75). The latter requires substrate shuttles (see p. 79.]

1. **Synthesis of 1,3-bisphosphoglycerate (1,3-BPG):** The oxidation of the aldehyde group of glyceraldehyde 3-phosphate to a carboxyl group is coupled to the attachment of P_i to the carboxyl group. The high-energy phosphate group at carbon 1 of 1,3-BPG conserves much of the free energy produced by the oxidation of glyceraldehyde 3-phosphate. The energy of this high-energy phosphate drives the synthesis of ATP in the next reaction of glycolysis.

2. **Mechanism of arsenic poisoning:** The toxicity of arsenic is explained primarily by the inhibition of enzymes such as *pyruvate dehydrogenase*, which require lipoic acid as a coenzyme (see p. 110). However, pentavalent arsenic (arsenate) also can prevent net ATP and NADH production by glycolysis, without inhibiting the pathway itself. The poison does so by competing with inorganic phosphate as a substrate for *glyceraldehyde 3-phosphate dehydrogenase*, forming a complex that spontaneously hydrolyzes to form 3-phosphoglycerate (see Figure 8.18). By bypassing the synthesis of and phosphate transfer from 1,3-BPG, the cell is deprived of energy usually obtained from the glycolytic pathway. [Note: Arsenic also replaces P_i on the F_1 domain of *ATP synthase* (see p. 78), resulting in formation of ADP-arsenate that is rapidly hydrolyzed.]

3. **Synthesis of 2,3-bisphosphoglycerate (2,3-BPG) in red blood cells:** Some of the 1,3-BPG is converted to 2,3-BPG by the action of *bisphosphoglycerate mutase* (see Figure 8.18). 2,3-BPG, which is found in only trace amounts in most cells, is present at high concentration in red blood cells (increases O_2 delivery, see p. 31). 2,3-BPG is hydrolyzed by a *phosphatase* to 3-phosphoglycerate, which is also an intermediate in glycolysis (see Figure 8.18). In the red blood cell, glycolysis is modified by inclusion of these "shunt" reactions.

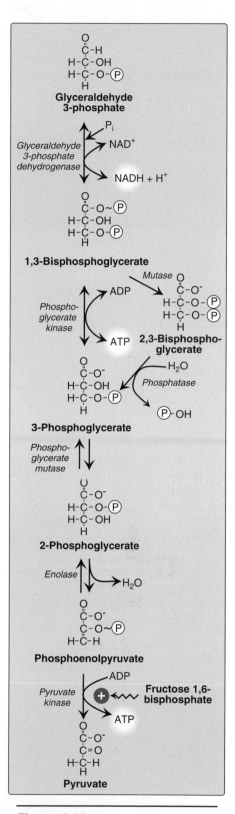

Figure 8.18
Energy generating phase: conversion of glyceraldehyde 3-phosphate to pyruvate.

G. Synthesis of 3-phosphoglycerate producing ATP

When 1,3-BPG is converted to 3-phosphoglycerate, the high-energy phosphate group of 1,3-BPG is used to synthesize ATP from ADP (see Figure 8.18). This reaction is catalyzed by *phosphoglycerate kinase*, which, unlike most other *kinases*, is physiologically reversible. Because two molecules of 1,3-BPG are formed from each glucose molecule, this *kinase* reaction replaces the two ATP molecules consumed by the earlier formation of glucose 6-phosphate and fructose 1,6-bisphosphate. [Note: This is an example of substrate-level phosphorylation, in which the energy needed for the production of a high-energy phosphate comes from a substrate rather than from the electron transport chain (see J. below and p. 113 for other examples).]

H. Shift of the phosphate group from carbon 3 to carbon 2

The shift of the phosphate group from carbon 3 to carbon 2 of phosphoglycerate by *phosphoglycerate mutase* is freely reversible (see Figure 8.18).

I. Dehydration of 2-phosphoglycerate

The dehydration of 2-phosphoglycerate by *enolase* redistributes the energy within the 2-phosphoglycerate molecule, resulting in the formation of phosphoenolpyruvate (PEP), which contains a high-energy enol phosphate (see Figure 8.18). The reaction is reversible despite the high-energy nature of the product.

J. Formation of pyruvate producing ATP

The conversion of PEP to pyruvate is catalyzed by *pyruvate kinase*, the third irreversible reaction of glycolysis. The equilibrium of the *pyruvate kinase* reaction favors the formation of ATP (see Figure 8.18). [Note: This is another example of substrate-level phosphorylation.]

1. **Feed-forward regulation:** In liver, *pyruvate kinase* is activated by fructose 1,6-bisphosphate, the product of the *phosphofructokinase* reaction. This feed-forward (instead of the more usual feedback) regulation has the effect of linking the two *kinase* activities: increased *phosphofructokinase* activity results in elevated levels of fructose 1,6-bisphosphate, which activates *pyruvate kinase*.

2. **Covalent modulation of pyruvate kinase:** Phosphorylation by a *cAMP-dependent protein kinase* leads to inactivation of *pyruvate kinase* in the liver (Figure 8.19). When blood glucose levels are low, elevated glucagon increases the intracellular level of cAMP, which causes the phosphorylation and inactivation of *pyruvate kinase*. Therefore, PEP is unable to continue in glycolysis, but instead enters the gluconeogenesis pathway. This, in part, explains the observed inhibition of hepatic glycolysis and stimulation of gluconeogenesis by glucagon. Dephosphorylation of *pyruvate kinase* by a *phosphoprotein phosphatase* results in reactivation of the enzyme.

3. **Pyruvate kinase deficiency:** The normal, mature erythrocyte lacks mitochondria and is, therefore, completely dependent on glycolysis for production of ATP. This high-energy compound is required to meet the metabolic needs of the red blood cell, and also to fuel the pumps necessary for the maintenance of the biconcave, flexi-

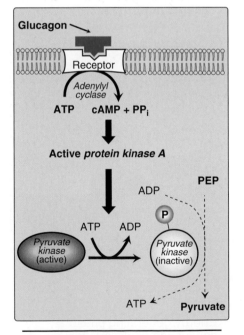

Figure 8.19
Covalent modification of hepatic *pyruvate kinase* results in inactivation of enzyme.

ble shape of the cell, which allows it to squeeze through narrow capillaries. The anemia observed in glycolytic enzyme deficiencies is a consequence of the reduced rate of glycolysis, leading to decreased ATP production. The resulting alterations in the red blood cell membrane lead to changes in the shape of the cell and, ultimately, to phagocytosis by the cells of the reticuloendothelial system, particularly macrophages of the spleen. The premature death and lysis of red blood cells results in hemolytic anemia. Among patients exhibiting the rare genetic defects of glycolytic enzymes, about 95% show a deficiency in *pyruvate kinase*, and 4% exhibit *phosphoglucose isomerase* deficiency. *PK* deficiency is restricted to the erythrocytes, and produces mild to severe chronic hemolytic anemia (erythrocyte destruction), with the severe form requiring regular cell transfusions. The severity of the disease depends both on the degree of enzyme deficiency (generally 5–25% of normal levels), and on the extent to which the individual's red blood cells compensate by synthesizing increased levels of 2,3-BPG (see p. 31). Almost all individuals with *PK* deficiency have a mutant enzyme that shows abnormal properties—most often altered kinetics (Figure 8.20).

> *Pyruvate kinase* deficiency is the second most common cause (after *glucose 6-phosphate dehydrogenase* deficiency) of enzyme deficiency-related nonspherocytic hemolytic anemia.

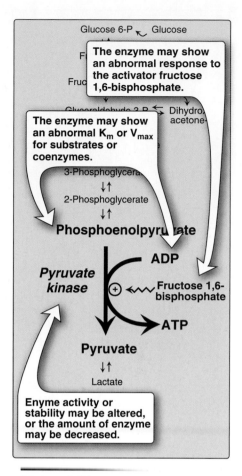

Figure 8.20
Alterations observed with various mutant forms of *pyruvate kinase*.

K. Reduction of pyruvate to lactate

Lactate, formed by the action of *lactate dehydrogenase*, is the final product of anaerobic glycolysis in eukaryotic cells (Figure 8.21). The formation of lactate is the major fate for pyruvate in lens and cornea of the eye, kidney medulla, testes, leukocytes and red blood cells, because these are all poorly vascularized and/or lack mitochondria.

1. **Lactate formation in muscle:** In exercising skeletal muscle, NADH production (by *glyceraldehyde 3-phosphate dehydrogenase* and by the three NAD^+-linked *dehydrogenases* of the citric acid cycle, see p. 112) exceeds the oxidative capacity of the respiratory chain. This results in an elevated $NADH/NAD^+$ ratio, favoring reduction of pyruvate to lactate. Therefore, during intense exercise, lactate accumulates in muscle, causing a drop in the intracellular pH, potentially resulting in cramps. Much of this lactate eventually diffuses into the bloodstream, and can be used by the liver to make glucose (see p. 118).

2. **Lactate consumption:** The direction of the *lactate dehydrogenase* reaction depends on the relative intracellular concentrations of pyruvate and lactate, and on the ratio of $NADH/NAD^+$ in the cell. For example, in liver and heart, the ratio of $NADH/NAD^+$ is lower than in exercising muscle. These tissues oxidize lactate (obtained from the blood) to pyruvate. In the liver, pyruvate is either converted to glucose by gluconeogenesis or oxidized in the TCA cycle. Heart muscle exclusively oxidizes lactate to CO_2 and H_2O via the citric acid cycle.

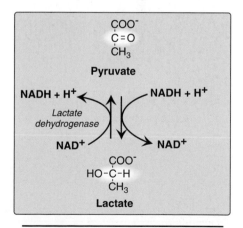

Figure 8.21
Interconversion of pyruvate and lactate.

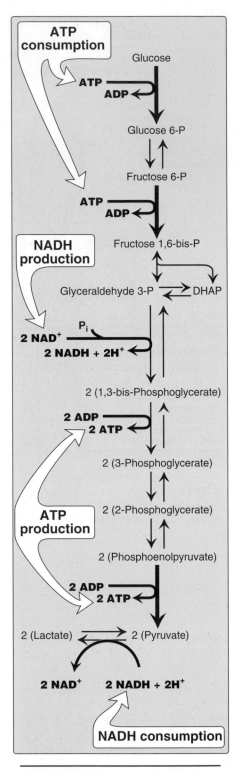

Figure 8.22
Summary of anaerobic glycolysis.
Reactions involving the production
or consumption of ATP or NADH
are indicated. The three irreversible
reactions of glycolysis are shown
with thick arrows. DHAP =
dihydroxyacetone phosphate.

3. **Lactic acidosis:** Elevated concentrations of lactate in the plasma, termed lactic acidosis, occur when there is a collapse of the circulatory system, such as in myocardial infarction, pulmonary embolism, and uncontrolled hemorrhage, or when an individual is in shock. The failure to bring adequate amounts of oxygen to the tissues results in impaired oxidative phosphorylation and decreased ATP synthesis. To survive, the cells use anaerobic glycolysis as a backup system for generating ATP, producing lactic acid as the endproduct. [Note: Production of even meager amounts of ATP may be life-saving during the period required to reestablish adequate blood flow to the tissues.] The excess oxygen required to recover from a period when the availability of oxygen has been inadequate is termed the oxygen debt.

> The oxygen debt is often related to patient morbidity or mortality. In many clinical situations, measuring the blood levels of lactic acid allows the rapid, early detection of oxygen debt in patients and the monitoring of their recovery.

L. Energy yield from glycolysis

Despite the production of some ATP during glycolysis, the end products, pyruvate or lactate, still contain most of the energy originally contained in glucose. The TCA cycle is required to release that energy completely (see p. 109).

1. **Anaerobic glycolysis:** Two molecules of ATP are generated for each molecule of glucose converted to two molecules of lactate (Figure 8.22). There is no net production or consumption of NADH.

2. **Aerobic glycolysis:** The direct consumption and formation of ATP is the same as in anaerobic glycolysis—that is, a net gain of two ATP per molecule of glucose. Two molecules of NADH are also produced per molecule of glucose. Ongoing aerobic glycolysis requires the oxidation of most of this NADH by the electron transport chain, producing approximately three ATP for each NADH molecule entering the chain (see p. 77). [Note: NADH cannot cross the inner mitochondrial membrane, and substrate shuttles are required (see p. 79).]

VI. HORMONAL REGULATION OF GLYCOLYSIS

The regulation of glycolysis by allosteric activation or inhibition, or the phosphorylation/dephosphorylation of rate-limiting enzymes, is short-term—that is, they influence glucose consumption over periods of minutes or hours. Superimposed on these moment-to-moment effects are slower, and often more profound, hormonal influences on the amount of enzyme protein synthesized. These effects can result in 10-fold to 20-fold increases in enzyme activity that typically occur over hours to days. Although the current focus is on glycolysis, reciprocal changes occur in the rate-limiting enzymes of gluconeogenesis, which are described in

Chapter 10 (see p. 117). Regular consumption of meals rich in carbohydrate or administration of insulin initiates an increase in the amount of *glucokinase, phosphofructokinase,* and *pyruvate kinase* in liver (Figure 8.23). These changes reflect an increase in gene transcription, resulting in increased enzyme synthesis. High activity of these three enzymes favors the conversion of glucose to pyruvate, a characteristic of the well-fed state (see p. 321). Conversely, gene transcription and synthesis of *glucokinase, phosphofructokinase,* and *pyruvate kinase* are decreased when plasma glucagon is high and insulin is low, for example, as seen in fasting or diabetes.

VII. ALTERNATE FATES OF PYRUVATE

A. Oxidative decarboxylation of pyruvate

Oxidative decarboxylation of pyruvate by *pyruvate dehydrogenase complex* is an important pathway in tissues with a high oxidative capacity, such as cardiac muscle (Figure 8.24). *Pyruvate dehydrogenase* irreversibly converts pyruvate, the end product of glycolysis, into acetyl CoA, a major fuel for the TCA cycle (see p. 109) and the building block for fatty acid synthesis (see p. 183).

B. Carboxylation of pyruvate to oxaloacetate

Carboxylation of pyruvate to oxaloacetate (OAA) by *pyruvate carboxylase* is a biotin-dependent reaction (see Figure 8.24). This reaction is important because it replenishes the citric acid cycle intermediates, and provides substrate for gluconeogenesis (see p. 118).

C. Reduction of pyruvate to ethanol (microorganisms)

The conversion of pyruvate to ethanol occurs by the two reactions summarized in Figure 8.24. The decarboxylation of pyruvate by *pyruvate decarboxylase* occurs in yeast and certain other microorganisms, but not in humans. The enzyme requires thiamine pyrophosphate as a coenzyme, and catalyzes a reaction similar to that described for *pyruvate dehydrogenase* (see p. 110).

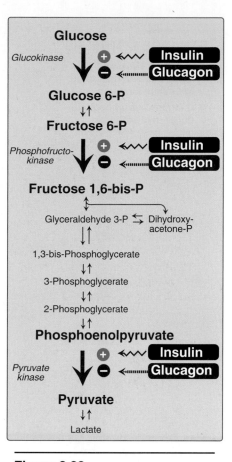

Figure 8.23
Effect of insulin and glucagon on the synthesis of key enzymes of glycolysis in liver.

VIII. CHAPTER SUMMARY

Most pathways can be classified as either **catabolic** (**degrade** complex molecules to a few simple products) or **anabolic** (**synthesize** complex end products from simple precursors). **Catabolic reactions** also **capture chemical energy** in the form of **ATP** from the degradation of energy-rich molecules. **Anabolic reactions require energy**, which is generally provided by the breakdown of ATP. The rate of a metabolic pathway can respond to **regulatory signals**, for example, **allosteric activators** or **inhibitors**, that arise from **within the cell**. Signaling **between cells** provides for the integration of metabolism. The most important route of this communication is **chemical signaling** between cells, for example, by **hormones** or **neurotransmitters**. **Second messenger molecules** convey the intent of a chemical signal (hormone or neurotransmitter) to appropriate intracellular responders. **Adenylyl cyclase** is a membrane-bound enzyme that synthesizes **cAMP** in response to chemical signals, such

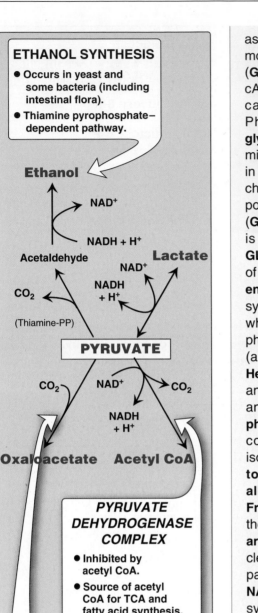

ETHANOL SYNTHESIS

- Occurs in yeast and some bacteria (including intestinal flora).
- Thiamine pyrophosphate–dependent pathway.

Ethanol

NAD$^+$

NADH + H$^+$

Acetaldehyde

CO$_2$

(Thiamine-PP)

Lactate

NAD$^+$

NADH + H$^+$

PYRUVATE

CO$_2$ NAD$^+$ CO$_2$

NADH + H$^+$

Oxaloacetate   Acetyl CoA

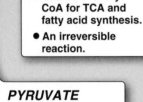

PYRUVATE DEHYDROGENASE COMPLEX

- Inhibited by acetyl CoA.
- Source of acetyl CoA for TCA and fatty acid synthesis.
- An irreversible reaction.

PYRUVATE CARBOXYLASE

- Activated by acetyl CoA.
- Replenishes intermediates of the TCA cycle.
- Provides substrates for gluconeogenesis.
- An irreversible reaction.

Figure 8.24
Summary of the metabolic fates of pyruvate.

as the hormones **glucagon** and **epinephrine**. Following binding of a hormone to its **cell-surface receptor**, a GTP-dependent regulatory protein (**G protein**) is activated that, in turn, activates **adenylyl cyclase**. The cAMP produced activates a **protein kinase**, which phosphorylates a cadre of enzymes, causing their activation or deactivation. Phosphorylation is reversed by **protein phosphatases**. **Aerobic glycolysis**, in which **pyruvate** is the end product, occurs in cells with mitochondria and an adequate supply of oxygen. **Anaerobic glycolysis**, in which **lactic acid** is the end product, occurs in cells that lack mitochondria, or in cells deprived of sufficient oxygen. Glucose is transported across membranes by one of 14 **glucose transporter isoforms** (**GLUTs**). **GLUT-1** is abundant in **erythrocytes** and **brain**, **GLUT-4** (which is **insulin-dependent**) is found in **muscle** and **adipose tissue**, and **GLUT-2** is found in **liver** and the **β cells** of the pancreas. The conversion of glucose to pyruvate (**glycolysis**, Figure 8.25) occurs in two stages: an **energy investment phase** in which phosphorylated intermediates are synthesized at the expense of ATP, and an **energy generation phase**, in which ATP is produced. In the energy investment phase, glucose is phosphorylated by **hexokinase** (found in **most tissues**) or **glucokinase** (a hexokinase found in **liver cells** and the **β cells** of the pancreas). **Hexokinase** has a **high affinity** (**low K$_m$**) and a **small V$_{max}$** for glucose, and is **inhibited** by **glucose 6-phosphate**. **Glucokinase** has a **large K$_m$** and a **large V$_{max}$** for glucose. It is indirectly **inhibited** by **fructose 6-phosphate** and **activated** by **glucose**, and the **transcription** of the glucokinase gene is **enhanced by insulin**. Glucose 6-phosphate is isomerized to fructose 6-phosphate, which is phosphorylated to **fructose 1,6-bisphosphate** by **phosphofructokinase**. This enzyme is **allosterically inhibited** by **ATP** and **citrate**, and **activated** by **AMP**. **Fructose 2,6-bisphosphate**, whose synthesis is **activated** by **insulin**, is the most potent allosteric activator of this enzyme. A total of **two ATP are used** during this phase of glycolysis. Fructose 1,6-bisphosphate is cleaved to form two trioses that are further metabolized by the glycolytic pathway, forming pyruvate. During these reactions, **four ATP** and **two NADH are produced** from ADP and NAD$^+$. The final step in pyruvate synthesis from phosphoenolpyruvate is catalyzed by **pyruvate kinase**. This enzyme is **allosterically activated** by **fructose 1,6-bisphosphate**, and **hormonally activated** by **insulin** and **inhibited** by **glucagon** via the **cAMP pathway**. **Pyruvate kinase deficiency** accounts for 95% of all inherited defects in glycolytic enzymes. It is restricted to **erythrocytes**, and causes mild to severe **chronic hemolytic anemia**. In **anaerobic glycolysis**, NADH is reoxidized to NAD$^+$ by the **conversion of pyruvate to lactic acid**. This occurs in cells, such as **erythrocytes**, that have few or no mitochondria, and in tissues, such as **exercising muscle**, where production of NADH exceeds the oxidative capacity of the respiratory chain. Elevated concentrations of lactate in the plasma (**lactic acidosis**) occur when there is a **collapse of the circulatory system**, or when an individual is in **shock**. Pyruvate can be: 1) **oxidatively decarboxylated** by **pyruvate dehydrogenase**, producing **acetyl CoA**; 2) **carboxylated** to **oxaloacetate** (a TCA cycle intermediate) by **pyruvate carboxylase**; or 3) **reduced** by microorganisms to **ethanol** by **pyruvate decarboxylase**.

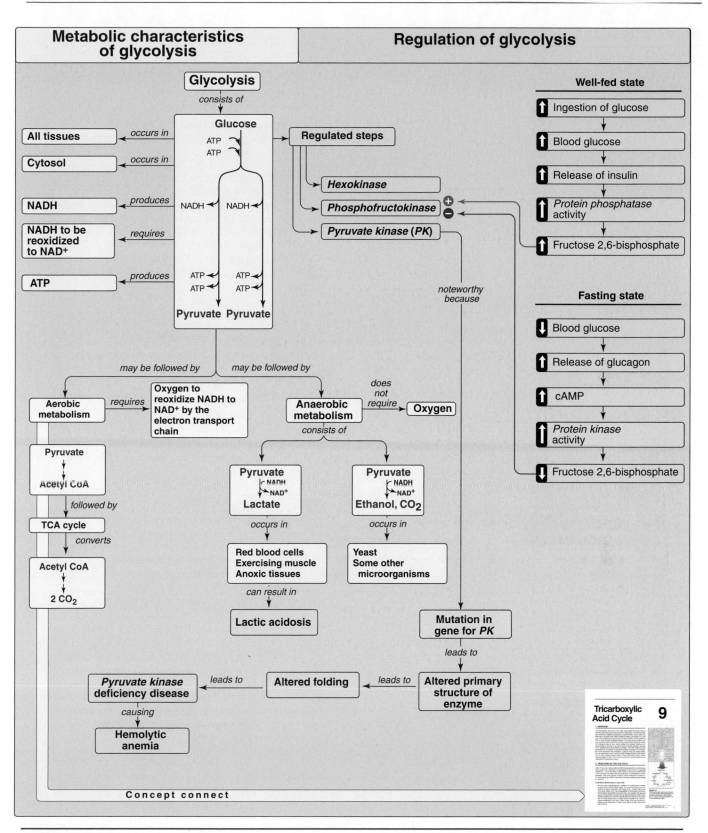

Figure 8.25
Key concept map for glycolysis.

Study Questions

Choose the ONE best answer.

8.1 Which one of the following statements concerning glycolysis is correct?

A. The conversion of glucose to lactate requires the presence of oxygen.

B. Hexokinase is important in hepatic glucose metabolism only in the absorptive period following consumption of a carbohydrate-containing meal.

C. Fructose 2,6-bisphosphate is a potent inhibitor of phosphofructokinase.

D. The regulated reactions are also the irreversible reactions.

E. The conversion of glucose to lactate yields two ATP and two NADH.

Correct answer = D. Hexokinase, phosphofructokinase, and pyruvate kinase are all irreversible and are the regulated steps in glycolysis. The conversion of glucose to lactate (anaerobic glycolysis) is a process that does not involve a net oxidation or reduction and, thus, oxygen is not required. Glucokinase (not hexokinase) is important in hepatic glucose metabolism only in the absorptive period following consumption of a carbohydrate-containing meal. Fructose 2,6-bisphosphate is a potent activator (not inhibitor) of phosphofructokinase. The conversion of glucose to lactate yields two ATP but no net production of NADH.

8.2 The reaction catalyzed by phosphofructokinase-1:

A. is activated by high concentrations of ATP and citrate.

B. uses fructose 1-phosphate as substrate.

C. is the rate-limiting reaction of the glycolytic pathway.

D. is near equilibrium in most tissues.

E. is inhibited by fructose 2,6-bisphosphate.

Correct answer = C. Phosphofructokinase-1 is the pace-setting enzyme of glycolysis. It is inhibited by ATP and citrate, uses fructose 6-phosphate as substrate, and catalyzes a reaction that is far from equilibrium. The reaction is activated by fructose 2,6-bisphosphate.

8.3 Compared with the resting state, vigorously contracting skeletal muscle shows:

A. an increased conversion of pyruvate to lactate.

B. decreased oxidation of pyruvate to CO_2 and water.

C. a decreased NADH/NAD^+ ratio.

D. a decreased concentration of AMP.

E. decreased levels of fructose 2,6-bisphosphate.

Correct answer = A. Vigorously contracting muscle shows an increased formation of lactate and an increased rate of pyruvate oxidation compared with resting skeletal muscle. The levels of AMP and NADH increase, whereas change in the concentration of fructose 2,6-bisphosphate is not a key regulatory factor in skeletal muscle.

8.4 A 43-year-old man presented with symptoms of weakness, fatigue, shortness of breath, and dizziness. His hemoglobin level was less than 7 g/dl (normal for a male being greater than 13.5 g/dl). Red blood cells isolated from the patient showed abnormally low level of lactate production. A deficiency of which one of the following enzymes would be the most likely cause of this patient's anemia?

A. Phosphoglucose isomerase

B. Phosphofructokinase

C. Pyruvate kinase

D. Hexokinase

E. Lactate dehydrogenase

Correct answer = C. Decreased lactate production in the erythrocyte indicates a defect in glycolysis. Among patients exhibiting genetic defects of glycolytic enzymes, about 95% show a deficiency in pyruvate kinase. Pyruvate kinase deficiency is the second most common cause (after glucose 6-phosphate dehydrogenase deficiency) of enzyme deficiency–related hemolytic anemia.

Tricarboxylic Acid Cycle

9

I. OVERVIEW

The tricarboxylic acid cycle (TCA cycle, also called the Krebs cycle or the citric acid cycle) plays several roles in metabolism. It is the final pathway where the oxidative metabolism of carbohydrates, amino acids, and fatty acids converge, their carbon skeletons being converted to CO_2. This oxidation provides energy for the production of the majority of ATP in most animals, including humans. The cycle occurs totally in the mitochondria and is, therefore, in close proximity to the reactions of electron transport (see p. 73), which oxidize the reduced coenzymes produced by the cycle. The TCA cycle is an aerobic pathway, because O_2 is required as the final electron acceptor. Most of the body's catabolic pathways converge on the TCA cycle (Figure 9.1). Reactions such as the catabolism of some amino acids generate intermediates of the cycle and are called anaplerotic reactions. The citric acid cycle also supplies intermediates for a number of important synthetic reactions. For example, the cycle functions in the formation of glucose from the carbon skeletons of some amino acids, and it provides building blocks for the synthesis of some amino acids (see p. 267) and heme (see p. 278). Therefore, this cycle should not be viewed as a closed circle, but instead as a traffic circle with compounds entering and leaving as required.

II. REACTIONS OF THE TCA CYCLE

In the TCA cycle, oxaloacetate is first condensed with an acetyl group from acetyl coenzyme A (CoA), and then is regenerated as the cycle is completed (Figure 9.1). Thus, the entry of one acetyl CoA into one round of the TCA cycle does not lead to the net production or consumption of intermediates. [Note: Two carbons entering the cycle as acetyl CoA are balanced by two CO_2 exiting.]

A. Oxidative decarboxylation of pyruvate

Pyruvate, the endproduct of aerobic glycolysis, must be transported into the mitochondrion before it can enter the TCA cycle. This is accomplished by a specific pyruvate transporter that helps pyruvate cross the inner mitochondrial membrane. Once in the matrix, pyruvate is converted to acetyl CoA by the *pyruvate dehydrogenase complex*, which is a multienzyme complex. Strictly speaking, the *pyruvate dehydrogenase complex* is not part of the TCA cycle proper, but is a major source of acetyl CoA—the two-carbon substrate for the cycle.

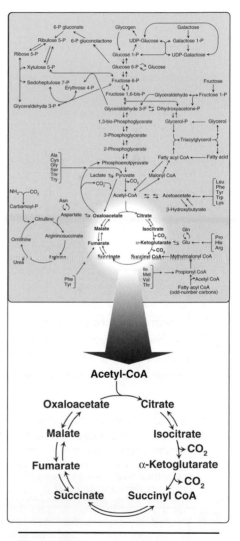

Figure 9.1
The tricarboxylic acid cycle shown as a part of the central pathways of energy metabolism. (See Figure 8.2, p. 92 for a more detailed view of the metabolic map.)

1. **Component enzymes:** The *pyruvate dehydrogenase complex* (*PDH complex*) is a multimolecular aggregate of three enzymes, *pyruvate dehydrogenase* (*PDH* or E_1, also called a *decarboxylase*), *dihydrolipoyl transacetylase* (E_2), and *dihydrolipoyl dehydrogenase* (E_3). Each catalyzes a part of the overall reaction (Figure 9.2). Their physical association links the reactions in proper sequence without the release of intermediates. In addition to the enzymes participating in the conversion of pyruvate to acetyl CoA, the complex also contains two tightly bound regulatory enzymes, *pyruvate dehydrogenase kinase* and *pyruvate dehydrogenase phosphatase*.

2. **Coenzymes:** The *PDH complex* contains five coenzymes that act as carriers or oxidants for the intermediates of the reactions shown in Figure 9.2. E_1 requires thiamine pyrophosphate (TPP), E_2 requires lipoic acid and CoA, and E_3 requires FAD and NAD^+.

> Deficiencies of thiamine or niacin can cause serious central nervous system problems. This is because brain cells are unable to produce sufficient ATP (via the TCA cycle) if the *PDH complex* is inactive. Wernicke-Korsakoff, an encephalopathy-psychosis syndrome due to thiamine deficiency, may be seen with alcohol abuse.

3. **Regulation of the pyruvate dehydrogenase complex:** Covalent modification by the two regulatory enzymes that are part of the complex alternately activate and inactivate E_1 (*PDH*). The cyclic AMP-independent *PDH kinase* phosphorylates and, thereby, inhibits E_1, whereas *PDH phosphatase* dephosphorylates and

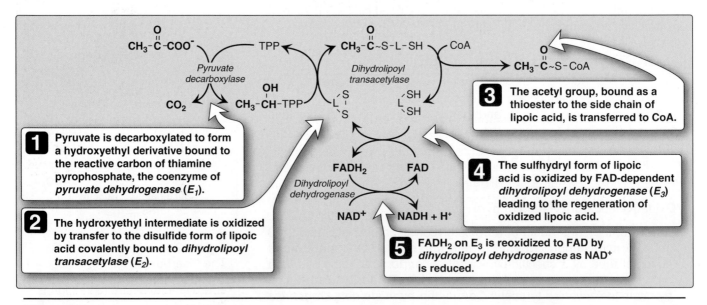

Figure 9.2
Mechanism of action of the *pyruvate dehydrogenase complex*. TPP = thiamine pyrophosphate; L = lipoic acid.

activates E_1 (Figure 9.3). The *kinase* itself is allosterically activated by ATP, acetyl CoA, and NADH. Therefore, in the presence
of these high-energy signals, the *PDH complex* is turned off.
Pyruvate is a potent inhibitor of *PDH kinase*. Therefore, if pyruvate
concentrations are elevated, E_1 will be maximally active. Calcium
is a strong activator of *PDH phosphatase*, stimulating E_1 activity.
This is particularly important in skeletal muscle, where release of
Ca^{2+} during contraction stimulates the *PDH complex*, and thereby
energy production. [Note: Although covalent regulation by the
kinase and *phosphatase* is key, the complex is also subject to
product (NADH, acetyl CoA) inhibition.]

4. **Pyruvate dehydrogenase deficiency:** A deficiency in the E_1 component of the *PDH complex*, although rare, is the most common
biochemical cause of congenital lactic acidosis. This enzyme deficiency results in an inability to convert pyruvate to acetyl CoA,
causing pyruvate to be shunted to lactic acid via *lactate dehydrogenase* (see p. 103). This causes particular problems for the
brain, which relies on the TCA cycle for most of its energy, and is
particularly sensitive to acidosis. Symptoms are variable and
include neurodegeneration, muscle spasticity and, in the neonatal
onset form, early death. The E_1 defect is X-linked, but because of
the importance of the enzyme in the brain, it affects both males
and females. Therefore, the defect is classified as X-linked dominant. There is no proven treatment for *pyruvate dehydrogenase*
deficiency: however, dietary restriction of carbohydrate and supplementation with TPP may reduce symptoms in select patients.

Leigh syndrome (subacute necrotizing encephalo-
myelopathy) is a rare, progressive neurological
disorder that is the result of defects in mitochondrial ATP production, primarily as a result of
mutations in the *PDH complex*, the electron
transport chain, or *ATP synthase*. Both nuclear
and mtDNA can be affected.

5. **Mechanism of arsenic poisoning:** As previously described (see
p. 101), arsenic can interfere with glycolysis at the *glyceraldehyde
3-phosphate* step, thereby decreasing ATP production. "Arsenic
poisoning" is, however, due primarily to inhibition of enzymes that
require lipoic acid as a coenzyme, including E_2 of the *PDH complex*, α-*ketoglutarate dehydrogenase* (see below), and *branched-
chain α-keto acid dehydrogenase* (see p. 266). Arsenite (the
trivalent form of arsenic) forms a stable complex with the thiol
(–SH) groups of lipoic acid, making that compound unavailable to
serve as a coenzyme. When it binds to lipoic acid in the *PDH
complex*, pyruvate (and consequently lactate) accumulates. Like
pyruvate dehydrogenase deficiency, this particularly affects the
brain, causing neurologic disturbances and death.

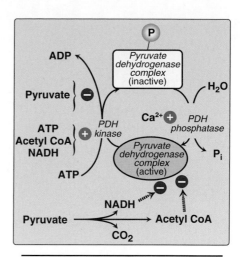

Figure 9.3
Regulation of *pyruvate
dehydrogenase complex.*
[▬▬▶ denotes product inhibition.]

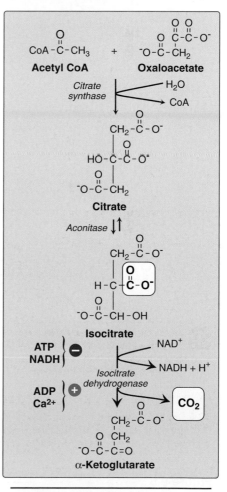

Figure 9.4
Formation of α-ketoglutarate from
acetyl CoA and oxaloacetate.

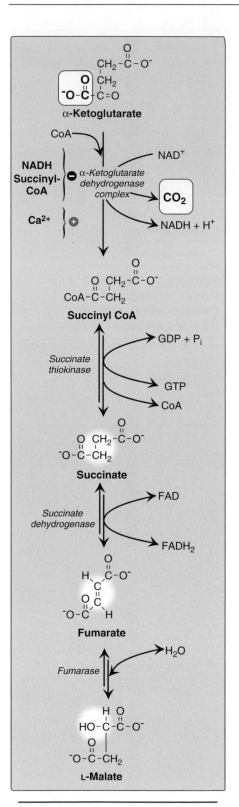

Figure 9.5
Formation of malate from
α-ketoglutarate.

B. Synthesis of citrate from acetyl CoA and oxaloacetate

The condensation of acetyl CoA and oxaloacetate to form citrate (a tricarboxylic acid) is catalyzed by *citrate synthase* (Figure 9.4). This aldol condensation has an equilibrium far in the direction of citrate synthesis. In humans, *citrate synthase* is not an allosteric enzyme. It is inhibited by its product, citrate. Substrate availability is another means of regulation for *citrate synthase*. The binding of oxaloacetate causes a conformational change in the enzyme that generates a binding site for acetyl CoA. [Note: Citrate, in addition to being an intermediate in the TCA cycle, provides a source of acetyl CoA for the cytosolic synthesis of fatty acids (see p. 183). Citrate also inhibits *phosphofructokinase*, the rate-limiting enzyme of glycolysis (see p. 99), and activates *acetyl CoA carboxylase* (the rate-limiting enzyme of fatty acid synthesis; see p. 183).]

C. Isomerization of citrate

Citrate is isomerized to isocitrate by *aconitase*, an Fe-S protein (see Figure 9.4). [Note: *Aconitase* is inhibited by fluoroacetate, a compound that is used as a rat poison. Fluoroacetate is converted to fluoroacetyl CoA, which condenses with oxaloacetate to form fluorocitrate—a potent inhibitor of *aconitase*—resulting in citrate accumulation.]

D. Oxidation and decarboxylation of isocitrate

Isocitrate dehydrogenase catalyzes the irreversible oxidative decarboxylation of isocitrate, yielding the first of three NADH molecules produced by the cycle, and the first release of CO_2 (see Figure 9.4). This is one of the rate-limiting steps of the TCA cycle. The enzyme is allosterically activated by ADP (a low-energy signal) and Ca^{2+}, and is inhibited by ATP and NADH, whose levels are elevated when the cell has abundant energy stores.

E. Oxidative decarboxylation of α-ketoglutarate

The conversion of α-ketoglutarate to succinyl CoA is catalyzed by the *α-ketoglutarate dehydrogenase complex*, a multimolecular aggregate of three enzymes (Figure 9.5). The mechanism of this oxidative decarboxylation is very similar to that used for the conversion of pyruvate to acetyl CoA by the *PDH complex*. The reaction releases the second CO_2 and produces the second NADH of the cycle. The coenzymes required are thiamine pyrophosphate, lipoic acid, FAD, NAD^+, and CoA. Each functions as part of the catalytic mechanism in a way analogous to that described for the *PDH complex* (see p. 110). The equilibrium of the reaction is far in the direction of succinyl CoA—a high-energy thioester similar to acetyl CoA. *α-Ketoglutarate dehydrogenase complex* is inhibited by its products, NADH and succinyl CoA, and activated by Ca^{2+}. However, it is not regulated by phosphorylation/dephosphorylation reactions as described for *PDH complex*. [Note: α-Ketoglutarate is also produced by the oxidative deamination (see p. 252) or transamination of the amino acid, glutamate (see p. 250).]

F. Cleavage of succinyl CoA

Succinate thiokinase (also called *succinyl CoA synthetase*—named for the reverse reaction) cleaves the high-energy thioester bond of succinyl CoA (see Figure 9.5). This reaction is coupled to phosphorylation of guanosine diphosphate (GDP) to guanosine triphosphate (GTP). GTP and ATP are energetically interconvertible by the *nucleoside diphosphate kinase* reaction:

$$GTP + ADP \rightleftarrows GDP + ATP$$

The generation of GTP by *succinate thiokinase* is another example of substrate-level phosphorylation (see p. 102). [Note: Succinyl CoA is also produced from propionyl CoA derived from the metabolism of fatty acids with an odd number of carbon atoms (see p. 193), and from the metabolism of several amino acids (see pp. 265–266).]

G. Oxidation of succinate

Succinate is oxidized to fumarate by *succinate dehydrogenase*, as FAD (its coenzyme) is reduced to $FADH_2$ (see Figure 9.5). *Succinate dehydrogenase* is the only enzyme of the TCA cycle that is embedded in the inner mitochondrial membrane. As such, it functions as Complex II of the electron transport chain (see p. 75). [Note: FAD, rather than NAD^+, is the electron acceptor because the reducing power of succinate is not sufficient to reduce NAD^+.]

H. Hydration of fumarate

Fumarate is hydrated to malate in a freely reversible reaction catalyzed by *fumarase* (also called *fumarate hydratase*, see Figure 9.5). [Note: Fumarate is also produced by the urea cycle (see p. 254), in purine synthesis (see p. 294), and during catabolism of the amino acids, phenylalanine and tyrosine (see p. 263).]

I. Oxidation of malate

Malate is oxidized to oxaloacetate by *malate dehydrogenase* (Figure 9.6). This reaction produces the third and final NADH of the cycle. The ΔG^0 of the reaction is positive, but the reaction is driven in the direction of oxaloacetate by the highly exergonic *citrate synthase* reaction. [Note: Oxaloacetate is also produced by the transamination of the amino acid, aspartic acid (see p. 250).]

III. ENERGY PRODUCED BY THE TCA CYCLE

Two carbon atoms enter the cycle as acetyl CoA and leave as CO_2. The cycle does not involve net consumption or production of oxaloacetate or of any other intermediate. Four pairs of electrons are transferred during one turn of the cycle: three pairs of electrons reducing three NAD^+ to NADH and one pair reducing FAD to $FADH_2$. Oxidation of one NADH by the electron transport chain leads to formation of approximately three ATP, whereas oxidation of $FADH_2$ yields approximately two ATP (see p. 77). The total yield of ATP from the oxidation of one acetyl CoA is shown in Figure 9.7. Figure 9.8 summarizes the reactions of the TCA cycle.

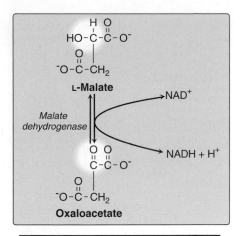

Figure 9.6
Formation of oxaloacetate from malate.

Energy producing reaction	Number of ATP produced
3 NADH ⟶ 3 NAD⁺	9
FADH₂ ⟶ FAD	2
GDP + Pᵢ ⟶ GTP	1
	12 ATP/acetyl CoA oxidized

Figure 9.7
Number of ATP molecules produced from the oxidation of one molecule of acetyl CoA (using both substrate-level and oxidative phosphorylation).

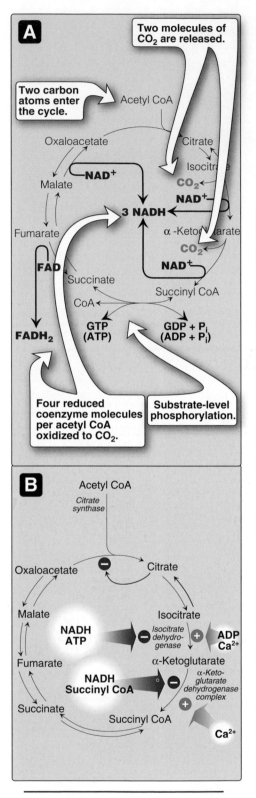

IV. REGULATION OF THE TCA CYCLE

In contrast to glycolysis, which is regulated primarily by *phosphofructo-kinase,* the TCA cycle is controlled by the regulation of several enzyme activities (see Figure 9.8). The most important of these regulated enzymes are those that catalyze reactions with highly negative ΔG^0: *citrate synthase, isocitrate dehydrogenase,* and *α-ketoglutarate dehydrogenase complex.* Reducing equivalents needed for oxidative phosphorylation are generated by the *pyruvate dehydrogenase complex* and the TCA cycle, and both processes are upregulated in response to a rise in ADP.

V. CHAPTER SUMMARY

Pyruvate is **oxidatively decarboxylated** by **pyruvate dehydrogenase (PDH) complex**, producing **acetyl CoA**, which is the major fuel for the tricarboxylic acid cycle (TCA cycle, Figure 9.9). This multienzyme complex requires five coenzymes: **thiamine pyrophosphate, lipoic acid, FAD, NAD+**, and **coenzyme A**. PDH complex is regulated by covalent modification of E_1 (pyruvate dehydrogenase, PDH) by PDH kinase and PDH phosphatase: phosphorylation inhibits PDH. PDH kinase is allosterically activated by ATP, acetyl CoA, and NADH and inhibited by pyruvate; the phosphatase is activated by Ca^{2+}. **Pyruvate dehydrogenase deficiency** is the most common biochemical cause of **congenital lactic acidosis**. The central nervous system is particularly affected in this is **X-linked dominant** disorder. **Arsenic poisoning** causes inactivation of PDH complex by binding to lipoic acid. **Citrate** is synthesized from **oxaloacetate** and **acetyl CoA** by **citrate synthase**. This enzyme is subject to product inhibition by citrate. Citrate is isomerized to **isocitrate** by **aconitase**. **Isocitrate** is oxidized and decarboxylated by **isocitrate dehydrogenase** to **α-ketoglutarate**, producing **CO$_2$** and **NADH**. The enzyme is inhibited by ATP and NADH, and activated by ADP and Ca^{2+}. **α-Ketoglutarate** is oxidatively decarboxylated to **succinyl CoA** by the **α-ketoglutarate dehydrogenase complex**, producing **CO$_2$** and **NADH**. The enzyme is very similar to pyruvate dehydrogenase and uses the same coenzymes. α-Ketoglutarate dehydrogenase complex is activated by calcium and inhibited by NADH and succinyl CoA, but is not covalently regulated. **Succinyl CoA** is cleaved by **succinate thiokinase** (also called **succinyl CoA synthetase**), producing **succinate** and **GTP**. This is an example of **substrate-level phosphorylation**. **Succinate** is oxidized to **fumarate** by **succinate dehydrogenase**, producing **FADH$_2$**. **Fumarate** is hydrated to **malate** by **fumarase (fumarate hydratase)**, and **malate** is oxidized to **oxaloacetate** by **malate dehydrogenase**, producing **NADH**. **Three NADH, one FADH$_2$**, and **one GTP** (whose terminal phosphate can be transferred to ADP by nucleoside diphosphate kinase, producing ATP) are produced by one round of the TCA cycle. The generation of acetyl CoA by the oxidation of pyruvate via the PDH complex also produces an NADH. Oxidation of these NADHs and FADH$_2$ by the electron transport chain yields 14 ATP. An additional ATP (GTP) comes from substrate level phosphorylation in the TCA cycle. Therefore, a total of 15 ATPs are produced from the complete mitochondrial oxidation of pyruvate to CO$_2$.

Figure 9.8
A. Production of reduced coenzymes, ATP, and CO$_2$ in the citric acid cycle.
B. Inhibitors and activators of the cycle.

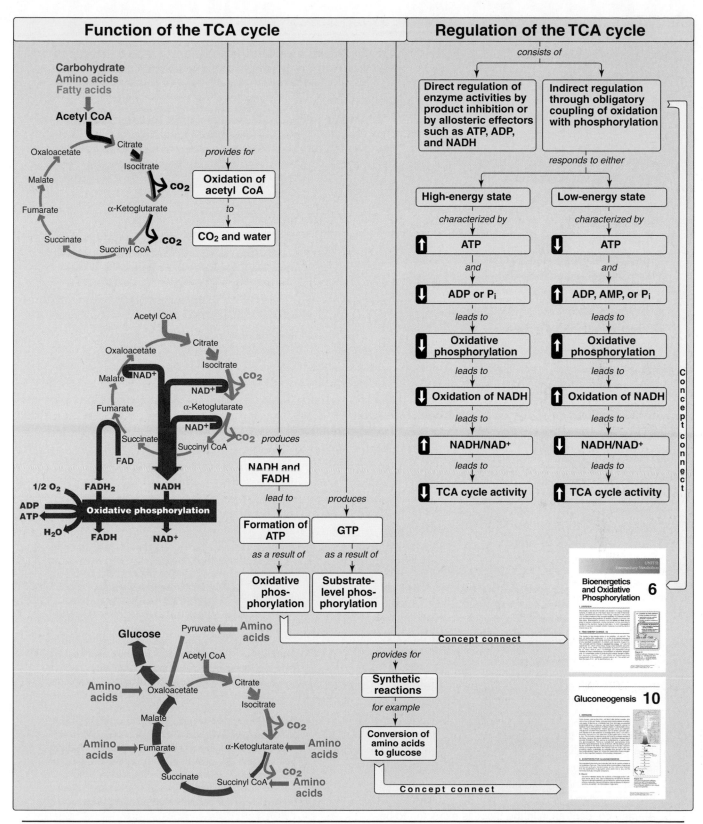

Figure 9.9
Key concept map for the tricarboxylic acid (TCA) cycle.

Study Questions

Choose the ONE correct answer.

9.1 The conversion of pyruvate to acetyl CoA and CO_2:

A. is reversible.

B. involves the participation of lipoic acid.

C. is activated when pyruvate dehydrogenase (PDH, E_1) of the pyruvate dehydrogenase complex is phosphorylated by PDH kinase in the presence of ATP.

D. occurs in the cytosol.

E. depends on the coenzyme biotin.

> Correct answer = B. Lipoic acid is an intermediate acceptor of the acetyl group formed in the reaction. Pyruvate dehydrogenase complex catalyzes an irreversible reaction that is inhibited when the PDH (E1) component is phosphorylated. The enzyme complex is located in the mitochondrial matrix. Biotin is utilized by carboxylases.

9.2 Which one of the following conditions decreases the oxidation of acetyl CoA by the citric acid cycle?

A. A low ATP/ADP ratio

B. A low NADH concentration due to rapid oxidation to NAD^+ through the respiratory chain

C. A low NAD^+/NADH ratio

D. A high concentration of AMP

E. A low GTP/GDP ratio

> Correct answer = C. A low NAD^+/NADH ratio limits the rates of the NAD^+-requiring dehydrogenases. A low ATP/ADP or GTP/GDP ratio stimulates the cycle. AMP does not directly affect the cycle.

9.3 The following is the sum of three steps in the citric acid cycle.

$$A + B + FAD + H_2O \rightarrow C + FADH_2 + NADH$$

Choose the lettered answer that corresponds to the missing "A", "B", and "C" in the equation.

	Reactant A	Reactant B	Reactant C
A.	Succinyl CoA	GDP	Succinate
B.	Succinate	NAD^+	Oxaloacetate
C.	Fumarate	NAD^+	Oxaloacetate
D.	Succinate	NAD^+	Malate
E.	Fumarate	GTP	Malate

> Correct answer = B. Succinate + NAD^+ + FAD $\rightarrow$ oxaloacetate + NADH + $FADH_2$

9.4 A 1-month-old male showed abnormalities of the nervous system and lactic acidosis. Enzyme assay for pyruvate dehydrogenase (PDH) activity on extracts of cultured skin fibroblasts showed 5% of normal activity, with a low concentration (1×10^{-4} mM) of thiamine pyrophosphate (TPP), but 80% of normal activity when the assay contained a high (0.4 mM) concentration of TPP. Which one of the following statements concerning this patient is most correct?

A. Elevated levels of lactate and pyruvate in the blood reliably predict the presence of PDH deficiency.

B. The patient is expected to show disturbances in fatty acid degradation.

C. A diet consisting of high carbohydrate intake would be expected to be beneficial in this patient.

D. Alanine concentration in the blood is expected to be less than normal.

E. Administration of thiamine is expected to reduce his serum lactate concentration and improve his clinical symptoms.

> Correct answer = E. The patient appears to have a thiamine-responsive PDH deficiency. The enzyme fails to bind thiamine pyrophosphate at low concentration, but shows significant activity at a high concentration of the coenzyme. This mutation, which affects the K_m of the enzyme for the coenzyme, is present in some, but not all, cases of PDH deficiency. All inborn errors of PDH are associated with elevated levels of lactate, pyruvate, and alanine (the transamination product of pyruvate). Patients routinely show neuroanatomic defects, developmental delay, and often early death. Elevated lactate and pyruvate are also observed in pyruvate carboxylase deficiency, another rare defect in pyruvate metabolism. Because PDH is an integral part of carbohydrate metabolism, a diet low in carbohydrates would be expected to blunt the effects of the enzyme deficiency. By contrast, fatty acid degradation occurs via conversion to acetyl CoA by β-oxidation, a process that does not involve pyruvate as an intermediate. Thus, fatty acid metabolism is not disturbed in this enzyme deficiency.

Gluconeogenesis 10

I. OVERVIEW

Some tissues, such as the brain, red blood cells, kidney medulla, lens and cornea of the eye, testes, and exercising muscle, require a continuous supply of glucose as a metabolic fuel. Liver glycogen, an essential postprandial source of glucose, can meet these needs for only 10–18 hours in the absence of dietary intake of carbohydrate (see p. 329). During a prolonged fast, however, hepatic glycogen stores are depleted, and glucose is formed from precursors such as lactate, pyruvate, glycerol (derived from the backbone of triacylglycerols, see p. 190), and α-ketoacids (derived from the catabolism of glucogenic amino acids, see p. 261). The formation of glucose does not occur by a simple reversal of glycolysis, because the overall equilibrium of glycolysis strongly favors pyruvate formation. Instead, glucose is synthesized by a special pathway, gluconeogenesis, that requires both mitochondrial and cytosolic enzymes. During an overnight fast, approximately 90% of gluconeogenesis occurs in the liver, with the kidneys providing 10% of the newly synthesized glucose molecules. However, during prolonged fasting, the kidneys become major glucose-producing organs, contributing an estimated 40% of the total glucose production. Figure 10.1 shows the relationship of gluconeogenesis to other important reactions of intermediary metabolism.

II. SUBSTRATES FOR GLUCONEOGENESIS

Gluconeogenic precursors are molecules that can be used to produce a net synthesis of glucose. They include intermediates of glycolysis and the tricarboxylic acid (TCA) cycle. Glycerol, lactate, and the α-keto acids obtained from the transamination of glucogenic amino acids are the most important gluconeogenic precursors.

A. Glycerol

Glycerol is released during the hydrolysis of triacylglycerols in adipose tissue (see p. 190), and is delivered by the blood to the liver. Glycerol is phosphorylated by *glycerol kinase* to glycerol phosphate, which is oxidized by *glycerol phosphate dehydrogenase* to dihydroxyacetone phosphate—an intermediate of glycolysis. [Note: Adipocytes cannot phosphorylate glycerol because they essentially lack *glycerol kinase*.]

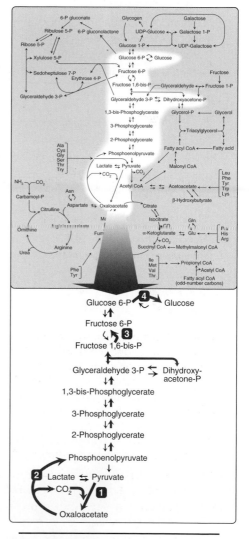

Figure 10.1
The gluconeogenesis pathway shown as part of the essential pathways of energy metabolism. The numbered reactions are unique to gluconeogenesis. (See Figure 8.2, p. 92, for a more detailed map of metabolism.)

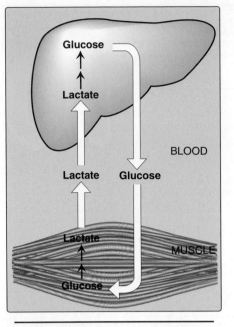

Figure 10.2
The Cori cycle.

B. Lactate

Lactate is released into the blood by exercising skeletal muscle, and by cells that lack mitochondria, such as red blood cells. In the Cori cycle, bloodborne glucose is converted by exercising muscle to lactate, which diffuses into the blood. This lactate is taken up by the liver and reconverted to glucose, which is released back into the circulation (Figure 10.2).

C. Amino acids

Amino acids derived from hydrolysis of tissue proteins are the major sources of glucose during a fast. α-Ketoacids, such as α-keto-glutarate, are derived from the metabolism of glucogenic amino acids (see p. 261). These α-ketoacids can enter the TCA cycle and form oxaloacetate (OAA)—a direct precursor of phosphoenol-pyruvate (PEP). [Note: Acetyl coenzyme A (CoA) and compounds that give rise only to acetyl CoA (for example, acetoacetate and amino acids such as lysine and leucine) cannot give rise to a net synthesis of glucose. This is due to the irreversible nature of the *pyruvate dehydrogenase* reaction, which converts pyruvate to acetyl CoA (see p. 109). These compounds give rise instead to ketone bodies (see p. 195) and are therefore termed ketogenic.]

III. REACTIONS UNIQUE TO GLUCONEOGENESIS

Seven glycolytic reactions are reversible and are used in the synthesis of glucose from lactate or pyruvate. However, three of the reactions are irreversible and must be circumvented by four alternate reactions that energetically favor the synthesis of glucose. These reactions, unique to gluconeogenesis, are described below.

A. Carboxylation of pyruvate

The first "roadblock" to overcome in the synthesis of glucose from pyruvate is the irreversible conversion in glycolysis of PEP to pyruvate by *pyruvate kinase*. In gluconeogenesis, pyruvate is first carboxylated by *pyruvate carboxylase* to OAA, which is then converted to PEP by the action of *PEP-carboxykinase* (Figure 10.3).

1. **Biotin is a coenzyme:** *Pyruvate carboxylase* requires biotin (see p. 381) covalently bound to the ε-amino group of a lysine residue in the enzyme (see Figure 10.3). Hydrolysis of ATP drives the formation of an enzyme–biotin–CO_2 intermediate. This high-energy complex subsequently carboxylates pyruvate to form OAA. [Note: This reaction occurs in the mitochondria of liver and kidney cells, and has two purposes: to provide an important substrate for gluconeogenesis, and to provide OAA that can replenish the TCA cycle intermediates that may become depleted, depending on the synthetic needs of the cell. Muscle cells also contain *pyruvate carboxylase*, but use the OAA produced only for the latter purpose—they do not synthesize glucose.]

> *Pyruvate carboxylase* is one of several *carboxylases* that require biotin. Others include *acetyl CoA carboxylase* (p. 183), *propionyl CoA carboxylase* (p. 194), and *methylcrotonyl CoA carboxylase* (p. 266).

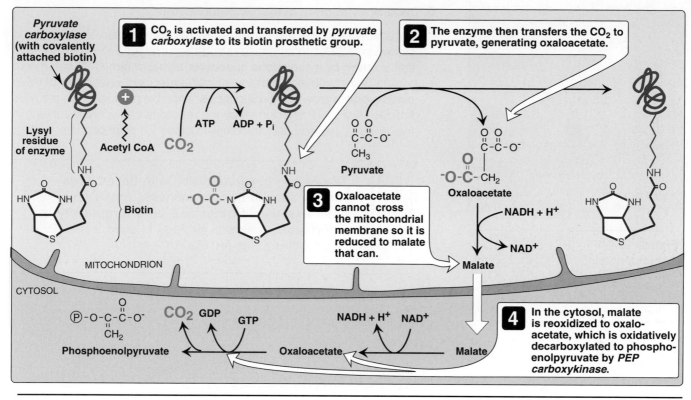

Figure 10.3
Activation and transfer of CO_2 to pyruvate, followed by transport of oxaloacetate to the cytosol and subsequent decarboxylation. Alternatively, OAA can be converted to PEP that is transported out of the mitochondria.

2. **Allosteric regulation:** *Pyruvate carboxylase* is allosterically activated by acetyl CoA. Elevated levels of acetyl CoA in mitochondria signal a metabolic state in which the increased synthesis of OAA is required. For example, this occurs during fasting, when OAA is used for the synthesis of glucose by gluconeogenesis in the liver and kidney. Conversely, at low levels of acetyl CoA, *pyruvate carboxylase* is largely inactive, and pyruvate is primarily oxidized by the *pyruvate dehydrogenase complex* to produce acetyl CoA that can be further oxidized by the TCA cycle (see p. 109).

B. Transport of oxaloacetate to the cytosol

OAA must be converted to PEP for gluconeogenesis to continue. The enzyme that catalyzes this conversion is found in both the mitochondria and the cytosol in humans. The PEP that is generated in the mitochondria is transported to the cytosol by a specific transporter, whereas that generated in the cytosol requires the transport of OAA from the mitochondria to the cytosol. However, OAA is unable to directly cross the inner mitochondrial membrane; it must first be reduced to malate by mitochondrial *malate dehydrogenase*. Malate can be transported from the mitochondria to the cytosol, where it is reoxidized to oxaloacetate by cytosolic *malate dehydrogenase* as NAD^+ is reduced (see Figure 10.3). The NADH produced is used in the reduction of 1,3-BPG to glyceraldehyde 3-phosphate (see p. 101), a step common to both glycolysis and gluconeogenesis.

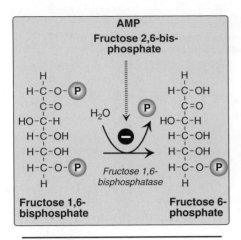

Figure 10.4
Dephosphorylation of fructose 1,6-bisphosphate.

C. Decarboxylation of cytosolic oxaloacetate

Oxaloacetate is decarboxylated and phosphorylated to PEP in the cytosol by *PEP-carboxykinase* (also referred to as *PEPCK*). The reaction is driven by hydrolysis of guanosine triphosphate (GTP, see Figure 10.3). The combined actions of *pyruvate carboxylase* and *PEP-carboxykinase* provide an energetically favorable pathway from pyruvate to PEP. Then, PEP is acted on by the reactions of glycolysis running in the reverse direction until it becomes fructose 1,6-bisphosphate.

> The pairing of carboxylation with decarboxylation, as seen in gluconeogenesis, drives reactions that would otherwise be energetically unfavorable. A similar strategy is used in fatty acid synthesis (see pp. 183–184).

D. Dephosphorylation of fructose 1,6-bisphosphate

Hydrolysis of fructose 1,6-bisphosphate by *fructose 1,6-bisphosphatase* bypasses the irreversible *phosphofructokinase-1* reaction, and provides an energetically favorable pathway for the formation of fructose 6-phosphate (Figure 10.4). This reaction is an important regulatory site of gluconeogenesis.

1. **Regulation by energy levels within the cell:** *Fructose 1,6-bisphosphatase* is inhibited by elevated levels of adenosine monophosphate (AMP), which signal an "energy-poor" state in the cell.

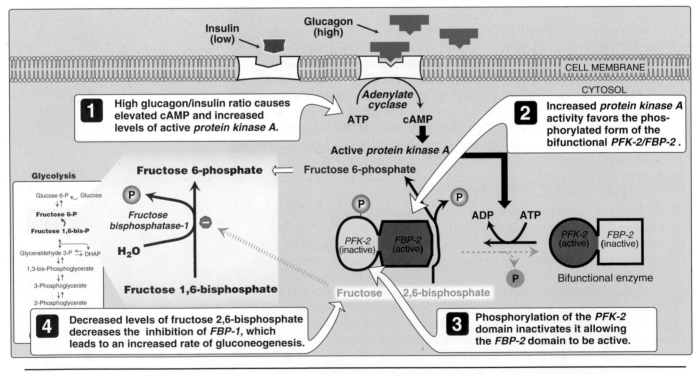

Figure 10.5
Effect of elevated glucagon on the intracellular concentration of fructose 2,6-bisphosphate in the liver.
PFK-2 = phosphofructokinase-2; FBP-2 = fructose bisphosphatase-2.

Conversely, high levels of ATP and low concentrations of AMP stimulate gluconeogenesis, an energy-requiring pathway.

2. **Regulation by fructose 2,6-bisphosphate:** *Fructose 1,6-bisphosphatase*, found in liver and kidney, is inhibited by fructose 2,6-bisphosphate, an allosteric effector whose concentration is influenced by the level of circulating glucagon (Figure 10.5). [Note: The signals that inhibit (low energy, high fructose 2,6-bisphosphate) or favor (high energy, low fructose 2,6-bisphosphate) gluconeogenesis have the opposite effect on glycolysis, providing reciprocal control of the pathways that synthesize and oxidize glucose (see p. 100).]

E. Dephosphorylation of glucose 6-phosphate

Hydrolysis of glucose 6-phosphate by *glucose 6-phosphatase* bypasses the irreversible *hexokinase* reaction, and provides an energetically favorable pathway for the formation of free glucose (Figure 10.6). Liver and kidney are the only organs that release free glucose from glucose 6-phosphate. This process actually requires two proteins: *glucose 6-phosphate translocase*, which transports glucose 6-phosphate across the endoplasmic reticulum (ER) membrane, and the ER enzyme, *glucose 6-phosphatase* (found only in gluconeogenic cells), which removes the phosphate, producing free glucose (see Figure 10.6). [Note: These proteins are also required for the final step of glycogen degradation (see p. 130). Type Ia glycogen storage disease (see p. 130), due to an inherited deficiency of *glucose 6-phosphatase*, is characterized by severe fasting hypoglycemia, because free glucose is unable to be produced from either gluconeogenesis or glycogenolysis.] Specific transporters are responsible for releasing free glucose and phosphate back into the cytosol and, for glucose, into blood. [Note: Muscle lacks *glucose 6-phosphatase*, and therefore muscle glycogen can not be used to maintain blood glucose levels.]

F. Summary of the reactions of glycolysis and gluconeogenesis

Of the 11 reactions required to convert pyruvate to free glucose, seven are catalyzed by reversible glycolytic enzymes (Figure 10.7). The irreversible reactions of glycolysis catalyzed by *hexokinase*, *phosphofructokinase-1*, and *pyruvate kinase* are circumvented by *glucose 6-phosphatase*, *fructose 1,6-bisphosphatase*, and *pyruvate carboxylase/PEP-carboxykinase*. In gluconeogenesis, the equilibria of the seven reversible reactions of glycolysis are pushed in favor of glucose synthesis as a result of the essentially irreversible formation of PEP, fructose 6-phosphate, and glucose catalyzed by the gluconeogenic enzymes. [Note: The stoichiometry of gluconeogenesis from pyruvate couples the cleavage of six high-energy phosphate bonds and the oxidation of two NADH with the formation of each molecule of glucose (see Figure 10.7).]

IV. REGULATION OF GLUCONEOGENESIS

The moment-to-moment regulation of gluconeogenesis is determined primarily by the circulating level of glucagon, and by the availability of gluconeogenic substrates. In addition, slow adaptive changes in

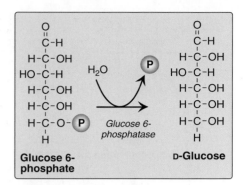

Figure 10.6
Dephosphorylation of glucose 6-phosphate allows release of free glucose from liver and kidney into blood.

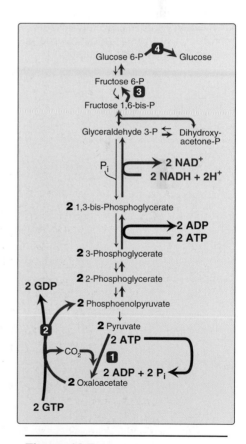

Figure 10.7
Summary of the reactions of glycolysis and gluconeogenesis, showing the energy requirements of gluconeogenesis.

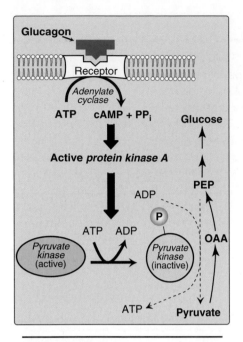

Figure 10.8
Covalent modification of *pyruvate kinase* results in inactivation of the enzyme. OAA = oxaloacetate. [Note: Only the hepatic isozyme is subject to covalent regulation.]

enzyme activity result from an alteration in the rate of enzyme synthesis or degradation, or both. [Note: Hormonal control of the glucoregulatory system is presented in Chapter 23.]

A. Glucagon

This hormone from the α cells of pancreatic islets (see p. 313) stimulates gluconeogenesis by three mechanisms.

1. **Changes in allosteric effectors:** Glucagon lowers the level of fructose 2,6-bisphosphate, resulting in activation of *fructose 1,6-bisphosphatase* and inhibition of *phosphofructokinase-1,* thus favoring gluconeogenesis over glycolysis (see Figure 10.5). [Note: See p. 100 for the role of fructose 2,6-bisphosphate in the regulation of glycolysis.]

2. **Covalent modification of enzyme activity:** Glucagon binds its G protein-coupled receptor (see p. 95) and, via an elevation in cyclic AMP (cAMP) level and *cAMP-dependent protein kinase* activity, stimulates the conversion of hepatic *pyruvate kinase* to its inactive (phosphorylated) form. This decreases the conversion of PEP to pyruvate, which has the effect of diverting PEP to the synthesis of glucose (Figure 10.8).

3. **Induction of enzyme synthesis:** Glucagon increases the transcription of the gene for *PEP-carboxykinase*, thereby increasing the availability of this enzyme as levels of its substrate rise during fasting. [Note: Insulin causes decreased transcription of the mRNA for this enzyme.]

B. Substrate availability

The availability of gluconeogenic precursors, particularly glucogenic amino acids, significantly influences the rate of hepatic glucose synthesis. Decreased levels of insulin favor mobilization of amino acids from muscle protein, and provide the carbon skeletons for gluconeogenesis. In addition, ATP and NADH, coenzymes-cosubstrates required for gluconeogenesis, are primarily provided by the catabolism of fatty acids.

C. Allosteric activation by acetyl CoA

Allosteric activation of hepatic *pyruvate carboxylase* by acetyl CoA occurs during fasting. As a result of increased lipolysis in adipose tissue, the liver is flooded with fatty acids (see p. 330). The rate of formation of acetyl CoA by β-oxidation of these fatty acids exceeds the capacity of the liver to oxidize it to CO_2 and H_2O. As a result, acetyl CoA accumulates and leads to activation of *pyruvate carboxylase*. [Note: Acetyl CoA inhibits *pyruvate dehydrogenase* (by activating *PDH kinase,* see p. 111). Thus, this single compound can divert pyruvate toward gluconeogenesis and away from the TCA cycle.]

D. Allosteric inhibition by AMP

Fructose 1,6-bisphosphatase is inhibited by AMP—a compound that activates *phosphofructokinase-1*. This results in a reciprocal regulation of glycolysis and gluconeogenesis seen previously with fructose 2,6-bisphosphate (see p. 121). [Note: Elevated AMP thus stimulates pathways that oxidize nutrients to provide energy for the cell.]

V. CHAPTER SUMMARY

Gluconeogenic precursors include the **intermediates of glycolysis** and the **citric acid cycle**, **glycerol** released during the hydrolysis of triacylglycerols in adipose tissue, **lactate** released into the blood by cells that lack mitochondria and by exercising skeletal muscle, and **α-ketoacids** derived from the metabolism of glucogenic amino acids (Figure 10.9). Seven of the reactions of glycolysis are reversible and are used for gluconeogenesis in the liver and kidneys. Three reactions are **physiologically irreversible** and must be circumvented. These reactions are catalyzed by the glycolytic enzymes **pyruvate kinase**, **phosphofructokinase**, and **hexokinase**. **Pyruvate** is converted to oxaloacetate (OAA) and then to **phosphoenolpyruvate (PEP)** by **pyruvate carboxylase** and **PEP-carboxykinase**. The carboxylase requires **biotin** and **ATP**, and is allosterically activated by **acetyl CoA**. PEP-carboxykinase requires **GTP**. The transcription of its mRNA is increased by glucagon and decreased by insulin. **Fructose 1,6-bisphosphate** is converted to **fructose 6-phosphate** by **fructose 1,6-bisphosphatase**. This enzyme is **inhibited** by elevated levels of **AMP** and **activated** when **ATP** levels are elevated. The enzyme is also **inhibited** by **fructose 2,6-bisphosphate**, the primary allosteric activator of glycolysis. **Glucose 6-phosphate** is converted to **glucose** by **glucose 6-phosphatase**. This enzyme of the ER is required for the final step in gluconeogenesis, as well as hepatic and renal glycogen degradation. A deficiency of this enzyme results in severe, fasting hypoglycemia.

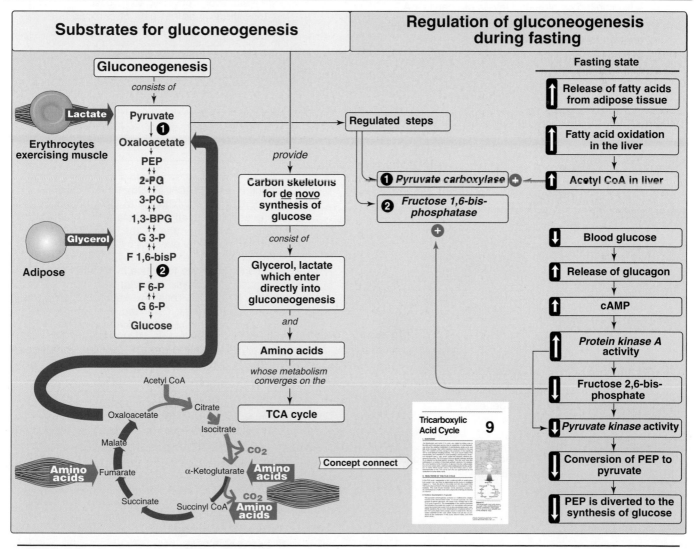

Figure 10.9
Key concept map for gluconeogenesis.

Study Questions

Choose the ONE correct answer.

10.1 The synthesis of glucose from pyruvate by gluconeogenesis:

A. occurs exclusively in the cytosol.

B. is inhibited by an elevated level of glucagon.

C. requires the participation of biotin.

D. involves lactate as an intermediate.

E. requires the oxidation/reduction of FAD.

> Correct answer = C. Biotin is the coenzyme-
> prosthetic group of pyruvate carboxylase. The
> carboxylation of pyruvate occurs in the mito-
> chondria. Glucagon stimulates gluconeogenesis.
> Lactate is not an intermediate in the conversion
> of pyruvate to glucose; however, pyruvate can
> be produced from lactate. FAD is not involved in
> gluconeogenesis.

10.2 Which one of the following statements concerning
gluconeogenesis is correct?

A. It occurs in muscle.

B. It is stimulated by fructose 2,6-bisphosphate.

C. It is inhibited by elevated levels of acetyl CoA.

D. It is important in maintaining blood glucose during
the normal overnight fast.

E. It uses carbon skeletons provided by degradation
of fatty acids.

> Correct answer = D. During the overnight fast,
> glycogen is partially depleted and gluconeo-
> genesis provides blood glucose. Gluconeo-
> genesis is inhibited by fructose 2,6-bisphosphate
> and stimulated by elevated levels of acetyl CoA.
> Degradation of fatty acids yields acetyl CoA,
> which cannot be converted to glucose. This is
> because there is no net gain of carbons from
> acetyl CoA in the TCA cycle, and the PDH reac-
> tion is physiologically irreversible. Carbon skele-
> tons of most amino acids are, however,
> gluconeogenic.

10.3 Which one of the following reactions is unique to gluconeogenesis?

A. Lactate → pyruvate

B. Phosphoenolpyruvate → pyruvate

C. Oxaloacetate → phosphoenolpyruvate

D. Glucose 6-phosphate → fructose 6-phosphate

E. 1,3-Bis-phosphoglycerate → 3-phosphoglycerate

> Correct answer = C. The other reactions are
> common to both gluconeogenesis and glycolysis.

10.4 The metabolism of ethanol by alcohol dehydrogenase (ADH) produces NADH. What effect is the
change in the NAD+/NADH expected to have on gluconeogenesis? Explain.

> The increase in NADH as ethanol is oxidized,
> will decrease the availability of OAA because
> the reversible oxidation of malate to OAA by
> malate dehydrogenase of the TCA cycle is
> driven in the reverse direction by the high avail-
> ability of NADH. Additionally, the reversible
> reduction of pyruvate to lactate by lactate dehy-
> drogenase of glycolysis is driven in the forward
> direction by NADH. Thus, two important gluco-
> neogenic substrates, OAA and pyruvate, are
> decreased as a result of the increase in NADH
> during ethanol metabolism. This will result in a
> decrease in gluconeogenesis.

10.5 Given that acetyl CoA cannot be a substrate for gluconeogenesis, why is its production in fatty acid oxidation essential for gluconeogenesis?

> Acetyl CoA inhibits pyruvate dehydrogenase and
> activates pyruvate carboxylase, pushing pyru-
> vate to gluconeogenesis.

10.6 What effect does AMP have on gluconeogenesis and
glycolysis? What enzymes are affected?

> AMP inhibits gluconeogenesis through inhibition
> of fructose 1,6-bisphosphatase and favors glycol-
> ysis through activation of phosphofructokinase-1.
> (Fructose 2,6-bisphosphate has a similar effect
> on these enzymes.)

Glycogen Metabolism

11

I. OVERVIEW

A constant source of blood glucose is an absolute requirement for human life. Glucose is the greatly preferred energy source for the brain, and the required energy source for cells with few or no mitochondria, such as mature erythrocytes. Glucose is also essential as an energy source for exercising muscle, where it is the substrate for anaerobic glycolysis. Blood glucose can be obtained from three primary sources: the diet, degradation of glycogen, and gluconeogenesis. Dietary intake of glucose and glucose precursors, such as starch, monosaccharides, and disaccharides, is sporadic and, depending on the diet, is not always a reliable source of blood glucose. In contrast, gluconeogenesis (see p. 117) can provide sustained synthesis of glucose, but it is somewhat slow in responding to a falling blood glucose level. Therefore, the body has developed mechanisms for storing a supply of glucose in a rapidly mobilizable form, namely, glycogen. In the absence of a dietary source of glucose, this sugar is rapidly released from liver and kidney glycogen. Similarly, muscle glycogen is extensively degraded in exercising muscle to provide that tissue with an important energy source. When glycogen stores are depleted, specific tissues synthesize glucose de novo, using amino acids from the body's proteins as a primary source of carbons for the gluconeogenic pathway. Figure 11.1 shows the reactions of glycogen synthesis and degradation as part of the essential pathways of energy metabolism.

II. STRUCTURE AND FUNCTION OF GLYCOGEN

The main stores of glycogen in the body are found in skeletal muscle and liver, although most other cells store small amounts of glycogen for their own use. The function of muscle glycogen is to serve as a fuel reserve for the synthesis of adenosine triphosphate (ATP) during muscle contraction. That of liver glycogen is to maintain the blood glucose concentration, particularly during the early stages of a fast (Figure 11.2, and see p. 329).

A. Amounts of liver and muscle glycogen

Approximately 400 g of glycogen make up 1–2% of the fresh weight of resting muscle, and approximately 100 g of glycogen make up to 10% of the fresh weight of a well-fed adult liver. What limits the production of glycogen at these levels is not clear. However, in some

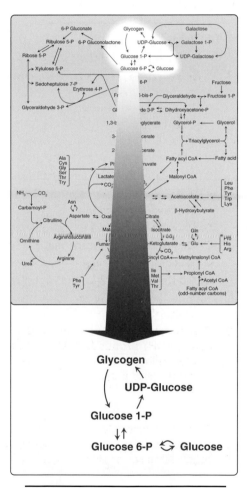

Figure 11.1
Glycogen synthesis and degradation shown as a part of the essential reactions of energy metabolism (see Figure 8.2, p. 92, for a more detailed view of the overall reactions of metabolism).

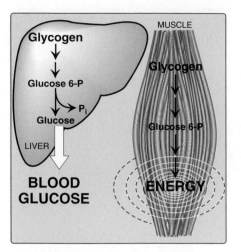

Figure 11.2
Functions of muscle and liver glycogen.

glycogen storage diseases (see Figure 11.8), the amount of glycogen in the liver and/or muscle can be significantly higher.

B. Structure of glycogen

Glycogen is a branched-chain polysaccharide made exclusively from α-D-glucose. The primary glycosidic bond is an α(1→4) linkage. After an average of eight to ten glucosyl residues, there is a branch containing an α(1→6) linkage (Figure 11.3). A single molecule of glycogen can have a molecular mass of up to 10^8 daltons. These molecules exist in discrete cytoplasmic granules that also contain most of the enzymes necessary for glycogen synthesis and degradation.

C. Fluctuation of glycogen stores

Liver glycogen stores increase during the well-fed state (see p. 323), and are depleted during a fast (see p. 329). Muscle glycogen is not affected by short periods of fasting (a few days) and is only moderately decreased in prolonged fasting (weeks). Muscle glycogen is synthesized to replenish muscle stores after they have been depleted following strenuous exercise. [Note: Glycogen synthesis and degradation are cytosolic processes that go on continuously. The differences between the rates of these two processes determine the levels of stored glycogen during specific physiologic states.]

III. SYNTHESIS OF GLYCOGEN (GLYCOGENESIS)

Glycogen is synthesized from molecules of α-D-glucose. The process occurs in the cytosol, and requires energy supplied by ATP (for the phosphorylation of glucose) and uridine triphosphate (UTP).

A. Synthesis of UDP-glucose

α-D-Glucose attached to uridine diphosphate (UDP) is the source of all the glucosyl residues that are added to the growing glycogen molecule. UDP-glucose (Figure 11.4) is synthesized from glucose 1-phosphate and UTP by *UDP-glucose pyrophosphorylase* (Figure 11.5). The high-energy bond in pyrophosphate (PP$_i$), the second product of the reaction, is hydrolyzed to two inorganic phosphates (P$_i$) by *pyrophosphatase*, which ensures that the *UDP-glucose pyrophosphorylase* reaction proceeds in the direction of UDP-glucose production. [Note: Glucose 6-phosphate is converted to glucose 1-phosphate by *phosphoglucomutase*. Glucose 1,6-bisphosphate is an obligatory intermediate in this reaction (Figure 11.6).]

B. Synthesis of a primer to initiate glycogen synthesis

Glycogen synthase is responsible for making the α(1→4) linkages in glycogen. This enzyme cannot initiate chain synthesis using free glucose as an acceptor of a molecule of glucose from UDP-glucose. Instead, it can only elongate already existing chains of glucose. Therefore, a fragment of glycogen can serve as a primer in cells whose glycogen stores are not totally depleted. In the absence of a

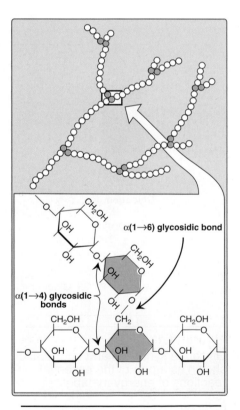

Figure 11.3
Branched structure of glycogen, showing α(1→ 4) and α(1→ 6) glycosidic bonds.

glycogen fragment, a protein, called *glycogenin*, can serve as an acceptor of glucose residues from UDP-glucose (see Figure 11.5). The side chain hydroxyl group of a specific tyrosine serves as the site at which the initial glucosyl unit is attached. The reaction is catalyzed by *glycogenin* itself via autoglucosylation; thus, *glycogenin* is an enzyme. *Glycogenin* then catalyzes the transfer of the next few molecules of glucose from UDP-glucose, producing a short, $\alpha(1\rightarrow4)$-linked glucosyl chain. This short chain serves as a primer that is able to be elongated by *glycogen synthase* as described below [Note: *Glycogenin* stays associated with and forms the core of a glycogen granule.]

C. Elongation of glycogen chains by glycogen synthase

Elongation of a glycogen chain involves the transfer of glucose from UDP-glucose to the nonreducing end of the growing chain, forming a new glycosidic bond between the anomeric hydroxyl of carbon 1 of the activated glucose and carbon 4 of the accepting glucosyl residue (see Figure 11.5). [Note: The nonreducing end of a carbohydrate chain is one in which the anomeric carbon of the terminal sugar is linked by a glycosidic bond to another compound, making the terminal sugar nonreducing (see p. 84).] The enzyme responsible for making the $\alpha(1\rightarrow4)$ linkages in glycogen is *glycogen synthase*. [Note: The UDP released when the new $\alpha(1\rightarrow4)$ glycosidic bond is made can be phosphorylated to UTP by *nucleoside diphosphate kinase* (UDP + ATP $\rightleftarrows$ UTP + ADP, see p. 296).]

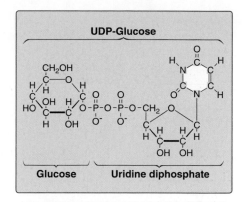

Figure 11.4
The structure of UDP-glucose, a nucleotide sugar.

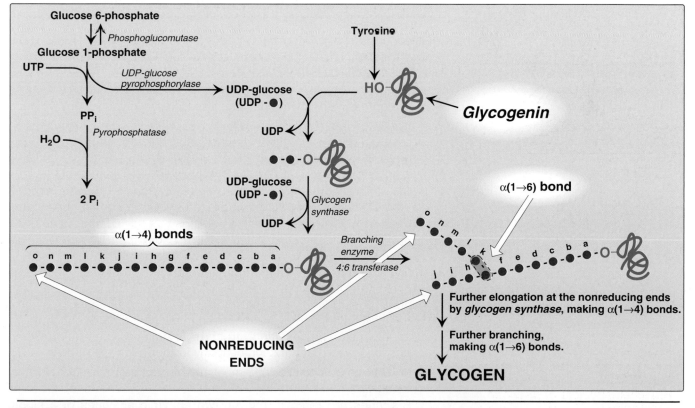

Figure 11.5
Glycogen synthesis.

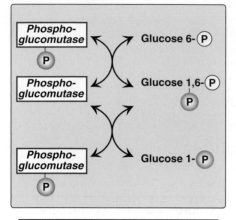

Figure 11.6
Interconversion of glucose 6-phosphate and glucose 1-phosphate by *phosphoglucomutase*.

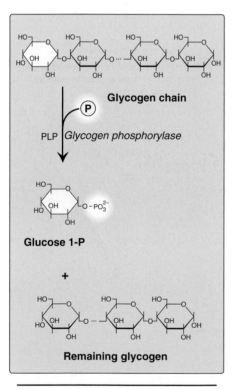

Figure 11.7
Cleavage of an α(1→4)-glycosidic bond. PLP= pyridoxal phosphate.

D. Formation of branches in glycogen

If no other synthetic enzyme acted on the chain, the resulting structure would be a linear (unbranched) molecule of glucosyl residues attached by α(1→4) linkages. Such a compound is found in plant tissues, and is called amylose. In contrast, glycogen has branches located, on average, eight glucosyl residues apart, resulting in a highly branched, tree-like structure (see Figure 11.3) that is far more soluble than the unbranched amylose. Branching also increases the number of nonreducing ends to which new glucosyl residues can be added (and also, as described later, from which these residues can be removed), thereby greatly accelerating the rate at which glycogen synthesis can occur, and dramatically increasing the size of the molecule.

1. **Synthesis of branches:** Branches are made by the action of the branching enzyme, *amylo-α(1→4) → α(1→6)-transglucosidase*. This enzyme removes a chain of six to eight glucosyl residues from the nonreducing end of the glycogen chain, breaking an α(1→4) bond to another residue on the chain, and attaches it to a non-terminal glucosyl residue by an α(1→6) linkage, thus functioning as a *4:6 transferase*. The resulting new, nonreducing end (see "j" in Figure 11.5), as well as the old nonreducing end from which the six to eight residues were removed (see "o" in Figure 11.5), can now be further elongated by *glycogen synthase*.

2. **Synthesis of additional branches:** After elongation of these two ends has been accomplished by *glycogen synthase*, their terminal six to eight glucosyl residues can be removed and used to make additional branches.

IV. DEGRADATION OF GLYCOGEN (GLYCOGENOLYSIS)

The degradative pathway that mobilizes stored glycogen in liver and skeletal muscle is not a reversal of the synthetic reactions. Instead, a separate set of cytosolic enzymes is required. When glycogen is degraded, the primary product is glucose 1-phosphate, obtained by breaking α(1→4) glycosidic bonds. In addition, free glucose is released from each α(1→6)-linked glucosyl residue.

A. Shortening of chains

Glycogen phosphorylase sequentially cleaves the α(1→4) glycosidic bonds between the glucosyl residues at the nonreducing ends of the glycogen chains by simple phosphorolysis (producing glucose 1-phosphate) until four glucosyl units remain on each chain before a branch point (Figure 11.7). [Note: This enzyme contains a molecule of covalently bound pyridoxal phosphate (PLP) that is required as a coenzyme.] The resulting structure is called a limit dextrin, and *phosphorylase* cannot degrade it any further (Figure 11.8).

B. Removal of branches

Branches are removed by the two enzymic activities of a single bifunctional protein, the debranching enzyme (see Figure 11.8). First, *oligo-α(1→4)→α(1→4)-glucan transferase* activity removes the

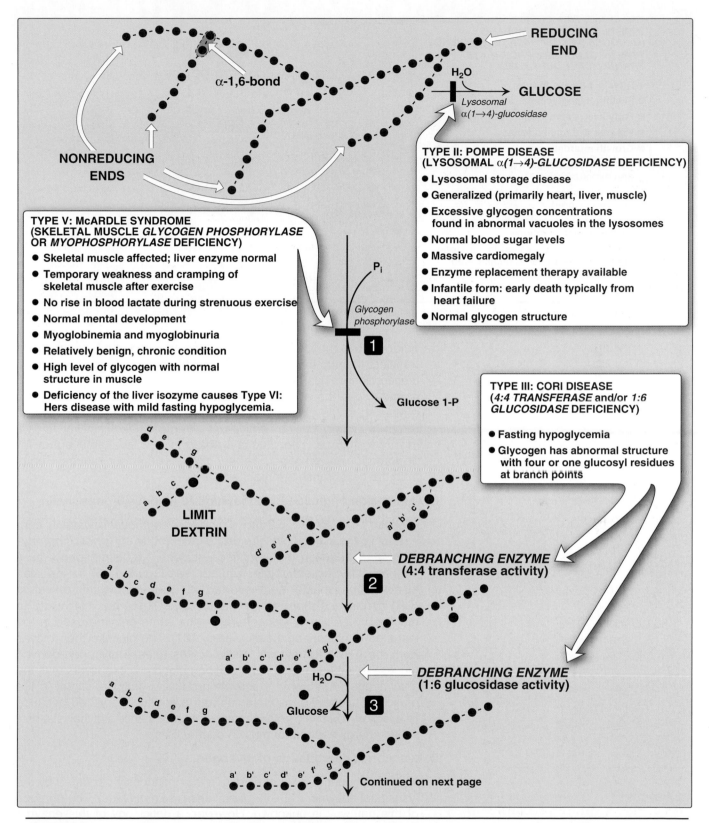

Figure 11.8
Glycogen degradation, showing some of the glycogen storage diseases (GSD). [Note: A GSD can also be caused by defects in *branching enzyme*, an enzyme of synthesis, resulting in Type IV: Andersen disease and causing death in early childhood.](*Continued on next page.*)

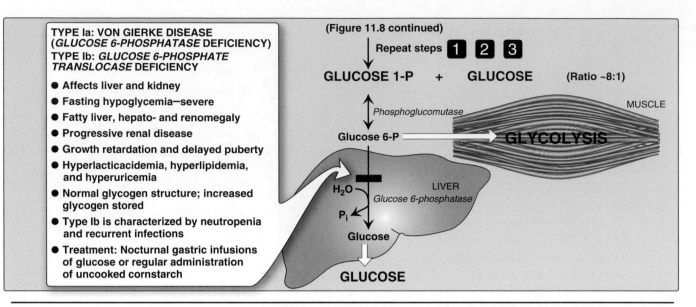

**TYPE Ia: VON GIERKE DISEASE
(*GLUCOSE 6-PHOSPHATASE* DEFICIENCY)
TYPE Ib: *GLUCOSE 6-PHOSPHATE
TRANSLOCASE* DEFICIENCY**

- Affects liver and kidney
- Fasting hypoglycemia—severe
- Fatty liver, hepato- and renomegaly
- Progressive renal disease
- Growth retardation and delayed puberty
- Hyperlacticacidemia, hyperlipidemia, and hyperuricemia
- Normal glycogen structure; increased glycogen stored
- Type Ib is characterized by neutropenia and recurrent infections
- Treatment: Nocturnal gastric infusions of glucose or regular administration of uncooked cornstarch

(Figure 11.8 continued)

Repeat steps **1** **2** **3**

GLUCOSE 1-P   +   GLUCOSE   (Ratio ~8:1)

Phosphoglucomutase

MUSCLE

Glucose 6-P   →   **GLYCOLYSIS**

H_2O

LIVER

Glucose 6-phosphatase

P_i

Glucose

GLUCOSE

Figure 11.8 (*Continued*)

outer three of the four glucosyl residues attached at a branch. It next transfers them to the nonreducing end of another chain, lengthening it accordingly. Thus, an $\alpha(1\rightarrow4)$ bond is broken and an $\alpha(1\rightarrow4)$ bond is made, and the enzyme functions as a *4:4 transferase*. Next, the remaining single glucose residue attached in an $\alpha(1\rightarrow6)$ linkage is removed hydrolytically by *amylo-$\alpha(1\rightarrow6)$-glucosidase* activity, releasing free glucose. The glucosyl chain is now available again for degradation by *glycogen phosphorylase* until four glucosyl units from the next branch are reached.

C. Conversion of glucose 1-phosphate to glucose 6-phosphate

Glucose 1-phosphate, produced by *glycogen phosphorylase*, is converted in the cytosol to glucose 6-phosphate by *phosphoglucomutase*—a reaction that produces glucose 1,6-bisphosphate as a temporary but essential intermediate (see Figure 11.6). In the liver, glucose 6-phosphate is transported into the endoplasmic reticulum (ER) by *glucose 6-phosphate translocase*. There it is converted to glucose by *glucose 6-phosphatase*—the same enzyme used in the last step of gluconeogenesis (see p. 121). The glucose then moves from the ER to the cytosol. Hepatocytes release glycogen-derived glucose into the blood to help maintain blood glucose levels until the gluconeogenic pathway is actively producing glucose. [Note: In the muscle, glucose 6-phosphate cannot be dephosphorylated because of a lack of *glucose 6-phosphatase*. Instead, it enters glycolysis, providing energy needed for muscle contraction.]

D. Lysosomal degradation of glycogen

A small amount (1–3%) of glycogen is continuously degraded by the lysosomal enzyme, $\alpha(1\rightarrow4)$-*glucosidase* (*acid maltase*). The purpose of this pathway is unknown. However, a deficiency of this enzyme causes accumulation of glycogen in vacuoles in the lysosomes, resulting in the serious glycogen storage disease Type II: Pompe disease (see Figure 11.8). [Note: Type II: Pompe disease is the only glycogen storage disease that is a lysosomal storage disease.]

> Lysosomal storage diseases are genetic disorders characterized by the accumulation of abnormal amounts of carbohydrates or lipids primarily due to their decreased lysosomal degradation.

V. REGULATION OF GLYCOGEN SYNTHESIS AND DEGRADATION

Because of the importance of maintaining blood glucose levels, the synthesis and degradation of its glycogen storage form are tightly regulated. In the liver, glycogenesis accelerates during periods when the body has been well fed, whereas glycogenolysis accelerates during periods of fasting. In skeletal muscle, glycogenolysis occurs during active exercise, and glycogenesis begins as soon as the muscle is again at rest. Regulation of glycogen synthesis and degradation is accomplished on two levels. First, *glycogen synthase* and *glycogen phosphorylase* are hormonally regulated to meet the needs of the body as a whole. Second, the pathways of glycogen synthesis and degradation are allosterically controlled to meet the needs of a particular tissue.

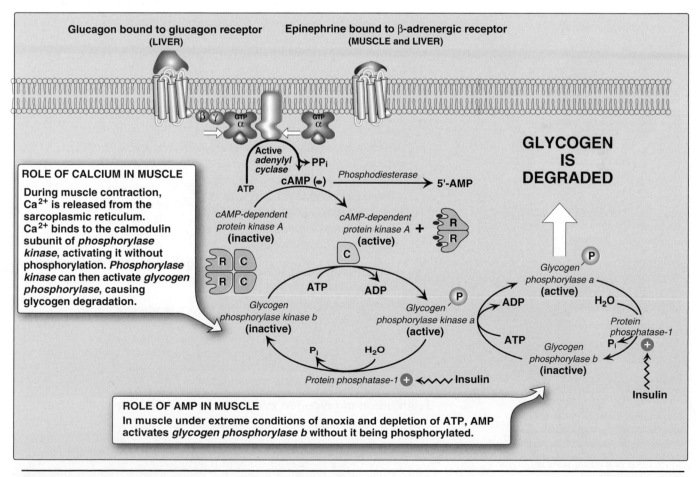

Figure 11.9
Stimulation and inhibition of glycogen degradation.

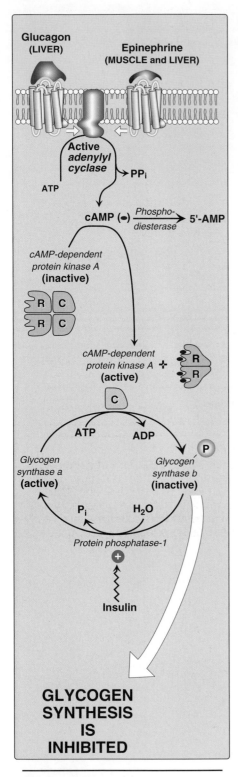

Figure 11.10
Hormonal regulation of glycogen synthesis. [Note: In contrast to *glycogen phosphorylase*, *glycogen synthase* is inactivated by phosphorylation.]

A. Activation of glycogen degradation by cAMP-directed pathway

The binding of hormones, such as glucagon or epinephrine, to plasma membrane G protein-coupled receptors (GPCR) signals the need for glycogen to be degraded—either to elevate blood glucose levels or to provide energy for exercising muscle.

1. **Activation of protein kinase A:** Binding of glucagon or epinephrine to their specific hepatocyte GPCR, or of epinephrine to specific myocyte GPCR, results in the G protein-mediated activation of *adenylyl cyclase*. This enzyme catalyzes the synthesis of cAMP, which activates *cAMP-dependent protein kinase A* (*PKA*), as described on page 95. *PKA* is a tetramer, having two regulatory subunits (R) and two catalytic subunits (C). cAMP binds to the regulatory subunit dimer, releasing individual catalytic subunits that are active (Figure 11.9). *PKA* then phosphorylates several enzymes of glycogen metabolism, affecting their activity. [Note: When cAMP is removed, the inactive tetramer, R_2C_2, is again formed.]

2. **Activation of phosphorylase kinase:** *Phosphorylase kinase* exists in two forms: an inactive "b" form and an active "a" form. Active *PKA* phosphorylates the inactive "b" form of *phosphorylase kinase*, producing the active "a" form (see Figure 11.9). [Note: The phosphorylated enzyme can be inactivated by the hydrolytic removal of its phosphate by *protein phosphatase-1*. This enzyme is activated by a signal cascade initiated by insulin (see p. 311). Insulin also activates the *phosphodiesterase* that degrades cAMP, thus opposing the effects of glucagon and epinephrine.]

3. **Activation of glycogen phosphorylase:** *Glycogen phosphorylase* also exists in two forms: the dephosphorylated, inactive "b" form and the phosphorylated, active "a" form. Active *phosphorylase kinase* phosphorylates *glycogen phosphorylase b* to its active "a" form, which then begins glycogenolysis (see Figure 11.9). *Phosphorylase a* is reconverted to *phosphorylase b* by the hydrolysis of its phosphate by *protein phosphatase-1*. [Note: *Protein phosphatase-1* is inactivated by inhibitor proteins that bind in response to their phosphorylation and activation by *PKA*.]

4. **Summary of the regulation of glycogen degradation:** The cascade of reactions listed above results in glycogenolysis. The large number of sequential steps serves to amplify the effect of the hormonal signal, that is, a few hormone molecules binding to their receptors result in a number of *protein kinase A* molecules being activated that can each activate many *phosphorylase kinase* molecules. This causes the production of many active *glycogen phosphorylase a* molecules that can degrade glycogen.

B. Inhibition of glycogen synthesis by a cAMP-directed pathway

The regulated enzyme in glycogenesis is *glycogen synthase*. It also exists in two forms, the active "a" form and the inactive "b" form. However, for *glycogen synthase*, in contrast to *phosphorylase kinase* and *glycogen phosphorylase*, the active form is dephosphorylated whereas the inactive form is phosphorylated (Figure 11.10). *Glycogen synthase a* is converted to the inactive "b" form by phosphorylation at several sites on the enzyme, with the level of inactivation proportional to its degree of phosphorylation. This conversion process is catalyzed by several different *protein kinases* that are regulated by cAMP or other signaling mechanisms (see C below). *Glycogen synthase b* can be reconverted to the "a" form by *protein phosphatase-1*, which removes the phosphate groups hydrolytically.

C. Allosteric regulation of glycogen synthesis and degradation

In addition to hormonal signals, *glycogen synthase* and *glycogen phosphorylase* respond to the levels of metabolites and energy needs of the cell. Glycogenesis is stimulated when substrate availability and energy levels are high, whereas glycogenolysis is increased when glucose and energy levels are low. This allosteric regulation allows a rapid response to the needs of a cell, and can override the effects of hormone-mediated covalent regulation.

1. Regulation of glycogen synthesis and degradation in the well-fed state:

In the well-fed state, *glycogen synthase b* in both liver and muscle is allosterically activated by glucose 6-phosphate which is present in elevated concentrations (Figure 11.11). In contrast, *glycogen phosphorylase a* is allosterically inhibited by glucose 6-phosphate, as well as by ATP, a high-energy signal in the cell. [Note: In liver, but not muscle, non-phosphorylated glucose is also an allosteric inhibitor of *glycogen phosphorylase a*, making it a better substrate for *protein phosphatase-1*.]

2. Activation of glycogen degradation by calcium:

Ca^{2+} is released into the cytoplasm in muscle in response to neural stimulation and in liver in response to epinephrine binding to α_1-adrenergic receptors. The Ca^{2+} binds to calmodulin, the most widely distributed member of a family of small, calcium-binding proteins. The binding of four molecules of Ca^{2+} to calmodulin triggers a conformational change such that the activated Ca^{2+}-calmodulin complex binds to and activates protein molecules—often enzymes—that are inactive in the absence of this complex (see Figure 11.12). Thus, calmodulin functions as an essential subunit of many complex proteins. One such protein is *phosphorylase kinase b*, which is activated by the Ca^{2+}-calmodulin complex without the need for the *kinase* to be phosphorylated by *PKA*. [Note: Epinephrine at β-adrenergic receptors signals through a rise in cAMP, not calcium (see p. 131).]

a. Calcium activation of muscle phosphorylase kinase:

During muscle contraction, there is a rapid and urgent need for ATP. This energy is supplied by the degradation of muscle glycogen to glucose, which can then enter glycolysis. Nerve impulses cause membrane depolarization, which promotes Ca^{2+} release from the sarcoplasmic reticulum into the sarcoplasm of myocytes. The Ca^{2+} binds calmodulin and the complex activates muscle *phosphorylase kinase b* (see Figure 11.9).

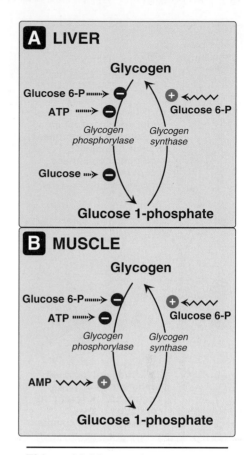

Figure 11.11
Allosteric regulation of glycogen synthesis and degradation.
A. Liver. B. Muscle. [Note: Ca^{2+} indirectly activates phosphorylase in both muscle and liver by directly activating *phosphorylase kinase*.]

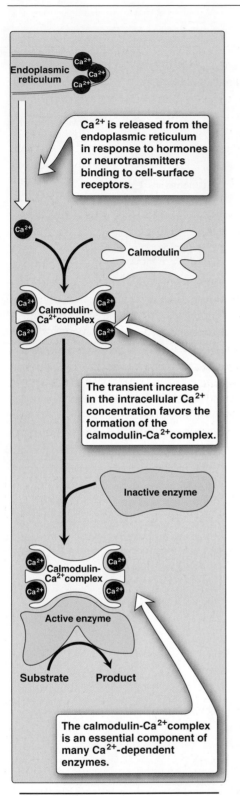

Figure 11.12
Calmodulin mediates many effects of intracellular calcium.

b. Calcium activation of liver phosphorylase kinase: During "fight or flight" situations, epinephrine is released from the adrenal medulla and signals the need for blood glucose. This glucose initially comes from hepatic glycogenolysis. Binding of epinephrine to hepatocyte α-adrenergic G protein-coupled receptors activates a phospholipid-dependent cascade (see p. 205) that results in movement of Ca^{2+} from the ER into the cytoplasm. A Ca^{2+}-calmodulin complex forms and activates hepatic *phosphorylase kinase b*. [Note: The released Ca^{2+} also helps to activate *protein kinase C* that can phosphorylate (thus inactivate) *glycogen synthase a*.]

3. Activation of glycogen degradation in muscle by AMP: Muscle *glycogen phosphorylase* is active in the presence of the high AMP concentrations that occur in the muscle under extreme conditions of anoxia and ATP depletion. AMP binds to *glycogen phosphorylase b*, causing its activation without phosphorylation (see Figure 11.9). [Note: Recall that AMP also activates *PFK-1* of glycolysis (see p. 99).]

VI. GLYCOGEN STORAGE DISEASES

These are a group of genetic diseases that result from a defect in an enzyme required for glycogen synthesis or degradation. They result either in formation of glycogen that has an abnormal structure, or in the accumulation of excessive amounts of normal glycogen in specific tissues as a result of impaired degradation. A particular enzyme may be defective in a single tissue, such as liver (resulting in hypoglycemia) or muscle (muscle weakness), or the defect may be more generalized, affecting liver, muscle, kidney, intestine, and myocardium. The severity of the glycogen storage diseases (GSDs) ranges from fatal in infancy to mild disorders that are not life-threatening. Some of the more prevalent GSDs are illustrated in Figure 11.8.

VII. CHAPTER SUMMARY

The **main stores** of glycogen in the body are found in **skeletal muscle**, where they serve as a **fuel reserve** for the synthesis of ATP during **muscle contraction**, and in the **liver**, where they are used to **maintain the blood glucose** concentration, particularly during the **early stages of a fast**. Glycogen is a **highly branched** polymer of α-D-glucose. The primary glycosidic bond is an **α(1→4) linkage**. After about eight to ten glucosyl residues, there is a **branch** containing an **α(1→6) linkage**. **UDP-glucose**, the **building block** of glycogen, is synthesized from **glucose 1-phosphate** and **UTP** by **UDP-glucose pyrophosphorylase** (Figure 11.13). Glucose from UDP-glucose is transferred to the nonreducing ends of glycogen chains by primer-requiring **glycogen synthase**, which makes α(1→4) linkages. The primer is made by glycogenin. **Branches** are formed by **amylo-α(1→4)→α(1→6)-transglucosidase**, which transfers a chain of six to eight glucosyl residues from the nonreducing end of the glycogen chain (**breaking an α(1→4) linkage**), and attaches it with an **α(1→6) linkage** to another residue in the chain.

PLP-requiring **glycogen phosphorylase** cleaves the α(1→4) **bonds** between glucosyl residues at the **nonreducing ends** of the glycogen chains, producing **glucose 1-phosphate**. This sequential degradation continues until four glucosyl units remain on each chain before a branch point. The resulting structure is called a **limit dextrin** that is degraded by the bifunctional debranching enzyme. **Oligo-α(1→4)→α(1→4)-glucan transferase** (common name, **glucosyl 4:4 transferase**) removes the outer three of the four glucosyl residues attached at a branch, and transfers them to the nonreducing end of another chain where they can be converted to glucose 1-phosphate by glycogen phosphorylase. Next, the remaining single glucose residue attached in an α(1→4) linkage is removed hydrolytically by the **amylo-(1→6) glucosidase** activity of debranching enzyme, releasing **free glucose**. **Glucose 1-phosphate** is converted to **glucose 6-phosphate** by **phosphoglucomutase**. In the **muscle**, glucose 6-phosphate enters glycolysis. In the **liver**, the phosphate is removed by **glucose 6-phosphatase**, releasing **free glucose** that can be used to maintain blood glucose levels at the beginning of a fast. A **deficiency** of the **phosphatase** causes **glycogen storage disease Type 1a** (**Von Gierke disease**). This disease results in an inability of the liver to provide free glucose to the body during a fast. It affects both glycogen degradation and gluconeogenesis. Glycogen synthesis and degradation are reciprocally regulated to meet whole-body needs by the same hormonal signals, namely, an **elevated insulin** level results in overall **increased glycogenesis** and **decreased glycogenolysis**, whereas an **elevated glucagon** (or **epinephrine**) level causes **increased glycogenolysis** and **decreased glycogenesis**. Key enzymes are phosphorylated by a family of **protein kinases**, some of which are **cAMP-dependent** (a compound increased by glucagon and epinephrine). Phosphate groups are removed by protein phosphatase-1 (activated when insulin levels are elevated). **Glycogen synthase, phosphorylase kinase** and **phosphorylase** are also **allosterically regulated** to meet tissues needs. In the well-fed state, **glycogen synthase** is **activated** by **glucose 6-phosphate**, but **glycogen phosphorylase** is inhibited by **glucose 6-phosphate**, as well as by **ATP**. In the liver, glucose also serves an an allosteric inhibitor of glycogen phosphorylase. The **Ca²⁺** released from the endoplasmic reticulum in muscle during exercise and in liver in response to epinephrine **activates phosphorylase kinase** by binding to the enzyme's **calmodulin** subunit. This allows the enzyme to activate **glycogen phosphorylase**, thereby causing glycogen degradation.

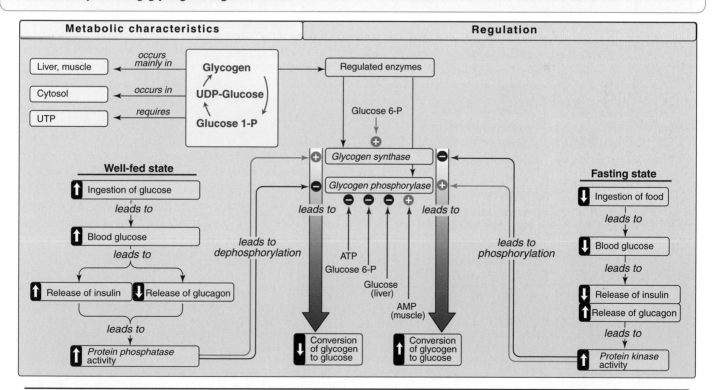

Figure 11.13
Key concept map for glycogen metabolism in liver. [Note: *Glycogen phosphorylase* is phosphorylated by *phosphorylase kinase,* the "b" form of which can be activated by Ca²⁺.]

Study Questions

Choose the ONE correct answer.

11.1 A 2-year-old boy was brought into the emergency room, suffering from severe fasting hypoglycemia. On physical examination, he was found to have hepatomegaly. Laboratory tests indicated that he also had hyperlacticacidemia and hyperuricemia. A liver biopsy indicated that hepatocytes contained greater than normal amounts of glycogen that was of normal structure. Enzyme assay likely confirmed a deficiency in which of the following enzymes?

A. Glycogen synthase

B. Glycogen phosphorylase

C. Glucose 6-phosphatase

D. Amylo-α(1→6)-glucosidase

E. Amylo-α(1→4)→α(1→6)-transglucosidase

Correct answer = C. A deficiency of glucose 6-phosphatase (Von Gierke disease) prevents the liver from releasing free glucose into the blood, causing severe fasting hypoglycemia, hyperlacticacidemia, and hyperuricemia. A deficiency of glycogen phosphorylase would result in a decrease in glycogen degradation, causing fasting hypoglycemia, but not the other symptoms. A deficiency of glycogen synthase would result in lower amounts of stored glycogen. Amylo-α(1→6)-glucosidase removes single glucosyl residues attached to the glycogen chain through an α(1→6)-glycosidic bond. A deficiency in this enzyme would result in a decreased ability of the cell to completely degrade glycogen branches. Amylo-α(1→4)→α(1→6)-transglucosidase deficiency would decrease the ability of the cell to make branches.

11.2 The hormones, epinephrine and glucagon have which one of the following effects on glycogen metabolism in the liver?

A. The net synthesis of glycogen is increased.

B. Glycogen phosphorylase is phosphorylated and active, whereas glycogen synthase is phosphorylated and inactive.

C. Both glycogen phosphorylase and glycogen synthase are activated by phosphorylation but at significantly different rates.

D. Glycogen phosphorylase is inactivated by a rise in Ca^{2+}, whereas glycogen synthase is activated.

E. cAMP-dependent protein kinase A is activated, whereas phosphorylase kinase is inactivated.

Correct answer = B. Epinephrine and glucagon both cause increased glycogen degradation in the liver through covalent modification (phosphorylation) of key enzymes of glycogen metabolism. Glycogen phosphorylase is phosphorylated and active ("a" form), whereas glycogen synthase is phosphorylated and inactive ("b" form). cAMP-dependent protein kinase A is active and phosphorylates (and activates) its substrate, phosphorylase kinase. It is phosphorylase kinase a that directly phosphorylates and activates phosphorylase.

11.3 In contracting skeletal muscle, a sudden elevation of the cytosolic Ca^{2+} concentration will result in:

A. activation of cAMP-dependent protein kinase A.

B. dissociation of cAMP-dependent protein kinase A into catalytic and regulatory subunits.

C. inactivation of phosphorylase kinase caused by the action of protein phosphatase-1.

D. direct activation of phosphorylase kinase b.

E. direct activation of glycogen phosphorylase b.

F. conversion of cAMP to AMP by phosphodiesterase.

Correct answer = D. Ca^{2+} released from the sarcoplasmic reticulum during exercise binds to the calmodulin subunit of phosphorylase kinase, thereby allosterically activating the "b" form of this enzyme. The other choices are not caused by an elevation of cytosolic calcium.

11.4 Explain why the hypoglycemia seen with Type Ia glycogen storage disease (glucose 6-phosphatase deficiency) is severe, whereas that seen with Type VI (liver phosphorylase deficiency) is mild.

With Type Ia, the liver is unable to generate free glucose either from glycogenolysis or gluconeogenesis because both processes produce glucose 6-phosphate. With Type VI, liver is still able to produce free glucose from gluconeogenesis; glycogenolysis, however, is inhibited.

Metabolism of Monosaccharides and Disaccharides

12

I. OVERVIEW

Glucose is the most common monosaccharide consumed by humans, and its metabolism has been discussed extensively. However, two other monosaccharides—fructose and galactose—occur in significant amounts in the diet (primarily in disaccharides), and make important contributions to energy metabolism. In addition, galactose is an important component of cell structural carbohydrates. Figure 12.1 shows the metabolism of fructose and galactose as part of the essential pathways of energy metabolism in the body.

II. FRUCTOSE METABOLISM

About 10% of the calories contained in the Western diet are supplied by fructose (approximately 55 g/day). The major source of fructose is the disaccharide sucrose, which, when cleaved in the intestine, releases equimolar amounts of fructose and glucose. Fructose is also found as a free monosaccharide in many fruits, in honey, and in high-fructose corn syrup (55% fructose/45% glucose typically), which is used to sweeten soft drinks and many foods. Entry of fructose into cells is not insulin-dependent (unlike that of glucose into certain tissues, see p. 97), and, in contrast to glucose, fructose does not promote the secretion of insulin.

A. Phosphorylation of fructose

For fructose to enter the pathways of intermediary metabolism, it must first be phosphorylated (Figure 12.2). This can be accomplished by either *hexokinase* or *fructokinase* (also called *ketohexokinase*). *Hexokinase* phosphorylates glucose in most cells of the body (see p. 98), and several additional hexoses can serve as substrates for this enzyme. However, it has a low affinity (that is, a high K_m, see p. 59) for fructose. Therefore, unless the intracellular concentration of fructose becomes unusually high, the normal presence of saturating concentrations of glucose means that little fructose is converted to fructose 6-phosphate by *hexokinase*. *Fructokinase* provides the primary mechanism for fructose phosphorylation (see Figure 12.2). It is found in the liver (which processes most of the dietary fructose), kidney, and the small intestinal mucosa, and converts fructose to fructose 1-phosphate, using ATP as the phosphate donor. [Note: These three tissues also contain *aldolase B*, discussed below.]

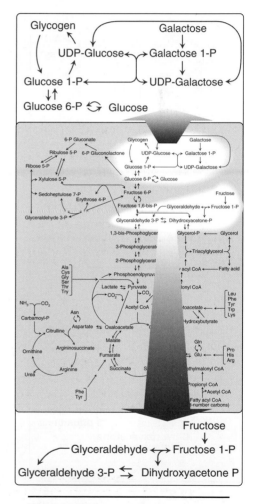

Figure 12.1
Galactose and fructose metabolism as part of the essential pathways of energy metabolism (see Figure 8.2, p. 92, for a more detailed view of the overall reactions of metabolism).

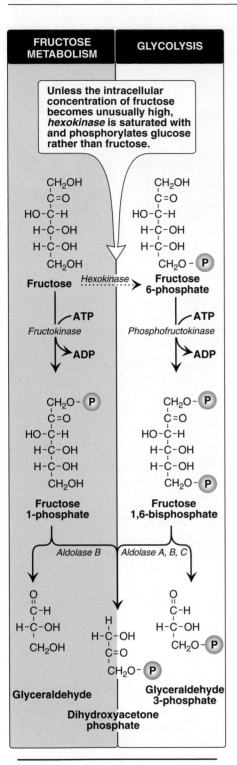

Figure 12.2
Phosphorylation products of fructose
and their cleavage.

B. Cleavage of fructose 1-phosphate

Fructose 1-phosphate is not phosphorylated to fructose 1,6-bis-phosphate as is fructose 6-phosphate (see p. 99), but is cleaved by *aldolase B* (also called *fructose 1-phosphate aldolase*) to dihydroxyacetone phosphate (DHAP) and glyceraldehyde. [Note: Humans express three *aldolases*, A, B and C, the products of three different genes. *Aldolase A* (found in most tissues), *aldolase B* (in liver), and *aldolase C* (in brain) all cleave fructose 1,6-bisphosphate produced during glycolysis to DHAP and glyceraldehyde 3-phosphate (see p. 100), but only *aldolase B* cleaves fructose 1-phosphate.] DHAP can directly enter glycolysis or gluconeogenesis, whereas glyceraldehyde can be metabolized by a number of pathways, as illustrated in Figure 12.3.

C. Kinetics of fructose metabolism

The rate of fructose metabolism is more rapid than that of glucose because the trioses formed from fructose 1-phosphate bypass *phosphofructokinase-1*—the major rate-limiting step in glycolysis (see p. 99).

D. Disorders of fructose metabolism

A deficiency of one of the key enzymes required for the entry of fructose into intermediary metabolic pathways can result in either a benign condition as a result of *fructokinase* deficiency (essential fructosuria), or a severe disturbance of liver and kidney metabolism as a result of *aldolase B* deficiency (hereditary fructose intolerance, HFI), which is estimated to occur in 1:20,000 live births (see Figure 12.3). The first symptoms of HFI appear when a baby is weaned from milk (see p. 142) and begins to be fed food containing sucrose or fructose. Fructose 1-phosphate accumulates, resulting in a drop in the level of inorganic phosphate (P_i) and, therefore, of ATP. As ATP falls, AMP rises. In the absence of P_i, AMP is degraded, causing hyperuricemia (and lactic acidosis, see p. 299). The decreased availability of hepatic ATP affects gluconeogenesis (causing hypoglycemia with vomiting), and protein synthesis (causing a decrease in blood clotting factors and other essential proteins). Kidney function may also be affected. Diagnosis of HFI can be made on the basis of fructose in the urine, enzyme assay or by DNA-based testing (see Chapter 33). In some states HFI is part of the newborn screening panel. With HFI, sucrose and sorbitol (a sugar alcohol), as well as fructose, must be removed from the diet to prevent liver failure and possible death. Individuals with HFI display an aversion to sweets and, consequently, have an absence of dental caries.

E. Conversion of mannose to fructose 6-phosphate

Mannose, the C-2 epimer of glucose (see p. 84), is an important component of glycoproteins (see p. 166). *Hexokinase* phosphorylates mannose, producing mannose 6-phosphate, which, in turn, is (reversibly) isomerized to fructose 6-phosphate by *phosphomannose isomerase*. [Note: There is little mannose in dietary carbohydrates. Most intracellular mannose is synthesized from fructose, or is preexisting mannose produced by the degradation of structural carbohydrates and salvaged by *hexokinase*.]

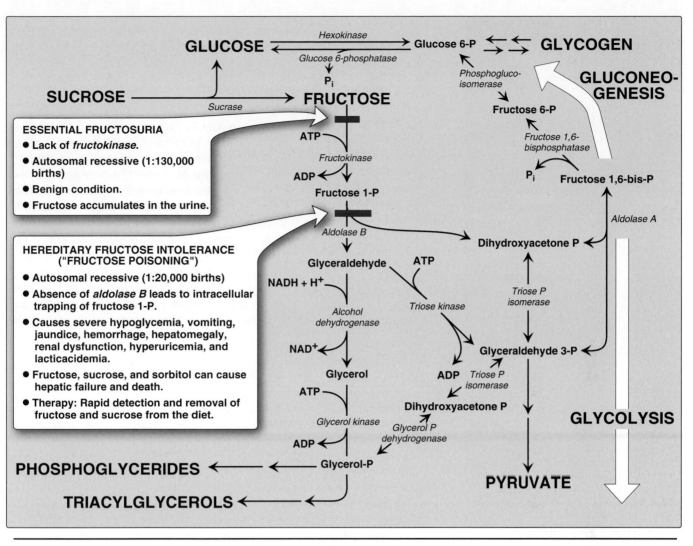

Figure 12.3
Summary of fructose metabolism.

F. Conversion of glucose to fructose via sorbitol

Most sugars are rapidly phosphorylated following their entry into cells. They are thereby trapped within the cells, because organic phosphates cannot freely cross membranes without specific transporters. An alternate mechanism for metabolizing a monosaccharide is to convert it to a polyol (sugar alcohol) by the reduction of an aldehyde group, thereby producing an additional hydroxyl group.

1. **Synthesis of sorbitol:** *Aldose reductase* reduces glucose, producing sorbitol (glucitol, Figure 12.4). This enzyme is found in many tissues, including the lens, retina, Schwann cells of peripheral nerves, liver, kidney, placenta, red blood cells, and in cells of the ovaries and seminal vesicles. In cells of the liver, ovaries, and seminal vesicles, there is a second enzyme, *sorbitol dehydrogenase,* which can oxidize the sorbitol to produce fructose (see Figure 12.4). The two-reaction pathway from glucose to fructose in the seminal vesicles is for the benefit of sperm cells, which use fructose as a major carbohydrate energy source. The pathway

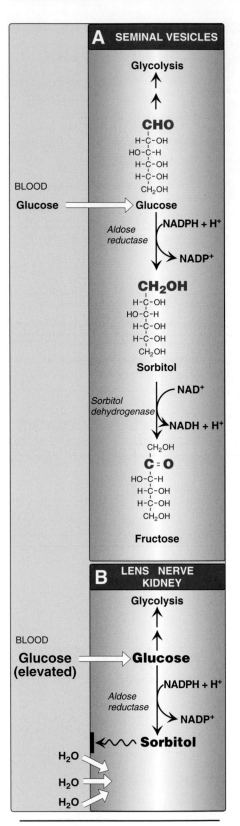

Figure 12.4
Sorbitol metabolism.

from sorbitol to fructose in the liver provides a mechanism by which any available sorbitol is converted into a substrate that can enter glycolysis or gluconeogenesis.

2. **The effect of hyperglycemia on sorbitol metabolism:** Because insulin is not required for the entry of glucose into the cells listed in the previous paragraph, large amounts of glucose may enter these cells during times of hyperglycemia, for example, in uncontrolled diabetes. Elevated intracellular glucose concentrations and an adequate supply of NADPH cause *aldose reductase* to produce a significant increase in the amount of sorbitol, which cannot pass efficiently through cell membranes and, therefore, remains trapped inside the cell (see Figure 12.4). This is exacerbated when *sorbitol dehydrogenase* is low or absent, for example, in retina, lens, kidney, and nerve cells. As a result, sorbitol accumulates in these cells, causing strong osmotic effects and, therefore, cell swelling as a result of water retention. Some of the pathologic alterations associated with diabetes can be attributed, in part, to this phenomenon, including cataract formation, peripheral neuropathy, and microvascular problems leading to nephropathy and retinopathy. (See p. 344 for a discussion of the complications of diabetes.)

III. GALACTOSE METABOLISM

The major dietary source of galactose is lactose (galactosyl β-1,4-glucose) obtained from milk and milk products. [Note: The digestion of lactose by *β-galactosidase* (*lactase*) of the intestinal mucosal cell membrane was discussed on p. 87.] Some galactose can also be obtained by lysosomal degradation of complex carbohydrates, such as glycoproteins and glycolipids, which are important membrane components. Like fructose, the entry of galactose into cells is not insulin-dependent.

A. Phosphorylation of galactose

Like fructose, galactose must be phosphorylated before it can be further metabolized. Most tissues have a specific enzyme for this purpose, *galactokinase*, which produces galactose 1-phosphate (Figure 12.5). As with other *kinases*, ATP is the phosphate donor.

B. Formation of UDP-galactose

Galactose 1-phosphate cannot enter the glycolytic pathway unless it is first converted to UDP-galactose (see Figure 12.5). This occurs in an exchange reaction, in which UDP-glucose reacts with galactose 1-phosphate, producing UDP-galactose and glucose 1-phosphate (Figure 12.6). The enzyme that catalyzes this reaction is *galactose 1-phosphate uridyltransferase* (*GALT*).

C. Use of UDP-galactose as a carbon source for glycolysis or gluconeogenesis

For UDP-galactose to enter the mainstream of glucose metabolism, it must first be converted to its C-4 epimer, UDP-glucose, by *UDP-hexose 4-epimerase*. This "new" UDP-glucose (produced from the original UDP-galactose) can then participate in many biosynthetic

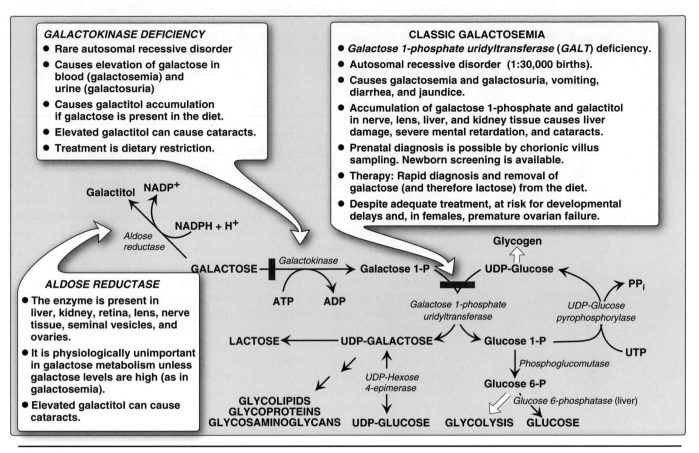

GALACTOKINASE DEFICIENCY
- **Rare autosomal recessive disorder**
- **Causes elevation of galactose in blood (galactosemia) and urine (galactosuria)**
- **Causes galactitol accumulation if galactose is present in the diet.**
- **Elevated galactitol can cause cataracts.**
- **Treatment is dietary restriction.**

CLASSIC GALACTOSEMIA
- *Galactose 1-phosphate uridyltransferase (GALT)* **deficiency.**
- **Autosomal recessive disorder (1:30,000 births).**
- **Causes galactosemia and galactosuria, vomiting, diarrhea, and jaundice.**
- **Accumulation of galactose 1-phosphate and galactitol in nerve, lens, liver, and kidney tissue causes liver damage, severe mental retardation, and cataracts.**
- **Prenatal diagnosis is possible by chorionic villus sampling. Newborn screening is available.**
- **Therapy: Rapid diagnosis and removal of galactose (and therefore lactose) from the diet.**
- **Despite adequate treatment, at risk for developmental delays and, in females, premature ovarian failure.**

ALDOSE REDUCTASE
- **The enzyme is present in liver, kidney, retina, lens, nerve tissue, seminal vesicles, and ovaries.**
- **It is physiologically unimportant in galactose metabolism unless galactose levels are high (as in galactosemia).**
- **Elevated galactitol can cause cataracts.**

Figure 12.5
Metabolism of galactose.

reactions, as well as being used in the *GALT* reaction described above. (See Figure 12.5 for a summary of this interconversion.) [Note: Rare deficiencies of the *epimerase* are known.]

D. Role of UDP-galactose in biosynthetic reactions

UDP-galactose can serve as the donor of galactose units in a number of synthetic pathways, including synthesis of lactose (see below), glycoproteins (see p. 166), glycolipids (see p. 210), and glycosaminoglycans (see p. 160). [Note: If galactose is not provided by the diet (for example, when it cannot be released from lactose as a result of a lack of *β-galactosidase* in people who are lactose-intolerant), all tissue requirements for UDP-galactose can be met by the action of *UDP-hexose 4-epimerase* on UDP-glucose, which is efficiently produced from glucose 1-phosphate (see Figure 12.5).]

E. Disorders of galactose metabolism

GALT is deficient in individuals with classic galactosemia (see Figure 12.5). In this disorder, galactose 1-phosphate and, therefore, galactose accumulate in cells. Physiologic consequences are similar to those found in hereditary fructose intolerance (see p. 138), but a broader spectrum of tissues is affected. The accumulated galactose is shunted into side pathways such as that of galactitol production.

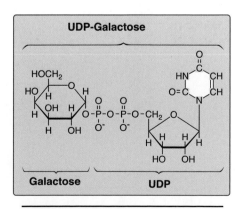

Figure 12.6
Structure of UDP-galactose.

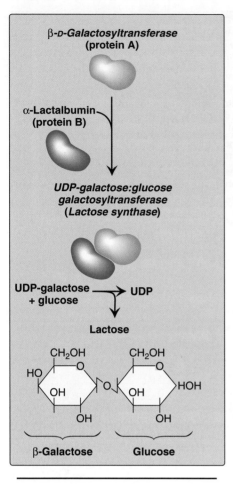

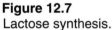

Figure 12.7
Lactose synthesis.

This reaction is catalyzed by *aldose reductase,* the same enzyme that converts glucose to sorbitol (see p. 139). [Note: A deficiency in *galactokinase* results in a less severe disorder of galactosemia metabolism, although cataracts are common (see Figure 12.5).]

IV. LACTOSE SYNTHESIS

Lactose is a disaccharide that consists of a molecule of β-galactose attached by a β(1→4) linkage to glucose. Therefore, lactose is galactosyl β(1→4)-glucose. Lactose, known as the "milk sugar," is produced by the mammary glands of most mammals. Therefore, milk and other dairy products are the dietary sources of lactose. Lactose is synthesized in the Golgi by *lactose synthase (UDP-galactose:glucose galactosyltransferase),* which transfers galactose from UDP-galactose to glucose, releasing UDP (Figure 12.7). This enzyme is composed of two proteins, A and B. Protein A is a *β-D-galactosyltransferase,* and is found in a number of body tissues. In tissues other than the lactating mammary gland, this enzyme transfers galactose from UDP-galactose to N-acetyl-D-glucosamine, forming the same β(1→4) linkage found in lactose, and producing N-acetyllactosamine—a component of the structurally important N-linked glycoproteins (see p. 167). In contrast, protein B is found only in lactating mammary glands. It is α-lactalbumin, and its synthesis is stimulated by the peptide hormone, prolactin. Protein B forms a complex with the enzyme, protein A, changing the specificity of that *transferase* so that lactose, rather than N-acetyllactosamine, is produced (see Figure 12.7).

V. CHAPTER SUMMARY

The major source of fructose is **sucrose**, which when cleaved releases equimolar amounts of fructose and glucose (Figure 12.8). Entry of fructose into cells is **insulin-independent**. Fructose is first phosphorylated to **fructose 1-phosphate** by **fructokinase**, and then cleaved by **aldolase B** to **dihydroxyacetone phosphate** and **glyceraldehyde**. These enzymes are found in the **liver**, **kidney**, and **small intestinal mucosa**. A **deficiency** of **fructokinase** causes a benign condition (**essential fructosuria**), but a **deficiency** of **aldolase B** causes **hereditary fructose intolerance (HFI)**, in which **severe hypoglycemia** and **liver failure** lead to **death** if fructose (and sucrose) in the diet is not severely limited. **Mannose**, an important component of **glycoproteins**, is phosphorylated by **hexokinase** to **mannose 6-phosphate**, which is reversibly isomerized to **fructose 6-phosphate** by **phosphomannose isomerase**. **Glucose** can be reduced to **sorbitol (glucitol)** by **aldose reductase** in many tissues, including the **lens**, **retina**, **Schwann cells**, **liver**, **kidney**, **ovaries**, and **seminal vesicles**. In cells of the **liver**, **ovaries**, and **seminal vesicles**, a second enzyme, **sorbitol dehydrogenase**, can oxidize sorbitol to produce **fructose**. **Hyperglycemia** results in the accumulation of sorbitol in those cells lacking sorbitol dehydrogenase. The resulting **osmotic events** cause cell swelling, and may contribute to the **cataract formation**, **peripheral** neuropathy, nephropathy, and retinopathy seen in diabetes. The major dietary source of galactose is lactose. The entry of galactose into cells is not insulin-dependent. Galactose is first phosphorylated by galactokinase (deficiency results in cataracts) to galactose 1-phosphate. This compound is converted to UDP-galactose by galactose 1-phosphate uridyltransferase (GALT), with the nucleotide supplied by UDP-glucose. A deficiency of this enzyme causes classic galactosemia. Galactose 1-phosphate accumulates, and excess galactose is converted to galactitol by aldose reductase. This causes liver damage, severe mental retardation, and cataracts. Treatment requires removal of galactose (and lactose) from the diet. For UDP-galactose to enter the mainstream of glucose metabolism, it must first be converted to UDP-glucose by UDP-hexose 4-epimerase. This enzyme can also be used to produce UDP-galactose from UDP-glucose when the former is required for the synthesis of structural carbohydrates. Lactose is a disaccharide that consists of galactose and glucose. Milk and other dairy products are the dietary sources of lactose. Lactose is synthesized by lactose synthase from UDP-galactose and glucose in the lactating mammary gland. The enzyme has two subunits, protein A (which is a galactosyl transferase found in most cells where it synthesizes N-acetyllactosamine) and protein B (α-lactalbumin, which is found only in the lactating mammary glands, and whose synthesis is stimulated by the peptide hormone, prolactin). When both subunits are present, the transferase produces lactose.

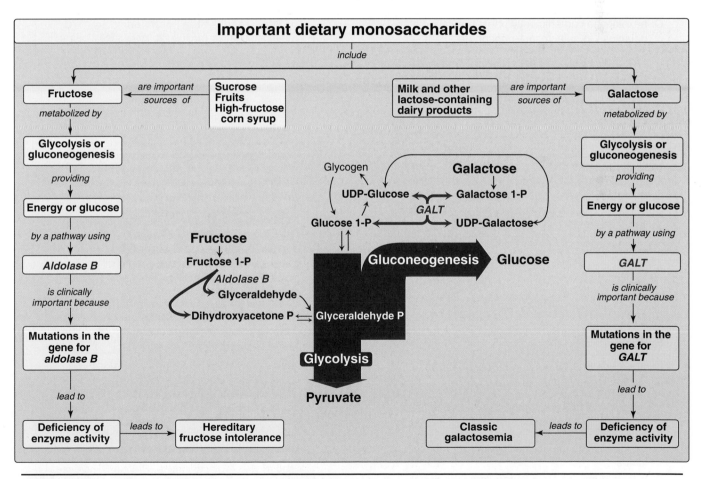

Figure 12.8
Key concept map for metabolism of fructose and galactose. [Note: *GALT* is *galactose 1-phosphate uridyltransferase.*]

Study Questions

Choose the ONE correct answer

12.1 Following the intravenous injection of lactose into a rat, none of the lactose is metabolized. However, ingestion of lactose leads to rapid metabolism of this disaccharide. The difference in these observations is a result of:

A. the presence of lactase in the serum.

B. the absence of hepatic galactokinase.

C. the absence of maltase in the serum.

D. the presence of lactase in the intestine.

Correct answer = D. Lactase and maltase are intestinal enzymes not found in the serum. Therefore, ingested lactose is degraded, but injected lactose is not. If hepatic galactokinase is absent, the galactose segment of the lactose is not metabolized, but the glucose segment of the lactose can still be metabolized.

12.2 A female with classic galactosemia due to GALT deficiency is able to produce lactose in breast milk because:

A. free (nonphosphorylated) galactose is the acceptor of glucose transferred by lactose synthase in the synthesis of lactose.

B. galactose can be produced from a glucose metabolite by epimerization.

C. hexokinase can efficiently phosphorylate dietary galactose to galactose 1-phosphate.

D. the enzyme deficient in galactosemia is activated by a hormone produced in the mammary gland.

E. galactose can be produced from fructose by isomerization.

Correct answer = B. UDP-hexose 4-epimerase converts UDP-glucose to UDP-galactose, thus providing the appropriate form of galactose for lactose synthesis. UDP-galactose, not free galactose, is the source of the galactose portion of lactose. Galactose is not converted to galactose 1-phosphate by hexokinase. Galactosemia is the result of a deficiency in GALT. Isomerization of fructose to galactose does not occur in the human body.

12.3 A 5-month-old boy is brought to his physician because of vomiting, night sweats, and tremors. History revealed that these symptoms began after fruit juices were introduced to his diet as he was being weaned off breast milk. The physical examination was remarkable for hepatomegaly. Tests on the baby's urine were positive for reducing sugar but negative for glucose. The infant most likely suffers from:

A. aldolase B deficiency.

B. fructokinase deficiency.

C. galactokinase deficiency.

D. β-galactosidase deficiency.

E. glucose 6-phosphatase deficiency.

Correct answer = A. The symptoms suggest fructose intolerance, a deficiency in aldolase B. Deficiencies in fructokinase or galactokinase result in relatively benign conditions characterized by elevated levels of fructose or galactose in the blood and urine. Deficiency in β–galactosidase (lactase) results in a decreased ability to degrade lactose (milk sugar). Congenital lactase deficiency is quite rare and would have presented much earlier in this baby, and with different symptoms. Typical lactase deficiency (adult hypolactasia) presents at a later age. The symptoms of glucose 6-phosphatase deficiency would result from fasting, and would not be related to ingestion of fruit juice.

12.4 Lactose synthesis is essential in the production of milk by mammary glands. In lactose synthesis:

A. galactose from galactose 1-P is transferred to glucose by galactosyltransferase (protein A), generating lactose.

B. protein A is used exclusively in the synthesis of lactose.

C. α-lactalbumin (protein B) regulates the sugar specificity of protein A by increasing its K_m for glucose.

D. protein B expression is stimulated by prolactin.

Correct answer = D. The expression of α-lactalbumin (protein B) is increased by the hormone, prolactin. UDP-galactose is the form used by the galactosyltransferase (protein A). Protein A is also involved in the synthesis of the amino sugar, N-acetyllactosamine. Protein B increases the affinity of protein A for glucose, and so decreases the K_m.

Pentose Phosphate Pathway and NADPH

13

I. OVERVIEW

The pentose phosphate pathway (also called the hexose monophosphate pathway, or 6-phosphogluconate pathway) occurs in the cytosol of the cell. It includes two, irreversible oxidative reactions, followed by a series of reversible sugar–phosphate interconversions (Figure 13.1). No ATP is directly consumed or produced in the cycle. Carbon 1 of glucose 6-phosphate is released as CO_2, and two NADPH are produced for each glucose 6-phosphate molecule entering the oxidative part of the pathway. The rate and direction of the reversible reactions of the pentose phosphate pathway are determined by the supply of and demand for intermediates of the cycle. The pathway provides a major portion of the body's NADPH, which functions as a biochemical reductant. It also produces ribose 5-phosphate, required for the biosynthesis of nucleotides (see p. 293), and provides a mechanism for the metabolic use of five-carbon sugars obtained from the diet or the degradation of structural carbohydrates in the body.

II. IRREVERSIBLE OXIDATIVE REACTIONS

The oxidative portion of the pentose phosphate pathway consists of three reactions that lead to the formation of ribulose 5-phosphate, CO_2, and two molecules of NADPH for each molecule of glucose 6-phosphate oxidized (Figure 13.2). This portion of the pathway is particularly important in the liver, lactating mammary glands, and adipose, which are active in the NADPH-dependent biosynthesis of fatty acids (see p. 186), in the testes, ovaries, placenta and adrenal cortex, which are active in the NADPH-dependent biosynthesis of steroid hormones (see p. 237), and in erythrocytes, which require NADPH to keep glutathione reduced (see p. 152).

A. Dehydrogenation of glucose 6-phosphate

Glucose 6-phosphate dehydrogenase (*G6PD*) catalyzes an irreversible oxidation of glucose 6-phosphate to 6-phosphogluconolactone in a reaction that is specific for $NADP^+$ as its coenzyme. The pentose phosphate pathway is regulated primarily at the *G6PD* reaction. NADPH is a potent competitive inhibitor of the enzyme,

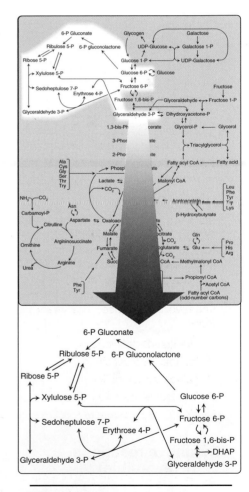

Figure 13.1
Hexose monophosphate pathway shown as a component of the metabolic map (see Figure 8.2, p. 92 for a more detailed view of the metabolic pathway).

and, under most metabolic conditions, the ratio of NADPH/NADP$^+$ is sufficiently high to substantially inhibit enzyme activity. However, with increased demand for NADPH, the ratio of NADPH/NADP$^+$ decreases and flux through the cycle increases in response to the enhanced activity of *G6PD*. Insulin upregulates expression of the gene for *G6PD*, and flux through the pathway increases in the well-fed state.

B. Formation of ribulose 5-phosphate

6-Phosphogluconolactone is hydrolyzed by *6-phosphogluconolactone hydrolase.* The reaction is irreversible and not rate-limiting. The oxidative decarboxylation of the product, 6-phosphogluconate is catalyzed by *6-phosphogluconate dehydrogenase.* This irreversible reaction produces a pentose sugar–phosphate (ribulose 5-phosphate), CO_2 (from carbon 1 of glucose), and a second molecule of NADPH (see Figure 13.2).

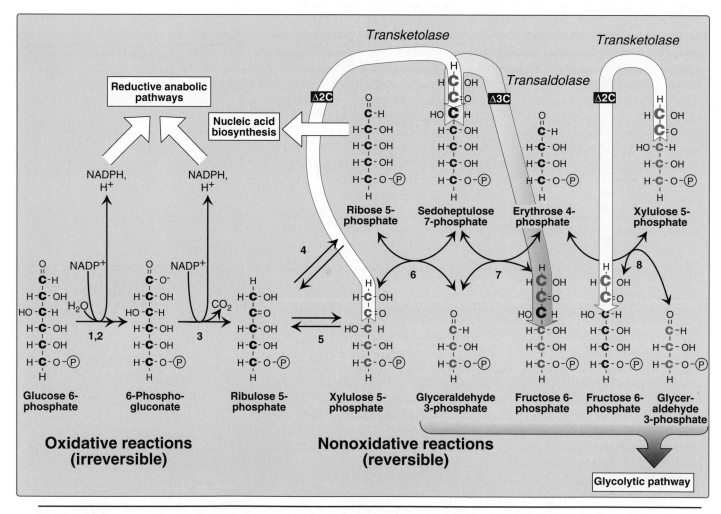

Figure 13.2

Reactions of the hexose monophosphate pathway. Enzymes numbered above are: 1,2) *glucose 6-phosphate dehydrogenase* and *6-phosphogluconolactone hydrolase*, 3) *6-phosphogluconate dehydrogenase*, 4) *ribose 5-phosphate isomerase*, 5) *phosphopentose epimerase*, 6) and 8) *transketolase* (coenzyme: thiamine pyrophosphate), and 7) *transaldolase*. Δ2C = two carbons are transferred in *transketolase* reactions; Δ3C = three carbons are transferred in the *transaldolase* reaction.

III. REVERSIBLE NONOXIDATIVE REACTIONS

The nonoxidative reactions of the pentose phosphate pathway occur in all cell types synthesizing nucleotides and nucleic acids. These reactions catalyze the interconversion of sugars containing three to seven carbons (see Figure 13.2). These reversible reactions permit ribulose 5-phosphate (produced by the oxidative portion of the pathway) to be converted either to ribose 5-phosphate (needed for nucleotide synthesis, see p. 293) or to intermediates of glycolysis—fructose 6-phosphate and glyceraldehyde 3-phosphate. For example, many cells that carry out reductive biosynthetic reactions have a greater need for NADPH than for ribose 5-phosphate. In this case, *transketolase* (which transfers two-carbon units in a thiamine pyrophosphate (TPP)-requiring reaction) and *transaldolase* (which transfers three-carbon units) convert the ribulose 5-phosphate produced as an endproduct of the oxidative reactions to glyceraldehyde 3-phosphate and fructose 6-phosphate, which are intermediates of glycolysis. In contrast, under conditions in which the demand for ribose for incorporation into nucleotides and nucleic acids is greater than the need for NADPH, the nonoxidative reactions can provide the biosynthesis of ribose 5-phosphate from glyceraldehyde 3-phosphate and fructose 6-phosphate in the absence of the oxidative steps (Figure 13.3).

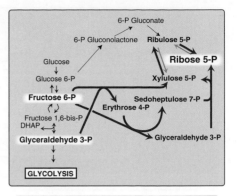

Figure 13.3
Formation of ribose 5-phosphate from intermediates of glycolysis.

> In addition to *transketolases*, thiamine pyrophosphate is required by the enzyme complexes *pyruvate dehydrogenase*, *α-ketoglutarate dehydrogenase* of the TCA cycle, and *branched-chain α-keto acid dehydrogenase* of branched-chain amino acid metabolism (see p. 266).

IV. USES OF NADPH

The coenzyme NADP$^+$ differs from NAD$^+$ only by the presence of a phosphate group on one of the ribose units (Figure 13.4). This seemingly small change in structure allows NADP$^+$ to interact with NADP$^+$-specific enzymes that have unique roles in the cell. For example, in the cytosol of hepatocytes the steady-state ratio of NADP$^+$/NADPH is approximately 0.1, which favors the use of NADPH in reductive biosynthetic reactions. This contrasts with the high ratio of NAD$^+$/NADH (approximately 1000), which favors an oxidative role for NAD$^+$. This section summarizes some important NADP$^+$ or NADPH-specific functions.

A. Reductive biosynthesis

NADPH can be thought of as a high-energy molecule, much in the same way as NADH. However, the electrons of NADPH are destined for use in reductive biosynthesis, rather than for transfer to oxygen as is the case with NADH (see p. 75). Thus, in the metabolic transformations of the pentose phosphate pathway, part of the energy of glucose 6-phosphate is conserved in NADPH—a molecule with a negative reduction potential (see p. 77) that, therefore, can be used in reactions requiring an electron donor.

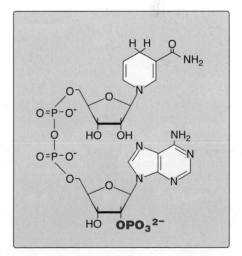

Figure 13.4
Structure of NADPH.

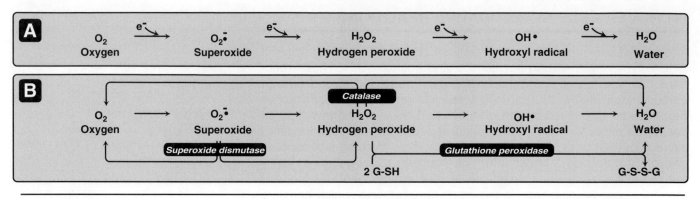

Figure 13.5
A. Formation of reactive intermediates from molecular oxygen. B. Actions of antioxidant enzymes. G-SH = reduced glutathione; G-S-S-G = oxidized glutathione.

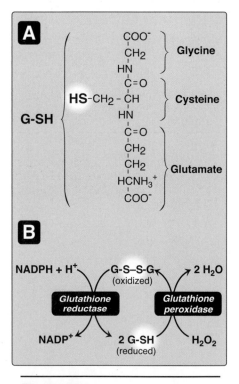

Figure 13.6
A. Structure of glutathione (G-SH).
[Note: Glutamate is linked to cysteine through a γ-carboxyl, rather than an α-carboxyl.] B. Glutathione-mediated reduction of hydrogen peroxide by NADPH.

B. Reduction of hydrogen peroxide

Hydrogen peroxide is one of a family of reactive oxygen species (ROS) that are formed from the partial reduction of molecular oxygen (Figure 13.5A). These compounds are formed continuously as by-products of aerobic metabolism, through reactions with drugs and environmental toxins, or when the level of antioxidants is diminished, all creating the condition of oxidative stress. The highly reactive oxygen intermediates can cause serious chemical damage to DNA, proteins, and unsaturated lipids, and can lead to cell death. These ROS have been implicated in a number of pathologic processes, including reperfusion injury, cancer, inflammatory disease, and aging. The cell has several protective mechanisms that minimize the toxic potential of these compounds.

1. **Enzymes that catalyze antioxidant reactions:** Reduced glutathione, a tripeptide-thiol (γ-glutamylcysteinylglycine) present in most cells, can chemically detoxify hydrogen peroxide (Figure 13.5B). This reaction, catalyzed by the selenium-requiring *glutathione peroxidase*, forms oxidized glutathione, which no longer has protective properties. The cell regenerates reduced glutathione in a reaction catalyzed by *glutathione reductase,* using NADPH as a source of reducing equivalents. Thus, NADPH indirectly provides electrons for the reduction of hydrogen peroxide (Figure 13.6). [Note: Erythrocytes are totally dependent on the pentose phosphate pathway for their supply of NADPH because, unlike other cell types, erythrocytes do not have an alternate source for this essential coenzyme.] Additional enzymes, such as *superoxide dismutase* and *catalase*, catalyze the conversion of other toxic oxygen intermediates to harmless products (see Figure 13.5B). As a group, these enzymes serve as a defense system to guard against the toxic effects of reactive oxygen species.

2. **Antioxidant chemicals:** A number of intracellular reducing agents, such as ascorbate (see p. 377), vitamin E (see p. 391), and β-carotene (see p. 382), are able to reduce and, thus, detoxify oxygen intermediates in the laboratory. Consumption of foods rich in these antioxidant compounds has been correlated with a

reduced risk for certain types of cancers, as well as decreased frequency of certain other chronic health problems. Thus, it is tempting to speculate that the effects of these compounds are, in part, an expression of their ability to quench the toxic effect of oxygen intermediates. However, clinical trials with antioxidants as dietary supplements have failed to show clear beneficial effects. In the case of dietary supplementation with β-carotene, the rate of lung cancer in smokers increased rather than decreased. Thus, the health-promoting effects of dietary fruits and vegetables probably reflects a complex interaction among many naturally occurring compounds, which has not been duplicated by consumption of isolated antioxidant compounds.

C. Cytochrome P450 monooxygenase system

Monooxygenases (*mixed function oxidases*) incorporate one atom from molecular oxygen into a substrate (creating a hydroxyl group), with the other atom being reduced to water. In the *cytochrome P450 monooxygenase* system, NADPH provides the reducing equivalents required by this series of reactions (Figure 13.7). This system performs different functions in two separate locations in cells. The overall reaction catalyzed by a cytochrome P450 enzyme is:

$$R\text{-}H + O_2 + NADPH + H^+ \rightarrow R\text{-}OH + H_2O + NADP^+$$

where R may be a steroid, drug, or other chemical. [Note: Cytochrome P450s (CYPs) are actually a superfamily of related, heme-containing *monooxygenase* enzymes that participate in a broad variety of reactions. The name P450 reflects the absorbance at 450 nm by the protein.]

1. **Mitochondrial system:** The function of the mitochondrial *cytochrome P450 monooxygenase* system found associated with the inner mitochondrial membrane is the biosynthesis of steroid hormones. In steroidogenic tissues, such as the placenta, ovaries, testes, and adrenal cortex, it is used to hydroxylate intermediates in the conversion of cholesterol to steroid hormones, a process that makes these hydrophobic compounds more water-soluble (see p. 237). The liver uses this same system in bile acid synthesis (see p. 224) and in the hydroxylation of cholecalciferol to 25-hydroxycholecalciferol (vitamin D_3, see p. 386), and the kidney uses it to hydroxylate vitamin D_3 to its biologically active 1,25-dihydroxylated form.

2. **Microsomal system:** An extremely important function of the microsomal *cytochrome P450 monooxygenase* system found associated with the membranes of the smooth endoplasmic reticulum (particularly in the liver) is the detoxification of foreign compounds (xenobiotics). These include numerous drugs and such varied pollutants as petroleum products and pesticides. The microsomal system can be used to hydroxylate these toxins, again using NADPH as the source of reducing equivalents. The purpose of these modifications is two-fold. First, it may itself activate or inactivate a drug or second, make a toxic compound more soluble, thus facilitating its excretion in the urine or feces. Frequently, however,

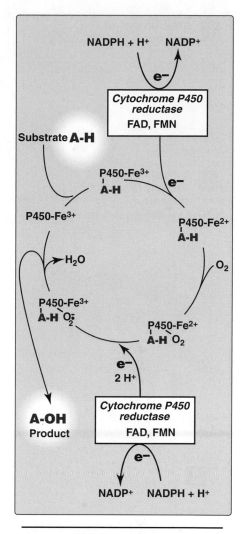

Figure 13.7
Cytochrome P450 monooxygenase cycle. Electrons move from NADPH to FAD to FMN and then to the heme iron.

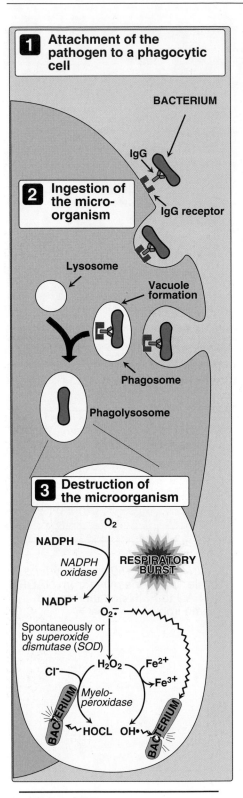

Figure 13.8
Phagocytosis and the oxygen-dependent pathway of microbial killing. IgG = the antibody immunoglobulin G.

the new hydroxyl group will serve as a site for conjugation with a polar molecule, such as glucuronic acid (see p. 161), which will significantly increase the compound's solubility.

D. Phagocytosis by white blood cells

Phagocytosis is the ingestion by receptor-mediated endocytosis of microorganisms, foreign particles, and cellular debris by cells such as neutrophils and macrophages (monocytes). It is an important body defense mechanism, particularly in bacterial infections. Neutrophils and monocytes are armed with both oxygen-independent and oxygen-dependent mechanisms for killing bacteria.

1. **Oxygen-independent mechanism:** Oxygen-independent mechanisms use pH changes in phagolysosomes and lysosomal enzymes to destroy pathogens.

2. **Oxygen-dependent system:** Oxygen-dependent mechanisms include the enzymes, *NADPH oxidase* and *myeloperoxidase* (*MPO*) that work together in killing bacteria (Figure 13.8). Overall, the *MPO* system is the most potent of the bactericidal mechanisms. An invading bacterium is recognized by the immune system and attacked by antibodies that bind it to a receptor on a phagocytic cell. After internalization of the microorganism has occurred, *NADPH oxidase*, located in the leukocyte cell membrane, is activated and reduces molecular oxygen from the surrounding tissue into superoxide ($O_2^{-\bullet}$), a free radical. The rapid consumption of molecular oxygen that accompanies formation of superoxide is referred to as the respiratory burst. [Note: Active *NADPH oxidase* is a membrane-associated complex containing a flavocytochrome plus additional peptides that translocate from the cytoplasm upon activation of the leukocyte. Electrons move from NADPH to O_2, via FAD and heme, generating $O_2^{-\bullet}$. Genetic deficiencies in *NADPH oxidase* cause chronic granulomatous disease (CGD) characterized by severe, persistent infections. and the formation of granulomas (nodular areas of inflammation) that sequester the bacteria that were not destroyed.] Next, superoxide is converted to hydrogen peroxide (a ROS), either spontaneously or catalyzed by *superoxide dismutase* (*SOD*). In the presence of *MPO*, a heme-containing lysosomal enzyme present within the phagolysosome, peroxide plus chloride ions are converted to hypochlorous acid (HOCl, the major component of household bleach), which kills the bacteria. The peroxide can also be partially reduced to the hydroxyl radical (OH•), a ROS, or be fully reduced to water by *catalase* or *glutathione peroxidase*. [Note: Deficiencies in *MPO* do not confer increased susceptibility to infection because peroxide from *NADPH oxidase* is bactericidal.]

E. Synthesis of nitric oxide

Nitric oxide (NO) is recognized as a mediator in a broad array of biologic systems. NO is the endothelium-derived relaxing factor, which causes vasodilation by relaxing vascular smooth muscle. NO also acts as a neurotransmitter, prevents platelet aggregation, and plays an essential role in macrophage function. [Note: NO is a free radical gas that is often confused with nitrous oxide (N_2O), the "laughing gas" that is used as an anesthetic and is chemically stable.] NO has a very short half-life in tissues (3–10 seconds) because it reacts with oxygen and superoxide, and then is converted into nitrates and nitrites including peroxynitrite ($O=NOO^-$), a reactive nitrogen species (RNS).

1. **Synthesis of NO:** Arginine, O_2, and NADPH are substrates for cytosolic *NO synthase* (Figure 13.9). Flavin mononucleotide (FMN), flavin adenine dinucleotide (FAD), heme, and tetrahydrobiopterin (see p. 268) are coenzymes for the enzyme, and NO and citrulline are products of the reaction. Three *NO synthases* have been identified. Two are constitutive (synthesized at a constant rate regardless of physiologic demand), Ca^{2+}-calmodulin-dependent enzymes. They are found primarily in endothelium (*eNOS*), and neural tissue (*nNOS*), and constantly produce low levels of NO. An inducible, Ca^{2+}-independent enzyme (*iNOS*) can be expressed in many cells, including hepatocytes, macrophages, monocytes, and neutrophils. The specific inducers for *iNOS* vary with cell type, and include tumor necrosis factor-α, bacterial endotoxins, and inflammatory cytokines. These compounds have been shown to promote synthesis of *iNOS*, which can result in large amounts of NO being produced over hours or even days.

2. **Actions of NO on vascular endothelium:** NO is an important mediator in the control of vascular smooth muscle tone. NO is synthesized by *eNOS* in endothelial cells, and diffuses to vascular smooth muscle, where it activates the cytosolic form of *guanylate cyclase* (also known as *guanylyl cyclase*) to form cGMP. [Note: This reaction is analogous to the formation of cAMP by *adenylate cyclase* (see p. 94), except that this *guanylate cyclase* is not membrane-associated.] The resultant rise in cGMP causes activation of *protein kinase G*, which phosphorylates Ca^{2+} channels, causing decreased entry of Ca^{2+} into smooth muscle cells. This decreases the calcium-calmodulin activation of *myosin light-chain kinase*, thereby decreasing smooth muscle contraction and favoring relaxation. Vasodilator nitrates, such as nitroglycerin and nitroprusside, are metabolized to nitric oxide, which causes relaxation of vascular smooth muscle and, therefore, lowers blood pressure. Thus, NO can be envisioned as an endogenous nitrovasodilator. [Note: Sildenafil citrate, used in the treatment of erectile dysfunction, inhibits the *phosphodiesterase* that inactivates cGMP.]

3. **Role of NO in mediating macrophage bactericidal activity:** In macrophages, *iNOS* activity is normally low, but synthesis of the enzyme is significantly stimulated by bacterial lipopolysaccharide and γ-interferon release in response to infection. Activated macrophages form superoxide radicals (see p. 150) that combine with NO to form intermediates that decompose, forming the highly bactericidal OH• radical.

4. **Other functions of NO:** NO is a potent inhibitor of platelet aggregation (by activating the cGMP pathway). It is also characterized as a neurotransmitter in the brain.

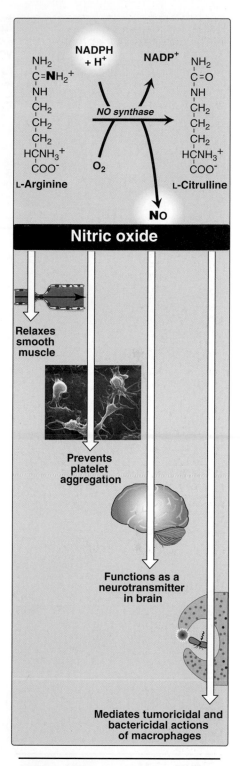

Figure 13.9
Synthesis and some of the actions of nitric oxide. [Note: FMN, FAD, heme, and tetrahydrobiopterin are additional coenzymes required by *NOS*.]

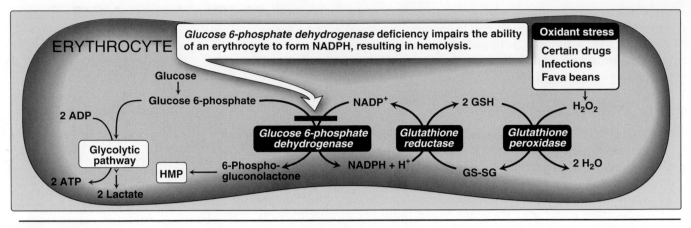

Figure 13.10
Pathways of glucose 6-phosphate metabolism in the erythrocyte. HMP = hexose monophosphate pathway.

V. GLUCOSE 6-P DEHYDROGENASE DEFICIENCY

Glucose 6-phosphate dehydrogenase (*G6PD*) deficiency is an inherited disease characterized by hemolytic anemia caused by the inability to detoxify oxidizing agents. *G6PD* deficiency is the most common disease-producing enzyme abnormality in humans, affecting more than 400 million individuals worldwide. This deficiency has the highest prevalence in the Middle East, tropical Africa and Asia, and parts of the Mediterranean. *G6PD* deficiency is X-linked, and is, in fact, a family of deficiencies caused by more than 400 different mutations in the gene coding for *G6PD*. Only some of these mutations cause clinical symptoms. [Note: In addition to hemolytic anemia, a clinical manifestation of *G6PD* deficiency is neonatal jaundice appearing 1–4 days after birth. The jaundice, which may be severe, typically results from increased production of unconjugated bilirubin (see p. 285).] The life span of individuals with a severe form of *G6PD* deficiency may be somewhat shortened as a result of complications arising from chronic hemolysis. This negative effect of *G6PD* deficiency has been balanced in evolution by an advantage in survival—an increased resistance to falciparum malaria shown by female carriers of the mutation. [Note: Sickle cell trait and β-thalassemia minor also confer resistance.]

A. Role of G6PD in red blood cells

Diminished *G6PD* activity impairs the ability of the cell to form the NADPH that is essential for the maintenance of the reduced glutathione pool. This results in a decrease in the cellular detoxification of free radicals and peroxides formed within the cell (Figure 13.10). Glutathione also helps maintain the reduced states of sulfhydryl groups in proteins, including hemoglobin. Oxidation of those sulfhydryl groups leads to the formation of denatured proteins that form insoluble masses (called Heinz bodies) that attach to the red cell membranes (Figure 13.11). Additional oxidation of membrane proteins causes the red cells to be rigid (less deformable), and they are removed from the circulation by macrophages in the spleen and liver. Although *G6PD* deficiency occurs in all cells of the affected individual, it is most severe in erythrocytes, where the pen-

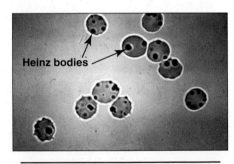

Figure 13.11
Heinz bodies in erythrocytes of a patient with *G6PD* deficiency.

tose phosphate pathway provides the only means of generating NADPH. Other tissues have alternative sources for NADPH production (such as *NADP+-dependent malate dehydrogenases*, see Figure 16.11, p. 187) that can keep glutathione reduced. The erythrocyte has no nucleus or ribosomes and cannot renew its supply of the enzyme. Thus, red blood cells are particularly vulnerable to enzyme variants with diminished stability.

B. Precipitating factors in G6PD deficiency

Most individuals who have inherited one of the many *G6PD* mutations do not show clinical manifestations, that is, they are asymptomatic. However, some patients with *G6PD* deficiency develop hemolytic anemia if they are treated with an oxidant drug, ingest fava beans, or contract a severe infection.

1. **Oxidant drugs:** Commonly used drugs that produce hemolytic anemia in patients with *G6PD* deficiency are best remembered from the mnemonic AAA—Antibiotics (for example, sulfamethoxazole and chloramphenicol), Antimalarials (for example, primaquine but not quinine), and Antipyretics (for example, acetanilid but not acetaminophen).

2. **Favism:** Some forms of *G6PD* deficiency, for example the Mediterranean variant, are particularly susceptible to the hemolytic effect of the fava (broad) bean, a dietary staple in the Mediterranean region. Favism, the hemolytic effect of ingesting fava beans, is not observed in all individuals with *G6PD* deficiency, but all patients with favism have *G6PD* deficiency.

3. **Infection:** Infection is the most common precipitating factor of hemolysis in *G6PD* deficiency. The inflammatory response to infection results in the generation of free radicals in macrophages, which can diffuse into the red blood cells and cause oxidative damage.

C. Properties of the variant enzymes

Almost all *G6PD* variants are caused by point mutations in the gene for *G6PD*. Some mutations do not disrupt the structure of the enzyme's active site and, hence, do not affect enzymic activity. However, many mutant enzymes show altered kinetic properties. For example, variant enzymes may show decreased catalytic activity, decreased stability, or an alteration of binding affinity for NADP+, NADPH, or glucose 6-phosphate. The severity of the disease usually correlates with the amount of residual enzyme activity in the patient's red blood cells. For example, variants can be classified as shown in Figure 13.12. *G6PD* A⁻ is the prototype of the moderate (Class III) form of the disease. The red cells contain an unstable but kinetically normal *G6PD*, with most of the enzyme activity present in the reticulocytes and younger erythrocytes (Figure 13.13). The oldest cells, therefore, have the lowest level of enzyme activity, and are preferentially removed in a hemolytic episode. *G6PD* Mediterranean is the prototype of a more severe (Class II) deficiency in which the enzyme has decreased stability resulting in decreased enzymic activity. Class I mutations (rare) are the most severe and are associated with chronic nonspherocytic anemia, which occurs even in the absence of oxidative stress.

Class	Clinical symptoms	Residual enzyme activity
I	Very severe (Chronic hemolytic anemia)	<10%
II	Severe (Episodic hemolytic anemia)	<10%
III	Moderate	10–60%
IV	None	>60%

Figure 13.12
Classification of *G6PD* deficiency variants. Note: Class V mutations (not shown in table) result in overproduction of *G6PD*.

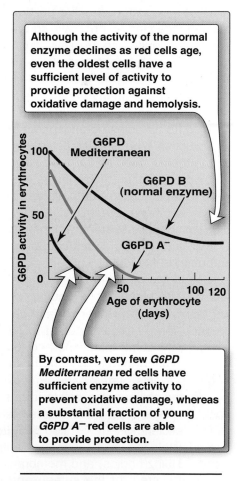

Although the activity of the normal enzyme declines as red cells age, even the oldest cells have a sufficient level of activity to provide protection against oxidative damage and hemolysis.

By contrast, very few *G6PD Mediterranean* red cells have sufficient enzyme activity to prevent oxidative damage, whereas a substantial fraction of young *G6PD A⁻* red cells are able to provide protection.

Figure 13.13
Decline of erythrocyte *G6PD* activity with cell age for the three most commonly encountered forms of the enzyme.

D. Molecular biology of G6PD

The cloning of the gene for *G6PD* and the sequencing of its DNA (see p. 467) have permitted the identification of mutations that cause *G6PD* deficiency. More than 400 different mutations or mutation combinations have been identified in this gene, a finding that explains the numerous biochemical variants that have been described. Most mutations that result in enzymic deficiency are missense mutations (see p. 433) in the coding region. Both *G6PD* A⁻ and *G6PD* Mediterranean represent mutant enzymes that differ from the respective normal variants by a single amino acid. Large deletions or frameshift mutations have not been identified, suggesting that complete absence of *G6PD* activity is probably lethal.

VI. CHAPTER SUMMARY

The pentose phosphate pathway includes two irreversible oxidative reactions followed by a series of reversible sugar–phosphate interconversions (Figure 13.14). No ATP is directly consumed or produced in the cycle. The NADPH-producing **oxidative portion** of the pentose phosphate pathway is particularly important in liver, mammary glands, and adipose, which are active in the biosynthesis of fatty acids; in the placenta, ovaries, testes, and adrenal cortex, which are active in the synthesis of steroid hormones; in erythrocytes, which require reduced glutathione. **Glucose 6-phosphate** is irreversibly converted to **ribulose 5-phosphate**, and **two NADPH** are produced. The regulated step is **glucose 6-phosphate dehydrogenase (G6PD)**, which is strongly **inhibited by NADPH**. **Reversible nonoxidative reactions** interconvert sugars. This part of the pathway is the **source of ribose 5-phosphate**, required for nucleotide and nucleic acid synthesis. Because the reactions are reversible, they can be entered from fructose 6-phosphate and glyceraldehyde 3-phosphate (glycolytic intermediates) if ribose is needed and glucose 6-phosphate dehydrogenase is inhibited. **NADPH** is a source of reducing equivalents in **reductive biosynthesis**, such as the production of fatty acids and steroids. It is also required for the **reduction of hydrogen peroxide**, providing the reducing equivalents required by **glutathione (GSH)**. GSH is used by **glutathione peroxidase** to reduce peroxide to water. The oxidized glutathione is reduced by **glutathione reductase**, using NADPH as the source of electrons. NADPH provides reducing equivalents for the mitochondrial **cytochrome P450 monooxygenase system**, which is used in steroid hormone synthesis in steroidogenic tissue, **bile acid synthesis** in liver, and **vitamin D activation in liver and kidney**. The microsomal system uses NADPH to **detoxify** foreign compounds (xenobiotics), such as drugs and a variety of pollutants. NADPH provides the reducing equivalents for phagocytes in the process of eliminating invading microorganisms. **NADPH oxidase** uses molecular oxygen and NADPH electrons to produce **superoxide radicals**, which, in turn, can be converted to peroxide by superoxide dismutase. **Myeloperoxidase** catalyzes the formation of bactericidal hypochlorous acid from peroxide and chloride ion. A genetic defect in NADPH oxidase causes **chronic granulomatous** disease characterized by severe, persistent, infections and formation of granulomas. NADPH is required for the synthesis of **nitric oxide (NO)**, an important molecule that causes **vasodilation** by relaxing vascular smooth muscle, acts as a **neurotransmitter**, prevents **platelet aggregation**, and helps mediate **macrophage bactericidal activity**. G6PD deficiency impairs the ability of the cell to form the NADPH that is essential for the maintenance of the reduced glutathione pool. The cells most affected are the **red blood cells** because they do not have additional sources of NADPH. G6PD deficiency is an X-linked **genetic disease** characterized by **hemolytic anemia**. **Free radicals** and **peroxides** formed within the cells cannot be neutralized, causing denaturation of cytosolic protein (for example, hemoglobin, forming Heinz bodies) and membrane proteins. The cells become rigid, and they are removed by the reticuloendothelial system of the spleen and liver. Babies with G6PD deficiency may experience **neonatal jaundice**. Hemolytic anemia can be caused by the production of free radicals and peroxides following the taking of **oxidant drugs**, ingestion of **fava beans**, or severe **infections**. The degree of severity of the anemia depends on the amount of residual enzyme. Class I mutations, the most severe, are associated with **chronic nonspherocytic anemia**. Class II mutations (for example, **G6PD Mediterranean**) are also severe. Class III mutations (such as **G6PD A⁻**) cause a more moderate form of the disease.

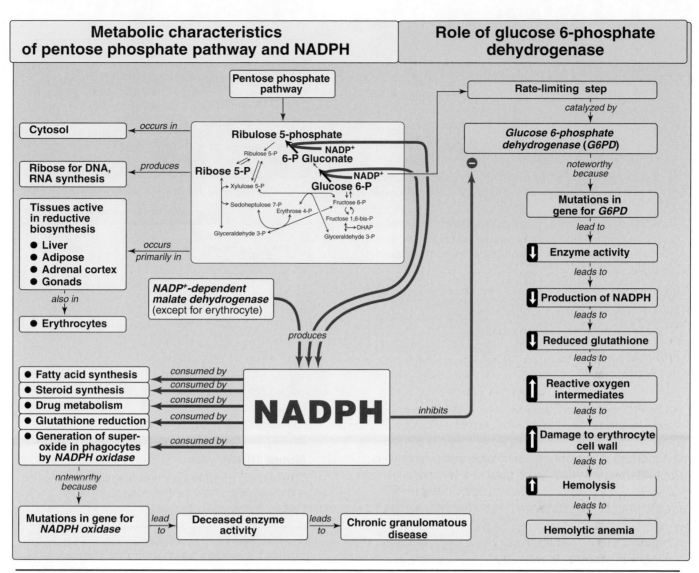

Figure 13.14
Key concept map for the pentose phosphate pathway and NADPH.

Study Questions

Choose the ONE correct answer.

13.1 In preparation for a trip to an area of India where malaria is endemic, a young man is given primaquine prophylactically. Soon thereafter, he develops a hemolytic condition. The most likely cause of the hemolysis is a less-than-normal level of which of the following?

A. Glucose 6-phosphate
B. Oxidized form of NAD
C. Reduced form of glutathione
D. Ribose 5-phosphate
E. Ribulose 5-phosphate

13.2 In male patients who are hemizygous for glucose 6-phosphate dehydrogenase (G6PD) deficiency, pathophysiologic consequences are more apparent in erythrocytes (RBC) than in other cells, such as in the liver. Which one of the following provides the most reasonable explanation for this different response by these individual tissue types?

A. Excess glucose 6-phosphate in the liver, but not in RBCs, can be channeled to glycogen, thus averting cellular damage.

B. Liver cells, in contrast to RBCs, have alternative mechanisms for supplying the NADPH required for keeping metabolic and cellular integrity.

C. Glucose 6-phosphatase activity in RBCs decreases the level of glucose 6-phosphate, thus resulting in cell damage. This does not happen in the hepatocyte.

D. Because RBCs do not have mitochondria, production of ATP required to keep cell integrity depends exclusively on the routing of glucose 6-phosphate to the pentose phosphate pathway.

E. The catalytic properties of the liver enzyme are significantly different than those of the RBC enzyme.

13.3 A G6PD A⁻ individual was treated with primaquine from day 0 to day 120 (Figure 13.15). Hemolysis occurred immediately after initiation of drug therapy, as indicated by progressive anemia, hemoglobinuria, and reticulocytosis. However, despite continued administration of the drug, the hemolysis spontaneously decreased and red cell survival improved with time. Red cell G6PD activity measured 2 months after termination of therapy was 10% of normal. Which one of the following statements about this patient is correct?

A. The patient will continue to be resistant to drug-induced hemolysis after 6 months or longer.

B. Erythrocytes in this patient exhibit a longer lifetime than in normal individuals.

C. During the period of peak hemolysis, erythrocytes from the patient will show no G6PD activity.

D. The intracellular concentration of NADPH in the patient's erythrocytes is greater than normal.

E. The patient shows increased bone marrow erythropoiesis.

Correct answer = B. Cellular damage is directly related to decreased ability of the cell to regenerate reduced glutathione, for which large amounts of NADPH are needed, and RBC have no other means of generating NADPH. Catalytic properties of G6PD in liver and RBCs are very similar. The pentose phosphate pathway does not generate ATP. RBCs do not have glucose 6-phosphatase.

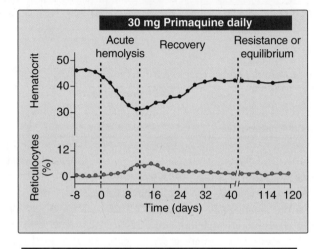

Figure 13.15

The course of primaquine-induced hemolysis in a patient with G6PD deficiency.

Correct answer = E. As red cells age, the activity of G6PD declines (see Figure 13.13). Despite this loss of enzyme activity, normal old red blood cells contain sufficient G6PD activity to generate NADPH and thereby sustain GSH levels in the face of oxidant stress. In contrast, the G6PD variants with hemolysis have much shorter half-lives. The clinical correlate of this age-related enzyme instability is that hemolysis in patients with G6PD A⁻ generally is mild and limited to the older deficient erythrocytes. The anemia is self-limited because the older, vulnerable population of erythrocytes is replaced by younger RBCs with sufficient G6PD activity to withstand an oxidative assault. Although red cell survival remains shortened as long as use of the drug continues, compensation by the erythroid marrow effectively abolishes the anemia in subjects with G6PD A⁻. The individual's continuing sensitivity to the effects of the drug is revealed by discontinuing the drug for several months to allow the rate of red cell production by the bone marrow to normalize; during this phase, the older red cells are able to survive, and the red cell population is rendered sensitive to drug-induced hemolysis.

Glycosaminoglycans, Proteoglycans, and Glycoproteins

14

I. OVERVIEW OF GLYCOSAMINOGLYCANS

Glycosaminoglycans are large complexes of negatively charged heteropolysaccharide chains. They are generally associated with a small amount of protein, forming proteoglycans, which typically consist of over 95% carbohydrate. [Note: This is in comparison to the glycoproteins, which consist primarily of protein with a small amount of carbohydrate (see p. 165).] Glycosaminoglycans have the special ability to bind large amounts of water, thereby producing the gel-like matrix that forms the basis of the body's ground substance, which, along with fibrous structural proteins such as collagen and elastin, and adhesive proteins such as fibronectin, make up the extracellular matrix (ECM). The hydrated glycosaminoglycans serve as a flexible support for the ECM, interacting with the structural and adhesive proteins, and as a molecular sieve, influencing movement of materials through the ECM. The viscous, lubricating properties of mucous secretions also result from the presence of glycosaminoglycans, which led to the original naming of these compounds as mucopolysaccharides.

II. STRUCTURE OF GLYCOSAMINOGLYCANS

Glycosaminoglycans (GAGs) are long, unbranched, heteropolysaccharide chains generally composed of a repeating disaccharide unit [acidic sugar–amino sugar]$_n$ (Figure 14.1). The amino sugar is either D-glucosamine or D-galactosamine, in which the amino group is usually acetylated, thus eliminating its positive charge. The amino sugar may also be sulfated on carbon 4 or 6 or on a nonacetylated nitrogen. The acidic sugar is either D-glucuronic acid or its C-5 epimer, L-iduronic acid (Figure 14.2). [Note: A single exception is keratan sulfate, in which galactose rather than an acidic sugar is present.] These acidic sugars contain carboxyl groups that are negatively charged at physiologic pH and, together with the sulfate groups, give GAGs their strongly negative nature.

A. Relationship between glycosaminoglycan structure and function

Because of their large number of negative charges, these heteropolysaccharide chains tend to be extended in solution. They repel each other, and are surrounded by a shell of water molecules. When brought together, they "slip" past each other, much as two magnets

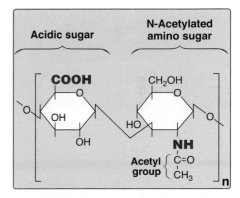

Figure 14.1
Repeating disaccharide unit.

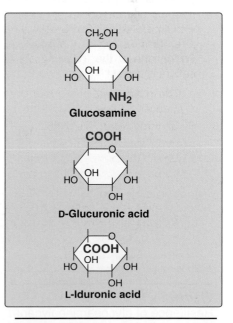

Figure 14.2
Some monosaccharide units found in glycosaminoglycans.

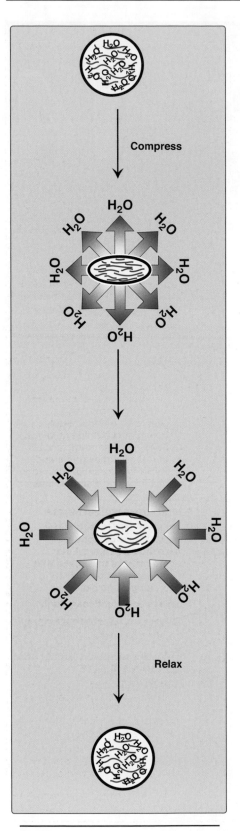

Figure 14.3
Resilience of glycosaminoglycans.

with the same polarity seem to slip past each other. This produces the "slippery" consistency of mucous secretions and synovial fluid. When a solution of glycosaminoglycans is compressed, the water is "squeezed out" and the glycosaminoglycans are forced to occupy a smaller volume. When the compression is released, the glycosaminoglycans spring back to their original, hydrated volume because of the repulsion of their negative charges. This property contributes to the resilience of synovial fluid and the vitreous humor of the eye (Figure 14.3).

B. Classification of the glycosaminoglycans

The six major classes of glycosaminoglycans are divided according to monomeric composition, type of glycosidic linkages, and degree and location of sulfate units. The structure of the glycosaminoglycans and their distribution in the body is illustrated in Figure 14.4.

C. Structure of proteoglycans

All of the glycosaminoglycans, except hyaluronic acid, are found covalently attached to protein, forming proteoglycan monomers.

1. **Structure of proteoglycan monomers:** A proteoglycan monomer found in cartilage consists of a core protein to which the linear glycosaminoglycan chains are covalently attached. These chains, which may each be composed of more than 100 monosaccharides, extend out from the core protein, and remain separated from each other because of charge repulsion. The resulting structure resembles a "bottle brush" (Figure 14.5). In cartilage proteoglycan, the species of glycosaminoglycans include chondroitin sulfate and keratan sulfate. [Note: Proteoglycans are now grouped into gene families that code for core proteins with common structural features. The aggrecan family (aggrecan, versecan, neurocan, and brevican), abundant in cartilage, is an example.]

2. **Linkage between the carbohydrate chain and the protein:** This linkage is most commonly through a trihexoside (galactose-galactose-xylose) and a serine residue, respectively. An O-glycosidic bond is formed between the xylose and the hydroxyl group of the serine (Figure 14.6).

3. **Proteoglycan aggregates:** The proteoglycan monomers associate with a molecule of hyaluronic acid to form proteoglycan aggregates. The association is not covalent, but occurs primarily through ionic interactions between the core protein and the hyaluronic acid. The association is stabilized by additional small proteins called link proteins (Figure 14.7).

III. SYNTHESIS OF GLYCOSAMINOGLYCANS

The polysaccharide chains are elongated by the sequential addition of alternating acidic and amino sugars donated by their UDP-derivatives. The reactions are catalyzed by a family of specific *glycosyltransferases*. The synthesis of the glycosaminoglycans is analogous to that of glycogen (see p. 126) except that the glycosaminoglycans are produced for export from the cell. Their synthesis occurs, therefore, primarily in the Golgi, rather than in the cytosol.

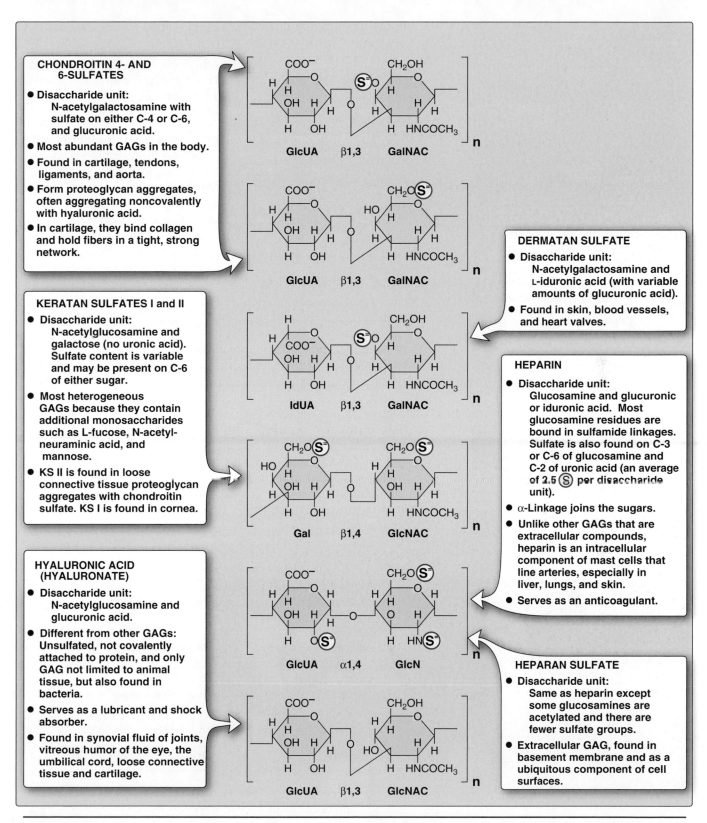

CHONDROITIN 4- AND 6-SULFATES

- Disaccharide unit: N-acetylgalactosamine with sulfate on either C-4 or C-6, and glucuronic acid.
- Most abundant GAGs in the body.
- Found in cartilage, tendons, ligaments, and aorta.
- Form proteoglycan aggregates, often aggregating noncovalently with hyaluronic acid.
- In cartilage, they bind collagen and hold fibers in a tight, strong network.

KERATAN SULFATES I and II

- Disaccharide unit: N-acetylglucosamine and galactose (no uronic acid). Sulfate content is variable and may be present on C-6 of either sugar.
- Most heterogeneous GAGs because they contain additional monosaccharides such as L-fucose, N-acetyl-neuraminic acid, and mannose.
- KS II is found in loose connective tissue proteoglycan aggregates with chondroitin sulfate. KS I is found in cornea.

HYALURONIC ACID (HYALURONATE)

- Disaccharide unit: N-acetylglucosamine and glucuronic acid.
- Different from other GAGs: Unsulfated, not covalently attached to protein, and only GAG not limited to animal tissue, but also found in bacteria.
- Serves as a lubricant and shock absorber.
- Found in synovial fluid of joints, vitreous humor of the eye, the umbilical cord, loose connective tissue and cartilage.

DERMATAN SULFATE

- Disaccharide unit: N-acetylgalactosamine and L-iduronic acid (with variable amounts of glucuronic acid).
- Found in skin, blood vessels, and heart valves.

HEPARIN

- Disaccharide unit: Glucosamine and glucuronic or iduronic acid. Most glucosamine residues are bound in sulfamide linkages. Sulfate is also found on C-3 or C-6 of glucosamine and C-2 of uronic acid (an average of 2.5 S per disaccharide unit).
- α-Linkage joins the sugars.
- Unlike other GAGs that are extracellular compounds, heparin is an intracellular component of mast cells that line arteries, especially in liver, lungs, and skin.
- Serves as an anticoagulant.

HEPARAN SULFATE

- Disaccharide unit: Same as heparin except some glucosamines are acetylated and there are fewer sulfate groups.
- Extracellular GAG, found in basement membrane and as a ubiquitous component of cell surfaces.

Figure 14.4

Structure and distribution of glycosaminoglycans (GAGs). Sulfate groups (S) are shown in all possible positions. GlcUA = glucuronic acid; IdUA = iduronic acid; GalNAC = N-acetylgalactosamine; GlcNAC = N-acetylglucosamine; GlcN = glucosamine; Gal = galactose.

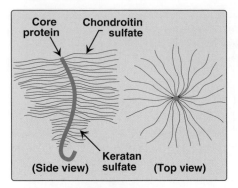

Figure 14.5
"Bottle-brush" model of a cartilage proteoglycan monomer.

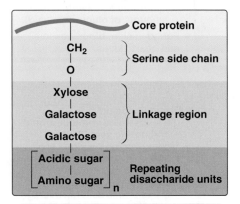

Figure 14.6
Linkage region of glycosamino-glycans.

A. Synthesis of amino sugars

Amino sugars are essential components of glycosaminoglycans, glycoproteins, glycolipids, and certain oligosaccharides, and are also found in some antibiotics. The synthetic pathway of amino sugars is very active in connective tissues, where as much as 20% of glucose flows through this pathway.

1. **N-Acetylglucosamine (GlcNAc) and N-acetylgalactosamine (GalNAc):** The monosaccharide fructose 6-phosphate is the precursor of GlcNAc, GalNAc, and the sialic acids, including N-acetylneuraminic acid (NANA, a nine-carbon, acidic monosaccharide). In each of these sugars, a hydroxyl group of the precursor is replaced by an amino group donated by glutamine (Figure 14.8). [Note: The amino groups are then almost always acetylated.] The UDP-derivatives of GlcNAc and GalNAc are synthesized by reactions analogous to those described for UDP-glucose synthesis (see p. 126). These nucleotide sugars are the activated forms of the monosaccharides that can be used to elongate the carbohydrate chains.

2. **N-Acetylneuraminic acid:** N-Acetylneuraminic acid (NANA) is a member of the family of sialic acids, each of which is acylated at a different site. These compounds are usually found as terminal carbohydrate residues of oligosaccharide side chains of glycoproteins, glycolipids, or, less frequently, of glycosaminoglycans. The carbons and nitrogens in NANA come from N-acetyl-mannosamine and phosphoenolpyruvate (an intermediate in the glycolytic pathway, see p. 102). [Note: Before NANA can be added to a growing oligosaccharide, it must be converted into its active form by reacting with cytidine triphosphate (CTP). The enzyme *CMP-NANA synthetase* catalyzes the reaction. This is the only nucleotide sugar in human metabolism in which the carrier nucleotide is a monophosphate.]

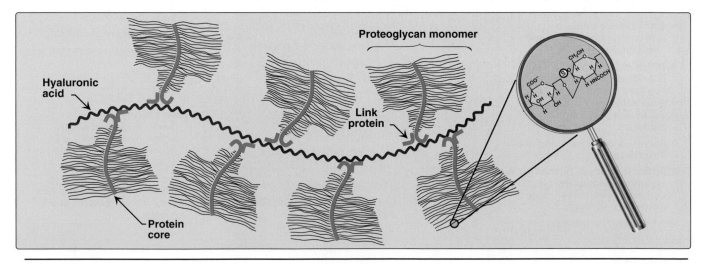

Figure 14.7
Proteoglycan aggregate.

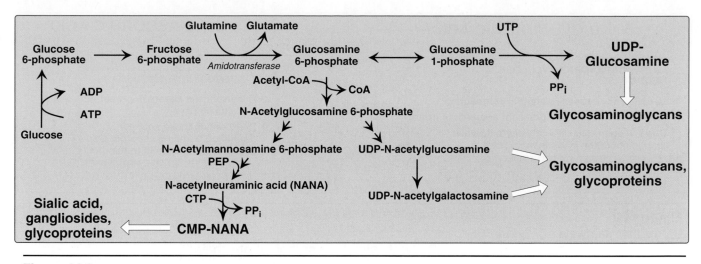

Figure 14.8
Synthesis of the amino sugars.

B. Synthesis of acidic sugars

D-Glucuronic acid, whose structure is that of glucose with an oxidized carbon 6 ($-CH_2OH \rightarrow -COOH$), and its C-5 epimer, L-iduronic acid, are essential components of glycosaminoglycans. Glucuronic acid is also required in detoxification reactions of a number of insoluble compounds, such as bilirubin (see p. 282), steroids, and several drugs, including morphine. In plants and mammals (other than guinea pigs and primates, including humans), glucuronic acid serves as a precursor of ascorbic acid (vitamin C). The uronic acid pathway also provides a mechanism by which dietary D-xylulose can enter the central metabolic pathways.

1. **Glucuronic acid:** Glucuronic acid can be obtained in small amounts from the diet. It can also be obtained from the intracellular lysosomal degradation of glycosaminoglycans, or via the uronic acid pathway. The endproduct of glucuronic acid metabolism in humans is D-xylulose 5-phosphate, which can enter the hexose monophosphate pathway and produce the glycolytic intermediates glyceraldehyde 3-phosphate and fructose 6-phosphate (Figure 14.9; see also Figure 13.2, p. 146). The active form of glucuronic acid that donates the sugar in glycosaminoglycan synthesis and other glucuronylating reactions is UDP-glucuronic acid, which is produced by oxidation of UDP-glucose (Figure 14.10).

2. **L-Iduronic acid synthesis:** Synthesis of L-iduronic acid residues occurs after D-glucuronic acid has been incorporated into the carbohydrate chain. *Uronosyl 5-epimerase* causes epimerization of the D- to the L-sugar.

C. Synthesis of the core protein

The core protein is synthesized on and enters the rough endoplasmic reticulum (RER). The protein is then glycosylated by bound *glycosyltransferases* located in the Golgi.

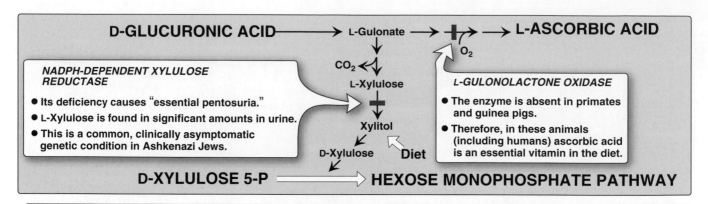

Figure 14.9
Uronic acid pathway.

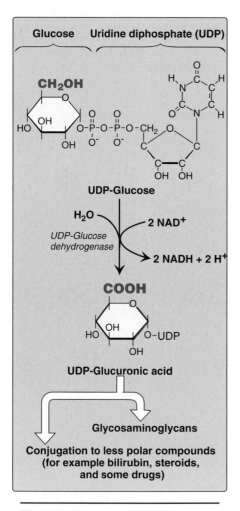

Figure 14.10
Oxidation of UDP-glucose to UDP-glucuronic acid.

D. Synthesis of the carbohydrate chain

Carbohydrate chain formation begins by synthesis of a short linkage region on the core protein on which carbohydrate chain synthesis will be initiated. The most common linkage region is formed by the transfer of a xylose from UDP-xylose to the hydroxyl group of a serine (or threonine) catalyzed by *xylosyltransferase*. Two galactose molecules are then added, completing the trihexoside. This is followed by sequential addition of alternating acidic and amino sugars (Figure 14.11), and epimerization of some D-glucuronyl to L-iduronyl residues.

E. Addition of sulfate groups

Sulfation of the carbohydrate chain occurs after the monosaccharide to be sulfated has been incorporated into the growing carbohydrate chain. The source of the sulfate is 3'-phosphoadenosyl-5'-phosphosulfate (PAPS, a molecule of AMP with a sulfate group attached to the 5'-phosphate). *Sulfotransferases* cause the sulfation of the carbohydrate chain at specific sites. [Note: An example of the synthesis of a sulfated glycosaminoglycan, chondroitin sulfate, is shown in Figure 14.11.] PAPS is also the sulfur donor in glycosphingolipid synthesis.

> A defect in the sulfation of the growing glycosaminoglycan chains results in one of several autosomal recessive disorders (chondrodystrophies) that affect the proper development and maintenance of the skeletal system.

IV. DEGRADATION OF GLYCOSAMINOGLYCANS

Glycosaminoglycans are degraded in lysosomes, which contain hydrolytic enzymes that are most active at a pH of approximately 5. [Note: Therefore, as a group, these enzymes are called *acid hydrolases*.] The low pH optimum is a protective mechanism that prevents the enzymes from destroying the cell should leakage occur into the cytosol where the pH is neutral. With the exception of keratan sulfate, which has a half-life of greater than 120 days, the glycosaminoglycans have a relatively short half-life, ranging from about 3 days for hyaluronic acid to 10 days for chondroitin and dermatan sulfate.

A. Phagocytosis of extracellular glycosaminoglycans

Because glycosaminoglycans are extracellular or cell-surface compounds, they must first be engulfed by an invagination of the cell membrane (phagocytosis), forming a vesicle inside of which the glycosaminoglycans are to be degraded. This vesicle then fuses with a lysosome, forming a single digestive vesicle in which the glycosaminoglycans are efficiently degraded (see p. 150 for a discussion of phagocytosis).

B. Lysosomal degradation of glycosaminoglycans

The lysosomal degradation of glycosaminoglycans requires a large number of *acid hydrolases* for complete digestion. First, the polysaccharide chains are cleaved by *endoglycosidases*, producing oligosaccharides. Further degradation of the oligosaccharides occurs sequentially from the nonreducing end of each chain (see p. 127), the last group (sulfate or sugar) added during synthesis being the first group removed. Examples of some of these enzymes and the bonds they hydrolyze are shown in Figure 14.12.

V. MUCOPOLYSACCHARIDOSES

The mucopolysaccharidoses are hereditary diseases (1:25,000 births) caused by a deficiency of any one of the lysosomal *hydrolases* normally involved in the degradation of heparan sulfate and/or dermatan sulfate (see Figure 14.12). They are progressive disorders characterized by accumulation of glycosaminoglycans in various tissues, causing a range of symptoms, such as skeletal and extracellular matrix deformities, and mental retardation. Children who are homozygous for any one of these diseases are apparently normal at birth, then gradually deteriorate. In severe cases, death occurs in childhood. All are autosomal recessive diseases except Hunter syndrome, which is X-linked. Incomplete lysosomal degradation of glycosaminoglycans results in the presence of oligosaccharides in the urine. These fragments can be used to diagnose the specific mucopolysaccharidosis by identifying the structure present on the nonreducing end of the oligosaccharide, as that residue would have been the substrate for the missing enzyme. Diagnosis is confirmed by measuring the patient's cellular level of the lysosomal *hydrolases*. Bone marrow and cord blood transplants have been used to treat Hurler and Hunter syndromes. Here the transplanted macrophages produce the enzymes needed to degrade glycosaminoglycans in the extracellular space. Enzyme replacement therapy (ERT) is currently available for both syndromes.

In addition to the degradation of glycosaminoglycans, lysosomal *endo-* and *exoglycosidases* are also involved in the degradation of glycoproteins (see p. 170) and glycolipids (see p. 210). Deficiencies in these enzymes result in the accumulation of partially degraded carbohydrates in the lysosomes, leading to cell and tissue damage.

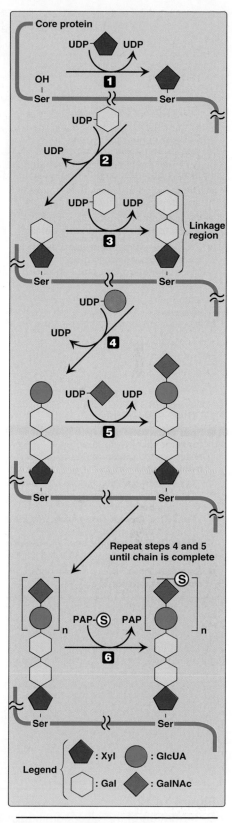

Figure 14.11
Synthesis of chondroitin sulfate.

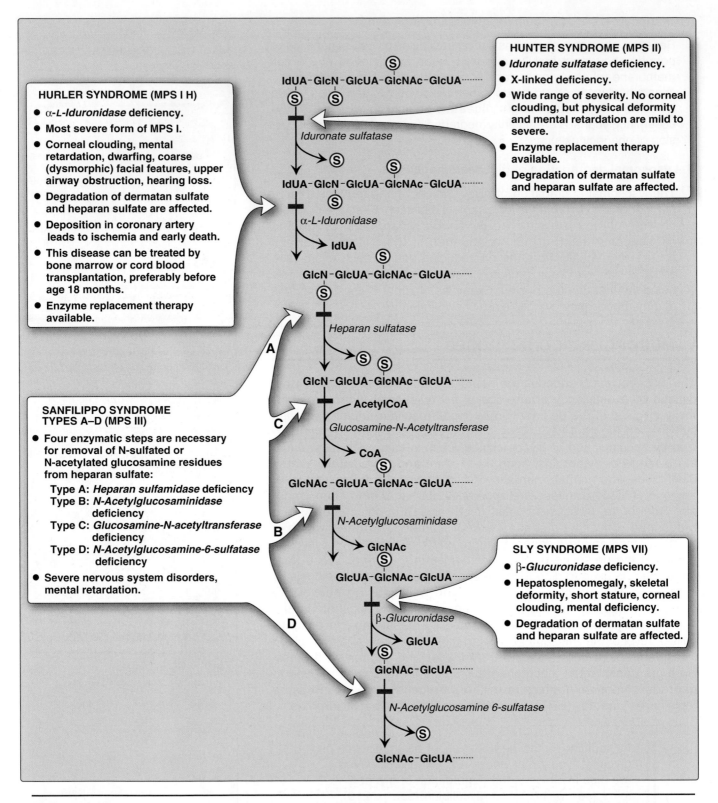

Figure 14.12
Degradation of the glycosaminoglycan heparan sulfate by lysosomal enzymes, indicating sites of enzyme deficiencies in some representative mucopolysaccharidoses. [Note: Deficiencies in the degradation of keratan sulfate result in Morquio syndrome, A and B.]

VI. OVERVIEW OF GLYCOPROTEINS

Glycoproteins are proteins to which oligosaccharides are covalently attached. They differ from the proteoglycans in that the length of the glycoprotein's carbohydrate chain is relatively short (usually two to ten sugar residues in length, although they can be longer), whereas it can be very long in the glycosaminoglycans (see p. 157). In addition, whereas glycosaminoglycans have diglucosyl repeat units, the carbohydrates of glycoproteins do not have serial repeats. The glycoprotein carbohydrate chains are often branched instead of linear, and may or may not be negatively charged. Glycoproteins contain highly variable amounts of carbohydrate. For example, immunoglobulin IgG, contains less than 4% of its mass as carbohydrate, whereas human gastric glycoprotein (mucin) contains more than 80% carbohydrate. Membrane-bound glycoproteins participate in a broad range of cellular phenomena, including cell surface recognition (by other cells, hormones, and viruses), cell surface antigenicity (such as the blood group antigens), and as components of the extracellular matrix and of the mucins of the gastrointestinal and urogenital tracts, where they act as protective biologic lubricants. In addition, almost all of the globular proteins present in human plasma are glycoproteins. (See Figure 14.13 for a summary of some of the functions of glycoproteins.)

VII. STRUCTURE OF GLYCOPROTEIN OLIGO-SACCHARIDES

The oligosaccharide components of glycoproteins are generally branched heteropolymers composed primarily of D-hexoses, with the addition in some cases of neuraminic acid, and of L-fucose—a 6-deoxyhexose.

A. Structure of the linkage between carbohydrate and protein

The oligosaccharide may be attached to the protein through an N- or an O-glycosidic link (see p. 86). In the former case, the sugar chain is attached to the amide group of an asparagine side chain, and in the latter case, to the hydroxyl group of either a serine or threonine R-group. [Note: In the case of collagen, there is an O-glycosidic linkage between galactose or glucose and the hydroxyl group of hydroxylysine (see p. 47).]

B. N- and O-linked oligosaccharides

A glycoprotein may contain only one type of glycosidic linkage (N- or O-linked), or may have both O- and N-linked oligosaccharides within the same molecule.

1. **O-Linked oligosaccharides:** The O-linked oligosaccharides may have one or more of a wide variety of sugars arranged in either a linear or a branched pattern. Many O-linked oligosaccharides are found in extracellular glycoproteins or as membrane glycoprotein components. For example, O-linked oligosaccharides on the surface of RBCs help provide the ABO blood group determinants.

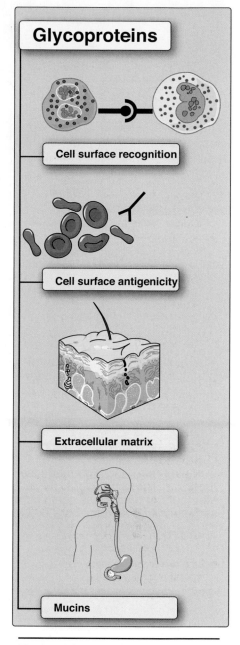

Glycoproteins

Cell surface recognition

Cell surface antigenicity

Extracellular matrix

Mucins

Figure 14.13
Functions of glycoproteins.

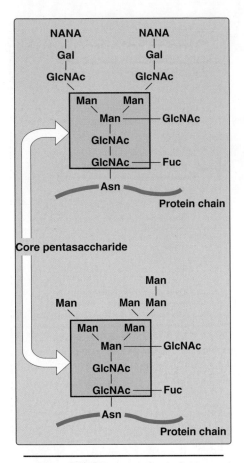

Figure 14.14
Complex (top) and high-mannose
(bottom) oligosaccharides. [Note:
Members of each class contain the
same pentasaccharide core.]

2. N-linked oligosaccharides: The N-linked oligosaccharides fall into two broad classes: complex oligosaccharides and high-mannose oligosaccharides. Both contain the same core pentasaccharide shown in Figure 14.14, but the complex oligosaccharides contain a diverse group of additional sugars, for example, N-acetyl-glucosamine (GlcNAc), L-fucose (Fuc), and N-acetylneuraminic acid (NANA), whereas the high-mannose oligosaccharides contain primarily mannose (Man).

VIII. SYNTHESIS OF GLYCOPROTEINS

Proteins destined to function in the cytoplasm are synthesized on free cytosolic ribosomes. However, proteins, including many glycoproteins, that are destined for cellular membranes, lysosomes, or to be exported from the cell, are synthesized on ribosomes attached to the RER. These proteins contain specific signal sequences that act as molecular "address labels," targeting the proteins to their proper destinations. An N-terminal hydrophobic sequence initially directs these proteins to the RER, allowing the growing polypeptide to be extruded into the lumen. The proteins are then transported via secretory vesicles to the Golgi complex, which acts as a sorting center (Figure 14.15). In the Golgi those glycoproteins that are to be secreted from the cell (or are targeted for lysosomes) are packaged into vesicles that fuse with the cell (or lysosomal) membrane and release their contents. Those that are destined to become components of the cell membrane are integrated into the Golgi membrane, which buds off, forming vesicles that add their membrane-bound glycoproteins to the cell membrane. [Note: The membrane glycoproteins are thus oriented with the carbohydrate portion on the outside of the cell (see Figure 14.15).]

A. Carbohydrate components of glycoproteins

The precursors of the carbohydrate components of glycoproteins are nucleotide sugars, which include UDP-glucose, UDP-galactose, UDP-N-acetylglucosamine, and UDP-N-acetylgalactosamine. In addition, GDP-mannose, GDP-L-fucose (which is synthesized from GDP-mannose), and CMP-N-acetylneuraminic acid may donate sugars to the growing chain. [Note: When NANA is present, the oligosaccharide has a negative charge at physiologic pH.] The oligosaccharides are covalently attached to specific amino acid R-groups of the protein, where the three-dimensional structure of the protein determines whether or not a specific amino acid R-group is glycosylated.

B. Synthesis of O-linked glycosides

The synthesis of the O-linked glycosides is very similar to that of the glycosaminoglycans (see p. 158). First, the protein to which the oligosaccharides are to be attached is synthesized on the RER, and extruded into its lumen. Glycosylation begins with the transfer of an N-acetylgalactosamine (from UDP-N-acetylgalactosamine) onto the R-group of a specific serine or threonine.

1. Role of glycosyltransferases: The *glycosyltransferases* responsible for the stepwise synthesis of the oligosaccharides are bound to the membranes of the Golgi apparatus. They act in a specific order, without using a template as is required for DNA, RNA, and protein synthesis (see Unit VI), but rather by recognizing the actual structure of the growing oligosaccharide as the appropriate substrate.

C. Synthesis of the N-linked glycosides

The synthesis of N-linked glycosides occurs in the lumen of the ER, and requires the participation of the phosphorylated form of dolichol (dolichol pyrophosphate), a lipid of the ER membrane (Figure 14.16). The initial product is processed in the ER and Golgi.

1. **Synthesis of dolichol-linked oligosaccharide:** First, as with the O-linked glycosides, the protein is synthesized on the RER and enters its lumen. However, the protein does not become glycosylated with individual sugars. Instead, a lipid-linked oligosaccharide is first constructed. This consists of dolichol (an ER membrane lipid 80–100 carbons long) attached through a pyrophosphate linkage to an oligosaccharide containing N-acetylglucosamine, mannose, and glucose. The sugars to be added sequentially to the dolichol by the membrane-bound *glycosyltransferases* are first N-acetylglucosamine, followed by mannose and glucose (see Figure 14.16). The entire 14-sugar oligosaccharide is then transferred from the dolichol to the amide N of an asparagine in the protein to be glycosylated by a *protein-oligosaccharide transferase* present in the ER.

Congenital disorders of glycosylation (CDG) are caused primarily by defects in the N-glycosylation of proteins, either oligosaccharide assembly (Type I) or processing (Type II).

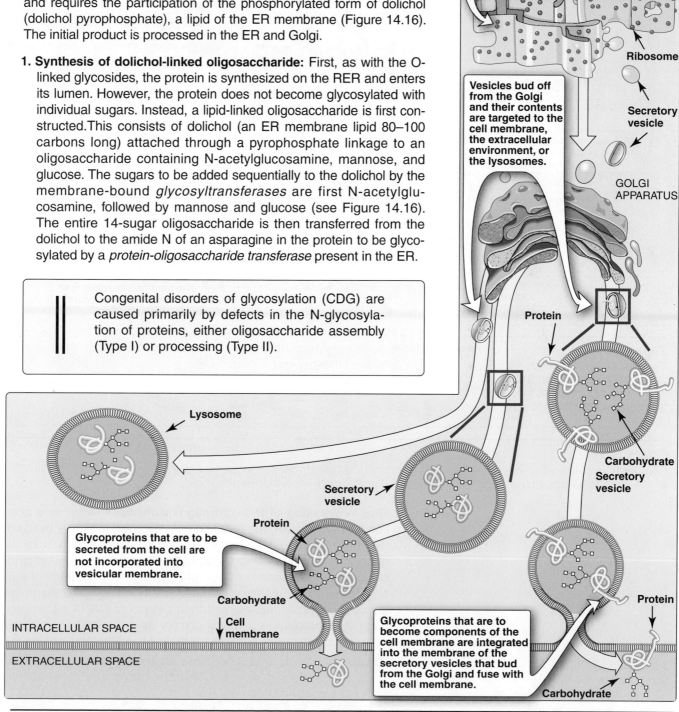

ROUGH ENDOPLASMIC RETICULUM (RER)
- RER is series of interconnected membrane-bound sacs.
- Ribosomes are bound to the cytosolic side of the membrane.

Ribosome

Secretory vesicle

Vesicles bud off from the Golgi and their contents are targeted to the cell membrane, the extracellular environment, or the lysosomes.

GOLGI APPARATUS

Protein

Carbohydrate

Secretory vesicle

Lysosome

Secretory vesicle

Protein

Glycoproteins that are to be secreted from the cell are not incorporated into vesicular membrane.

Carbohydrate

Cell membrane

INTRACELLULAR SPACE

EXTRACELLULAR SPACE

Glycoproteins that are to become components of the cell membrane are integrated into the membrane of the secretory vesicles that bud from the Golgi and fuse with the cell membrane.

Protein

Carbohydrate

Figure 14.15
Transport of glycoproteins through the Golgi apparatus and their subsequent release or incorporation into a lysosome or the cell membrane.

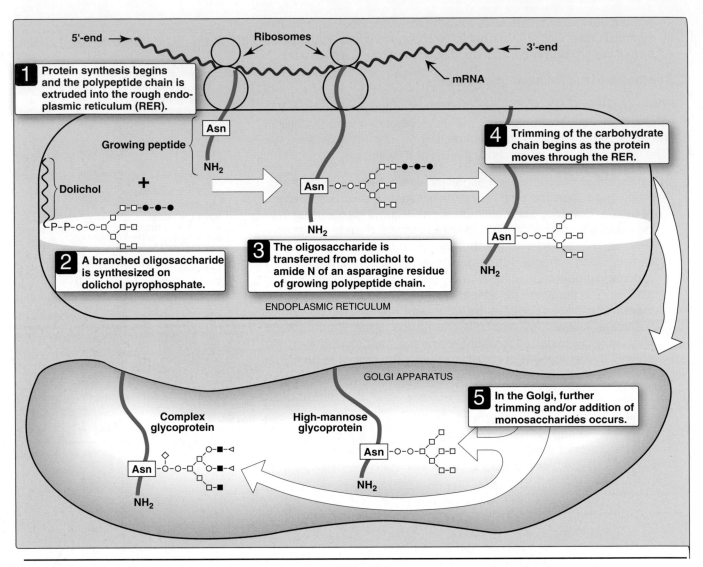

Figure 14.16
Synthesis of N-linked glycoproteins. ○ = N-acetylglucosamine; □ = mannose; ● = glucose;
■ = N-acetylgalactosamine; ◇ or ◁ for example, fucose or N-acetylneuraminic acid.

2. **Final processing of N-linked oligosaccharides:** After incorporation into the protein, the N-linked oligosaccharide is processed by the removal of specific mannosyl and glucosyl residues as the glycoprotein moves through the RER. Finally, the oligosaccharide chains are completed in the Golgi by addition of a variety of sugars (for example, N-acetylglucosamine, N-acetylgalactosamine, and additional mannoses, and then fucose or NANA as terminal groups) to produce a complex glycoprotein, or they are not processed further, leaving branched, mannose-containing chains in a high-mannose glycoprotein (see Figure 14.16). The ultimate fate of N-linked glycoproteins is the same as that of the O-linked, for example, they can be released by the cell, or become part of a cell membrane. In addition N-linked glycoproteins can be translocated to the lysosomes. [Note: Nonenzymatic glycosylation of proteins is known as glycation (see p. 345).]

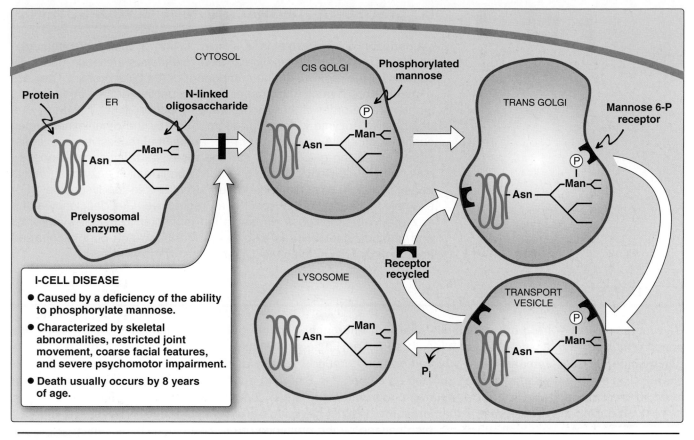

Figure 14.17
Mechanism for transport of N-linked glycoproteins to the lysosomes.

3. **Enzymes destined for lysosomes:** N-linked glycoproteins being processed through the Golgi can be phosphorylated at one or more specific mannosyl residues. Mannose 6-P receptors, located in the Golgi apparatus, bind the mannose 6-P residues of these targeted enzymes, which are then packaged into vesicles and sent to the lysosomes. I-cell disease is a rare syndrome in which the *acid hydrolase* enzymes normally found in lysosomes are absent, resulting in an accumulation of substrates normally degraded by lysosomal enzymes within these vesicles. [Note: I-cell disease is so-named because of the large inclusion bodies seen in cells of patients with this disease.] In addition, high amounts of lysosomal enzymes are found in the patient's plasma, suggesting that the targeting process to lysosomes (rather than the synthetic pathway of these enzymes) is deficient. It has been determined that individuals with I-cell disease are lacking the enzymic ability to phosphorylate the mannose residues of potential lysosomal enzymes, causing an incorrect targeting of these proteins to extracellular sites, rather than lysosomal vesicles (Figure 14.17). I-cell disease, a lysosomal storage disease, is characterized by skeletal abnormalities, restricted joint movement, coarse (dysmorphic) facial features, and severe psychomotor impairment. Death usually occurs by 8 years of age.

IX. LYSOSOMAL DEGRADATION OF GLYCOPROTEINS

Degradation of glycoproteins is similar to that of the glycosaminogly-cans (see p. 162). The lysosomal *acid hydrolases* are each generally specific for the removal of one component of the glycoprotein. They are primarily exoenzymes that remove their respective groups in sequence in the reverse order of their incorporation ("last on, first off"). If any one degradative enzyme is missing, degradation by the other exoenzymes cannot continue. A group of very rare, autosomal recessive genetic dis-eases called the glycoprotein storage diseases (oligosaccharidoses), caused by a deficiency of any one of the degradative enzymes, results in accumulation of partially degraded structures in the lysosomes. For example, α-mannosidosis type 1 is a progressive, fatal deficiency of the enzyme, α-*mannosidase*. Presentation is similar to Hurler syndrome, and immune deficiency is also seen. Mannose-rich oligosaccharide fragments appear in the urine. Diagnosis is by enzyme assay.

X. CHAPTER SUMMARY

Glycosaminoglycans are **long, negatively charged, unbranched, heteropolysaccharide chains** generally com-posed of a **repeating disaccharide unit** [acidic sugar–amino sugar]$_n$ (Figure 14.18). The **amino sugar** is either D-**glucosamine** or D-**galactosamine** in which the amino group is usually acetylated, thus eliminating its positive charge. The amino sugar may also be sulfated on carbon 4 or 6 or on a nonacetylated nitrogen. The **acidic sugar** is either D-**glucuronic acid** or its C-5 epimer, L-**iduronic acid**. These compounds **bind large amounts of water**, thereby producing the gel-like matrix that forms the basis of the body's **ground substance**. The viscous, lubricat-ing properties of **mucous secretions** are also caused by the presence of glycosaminoglycans, which led to the original naming of these compounds as **mucopolysaccharides**. As essential components of cell surfaces, gly-cosaminoglycans play an important role in mediating **cell–cell signaling** and **adhesion**. There are **six major classes** of glycosaminoglycans, including **chondroitin 4- and 6-sulfates**, **keratan sulfate**, **dermatan sulfate**, **hep-arin**, **heparan sulfate**, and **hyaluronic acid**. All of the glycosaminoglycans, except hyaluronic acid, are found covalently attached to protein, forming **proteoglycan monomers**, which consist of a **core protein** to which the lin-ear glycosaminoglycan chains are covalently attached. The proteoglycan monomers associate with a molecule of **hyaluronic acid** to form **proteoglycan aggregates**. Glycosaminoglycans are synthesized in the **Golgi**. The polysaccharide chains are elongated by the sequential addition of alternating acidic and amino sugars, donated by their **UDP-derivatives**. D-glucuronate maybe epimerized to L-iduronate. The last step in synthesis is sulfation of some of the amino sugars. The source of the sulfate is **3'-phosphoadenosyl-5'-phosphosulfate**. Glycosaminoglycans are **degraded** by **lysosomal hydrolases**. They are first broken down to oligosaccharides, which are degraded sequentially from the nonreducing end of each chain. A **deficiency** of any one of the hydro-lases results in a **mucopolysaccharidosis**. These are hereditary disorders in which glycosaminoglycans accumu-late in tissues, causing symptoms such as **skeletal** and **extracellular matrix deformities**, and **mental retardation**. Examples of these genetic diseases include **Hunter** and **Hurler syndromes**. **Glycoproteins** are proteins to which **oligosaccharides** are covalently attached. They differ from the proteoglycans in that the length of the glycopro-tein's carbohydrate chain is relatively short (usually two to ten sugar residues long, although they can be longer), may be branched, and does not contain serial disaccharide units. **Membrane-bound** glycoproteins participate in a broad range of cellular phenomena, including **cell surface recognition** (by other cells, hormones, and viruses), **cell surface antigenicity** (such as the blood group antigens), and as components of the **extracellular matrix** and of the **mucins** of the gastrointestinal and urogenital tracts, where they act as protective biologic lubricants. In addition, almost all of the globular proteins present in human plasma are glycoproteins. Glycoproteins are **syn-thesized** in the **endoplasmic reticulum** and the **Golgi**. The precursors of the carbohydrate components of glyco-proteins are **nucleotide sugars**. **O–linked glycoproteins** are synthesized in the Golgi by the sequential transfer of sugars from their nucleotide carriers to the protein. **N–linked glycoproteins** contain varying amounts of **mannose**.

They are synthesized by the transfer of a preformed oligosaccharide from its ER membrane lipid carrier, **dolichol**, to the protein. A deficiency in the phosphorylation of mannose residues in N–linked glycoprotein pre-enzymes destined for the lysosomes results in **I–cell disease**. Glycoproteins are degraded in lysosomes by acid hydrolases. A deficiency of any one of these enzymes results in a lysosomal **glycoprotein storage disease** (**oligosaccharidosis**), resulting in accumulation of partially degraded structures in the lysosome.

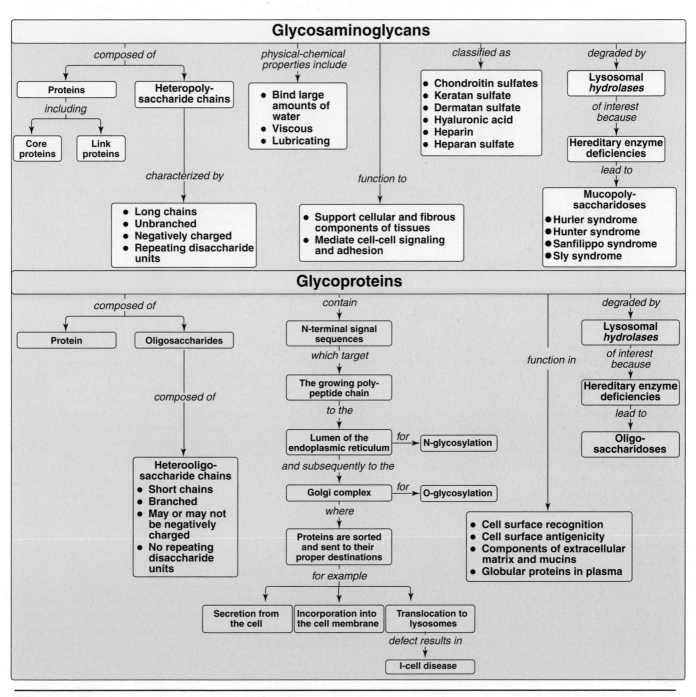

Figure 14.18
Key concept map for glycosaminoglycans and glycoproteins.

Study Questions

Choose the ONE correct answer.

14.1 Mucopolysaccharidoses are inherited lysosomal storage diseases. They are caused by:

A. an increased rate of synthesis of the carbohydrate component of proteoglycans.

B. the synthesis of polysaccharides with an altered structure.

C. defects in the degradation of the GAGs in proteoglycans.

D. the synthesis of abnormally small amounts of protein cores.

E. an insufficient amount of proteolytic enzymes.

Correct answer = C. In mucopolysaccharidoses, synthesis of proteoglycans is unaffected, both in terms of the structure and the amount of material synthesized. The diseases are caused by a deficiency of one of the lysosomal, hydrolytic enzymes responsible for the degradation of glycosaminoglycans (not the core protein).

14.2 The presence of the following compound in the urine of a patient suggests a deficiency in which one of the enzymes listed below?

$$
\begin{array}{ccc}
\text{Sulfate} & & \text{Sulfate} \\
| & & | \\
\text{GalNac}\!-\!\text{GlcUA}\!-\!\text{GalNAc}\!-\!
\end{array}
$$

A. Galactosidase

B. Glucosidase

C. Glucuronidase

D. Mannosidase

E. Sulfatase

Correct answer = E. Degradation of glycoproteins follows the rule "last on, first off." Because sulfation is the last step in the synthesis of this sequence, a sulfatase is required for the next step in the degradation of the compound shown.

14.3 An 8-month-old boy with coarse facial features, skeletal abnormalities, and delays in both growth and development is diagnosed with I-cell disease based on his presentation, and on histologic and biochemical testing. I-cell disease is the consequence of:

A. decreased production of cell-surface glycoproteins.

B. an inability to ubiquitinate proteins.

C. an inability to glycosylate proteins.

D. incorrect targeting of lysosomal proteins.

E. increased synthesis of proteoglycans.

Correct answer = D. I-cell disease is a lysosomal storage disease caused by a defect in the gene that initiates the synthesis of the mannose 6-phosphate signal that targets acid hydrolases to the lysosome, resulting in accumulation of materials within the lysosome due to decreased degradation. None of the other choices relate in any way to I-cell disease or lysosomal function.

14. 4 Distinguish between glycoproteins and proteoglycans.

Glycoproteins are proteins to which short, branched, oligosaccharide chains are attached. Proteoglycans consist of a core protein to which long, unbranched, glycosaminoglycan (GAG) chains are attached. GAGs are large complexes of negatively charged heteropolysaccharides composed of repeating [acidic sugar-amino sugar]n disaccharide units.

Metabolism of Dietary Lipids

15

I. OVERVIEW

Lipids are a heterogeneous group of water-insoluble (hydrophobic) organic molecules that can be extracted from tissues by nonpolar solvents (Figure 15.1). Because of their insolubility in aqueous solutions, body lipids are generally found compartmentalized, as in the case of membrane-associated lipids or droplets of triacylglycerol in white adipocytes, or transported in plasma in association with protein, as in lipoprotein particles (see p. 227), or on albumin. Lipids are a major source of energy for the body, and they also provide the hydrophobic barrier that permits partitioning of the aqueous contents of cells and subcellular structures. Lipids serve additional functions in the body, for example, some fat-soluble vitamins have regulatory or coenzyme functions, and the prostaglandins and steroid hormones play major roles in the control of the body's homeostasis. Not surprisingly, deficiencies or imbalances of lipid metabolism can lead to some of the major clinical problems encountered by physicians, such as atherosclerosis and obesity.

II. DIGESTION, ABSORPTION, SECRETION, AND UTILIZATION OF DIETARY LIPIDS

The average daily intake of lipids by U.S. adults is about 81 g, of which more than 90% is normally triacylglycerol (TAG, formerly called triglyceride). The remainder of the dietary lipids consists primarily of cholesterol, cholesteryl esters, phospholipids, and unesterified ("free") fatty acids. The digestion of dietary lipids is summarized in Figure 15.2.

A. Processing of dietary lipid in the stomach

The digestion of lipids begins in the stomach, catalyzed by an acid-stable *lipase* (*lingual lipase*) that originates from glands at the back of the tongue. TAG molecules, particularly those containing fatty acids of short- or medium-chain length (fewer than 12 carbons, such as are found in milk fat), are the primary target of this enzyme. These same TAGs are also degraded by a separate *gastric lipase*, secreted by the gastric mucosa. Both enzymes are relatively acid-

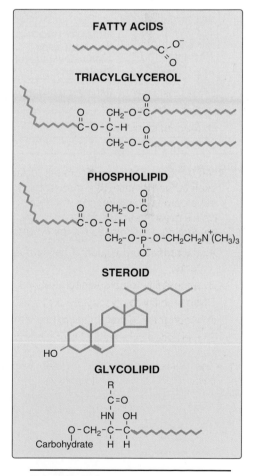

Figure 15.1
Structures of some common classes of lipids. Hydrophobic portions of the molecules are shown in orange.

173

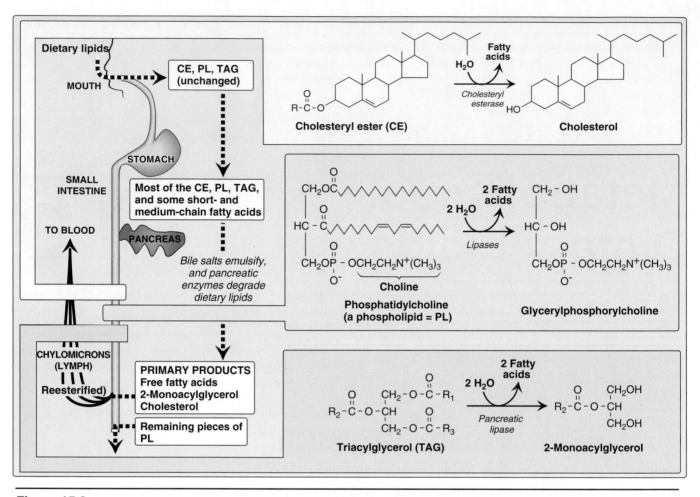

Figure 15.2
Overview of lipid digestion.

stable, with pH optimums of pH 4 to pH 6. These "*acid lipases*" play a particularly important role in lipid digestion in neonates, for whom milk fat is the primary source of calories. They also become important digestive enzymes in individuals with pancreatic insufficiency, such as those with cystic fibrosis (see below). *Lingual* and *gastric lipases* aid these patients in degrading TAG molecules (especially those with short- to medium-chain fatty acids) despite a near or complete absence of *pancreatic lipase* (see below).

1. **Cystic fibrosis (CF):** This is the most common lethal genetic disease in Caucasians of Northern European ancestry, and has a prevalence of about 1:3,000 births. This autosomal recessive disorder is caused by mutations to the gene for the CF transmembrane conductance regulator (CFTR) protein that functions as a chloride channel on epithelium. Defective CFTR results in decreased secretion of chloride and increased reabsorption of sodium and water. In the pancreas, the decreased hydration results in thickened secretions such that pancreatic enzymes are not able to reach the intestine, leading to pancreatic insufficiency. Treatment includes replacement of these enzymes and supplementation with fat-soluble vitamins. [Note: CF also causes chronic lung infections with progressive pulmonary disease.]

B. Emulsification of dietary lipid in the small intestine

The critical process of emulsification of dietary lipids occurs in the duodenum. Emulsification increases the surface area of the hydrophobic lipid droplets so that the digestive enzymes, which work at the interface of the droplet and the surrounding aqueous solution, can act effectively. Emulsification is accomplished by two complementary mechanisms, namely, use of the detergent properties of the bile salts, and mechanical mixing due to peristalsis. Bile salts, made in the liver and stored in the gallbladder, are derivatives of cholesterol (see p. 224). They consist of a sterol ring structure with a side chain to which a molecule of glycine or taurine is covalently attached by an amide linkage (Figure 15.3). These emulsifying agents interact with the dietary lipid particles and the aqueous duodenal contents, thereby stabilizing the particles as they become smaller, and preventing them from coalescing. A more complete discussion of bile salt metabolism is given on p. 225.

C. Degradation of dietary lipids by pancreatic enzymes

The dietary TAG, cholesteryl esters, and phospholipids are enzymically degraded ("digested") by pancreatic enzymes, whose secretion is hormonally controlled.

1. **TAG degradation:** TAG molecules are too large to be taken up efficiently by the mucosal cells of the intestinal villi. They are, therefore, acted upon by an *esterase*, *pancreatic lipase*, which preferentially removes the fatty acids at carbons 1 and 3. The primary products of hydrolysis are thus a mixture of 2-monoacylglycerol and free fatty acids (see Figure 15.2). [Note: This enzyme is found in high concentrations in pancreatic secretions (2–3% of the total protein present), and it is highly efficient catalytically, thus insuring that only severe pancreatic deficiency, such as that seen in cystic fibrosis, results in significant malabsorption of fat.] A second protein, *colipase*, also secreted by the pancreas, binds the *lipase* at a ratio of 1:1, and anchors it at the lipid-aqueous interface. *Colipase* restores activity to *lipase* in the presence of inhibitory substances like bile acids that bind the micelles. [Note: *Colipase* is secreted as the zymogen, procolipase, which is activated in the intestine by *trypsin*.] Orlistat, an antiobesity drug, inhibits *gastric* and *pancreatic lipases,* thereby decreasing fat absorption, resulting in loss of weight.[1]

2. **Cholesteryl ester degradation:** Most dietary cholesterol is present in the free (nonesterified) form, with 10–15% present in the esterified form. Cholesteryl esters are hydrolyzed by pancreatic *cholesteryl ester hydrolase* (*cholesterol esterase*), which produces cholesterol plus free fatty acids (see Figure 15.2). *Cholesteryl ester hydrolase* activity is greatly increased in the presence of bile salts.

3. **Phospholipid degradation:** Pancreatic juice is rich in the proenzyme of *phospholipase A$_2$* that, like procolipase, is activated by *trypsin* and, like *cholesteryl ester hydrolase*, requires bile salts for optimum activity. *Phospholipase A$_2$* removes one fatty acid from carbon 2 of a phospholipid, leaving a lysophospholipid. For example, phosphatidylcholine (the predominant phospholipid during digestion) becomes lysophosphatidylcholine. The remaining fatty

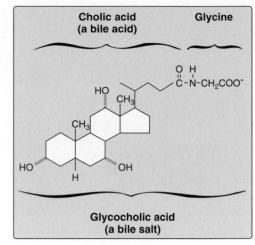

Figure 15.3
Structure of glycocholic acid.

[1]See Chapter 29 in *Lippincott's Illustrated Reviews: Pharmacology* for a discussion of orlistat.

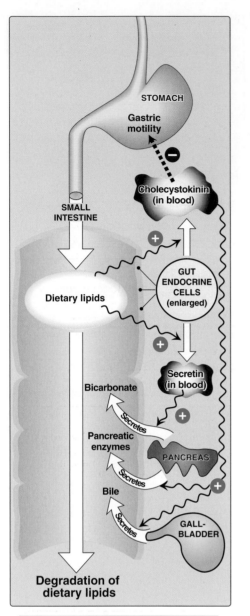

Figure 15.4
Hormonal control of lipid
digestion in the small intestine.

acid at carbon 1 can be removed by *lysophospholipase*, leaving a glycerylphosphoryl base (for example, glycerylphosphorylcholine, see Figure 15.2) that may be excreted in the feces, further degraded, or absorbed.

4. **Control of lipid digestion:** Pancreatic secretion of the hydrolytic enzymes that degrade dietary lipids in the small intestine is hormonally controlled (Figure 15.4). Cells in the mucosa of the lower duodenum and jejunum produce a small peptide hormone, cholecystokinin (CCK), in response to the presence of lipids and partially digested proteins entering these regions of the upper small intestine. CCK acts on the gallbladder (causing it to contract and release bile—a mixture of bile salts, phospholipids, and free cholesterol), and on the exocrine cells of the pancreas (causing them to release digestive enzymes). It also decreases gastric motility, resulting in a slower release of gastric contents into the small intestine (see p. 353). Other intestinal cells produce another small peptide hormone, secretin, in response to the low pH of the chyme entering the intestine. Secretin causes the pancreas and the liver to release a solution rich in bicarbonate that helps neutralize the pH of the intestinal contents, bringing them to the appropriate pH for digestive activity by pancreatic enzymes.

D. Absorption of lipids by intestinal mucosal cells (enterocytes)

Free fatty acids, free cholesterol, and 2-monoacylglycerol are the primary products of lipid digestion in the jejunum. These, plus bile salts and fat-soluble vitamins (A, D, E, and K), form mixed micelles—disk-shaped clusters of amphipathic lipids that coalesce with their hydrophobic groups on the inside and their hydrophilic groups on the outside. Mixed micelles are, therefore, soluble in the aqueous environment of the intestinal lumen (Figure 15.5). These particles approach the primary site of lipid absorption, the brush border membrane of the enterocytes (mucosal cell). This membrane is separated from the liquid contents of the intestinal lumen by an unstirred water layer that mixes poorly with the bulk fluid. The hydrophilic surface of the micelles facilitates the transport of the hydrophobic lipids through the unstirred water layer to the brush border membrane where they are absorbed. Bile salts are absorbed in the ileum. [Note: Relative to other dietary lipids, cholesterol is only poorly absorbed by the enterocytes. Drug therapy (for example, with ezetimibe[2]) can further reduce cholesterol absorption in the small intestine.] Short- and medium-chain length fatty acids do not require the assistance of mixed micelles for absorption by the intestinal mucosa.

E. Resynthesis of TAG and cholesteryl esters

The mixture of lipids absorbed by the enterocytes migrates to the endoplasmic reticulum where biosynthesis of complex lipids takes place. Fatty acids are first converted into their activated form by *fatty acyl-CoA synthetase* (*thiokinase*) (Figure 15.6). Using the fatty acyl CoA derivatives, the 2-monoacylglycerols absorbed by the enterocytes are converted to TAGs by the enzyme complex, *TAG synthase*. This complex synthesizes TAG by the consecutive actions of two enzyme activities—*acyl CoA:monoacylglycerol acyltrans-*

[2]See Chapter 21 in ***Lippincott's Illustrated Reviews: Pharmacology*** for a discussion of ezetimibe (Zetia).

ferase and *acyl CoA:diacylglycerol acyltransferase*. Lysophospholipids are reacylated to form phospholipids by a family of *acyltransferases*, and cholesterol is esterified to a fatty acid primarily by *acyl CoA:cholesterol acyltransferase* (see p. 232). [Note: Virtually all long-chain fatty acids entering the enterocytes are used in this fashion to form TAGs, phospholipids, and cholesteryl esters. Short- and medium-chain length fatty acids are not converted to their CoA derivatives, and are not reesterified to 2-monoacylglycerol. Instead, they are released into the portal circulation, where they are carried by serum albumin to the liver.]

F. Lipid malabsorption

Lipid malabsorption, resulting in increased lipid (including the fat-soluble vitamins and essential fatty acids, see p. 182) in the feces (that is, steatorrhea), can be caused by disturbances in lipid digestion and/or absorption (Figure 15.7). Such disturbances can result from several conditions, including CF (causing poor digestion) and shortened bowel (causing decreased absorption).

> The ability of short- and medium-chain length fatty acids to be taken up by enterocytes without the aid of mixed micelles has made them important in dietary therapy for individuals with malabsorption disorders.

G. Secretion of lipids from enterocytes

The newly resynthesized TAGs and cholesteryl esters are very hydrophobic, and aggregate in an aqueous environment. It is, therefore, necessary that they be packaged as particles of lipid droplets surrounded by a thin layer composed of phospholipids, unesterified cholesterol, and a molecule of the characteristic protein, apolipoprotein B-48 (see p. 228). This layer stabilizes the particle and increases its solubility, thereby preventing multiple particles from

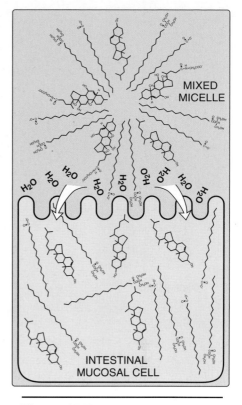

Figure 15.5
Absorption of lipids contained in a mixed micelle by an intestinal mucosal cell. [Note: The micelle itself is not taken up.]

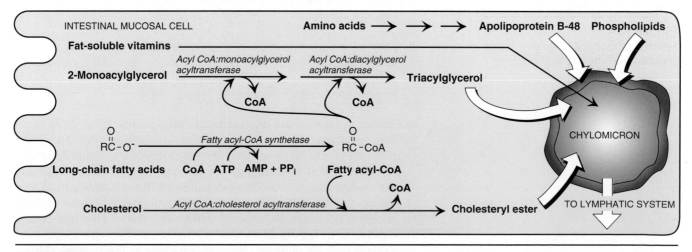

Figure 15.6
Assembly and secretion of chylomicrons by intestinal mucosal cells. [Note: Short- and medium-chain length fatty acids do not require incorporation into micelles and directly enter into the blood.]

coalescing. [Note: Microsomal TAG transfer protein is essential for the assembly of these TAG-rich apolipoprotein B–containing lipoprotein particles in the endoplasmic reticulum.] The particles are released by exocytosis from enterocytes into the lacteals (lymphatic vessels originating in the villi of the small intestine). The presence of these particles in the lymph after a lipid-rich meal gives it a milky appearance. This lymph is called chyle (as opposed to chyme—the name given to the semifluid mass of partially digested food that passes from the stomach to the duodenum), and the particles are named chylomicrons. Chylomicrons follow the lymphatic system to the thoracic duct, and are then conveyed to the left subclavian vein, where they enter the blood. The steps in the production of chylomicrons are summarized in Figure 15.6. (For a more detailed description of chylomicron structure and metabolism, see p. 228.)

H. Use of dietary lipids by the tissues

Triacylglycerol contained in chylomicrons is broken down primarily in the capillaries of skeletal muscle and adipose tissues, but also those of the heart, lung, kidney, and liver. Triacylglycerol in chylomicrons is degraded to free fatty acids and glycerol by *lipoprotein lipase*. This enzyme is synthesized primarily by adipocytes and muscle cells. It is secreted and becomes associated with the luminal surface of endothelial cells of the capillary beds of the peripheral tissues. [Note: Familial *lipoprotein lipase* deficiency (Type I hyperlipoproteinemia) is a rare, autosomal recessive disorder caused by a deficiency of *lipoprotein lipase* or its coenzyme, apolipoprotein C-II (see p. 228). The result is fasting chylomicronemia and hypertriacylglycerolemia.]

1. **Fate of free fatty acids:** The free fatty acids derived from the hydrolysis of TAG may either directly enter adjacent muscle cells or adipocytes, or they may be transported in the blood in association with serum albumin until they are taken up by cells. [Note: Serum albumin is a large protein secreted by the liver. It transports a number of primarily hydrophobic compounds in the circulation, including free fatty acids and some drugs.] Most cells can oxidize fatty acids to produce energy (see p. 190). Adipocytes can also reesterify free fatty acids to produce TAG molecules, which are stored until the fatty acids are needed by the body (see p. 188).

2. **Fate of glycerol:** Glycerol that is released from TAG is used almost exclusively by the liver to produce glycerol 3-phosphate, which can enter either glycolysis or gluconeogenesis by oxidation to dihydroxyacetone phosphate (see p. 190).

3. **Fate of the remaining chylomicron components:** After most of the TAG has been removed, the chylomicron remnants (which contain cholesteryl esters, phospholipids, apolipoproteins, fat-soluble vitamins, and some TAG) bind to receptors on the liver (see p. 230) and are then endocytosed. The remnants are then hydrolyzed to their component parts. Cholesterol and the nitrogenous bases of phospholipids (for example, choline) can be recycled by the body. [Note: If removal of remnants by the liver is decreased due to impaired binding to their receptor, they accumulate in the plasma. This is seen in Type III hyperlipoproteinemia (rare, also called familial dysbetalipoproteinemia, see p. 231).]

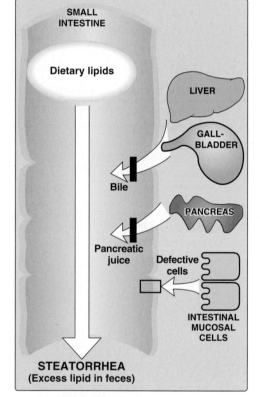

Figure 15.7
Possible causes of steatorrhea.

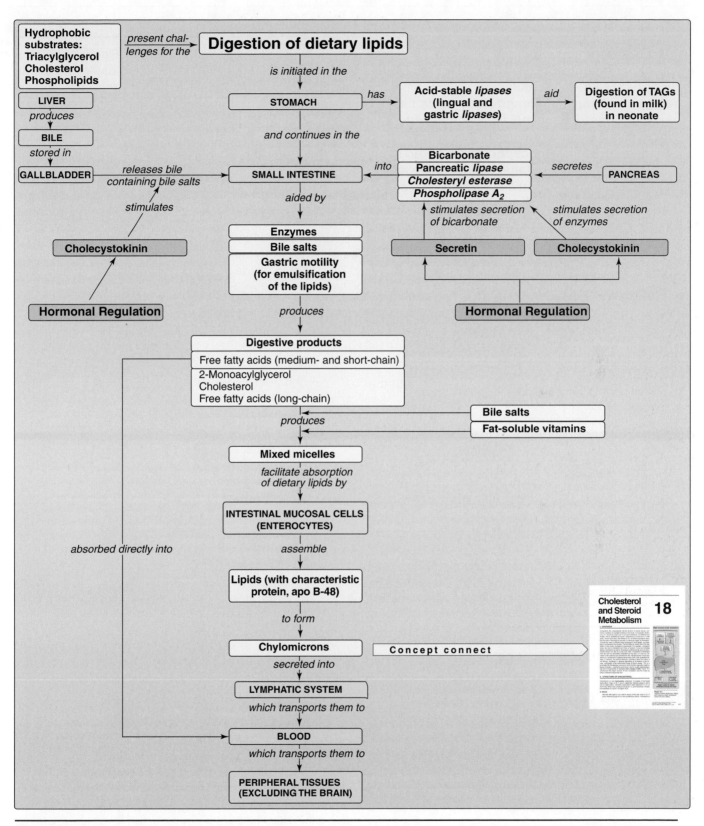

Figure 15.8
Key concept map for metabolism of dietary lipids. apo = apolipoprotein; TAGs = triacylglycerols.

III. CHAPTER SUMMARY

The digestion of **dietary lipids** begins in the **stomach** and continues in the **small intestine** (Figure 15.8). The **hydrophobic nature** of lipids requires that the dietary lipids—particularly those that contain long-chain length fatty acids (LCFA)—be **emulsified** for efficient degradation. Triacylglycerols (TAG) obtained from milk contain **short-** to **medium-chain length fatty acids** that can be degraded in the **stomach** by the acid lipases (**lingual lipase** and **gastric lipase**). Cholesteryl esters (CE), phospholipids (PL), and TAG containing LCFAs are degraded in the **small intestine** by enzymes secreted by the **pancreas**. The most important of these enzymes are **pancreatic lipase**, **phospholipase A₂**, and **cholesteryl esterase**. The dietary lipids are **emulsified** in the small intestine using **peristaltic action**, and **bile salts**, which serve as a detergent. The primary products resulting from enzymatic degradation of dietary lipid are **2-monoacylglycerol**, unesterified **cholesterol**, and **free fatty acids**. These compounds, plus the fat-soluble vitamins, form **mixed micelles** that facilitate the absorption of dietary lipids by **intestinal mucosal cells** (**enterocytes**). These cells resynthesize TAG, CE, and PL, and also synthesize protein (**apolipoprotein B-48**), all of which are then assembled with the fat-soluble vitamins into **chylomicrons**. These **serum lipoprotein** particles are released into the **lymph**, which carries them to the **blood**. Short- and medium chain fatty acids enter blood directly. Thus, dietary lipids are transported to the peripheral tissues. Problems with fat absorption cause steatorrhea. A deficiency in the ability to degrade chylomicron components, or remove their remnants after TAG has been removed, results in accumulation of these particles in blood.

Study Questions

15.1 Which one of the following statements about the digestion of lipids is correct?

   A. Lipid digestion begins with acid-stable lipases that primarily use TAG with long to very long-chain fatty acids as substrates.

   B. Large lipid droplets are emulsified (have their surface area increased) in the mouth through the act of chewing (mastication).

   C. Colipase facilitates the binding of bile salts to mixed micelles, maximizing the activity of pancreatic lipase.

   D. The peptide hormone secretin causes the gallbladder to contract and release bile.

   E. Patients with cystic fibrosis have difficulties with digestion because their thickened pancreatic secretions are less able to reach the small intestine, the primary site of lipid digestion.

   F. Formation of chylomicrons is independent of protein synthesis in the intestinal mucosa.

Correct answer = E. Patients with CF, a genetic disease due to a deficiency of functional CFTR, have thickened secretions that impede the flow of pancreatic enzymes into the duodenum. The acid-stable lipases, lingual and gastric lipase, use as substrates TAG with short to medium-chain fatty acids that are abundant in milk. Emulsification occurs through peristalsis that provides mechanical mixing, and bile salts that function as detergents. Colipase restores activity to pancreatic lipase in the presence of inhibitory bile acids that bind the micelles. CCK (cholecystokinin) is the hormone that causes contraction of the gallbladder and release of stored bile; secretin causes release of bicarbonate. Chylomicron formation requires synthesis of the protein apolipoprotein B-48.

15.2 Which one of the following statements about the absorption of lipids from the intestine is correct?

   A. Dietary triacylglycerol must be completely hydrolyzed to free fatty acids and glycerol before absorption.

   B. The TAG carried by chylomicrons is degraded to free fatty acids and glycerol by lipoprotein lipase on the endothelial surface of capillaries in muscle and adipose primarily.

   C. Fatty acids that contain ten carbons or less are absorbed and enter the circulation primarily via the lymphatic system.

   D. Deficiencies in the ability to absorb fat result in excessive amounts of chylomicrons in the blood.

Correct answer = B. The TAG in chylomicrons are degraded to fatty acids and glycerol by lipoprotein lipase on the endothelial surface of capillaries in muscle and adipose, thus providing a source of fatty acids to these tissues for degradation or storage. In the duodenum, TAG are degraded to 1 monoacylglycerol + 2 free fatty acids that get absorbed. Medium and short chain fatty acids enter directly into blood; they do not get packaged into chylomicrons. Chylomicrons contain dietary lipids that were digested and absorbed, thus a defect in fat absorption would result in decreased production of chylomicrons.

Fatty Acid and Triacylglycerol Metabolism

16

I. OVERVIEW

Fatty acids exist "free" in the body (that is, they are unesterified), and are also found as fatty acyl esters in more complex molecules, such as triacylglycerols. Low levels of free fatty acids occur in all tissues, but substantial amounts can sometimes be found in the plasma, particularly during fasting. Plasma free fatty acids (transported on serum albumin) are in route from their point of origin (triacylglycerol of adipose tissue or circulating lipoproteins) to their site of consumption (most tissues). Free fatty acids can be oxidized by many tissues—particularly liver and muscle—to provide energy. Fatty acids are also structural components of membrane lipids, such as phospholipids and glycolipids (see p. 201). Fatty acids are attached to certain intracellular proteins to enhance the ability of those proteins to associate with membranes (see p. 206). Fatty acids are also precursors of the hormone-like prostaglandins (see p. 213). Esterified fatty acids, in the form of triacylglycerols stored in adipose cells, serve as the major energy reserve of the body. Figure 16.1 illustrates the metabolic pathways of fatty acid synthesis and degradation, and their relationship to carbohydrate metabolism.

II. STRUCTURE OF FATTY ACIDS

A fatty acid consists of a hydrophobic hydrocarbon chain with a terminal carboxyl group that has a pK_a of about 4.8 (Figure 16.2). At physiologic pH, the terminal carboxyl group (–COOH) ionizes, becoming –COO⁻. This anionic group has an affinity for water, giving the fatty acid its amphipathic nature (having both a hydrophilic and a hydrophobic region). However, for long-chain fatty acids (LCFAs), the hydrophobic portion is predominant. These molecules are highly water-insoluble, and must be transported in the circulation in association with protein. More than 90% of the fatty acids found in plasma are in the form of fatty acid esters (primarily triacylglycerol, cholesteryl esters, and phospholipids) contained in circulating lipoprotein particles (see p. 227). Unesterified (free) fatty acids are transported in the circulation in association with albumin.

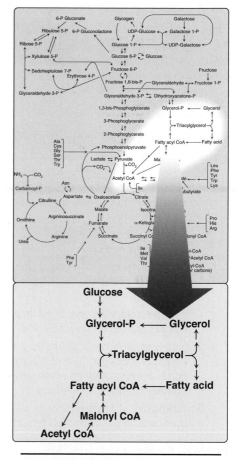

Figure 16.1
Triacylglycerol synthesis and degradation.

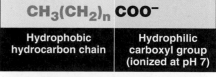

Figure 16.2
Structure of a fatty acid.

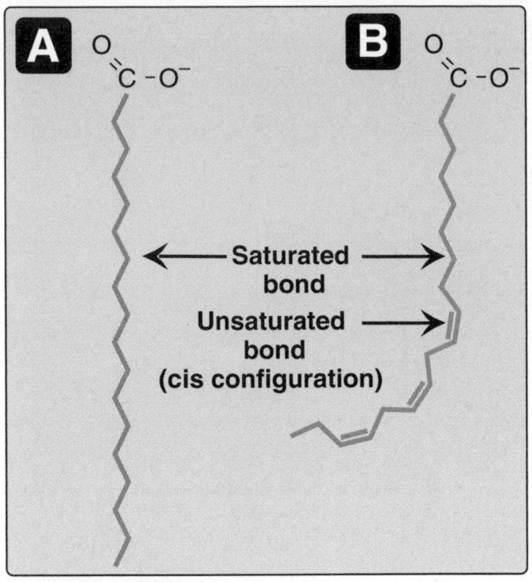

Figure 16.3
A saturated (A) and an unsaturated
(B) fatty acid. Orange denotes
hydrophobic portions of the
molecules. [Note: Cis double bonds
cause a fatty acid to "kink."]

Figure 16.4
Some fatty acids of physiologic
importance.

A. Saturation of fatty acids

Fatty acid chains may contain no double bonds—that is, be saturated—or contain one or more double bonds—that is, be mono- or polyunsaturated. When double bonds are present, they are nearly always in the cis rather than in the trans configuration. (See p. 363 for a discussion of the dietary occurrence of cis and trans unsaturated fatty acids.) The introduction of a cis double bond causes the fatty acid to bend or "kink" at that position (Figure 16.3). If the fatty acid has two or more double bonds, they are always spaced at three-carbon intervals. [Note: In general, addition of double bonds decreases the melting temperature (T_m) of a fatty acid, whereas increasing the chain length increases the T_m. Because membrane lipids typically contain LCFA, the presence of double bonds in some fatty acids helps maintain the fluid nature of those lipids.]

B. Chain lengths of fatty acids

The common names and structures of some fatty acids of physiologic importance are listed in Figure 16.4. The carbon atoms are numbered, beginning with the carboxyl carbon as carbon 1. The number before the colon indicates the number of carbons in the chain, and those after the colon indicate the numbers and positions (relative to the carboxyl end) of double bonds. For example, as shown in Figure 16.5A, arachidonic acid, 20:4(5,8,11,14), is 20 carbons long and has 4 double bonds (between carbons 5–6, 8–9, 11–12, and 14–15). [Note: Carbon 2, the carbon to which the carboxyl group is attached, is also called the α-carbon, carbon 3 is the β-carbon, and carbon 4 is the γ-carbon. The carbon of the terminal methyl group is called the ω-carbon regardless of the chain length.] The double bonds in a fatty acid can also be denoted relative to the ω (or methyl-terminal) end of the chain. Arachidonic acid is referred to as an ω-6 fatty acid acid (also an n-6, Figure 16.5A) because the terminal double bond is six bonds in from the ω end (Figure 16.5B). Another ω-6 fatty acid is the essential linoleic acid, 18:2(9,12). In contrast, α-linolenic acid, 18:3(9,12,15), is an essential ω-3 fatty acid. (See p. 363 for a discussion of the nutritional significance of ω-3 and ω-6 fatty acids.)

C. Essential fatty acids

Two fatty acids are dietary essentials in humans because of our inability to synthesize them: linoleic acid, which is the precursor of ω-6 arachidonic acid, the substrate for prostaglandin synthesis (see p. 213), and α-linolenic acid, the precursor of other ω-3 fatty acids important for growth and development. Plants provide us with the essential fatty acids. [Note: Arachidonic acid becomes essential if linoleic acid is deficient in the diet.]

Essential fatty acid deficiency can result in a scaly dermatitis (ichthyosis), as well as visual and neurologic abnormalities. Essential fatty acid deficiency, however, is rare.

III. DE NOVO SYNTHESIS OF FATTY ACIDS

A large proportion of the fatty acids used by the body is supplied by the diet. Carbohydrates and protein obtained from the diet in excess of the body's needs for these compounds can be converted to fatty acids, which are stored as triacylglycerols. (See p. 321 for a discussion of the metabolism of dietary nutrients in the well-fed state.) In adult humans, fatty acid synthesis occurs primarily in the liver and lactating mammary glands and, to a lesser extent, in adipose tissue. This cytosolic process incorporates carbons from acetyl coenzyme A (CoA) into the growing fatty acid chain, using adenosine triphosphate (ATP) and reduced nicotinamide adenine dinucleotide phosphate (NADPH).

A. Production of cytosolic acetyl CoA

The first step in de novo fatty acid synthesis is the transfer of acetate units from mitochondrial acetyl CoA to the cytosol. Mitochondrial acetyl CoA is produced by the oxidation of pyruvate (see p. 109), and by the catabolism of fatty acids (see p. 190), ketone bodies (see p. 196), and certain amino acids (see p. 266). The CoA portion of acetyl CoA, however, cannot cross the inner mitochondrial membrane; only the acetyl portion enters the cytosol. It does so as part of citrate produced by the condensation of oxaloacetate (OAA) and acetyl CoA (Figure 16.6). [Note: This process of translocation of citrate from the mitochondrion to the cytosol, where it is cleaved by *ATP-citrate lyase* to produce cytosolic acetyl CoA and OAA, occurs when the mitochondrial citrate concentration is high. This is observed when *isocitrate dehydrogenase* is inhibited by the presence of large amounts of ATP, causing citrate and isocitrate to accumulate (see p. 112). Therefore, cytosolic citrate may be viewed as a high-energy signal.] Because a large amount of ATP is needed for fatty acid synthesis, the increase in both ATP and citrate enhances this pathway.

B. Carboxylation of acetyl CoA to form malonyl CoA

The energy for the carbon-to-carbon condensations in fatty acid synthesis is supplied by the process of carboxylation and then decarboxylation of acetyl groups in the cytosol. The carboxylation of acetyl CoA to form malonyl CoA is catalyzed by *acetyl CoA carboxylase* (Figure 16.7), and requires CO_2 and ATP. The coenzyme is the vitamin, biotin, which is covalently bound to a lysyl residue of the *carboxylase* (see Figure 28.16).

1. **Short-term regulation of acetyl CoA carboxylase (ACC):** This carboxylation is both the rate-limiting and the regulated step in fatty acid synthesis (see Figure 16.7). The inactive form of *ACC* is a protomer (dimer). The enzyme undergoes allosteric activation by citrate, which causes dimers to polymerize, and allosteric inactivation by long-chain fatty acyl CoA (the end product of the pathway), which causes its depolymerization. A second mechanism of short-term regulation is by reversible phosphorylation. *AMP-activated protein kinase* (*AMPK*) phosphorylates and inactivates *ACC*. *AMPK* itself is allosterically activated by AMP and covalently activated by phosphorylation via several *kinases*. At least one of these

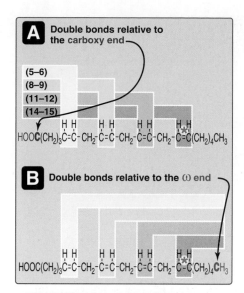

Figure 16.5
Arachidonic acid, illustrating the position of the double bonds. Arachidonic acid, 20:4(5,8,11,14) is an n-6 fatty acid because the double bond furthest from the carboxy end (carbon 1) is 14 carbons from that end: 20-14 = 6. It is also referred to as an ω-6 fatty acid because the terminal double bond is six bonds in from the ω end. Thus, the "ω" and "n" designations are equivalent (see ∗).

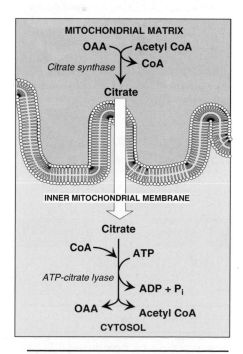

Figure 16.6
Production of cytosolic acetyl CoA.

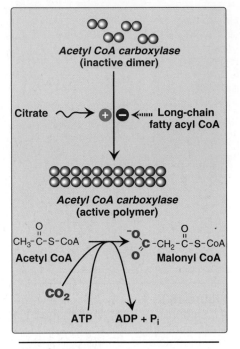

Figure 16.7
Allosteric regulation of malonyl CoA synthesis by *acetyl CoA carboxylase* (*ACC*). The carboxyl group contributed by dissolved CO_2 is shown in blue.

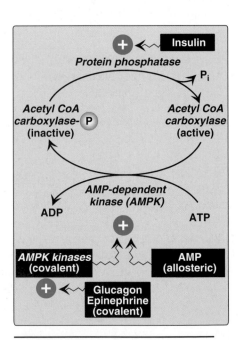

Figure 16.8
Covalent regulation (phosphorylation) of *acetyl CoA carboxylase* (*ACC*) by *AMP-dependent kinase* (*AMPK*), which itself is regulated both covalently and allosterically.

AMPK kinases is activated by *cAMP-dependent protein kinase A* (*PKA*). Thus, in the presence of counterregulatory hormones, such as epinephrine and glucagon, *ACC* is phosphorylated and, thereby, inactivated (Figure 16.8). In the presence of insulin, *ACC* is dephosphorylated and, thereby, activated. [Note: This is analogous to the regulation of *glycogen synthase*, see p. 131.]

2. **Long-term regulation of acetyl CoA carboxylase:** Prolonged consumption of a diet containing excess calories (particularly high-calorie, high-carbohydrate diets) causes an increase in *ACC* synthesis, thus increasing fatty acid synthesis. Conversely, a low-calorie or a high-fat diet causes a reduction in fatty acid synthesis by decreasing the synthesis of *ACC*. [Note: Synthesis of the *carboxylase* is upregulated by insulin via a sterol response element binding protein, SREBP-1. The function and regulation of SREBPs are described on p. 222. *Fatty acid synthase* (see below) is similarly regulated by diet and SREBP-1.] Metformin, used in the treatment of type 2 diabetes, lowers serum TAG through activation of *AMPK* resulting in inhibition of *ACC* activity (by phosphorylation) and inhibition of *ACC* and *fatty acid synthase* expression (by decreasing SREBP-1). Metformin also lowers blood glucose by increasing *AMPK*-mediated uptake of glucose by muscle.

C. Fatty acid synthase: a multifunctional enzyme in eukaryotes

The remaining series of reactions of fatty acid synthesis in eukaryotes is catalyzed by the multifunctional, dimeric enzyme, *fatty acid synthase* (*FAS*). Each *FAS* monomer is a multicatalytic polypeptide with seven different enzymic activities plus a domain that covalently binds a molecule of 4'-phosphopantetheine. [Note: 4'-Phosphopantetheine, a derivative of the vitamin pantothenic acid (see p. 381), carries acyl units on its terminal thiol (–SH) group during fatty acid synthesis. It also is a component of CoA.] In prokaryotes, *FAS* is a multienzyme complex, and the 4'-phosphopantetheine domain is a separate protein, referred to as the acyl carrier protein (ACP). ACP is used below to refer to the phosphopantetheine-containing domain of eukaryotic *FAS*. The reaction numbers in brackets below refer to Figure 16.9. [Note: The enzyme activities listed are separate catalytic domains present in each multicatalytic *FAS* monomer.]

[1] A molecule of acetate is transferred from acetyl CoA to the –SH group of the ACP. Domain: *Acetyl CoA-ACP acetyltransacylase.*

[2] Next, this two-carbon fragment is transferred to a temporary holding site, the thiol group of a cysteine residue on the enzyme.

[3] The now-vacant ACP accepts a three-carbon malonate unit from malonyl CoA. Domain: *Malonyl CoA-ACP transacylase.*

[4] The acetyl group on the cysteine residue condenses with the malonyl group on ACP as the CO_2 originally added by *acetyl CoA carboxylase* is released. The result is a four-carbon unit attached to the ACP domain. The loss of free energy from the decarboxylation drives the reaction. Domain: *3-Ketoacyl-ACP synthase.*

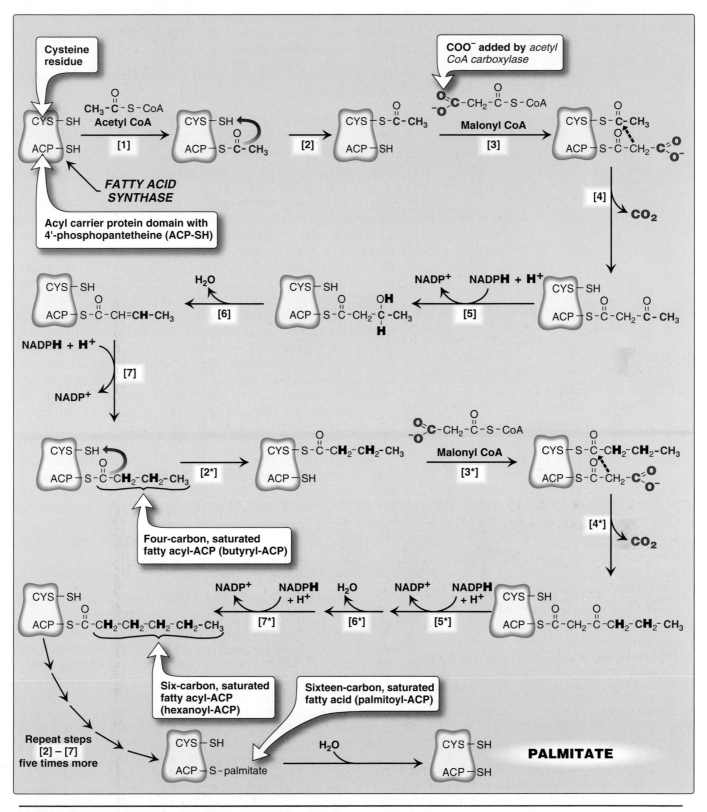

Figure 16.9
Synthesis of palmitate (16:0) by multifunctional *fatty acid synthase* (*FAS*). [Note: Numbers in brackets correspond to bracketed numbers in the text. A second repetition of the steps is indicated by numbers with an asterisk (*). Carbons provided directly by acetyl CoA are shown in red.]

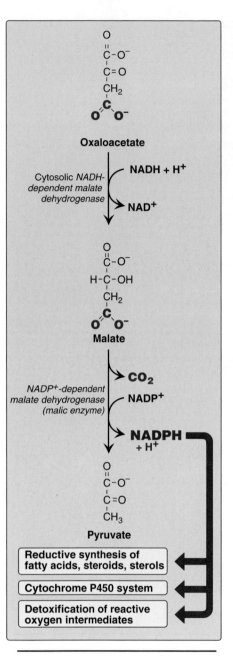

Figure 16.10
Cytosolic conversion of oxalo-acetate to pyruvate with the generation of NADPH. [Note: The pentose phosphate pathway is the primary source of the NADPH.]

The next three reactions convert the 3-ketoacyl group to the corresponding saturated acyl group by a pair of reductions requiring NADPH and a dehydration step.

[5] The keto group is reduced to an alcohol. Domain: *3-Ketoacyl-ACP reductase.*

[6] A molecule of water is removed to introduce a double bond between carbons 2 and 3 (the α- and β-carbons). Domain: *3-Hydroxyacyl-ACP dehydratase.*

[7] The double bond is reduced. Domain: *Enoyl-ACP reductase.*

The result of these seven steps is production of a four-carbon compound (butyryl) whose three terminal carbons are fully saturated, and which remains attached to the ACP. These seven steps are repeated, beginning with the transfer of the butyryl chain from the ACP to the Cys residue [2*], the attachment of a molecule of malonate to the ACP [3*], and the condensation of the two molecules liberating CO_2 [4*]. The carbonyl group at the β-carbon (carbon 3—the third carbon from the sulfur) is then reduced [5*], dehydrated [6*], and reduced [7*], generating hexanoyl-ACP. This cycle of reactions is repeated five more times, each time incorporating a two-carbon unit (derived from malonyl CoA) into the growing fatty acid chain at the carboxyl end. When the fatty acid reaches a length of 16 carbons, the synthetic process is terminated with palmitoyl-S-ACP. [Note: Shorter-length fatty acids are important end-products in the lactating mammary gland.] *Palmitoyl thioesterase* cleaves the thioester bond, releasing a fully saturated molecule of palmitate (16:0). [Note: All the carbons in palmitic acid have passed through malonyl CoA except the two donated by the original acetyl CoA, which are found at the methyl-group (ω) end of the fatty acid. This underscores the rate-limiting nature of the *acetyl CoA carboxylase* reaction.]

D. Major sources of the NADPH required for fatty acid synthesis

The hexose monophosphate pathway (see p. 145) is the major supplier of NADPH for fatty acid synthesis. Two NADPH are produced for each molecule of glucose that enters this pathway. The cytosolic conversion of malate to pyruvate, in which malate is oxidized and decarboxylated by cytosolic *malic enzyme* (*NADP⁺-dependent malate dehydrogenase*), also produces cytosolic NADPH (and CO_2, Figure 16.10). [Note: Malate can arise from the reduction of OAA by cytosolic *NADH-dependent malate dehydrogenase* (see Figure 16.10). One source of the cytosolic NADH required for this reaction is that produced during glycolysis (see p. 101). OAA, in turn, can arise from citrate. Recall from Figure 16.6 that citrate was shown to move from the mitochondria into the cytosol, where it is cleaved into acetyl CoA and OAA by *ATP-citrate lyase*.] A summary of the interrelationship between glucose metabolism and palmitate synthesis is shown in Figure 16.11.

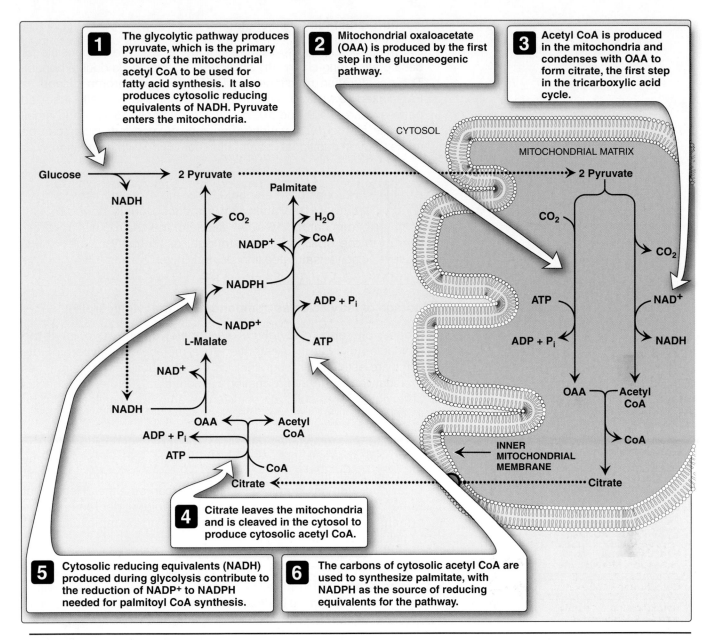

Figure 16.11
Interrelationship between glucose metabolism and palmitate synthesis.

E. Further elongation of fatty acid chains

Although palmitate, a 16-carbon, fully saturated long-chain length fatty acid (16:0), is the primary endproduct of *fatty acid synthase* activity, it can be further elongated by the addition of two-carbon units in the smooth endoplasmic reticulum (SER). Elongation requires a system of separate enzymes rather than a multifunctional enzyme. Malonyl CoA is the two-carbon donor and NADPH supplies the electrons. The brain has additional elongation capabilities, allowing it to produce the very-long-chain fatty acids (over 22 carbons) that are required for synthesis of brain lipids.

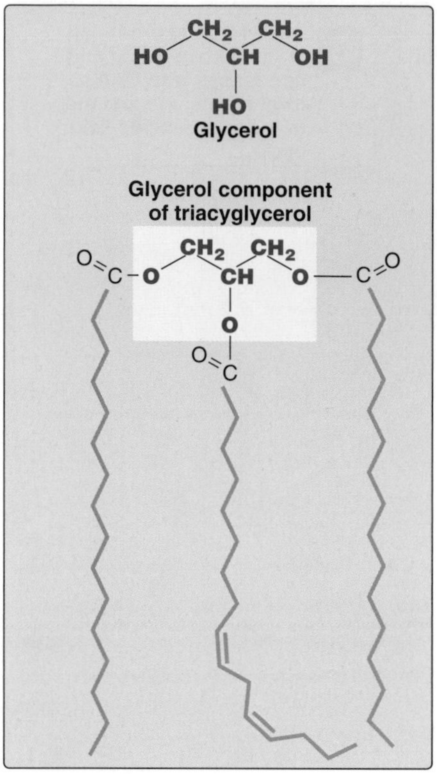

Figure 16.12
A triacylglycerol with an unsaturated fatty acid on carbon 2.

F. Desaturation of fatty acid chains

Enzymes (*desaturases*) also present in the SER are responsible for desaturating long-chain fatty acids (that is, adding cis double bonds). The desaturation reactions require NADH, cytochrome b_5 and its FAD-linked *reductase*. The first double bond is typically inserted between carbons 9 and 10, producing primarily 18:1(9) and small amounts of 16:1(9). A variety of polyunsaturated fatty acids can be made through additional desaturation combined with elongation.

> Humans have carbon 9, 6, 5 and 4 *desaturases*, but lack the ability to introduce double bonds from carbon 10 to the ω end of the chain. This is the basis for the nutritional essentiality of the polyunsaturated linoleic and linolenic acids.

G. Storage of fatty acids as components of triacylglycerols

Mono-, di-, and triacylglycerols consist of one, two, or three molecules of fatty acid esterified to a molecule of glycerol. Fatty acids are esterified through their carboxyl groups, resulting in a loss of negative charge and formation of "neutral fat." [Note: If a species of acylglycerol is solid at room temperature, it is called a "fat"; if liquid, it is called an "oil."]

1. **Structure of triacylglycerol (TAG):** The three fatty acids esterified to a glycerol molecule are usually not of the same type. The fatty acid on carbon 1 is typically saturated, that on carbon 2 is typically unsaturated, and that on carbon 3 can be either. Recall that the presence of the unsaturated fatty acid(s) decrease(s) the melting temperature (T_m) of the lipid. An example of a TAG molecule is shown in Figure 16.12.

2. **Storage of TAG:** Because TAGs are only slightly soluble in water and cannot form stable micelles by themselves, they coalesce within adipocytes to form oily droplets that are nearly anhydrous. These cytosolic lipid droplets are the major energy reserve of the body.

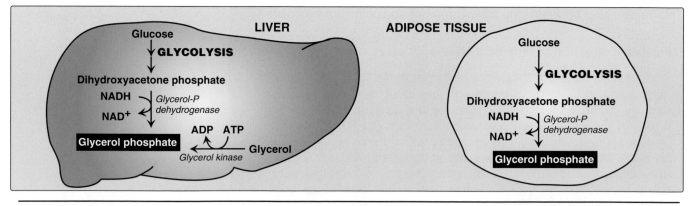

Figure 16.13
Pathways for production of glycerol phosphate in liver and adipose tissue.

3. **Synthesis of glycerol phosphate:** Glycerol phosphate is the initial acceptor of fatty acids during TAG synthesis. There are two pathways for glycerol phosphate production (Figure 16.13). In both liver (the primary site of TAG synthesis) and adipose tissue, glycerol phosphate can be produced from glucose, using first the reactions of the glycolytic pathway to produce dihydroxyacetone phosphate (DHAP, see p. 101). Next, DHAP is reduced by *glycerol phosphate dehydrogenase* to glycerol phosphate. A second pathway found in the liver, but not in adipose tissue, uses *glycerol kinase* to convert free glycerol to glycerol phosphate (see Figure 16.13). [Note: The glucose transporter in adipocytes (GLUT-4) is insulin-dependent (see p. 312). Thus, when plasma glucose—and, therefore, plasma insulin—levels are low, adipocytes have only a limited ability to synthesize glycerol phosphate, and cannot produce TAG.]

4. **Conversion of a free fatty acid to its activated form:** A fatty acid must be converted to its activated form (attached to CoA) before it can participate in metabolic processes such as TAG synthesis. This reaction, illustrated in Figure 15.6, is catalyzed by a family of *fatty acyl CoA synthetases* (*thiokinases*).

5. **Synthesis of a molecule of TAG from glycerol phosphate and fatty acyl CoA:** This pathway involves four reactions, shown in Figure 16.14. These include the sequential addition of two fatty acids from fatty acyl CoA, the removal of phosphate, and the addition of the third fatty acid.

H. Different fates of TAG in the liver and adipose tissue

In white adipose tissue, TAG is stored in a nearly anhydrous form as fat droplets in the cytosol of the cells. It serves as "depot fat," ready for mobilization when the body requires it for fuel. Little TAG is stored in the liver. Instead, most is exported, packaged with other lipids and apoproteins to form lipoprotein particles called very-low-density lipoproteins (VLDL). Nascent VLDL are secreted directly into the blood where they mature and function to deliver the endogenously derived lipids to the peripheral tissues. [Note: Recall that chylomicrons deliver primarily dietary (exogenously derived) lipids.] Plasma lipoproteins are discussed in Chapter 18.

IV. MOBILIZATION OF STORED FATS AND OXIDATION OF FATTY ACIDS

Fatty acids stored in adipose tissue, in the form of neutral TAG, serve as the body's major fuel storage reserve. TAGs provide concentrated stores of metabolic energy because they are highly reduced and largely anhydrous. The yield from the complete oxidation of fatty acids to CO_2 and H_2O is 9 kcal/g fat (as compared to 4 kcal/g protein or carbohydrate, see Figure 27.5). [Note: Fatty acids are also supplied to tissues by lipoproteins (see p. 228).]

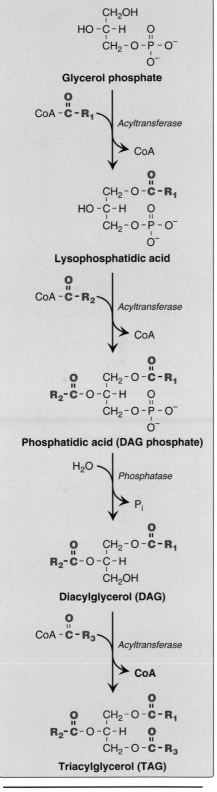

Figure 16.14
Synthesis of triacylglycerol.

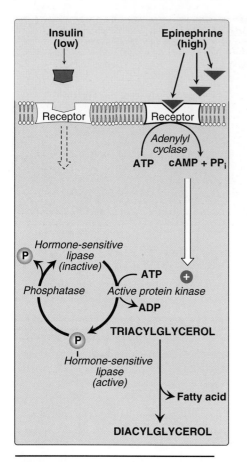

Figure 16.15
Hormonal regulation of triacylglycerol degradation in the adipocyte.

A. Release of fatty acids from TAG

The mobilization of stored fat requires the hydrolytic release of fatty acids and glycerol from their TAG form. This process is initiated by *hormone-sensitive lipase*, which removes a fatty acid from carbon 1 and/or carbon 3 of the TAG. Additional *lipases* specific for diacylglycerol or monoacylglycerol remove the remaining fatty acid(s).

1. **Activation of hormone-sensitive lipase (HSL):** This enzyme is activated when phosphorylated by a *3´,5´-cyclic AMP(cAMP)– dependent protein kinase.* 3´,5´-Cyclic AMP is produced in the adipocyte when one of several hormones (such as epinephrine or glucagon) binds to receptors on the cell membrane, and activates *adenylyl cyclase* (Figure 16.15). The process is similar to that of the activation of *glycogen phosphorylase* (see Figure 11.10). [Note: Because *acetyl CoA carboxylase* is inhibited by hormone-directed phosphorylation when the cAMP-mediated cascade is activated (see Figure 16.8), fatty acid synthesis is turned off when TAG degradation is turned on.] In the presence of high plasma levels of insulin and glucose, *HSL* is dephosphorylated, and becomes inactive.

2. **Fate of glycerol:** The glycerol released during TAG degradation cannot be metabolized by adipocytes because they apparently lack *glycerol kinase*. Rather, glycerol is transported through the blood to the liver, where it can be phosphorylated. The resulting glycerol phosphate can be used to form TAG in the liver, or can be converted to DHAP by reversal of the *glycerol phosphate dehydrogenase* reaction illustrated in Figure 16.13. DHAP can participate in glycolysis or gluconeogenesis.

3. **Fate of fatty acids:** The free (unesterified) fatty acids move through the cell membrane of the adipocyte, and bind to plasma albumin. They are transported to the tissues, enter cells, get activated to their CoA derivatives, and are oxidized for energy. Regardless of their levels, plasma free fatty acids (FFA) cannot be used for fuel by erythrocytes, which have no mitochondria. Brain, too, does not use fatty acids for energy, but the reasons are less clear. [Note: Over 50% of the fatty acids released from adipose TAG are reesterified to glycerol 3-phosphate. White adipose does not express *glycerol kinase*, and the phosphorylated glycerol is produced by glyceroneogenesis, an incomplete version of gluconeogenesis: pyruvate to PEP to OAA to DHAP to glycerol 3-phosphate. The process reduces plasma FFA, molecules associated with insulin resistance in type 2 diabetes and obesity (see p. 343).]

B. β-Oxidation of fatty acids

The major pathway for catabolism of fatty acids is a mitochondrial pathway called β-oxidation, in which two-carbon fragments are successively removed from the carboxyl end of the fatty acyl CoA, producing acetyl CoA, NADH, and $FADH_2$.

1. **Transport of long-chain fatty acids (LCFA) into the mitochondria:** After a LCFA enters a cell, it is converted in the cytosol to its CoA derivative by *long-chain fatty acyl CoA synthetase* (*thiokinase*), an enzyme of the outer mitochondrial membrane. Because β-oxida-

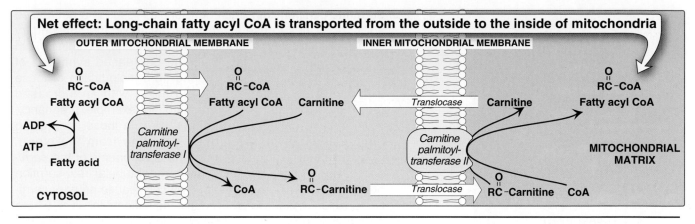

Figure 16.16
Carnitine shuttle. [Note: *Long-chain fatty acyl CoA synthetase* is in the outer mitochondrial membrane; active site faces the cytosol.]

tion occurs in the mitochondrial matrix, the fatty acid must be transported across the inner mitochondrial membrane that is impermeable to CoA. Therefore, a specialized carrier transports the long-chain acyl group from the cytosol into the mitochondrial matrix. This carrier is carnitine, and this rate-limiting transport process is called the carnitine shuttle (Figure 16.16).

a. **Steps in LCFA translocation:** First, the acyl group is transferred from CoA to carnitine by *carnitine palmitoyltransferase I* (*CPT-I*)—an enzyme of the outer mitochondrial membrane. [Note: *CPT-I* is also known as *CAT-I* for *carnitine acyltransferase I*.] This reaction forms acylcarnitine, and regenerates free CoA. Second, the acylcarnitine is transported into the mitochondrial matrix in exchange for free carnitine by *carnitine–acylcarnitine translocase*. *Carnitine palmitoyltransferase II* (*CPT-II*, or *CAT-II*)—an enzyme of the inner mitochondrial membrane—catalyzes the transfer of the acyl group from carnitine to CoA in the mitochondrial matrix, thus regenerating free carnitine.

b. **Inhibitor of the carnitine shuttle:** Malonyl CoA inhibits *CPT-I*, thus preventing the entry of long-chain acyl groups into the mitochondrial matrix. Therefore, when fatty acid synthesis is occurring in the cytosol (as indicated by the presence of malonyl CoA), the newly made palmitate cannot be transferred into the mitochondria and degraded. [Note: Muscle, though it does not synthesize fatty acids, contains the mitochondrial isoform of *acetyl CoA carboxylase* (*ACC2*), allowing muscle to regulate β-oxidation.] Fatty acid oxidation is also regulated by the acetyl CoA to CoA ratio: as the ratio increases, the CoA-requiring *thiolase* reaction decreases (Figure 16.17).

c. **Sources of carnitine:** Carnitine can be obtained from the diet, where it is found primarily in meat products. Carnitine can also be synthesized from the amino acids lysine and methionine by an enzymatic pathway found in the liver and kidney but not in skeletal or heart muscle. Therefore, these latter tissues are totally dependent on uptake of carnitine provided by endogenous synthesis or the diet, and distributed by the blood. [Note: Skeletal muscle contains about 97% of all carnitine in the body.]

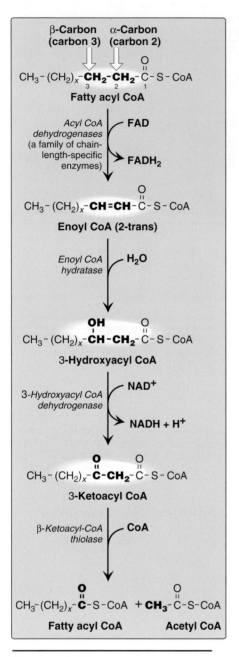

Figure 16.17
Enzymes involved in the β-oxidation of fatty acyl CoA. [Note: *Enoyl CoA hydratase* requires a trans double bond between carbon 2 and carbon 3.]

d. Carnitine deficiencies: Such deficiencies result in a decreased ability of tissues to use LCFA as a metabolic fuel. Secondary carnitine deficiency occurs in many situations, including: 1) in patients with liver disease causing decreased synthesis of carnitine; 2) in individuals suffering from malnutrition or those on strictly vegetarian diets; 3) in those with an increased requirement for carnitine as a result of, for example, pregnancy, severe infections, burns, or trauma; or 4) in those undergoing hemodialysis, which removes carnitine from the blood. Congenital deficiencies in one of the components of the *carnitine palmitoyltransferase* system, in renal tubular reabsorption of carnitine, or in carnitine uptake by cells cause primary carnitine deficiency. Genetic *CPT-I* deficiency affects the liver, where an inability to use LCFA for fuel greatly impairs that tissue's ability to synthesize glucose during a fast. This can lead to severe hypoglycemia, coma, and death. *CPT-II* deficiency occurs primarily in cardiac and skeletal muscle, where symptoms of carnitine deficiency range from cardiomyopathy to muscle weakness with myoglobinemia following prolonged exercise. [Note: This is an example of how the impaired flow of a metabolite from one cell compartment to another results in pathology.] Treatment includes avoidance of prolonged fasts, adopting a diet high in carbohydrate and low in LCFA, but supplemented with medium-chain fatty acids and carnitine.

2. **Entry of short- and medium-chain fatty acids into the mitochondria:** Fatty acids shorter than 12 carbons can cross the inner mitochondrial membrane without the aid of carnitine or the *CPT* system. Once inside the mitochondria, they are activated to their CoA derivatives by matrix enzymes, and are oxidized. [Note: Medium-chain fatty acids are plentiful in human milk. Because their oxidation is not dependent on *CPT-I*, it is not subject to inhibition by malonyl CoA.]

3. **Reactions of β-oxidation:** The first cycle of β-oxidation is shown in Figure 16.17. It consists of a sequence of four reactions involving the β-carbon (carbon 3) that results in shortening the fatty acid chain by two carbons. The steps include an oxidation that produces $FADH_2$, a hydration step, a second oxidation that produces NADH, and a thiolytic cleavage that releases a molecule of acetyl CoA. Each step is catalyzed by enzymes with chain-length specificity. These four steps are repeated for saturated fatty acids of even-numbered carbon chains (n/2) – 1 times (where n is the number of carbons), each cycle producing an acetyl group plus one NADH and one $FADH_2$. The final thiolytic cleavage produces two acetyl groups. [Note: Acetyl CoA is a positive allosteric effector of *pyruvate carboxylase* (see p. 119), thus linking fatty acid oxidation and gluconeogenesis.]

4. **Energy yield from fatty acid oxidation:** The energy yield from the β-oxidation pathway is high. For example, the oxidation of a molecule of palmitoyl CoA to CO_2 and H_2O produces 8 acetyl CoA, 7 NADH, and 7 $FADH_2$, from which 131 ATP can be generated; however, activation of the fatty acid requires 2 ATP. Thus, the net yield from palmitate is 129 ATP (Figure 16.18). A comparison of the processes of synthesis and degradation of long-chain saturated fatty acids with an even number of carbon atoms is provided in Figure 16.19.

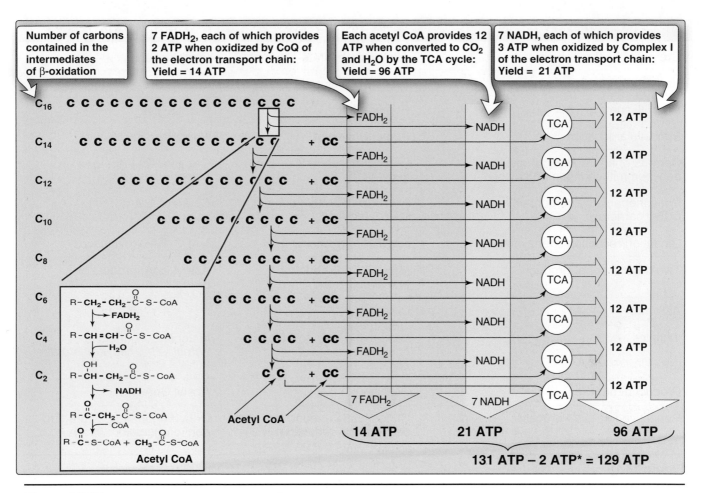

Figure 16.18
Summary of the energy yield from the oxidation of palmitoyl CoA (16 carbons). CC = acetyl CoA. *Activation of palmitate to palmitoyl CoA requires the equivalent of 2 ATP.

5. **Medium-chain fatty acyl CoA dehydrogenase (MCAD) deficiency:** In mitochondria, there are four *fatty acyl CoA dehydrogenase* species, each with a specificity for either short-, medium-, long-, or very-long-chain fatty acids. *MCAD* deficiency, an autosomal recessive disorder, is one of the most common inborn errors of metabolism, and the most common inborn error of fatty acid oxidation, being found in 1:14,000 births worldwide, with a higher incidence in Northern Europeans. It results in decreased ability to oxidize fatty acids with six to ten carbons (these accumulate and can be measured in urine), and severe hypoglycemia (because the tissues must increase their reliance on glucose). Treatment includes avoidance of fasting. *MCAD* deficiency has been identified as the cause of some cases originally reported as sudden infant death syndrome (SIDS) or Reye syndrome.

6. **Oxidation of fatty acids with an odd number of carbons:** The β-oxidation of a saturated fatty acid with an odd number of carbon atoms proceeds by the same reaction steps as that of fatty acids with an even number, until the final three carbons are reached. This compound, propionyl CoA, is metabolized by a three-step pathway (Figure 16.20). [Note: Propionyl CoA is also produced during the metabolism of certain amino acids (see Figure 20.10).]

	SYNTHESIS	DEGRADATION
Greatest flux through pathway	After carbohydrate-rich meal	In starvation
Hormonal state favoring pathway	High insulin/glucagon ratio	Low insulin/glucagon ratio
Major tissue site	Primarily liver	Muscle, liver
Subcellular location	Primarily cytosol	Primarily mitochondria
Carriers of acyl/acetyl groups between mitochondria and cytosol	Citrate (mitochondria to cytosol)	Carnitine (cytosol to mitochondria)
Phosphopantetheine-containing active carriers	Acyl carrier protein domain, coenzyme A	Coenzyme A
Oxidation/reduction coenzymers	NADPH (reduction)	NAD^+, FAD (oxidation)
Two-carbon donor/product	Malonyl CoA: donor of one acetyl group	Acetyl CoA: product of β-oxidation
Activator	Citrate	
Inhibitor	Long-chain fatty acyl CoA (inhibits *acetyl CoA carboxylase*)	Malonyl CoA (inhibits *carnitine palmitoyltransferase-I*)
Product of pathway	Palmitate	Acetyl CoA
Repetitive four-step process	Condensation, reduction dehydration, reduction	Dehydrogenation, hydration dehydrogenation, thiolysis

Figure 16.19
Comparison of the synthesis and degradation of long-chain, even-numbered, saturated fatty acids.

a. **Synthesis of D-methylmalonyl CoA:** First, propionyl CoA is carboxylated, forming D-methylmalonyl CoA. The enzyme *propionyl CoA carboxylase* has an absolute requirement for the coenzyme biotin, as do most other *carboxylases* (see p. 381).

b. **Formation of L-methylmalonyl CoA:** Next, the D-isomer is converted to the L-form by the enzyme, *methylmalonyl CoA racemase*.

c. **Synthesis of succinyl CoA:** Finally, the carbons of L-methylmalonyl CoA are rearranged, forming succinyl CoA, which can enter the tricarboxylic acid (TCA) cycle (see p. 109). [Note: This is the only example of a glucogenic precursor generated from fatty acid oxidation.] The enzyme, *methylmalonyl CoA mutase*, requires a coenzyme form of vitamin B_{12} (deoxyadenosylcobalamin) for its action. The *mutase* reaction is one of only two reactions in the body that require vitamin B_{12} (see p. 375). [Note: In patients with vitamin B_{12} deficiency, both propionate and methylmalonate are excreted in the urine. Two types of heritable methylmalonic acidemia and aciduria have been described: one in which the *mutase* is missing or deficient (or has reduced affinity for the coenzyme), and one in which the patient is unable to convert vitamin B_{12} into its coenzyme form. Either type results in metabolic acidosis, with developmental retardation seen in some patients.]

7. **Oxidation of unsaturated fatty acids:** The oxidation of unsaturated fatty acids provides less energy than that of saturated fatty acids because unsaturated fatty acids are less highly reduced and, therefore, fewer reducing equivalents can be produced from these structures. Oxidation of monounsaturated fatty acids, such as 18:1(9) (oleic acid) requires one additional enzyme, *3,2-enoyl CoA isomerase*, which converts the 3-trans derivative obtained after three rounds of β-oxidation to the 2-trans derivative required as a substrate by the *enoyl CoA hydratase.* Oxidation of polyunsaturated fatty acids, such as 18:2(9,12) (linoleic acid), requires an *NADPH-dependent 2,4-dienoyl CoA reductase* in addition to the *isomerase.*

8. **β-Oxidation in the peroxisome:** Very-long-chain fatty acids (VLCFA), or those 22 carbons long or longer, undergo a preliminary β-oxidation in peroxisomes. The shortened fatty acid (linked to carnitine) diffuses to a mitochondrion for further oxidation. In contrast to mitochondrial β-oxidation, the initial dehydrogenation in peroxisomes is catalyzed by an FAD-containing *acyl CoA oxidase.* The $FADH_2$ produced is oxidized by molecular oxygen, which is reduced to H_2O_2; thus, no ATP is generated by this step. The H_2O_2 is reduced to H_2O by *catalase* (see p. 148). [Note: Genetic defects either in the ability to target matrix proteins to peroxisomes (resulting in Zellweger syndrome—a peroxisomal biogenesis disorder) or in the ability to transport VLCFA across the peroxisomal membrane (resulting in X-linked adrenoleukodystrophy), lead to accumulation of VLCFA in the blood and tissues.]

C. α-Oxidation of fatty acids

Branched-chain, 20 carbon fatty acid, phytanic acid: This is not a substrate for *acyl CoA dehydrogenase* because of the methyl group on its β carbon (Figure 16.21). Instead, it is hydroxylated at the α-carbon by *phytanoyl CoA α-hydroxylase (PhyH)*, carbon 1 is released as CO_2, and the product, 19 carbon pristanic acid, is activated to its CoA derivative and undergoes β-oxidation. Refsum disease is a rare, autosomal recessive disorder caused by a deficiency of peroxisomal *PhyH*. This results in the accumulation of phytanic acid in the plasma and tissues. The symptoms are primarily neurologic, and the treatment involves dietary restriction to halt disease progression. [Note: ω-Oxidation (at the methyl terminus) also is known, and generates dicarboxylic acids. Normally a minor pathway of the ER, its up-regulation is seen with conditions such as MCAD deficiency that limit fatty acid β-oxidation.]

V. KETONE BODIES: AN ALTERNATE FUEL FOR CELLS

Liver mitochondria have the capacity to convert acetyl CoA derived from fatty acid oxidation into ketone bodies. The compounds categorized as ketone bodies are acetoacetate, 3-hydroxybutyrate (also called β-hydroxybutyrate), and acetone (a nonmetabolized side product, Figure 16.22). [Note: The two functional ketone bodies are actually organic acids.] Acetoacetate and 3-hydroxybutyrate are transported in the blood to the peripheral tissues. There they can be reconverted to acetyl CoA, which can be oxidized by the TCA cycle. Ketone bodies

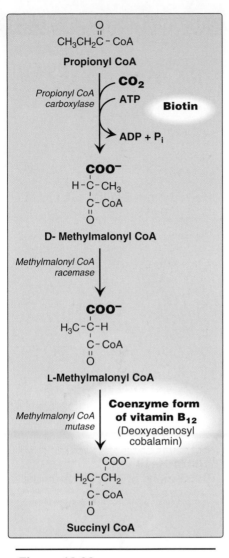

Figure 16.20
Metabolism of propionyl CoA.

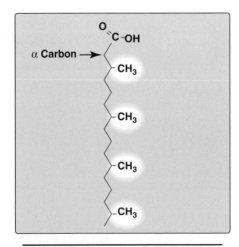

Figure 16.21
Phytanic acid—a branched-chain fatty acid.

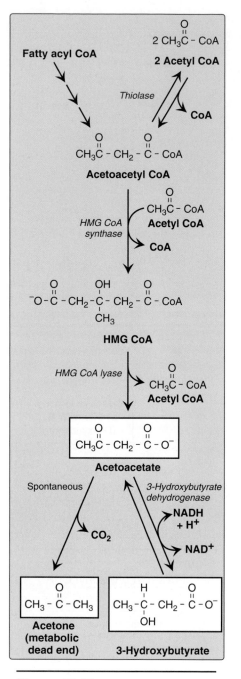

Figure 16.22
Synthesis of ketone bodies. HMG =
hydroxymethylglutaryl CoA.

are important sources of energy for the peripheral tissues because 1) they are soluble in aqueous solution and, therefore, do not need to be incorporated into lipoproteins or carried by albumin as do the other lipids; 2) they are produced in the liver during periods when the amount of acetyl CoA present exceeds the oxidative capacity of the liver; and 3) they are used in proportion to their concentration in the blood by extrahepatic tissues, such as the skeletal and cardiac muscle and renal cortex. Even the brain can use ketone bodies to help meet its energy needs if the blood levels rise sufficiently; thus, ketone bodies spare glucose.This is particularly important during prolonged periods of fasting (see p. 332). [Note: Disorders of fatty acid oxidation present with the general picture of hypoketosis (due to decreased availability of acetyl CoA) and hypoglycemia (due to increased reliance on glucose for energy.]

A. Synthesis of ketone bodies by the liver: ketogenesis

During a fast, the liver is flooded with fatty acids mobilized from adipose tissue. The resulting elevated hepatic acetyl CoA produced primarily by fatty acid degradation inhibits *pyruvate dehydrogenase* (see p. 111), and activates *pyruvate carboxylase* (see p. 119). The OAA thus produced is used by the liver for gluconeogenesis rather than for the TCA cycle. Therefore, acetyl CoA is channeled into ketone body synthesis. [Note: Fatty acid oxidation decreases the NAD^+ to NADH ratio, and the rise in NADH shifts OAA to malate (see p. 113). This pushes acetyl CoA away from gluconeogenesis and into ketogenesis (Figure 16.24).]

1. **Synthesis of 3-hydroxy-3-methylglutaryl (HMG) CoA:** The first synthetic step, formation of acetoacetyl CoA, occurs by reversal of the *thiolase* reaction of fatty acid oxidation (see Figure 16.17). Mitochondrial *HMG CoA synthase* combines a third molecule of acetyl CoA with acetoacetyl CoA to produce HMG CoA. [Note: HMG CoA is also a precursor of cholesterol (see p. 220). These pathways are separated by location in, and conditions of, the cell.] *HMG CoA synthase* is the rate-limiting step in the synthesis of ketone bodies, and is present in significant quantities only in the liver.

2. **Synthesis of the ketone bodies:** HMG CoA is cleaved to produce acetoacetate and acetyl CoA, as shown in Figure 16.22. Acetoacetate can be reduced to form 3-hydroxybutyrate with NADH as the hydrogen donor. Acetoacetate can also spontaneously decarboxylate in the blood to form acetone—a volatile, biologically nonmetabolized compound that can be released in the breath. The equilibrium between acetoacetate and 3-hydroxybutyrate is determined by the NAD^+/NADH ratio. Because this ratio is low during fatty acid oxidation, 3-hydroxybutyrate synthesis is favored. [Note: The generation of free CoA during ketogenesis allows fatty acid oxidation to continue.]

B. Use of ketone bodies by the peripheral tissues: ketolysis

Although the liver constantly synthesizes low levels of ketone bodies, their production becomes much more significant during fasting

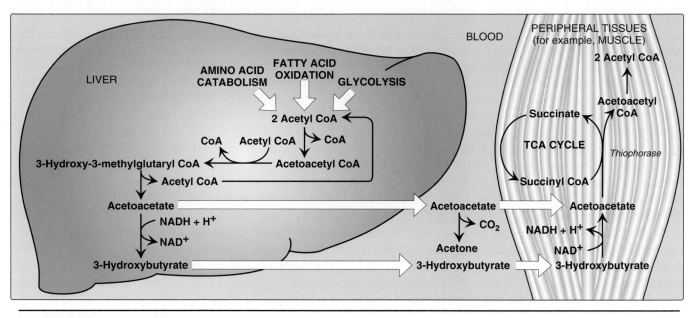

Figure 16.23
Ketone body synthesis in the liver and use in peripheral tissues. [Note: *Thiophorase* is also known as *succinyl CoA: acetoacetate CoA transferase.*]

when ketone bodies are needed to provide energy to the peripheral tissues. 3-Hydroxybutyrate is oxidized to acetoacetate by *3-hydroxybutyrate dehydrogenase*, producing NADH (Figure 16.23). Acetoacetate is then provided with a CoA molecule taken from succinyl CoA by *succinyl CoA:acetoacetate CoA transferase* (*thiophorase*). This reaction is reversible, but the product, acetoacetyl CoA, is actively removed by its conversion to two acetyl CoA. Extrahepatic tissues, including the brain but excluding cells lacking mitochondria (for example, red blood cells), efficiently oxidize acetoacetate and 3-hydroxybutyrate in this manner. In contrast, although the liver actively produces ketone bodies, it lacks *thiophorase* and, therefore, is unable to use ketone bodies as fuel.

C. Excessive production of ketone bodies in diabetes mellitus

When the rate of formation of ketone bodies is greater than the rate of their use, their levels begin to rise in the blood (ketonemia) and, eventually, in the urine (ketonuria). This is seen most often in cases of uncontrolled, type 1 diabetes mellitus. In diabetic individuals with severe ketosis, urinary excretion of the ketone bodies may be as high as 5,000 mg/24 hr, and the blood concentration may reach 90 mg/dl (versus less than 3 mg/dl in normal individuals). A frequent symptom of diabetic ketoacidosis is a fruity odor on the breath, which results from increased production of acetone. An elevation of the ketone body concentration in the blood results in acidemia. [Note: The carboxyl group of a ketone body has a pK_a of about 4. Therefore, each ketone body loses a proton (H^+) as it circulates in the blood, which lowers the pH of the body. Also, excretion of glucose and ketone bodies in the urine results in dehydration of the body. Therefore, the increased number of H^+, circulating in a decreased volume of plasma, can cause severe acidosis (ketoacidosis).] Ketoacidosis may also be seen in cases of fasting (see p. 330).

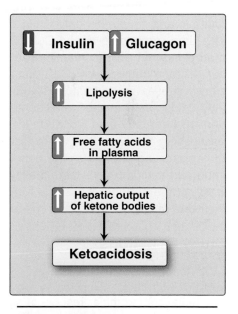

Figure 16.24
Mechanism of diabetic ketoacidosis seen in type 1 diabetes.

VI. CHAPTER SUMMARY

Generally a linear hydrocarbon chain with a terminal carboxyl group, a fatty acid can be **saturated** or **unsaturated**. Two fatty acids are essential (must be obtained from the diet): **linoleic** and **α-linolenic acids**. Fatty acids are synthesized in the cytosol of **liver** following a meal containing excess carbohydrate and protein. Carbons used to synthesize fatty acids are provided by **acetyl CoA**, energy by **ATP**, and reducing equivalents by **NADPH** (Figure 16.25). **Citrate** carries two-carbon acetyl units from the mitochondrial matrix to the cytosol. The regulated step in fatty acid synthesis is catalyzed by **acetyl CoA carboxylase**, which requires **biotin**. **Citrate** is the allosteric **activator** and **long-chain fatty acyl CoA** is the **inhibitor**. The enzyme can also be activated in the presence of **insulin** and inactivated by **AMPK** in response to **epinephrine**, **glucagon**, or a **rise in AMP**. The rest of the steps in fatty acid synthesis are catalyzed by the multifunctional enzyme, **fatty acid synthase**, which produces **palmitoyl CoA** from acetyl CoA and malonyl CoA, with NADPH (from the pentose phosphate pathway) as the source of reducing equivalents. Fatty acids can be elongated and desaturated in the ER. When fatty acids are required by the body for energy, adipose cell **hormone-sensitive lipase** (**activated** by **epinephrine** or **glucagon**, and **inhibited** by **insulin**) initiates degradation of stored triacylglycerol. Fatty acids are carried by **serum albumin** to the liver and peripheral tissues, where oxidation of the fatty acids provides energy. The **glycerol** backbone of the degraded triacylglycerol is carried by the blood to the **liver**, where it serves as an important **gluconeogenic precursor**. Fatty acid degradation (**β-oxidation**) occurs in **mitochondria**. The **carnitine shuttle** is required to transport LCFA from the cytosol to the mitochondrial matrix. A translocase and the enzymes **carnitine palmitoyltransferases I** and **II** are required. Carnitine palmitoyltransferase I is **inhibited** by **malonyl CoA**. This prevents fatty acids being synthesized in the cytosol from malonyl CoA from being transported into the mitochondria where they would be degraded. Once in the mitochondria, fatty acids are oxidized, producing acetyl CoA, NADH, and $FADH_2$. The first step in the β-oxidation pathway is catalyzed by one of a family of four acyl CoA dehydrogenases, each of which has a specificity for either short-, medium-, long-, or very-long-chain fatty acids. **Medium-chain fatty acyl CoA dehydrogenase (MCAD) deficiency** is one of the most common inborn errors of metabolism. It causes a decrease in fatty acid oxidation (process stops once a medium chain fatty acid is produced), resulting in hypoketonemia and severe hypoglycemia. Oxidation of fatty acids with an odd number of carbons proceeds two carbons at a time (producing acetyl CoA) until three carbons remain (**propionyl CoA**). This compound is converted to **methylmalonyl CoA** (a reaction requiring **biotin**), which is then converted to **succinyl CoA** (a gluconeogenic precursor) by methylmalonyl CoA mutase (requiring **vitamin B_{12}**). A genetic error in the mutase or vitamin B_{12} deficiency causes **methylmalonic acidemia** and **aciduria**. β-Oxidation of VLCFA and α-oxidation of branched-chain fatty acids occur in the peroxisome. ω-Oxidation occurs in the ER. Liver mitochondria can convert acetyl CoA derived from fatty acid oxidation into the ketone bodies, **acetoacetate** and **3-hydroxybutyrate**. Peripheral tissues possessing mitochondria can oxidize 3-hydroxybutyrate to acetoacetate, which can be reconverted to acetyl CoA, thus producing energy for the cell. Unlike fatty acids, ketone bodies are utilized by the **brain** and, therefore, are important fuels during a fast. The liver lacks the ability to degrade ketone bodies, and so synthesizes them specifically for the peripheral tissues. **Ketoacidosis** occurs when the rate of formation of ketone bodies is greater than their rate of use, as is seen in cases of uncontrolled, **type 1 diabetes mellitus**.

Study Questions

Choose the ONE correct answer.

16.1 Triacylglycerol molecules stored in adipose tissue represent the major reserve of substrate providing energy during a prolonged fast. During such a fast:

A. the stored fatty acids are released from adipose tissue into the plasma as components of the serum lipoprotein particle, VLDL.

B. free fatty acids are produced at a high rate in the plasma by the action of lipoprotein lipase on chylomicrons.

C. glycerol produced by the degradation of triacylglycerol is an important direct source of energy for adipocytes and fibroblasts.

D. hormone-sensitive lipase is phosphorylated and activated by a cAMP-activated protein kinase.

Correct answer = D. Hormone-sensitive lipase is phosphorylated by cAMP-activated protein kinase, which is itself activated by epinephrine or glucagon. Fatty acids released from adipose tissue are carried in the plasma by serum albumin, not VLDL. During a fast, the amount of circulating triacylglycerol (found in chylomicrons and VLDL) will be low. Therefore, there is little substrate for lipoprotein lipase. The glycerol produced during triacylglycerol degradation cannot be metabolized by adipocytes or fibroblasts, but rather must go to the liver where it can be phosphorylated (by glycerol kinase).

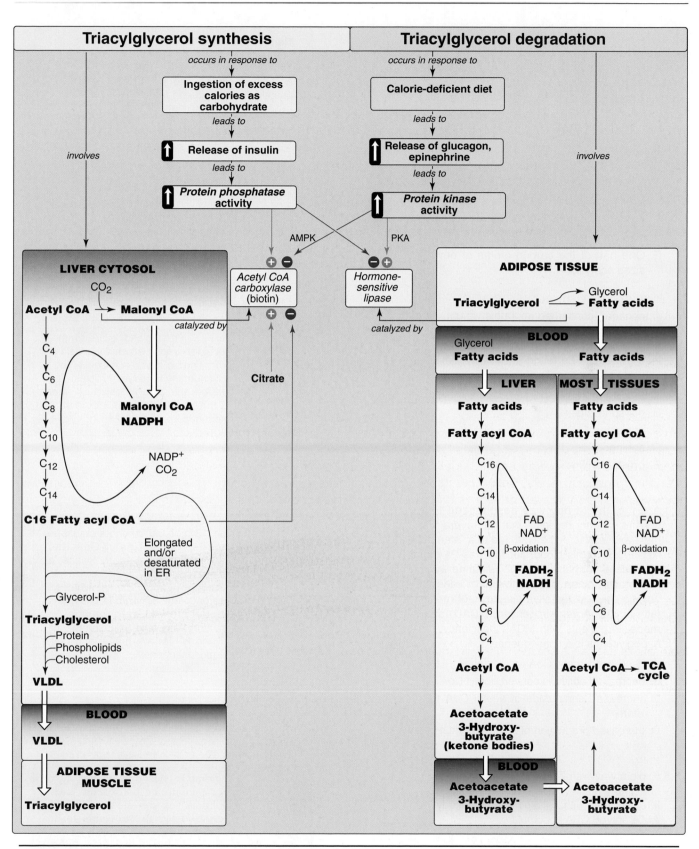

Figure 16.25
Key concept map for fatty acid and triacylglycerol metabolism.

16.2 A low level of carbon dioxide labeled with ^{14}C is accidentally released into the atmosphere surrounding industrial workers as they resume work following the lunch hour. Unknowingly, they breathe the contaminated air for 1 hour. Which of the following compounds will be radioactively labeled?

A. All of the carbon atoms of newly synthesized fatty acid.

B. About one half of the carbon atoms of newly synthesized fatty acids.

C. The carboxyl atom of newly synthesized fatty acids.

D. About one third of the carbons of newly synthesized malonyl CoA.

E. One half of the carbon atoms of newly synthesized acetyl CoA.

Correct answer = D. Malonyl CoA (three carbons) is synthesized from acetyl CoA (two carbons) by the addition of CO_2, using the enzyme acetyl CoA carboxylase. Because CO_2 is subsequently removed during fatty acid synthesis, the radioactive label will not appear at any position in newly synthesized fatty acids.

16.3 A teenager, concerned about his weight, attempts to maintain a fat-free diet for a period of several weeks. If his ability to synthesize various lipids were examined, he would be found to be most deficient in his ability to synthesize:

A. triacylglycerol.

B. phospholipids.

C. cholesterol.

D. sphingolipids.

E. prostaglandins.

Correct answer = E. Prostaglandins are synthesized from arachidonic acid. Arachidonic acid is synthesized from linoleic acid, an essential fatty acid obtained by humans from dietary lipids. The teenager would be able to synthesize all other compounds, but presumably in somewhat depressed amounts.

16.4 A 6-month-old boy was hospitalized following a seizure. History revealed that for several days prior, his appetite was decreased due to a "stomach virus". At admission, his blood glucose was 24 mg/dl (age-referenced normal is 60-100). His urine was negative for ketone bodies, but positive for a variety of dicarboxylic acids. A tentative diagnosis of medium-chain fatty acyl CoA dehydrogenase (MCAD) deficiency is made. In patients with MCAD deficiency, the fasting hypoglycemia is a consequence of:

A. decreased acetyl CoA production.

B. decreased ability to convert acetyl CoA to glucose.

C. increased conversion of acetyl CoA to acetoacetate.

D. increased production of ATP and NADH.

Correct answer = A. Impaired oxidation of fatty acids less than 12 carbons in length results in decreased production of acetyl CoA, the allosteric activator of pyruvate carboxylase, a gluconeogenic enzyme; thus, glucose levels fall. Acetyl CoA cannot be used for the net synthesis of glucose. Acetoacetate is a ketone body, and with MCAD deficiency ketogenesis is decreased. Impaired fatty acid oxidation means that less ATP and NADH are made, and both are needed for gluconeogenesis.

16.5 Explain why with Zellweger syndrome both very long chain fatty acids (VLCFA) and phytanic acid accumulate, whereas with X-linked adrenoleukodystrophy (X-ALD) only VLCFA accumulate.

Zellweger syndrome is caused by an inability to target matrix proteins to the peroxisome; thus, all peroxisomal activities are affected because functional peroxisomes are not able to be formed. In X-ALD, the defect is an inability to transport VLCFA into the peroxisome—other peroxisomal functions such as α oxidation are normal.

Complex Lipid Metabolism

17

I. OVERVIEW OF PHOSPHOLIPIDS

Phospholipids are polar, ionic compounds composed of an alcohol that is attached by a phosphodiester bridge to either diacylglycerol or sphingosine. Like fatty acids, phospholipids are amphipathic in nature, that is, each has a hydrophilic head (the phosphate group plus whatever alcohol is attached to it, for example, serine, ethanolamine, and choline, highlighted in blue in Figure 17.1A), and a long, hydrophobic tail (containing fatty acids or fatty acid–derived hydrocarbons, shown in orange in Figure 17.1A). Phospholipids are the predominant lipids of cell membranes. In membranes, the hydrophobic portion of a phospholipid molecule is associated with the nonpolar portions of other membrane constituents, such as glycolipids, proteins, and cholesterol. The hydrophilic (polar) head of the phospholipid extends outward, interacting with the intracellular or extracellular aqueous environment (see Figure 17.1A). Membrane phospholipids also function as a reservoir for intracellular messengers, and, for some proteins, phospholipids serve as anchors to cell membranes. Nonmembrane-bound phospholipids serve additional functions in the body, for example, as components of lung surfactant and essential components of bile, where their detergent properties aid in the solubilization of cholesterol.

II. STRUCTURE OF PHOSPHOLIPIDS

There are two classes of phospholipids: those that have glycerol as a backbone and those that contain sphingosine. Both classes are found as structural components of membranes, and both play a role in the generation of lipid-signaling molecules.

A. Glycerophospholipids

Phospholipids that contain glycerol are called glycerophospholipids (or phosphoglycerides). Glycerophospholipids constitute the major class of phospholipids. All contain (or are derivatives of) phosphatidic acid (diacylglycerol with a phosphate group on the third carbon, Figure 17.1B). Phosphatidic acid is the simplest phosphoglyceride, and is the precursor of the other members of this group.

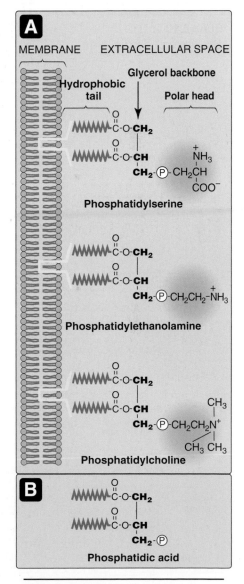

Figure 17.1
A. Structures of some glycerophospholipids. B. Phosphatidic acid. P = phosphate, PO_4^{1-}.

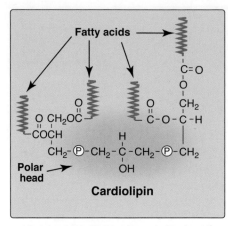

Figure 17.2
Structure of cardiolipin.

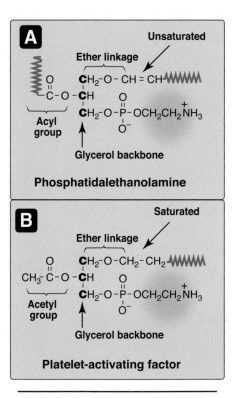

Figure 17.3
A. The plasmalogen phosphatidal-ethanolamine. B. Platelet-activating factor.

1. **Glycerophospholipids are formed from phosphatidic acid (PA) and an alcohol:** The phosphate group on PA can be esterified to another compound containing an alcohol group (see Figure 17.1). For example:

Serine	+ PA →	phosphatidylserine
Ethanolamine	+ PA →	phosphatidylethanolamine (cephalin)
Choline	+ PA →	phosphatidylcholine (lecithin)
Inositol	+ PA →	phosphatidylinositol
Glycerol	+ PA →	phosphatidylglycerol

2. **Cardiolipin:** Two molecules of PA esterified through their phosphate groups to an additional molecule of glycerol is called cardiolipin (diphosphatidylglycerol, Figure 17.2). Cardiolipin is found in bacteria and eukaryotes. In eukaryotes, cardiolipin is virtually exclusive to the inner mitochondrial membrane, where it appears to be required for the maintenance of certain respiratory complexes of the electron transport chain. [Note: Cardiolipin is antigenic, and is recognized by antibodies raised against <u>Treponema pallidum</u>, the bacterium that causes syphilis.]

3. **Plasmalogens:** When the fatty acid at carbon 1 of a glycerophospholipid is replaced by an unsaturated alkyl group attached by an ether (rather than by an ester) linkage to the core glycerol molecule, a plasmalogen is produced. For example, phosphatidalethanolamine (abundant in nerve tissue, Figure 17.3A) is the plasmalogen that is similar in structure to phosphatidylethanolamine. Phosphatidalcholine (abundant in heart muscle) is the other quantitatively significant ether lipid in mammals.

4. **Platelet-activating factor (PAF):** This is an unusual ether glycerophospholipid, with a saturated alkyl group in an ether link to carbon 1 and an acetyl residue (rather than a fatty acid) at carbon 2 of the glycerol backbone (Figure 17.3B). PAF is synthesized and released by a variety of cell types. It binds to surface receptors, triggering potent thrombotic and acute inflammatory events. For example, PAF activates inflammatory cells and mediates hypersensitivity, acute inflammatory, and anaphylactic reactions. It causes platelets to aggregate and degranulate, and neutrophils and alveolar macrophages to generate superoxide radicals (see p. 148 for a discussion of the role of superoxides in killing bacteria). [Note: PAF is one of the most potent bioactive molecules known, causing effects at concentrations as low as 10^{-12} mol/L.]

B. Sphingophospholipids: sphingomyelin

The backbone of sphingomyelin is the amino alcohol sphingosine, rather than glycerol (Figure 17.4). A long-chain fatty acid is attached to the amino group of sphingosine through an amide linkage, producing a ceramide, which can also serve as a precursor of glycolipids (see p. 209). The alcohol group at carbon 1 of sphingosine is esterified to phosphorylcholine, producing sphingomyelin, the only significant sphingophospholipid in humans. Sphingomyelin is an important constituent of the myelin of nerve fibers. [Note: The myelin sheath is a layered, membranous structure that insulates and protects neuronal fibers of the central nervous system.]

III. PHOSPHOLIPID SYNTHESIS

Glycerophospholipid synthesis involves either the donation of phosphatidic acid from CDP-diacylglycerol to an alcohol, or the donation of the phosphomonoester of the alcohol from CDP-alcohol to 1,2-diacylglycerol (Figure 17.5). [Note: CDP is the nucleotide cytidine diphosphate (see p. 292).] In both cases, the CDP-bound structure is considered an "activated intermediate," and cytidine monophosphate (CMP) is released as a side product of glycerophospholipid synthesis. A key concept in phosphoglyceride synthesis, therefore, is activation—either of diacylglycerol or the alcohol to be added—by linkage with CDP. [Note: This is similar in principle to the activation of sugars by their attachment to uridine diphosphate (UDP) (see p. 126).] The fatty acids esterified to the glycerol alcohol groups can vary widely, contributing to the heterogeneity of this group of compounds. Most phospholipids are synthesized in the smooth endoplasmic reticulum. From there, they are transported to the Golgi apparatus and then to membranes of organelles or the plasma membrane, or are secreted from the cell by exocytosis. [Note: Ether lipid synthesis occurs in peroxisomes.]

A. Synthesis of phosphatidic acid (PA)

PA is the precursor of many other phosphoglycerides. The steps in its synthesis from glycerol phosphate and two fatty acyl coenzyme A (CoA) molecules were illustrated in Figure 16.14, p. 189, in which PA is shown as a precursor of triacylglycerol.

> Essentially all cells except mature erythrocytes can synthesize phospholipids, whereas triacylglycerol synthesis occurs essentially only in liver, adipose tissue, lactating mammary glands, and intestinal mucosal cells.

B. Synthesis of phosphatidylethanolamine (PE) and phosphatidylcholine (PC)

PC and PE are the most abundant phospholipids in most eukaryotic cells. The primary route of their synthesis uses choline and ethanolamine obtained either from the diet or from the turnover of the body's phospholipids. [Note: In the liver, PC also can be synthesized from phosphatidylserine (PS) and PE (see below).]

1. **Synthesis of PE and PC from preexisting choline and ethanolamine:** These synthetic pathways involve the phosphorylation of choline or ethanolamine by *kinases*, followed by conversion to the activated form, CDP-choline or CDP-ethanolamine. Finally, choline-phosphate or ethanolamine-phosphate is transferred from the nucleotide (leaving CMP) to a molecule of diacylglycerol (see Figure 17.5).

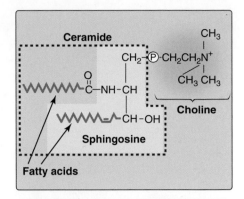

Figure 17.4
Structure of sphingomyelin, showing sphingosine (in green box) and ceramide components (in dashed box).

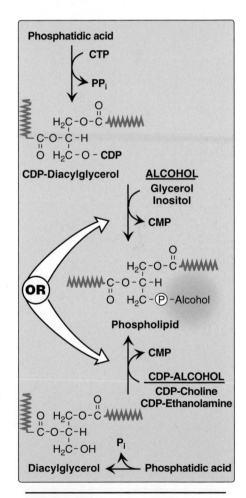

Figure 17.5
Activation of either diacylglycerol or an alcohol by linkage to a nucleoside diphosphate (CDP) promotes phospholipid synthesis.

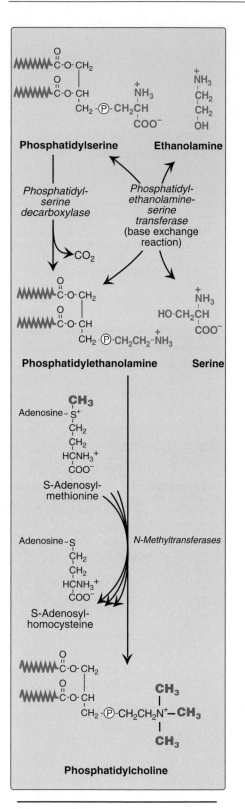

Figure 17.6
Synthesis of phosphatidylcholine from phosphatidylserine in the liver.

a. Significance of choline reutilization: The reutilization of choline is important because, whereas humans can synthesize choline <u>de novo</u>, the amount made is insufficient for our needs. Thus, choline is an essential dietary nutrient with an Adequate Intake (see p. 358) of 550 mg for men and 425 mg for women. [Note: Choline is also used for the synthesis of acetylcholine—a neurotransmitter.]

b. Role of PC in lung surfactant: The pathway described above is the principal pathway for the synthesis of dipalmitoyl-phosphatidylcholine (DPPC, or dipalmitoyl lecithin). In DPPC, positions 1 and 2 on the glycerol are occupied by palmitate. DPPC, made and secreted by Type II pneumocytes, is the major lipid component of lung surfactant—the extracellular fluid layer lining the alveoli. Surfactant serves to decrease the surface tension of this fluid layer, reducing the pressure needed to reinflate alveoli, thereby preventing alveolar collapse (atelectasis). [Note: Surfactant is a complex mixture of lipids (90%) and proteins (10%), with DPPC being the major component for reducing surface tension.] Respiratory distress syndrome (RDS) in preterm infants is associated with insufficient surfactant production and/or secretion, and is a significant cause of all neonatal deaths in Western countries.

> Lung maturity of the fetus can be gauged by determining the ratio of DPPC to sphingomyelin, usually written as the L (for lecithin)/S ratio, in amniotic fluid. A ratio of two or above is evidence of maturity, because it reflects the major shift from sphingomyelin to DPPC synthesis that occurs in the pneumocytes at about 32 weeks of gestation.

Lung maturation can be accelerated by giving the mother glucocorticoids shortly before delivery. Administration of natural or synthetic surfactant (by intratracheal instillation) is also used in the prevention and treatment of infant RDS. RDS due to an insufficient amount of surfactant can also occur in adults whose surfactant-producing pneumocytes have been damaged or destroyed, for example, by infection or trauma.

2. Synthesis of PC from phosphatidylserine (PS) in the liver: The liver requires a mechanism for producing PC, even when free choline levels are low, because it exports significant amounts of PC in the bile and as a component of serum lipoproteins. To provide the needed PC, PS is decarboxylated to PE by *PS decarboxylase*, an enzyme requiring pyridoxal phosphate as a coenzyme. PE then undergoes three methylation steps to produce PC, as illustrated in Figure 17.6. S-adenosylmethionine is the methyl group donor (see p. 264).

C. Phosphatidylserine (PS)

The primary pathway for synthesis of PS in mammalian tissues is provided by the base exchange reaction, in which the ethanolamine of PE is exchanged for free serine (see Figure 17.6). This reaction, although reversible, is used primarily to produce the PS required for membrane synthesis.

D. Phosphatidylinositol (PI)

PI is synthesized from free inositol and CDP-diacylglycerol as shown in Figure 17.5. PI is an unusual phospholipid in that it often contains stearic acid on carbon 1 and arachidonic acid on carbon 2 of the glycerol. PI, therefore, serves as a reservoir of arachidonic acid in membranes and, thus, provides the substrate for prostaglandin synthesis when required (see p. 213 for a discussion of these compounds).

1. **Role of PI in signal transmission across membranes:** The phosphorylation of membrane-bound phosphatidylinositol produces polyphosphoinositides, for example, phosphatidylinositol 4,5-bisphosphate (PIP_2, Figure 17.7). The degradation of PIP_2 by *phospholipase C* occurs in response to the binding of a variety of neurotransmitters, hormones, and growth factors to receptors on the cell membrane (Figure 17.8). The products of this degradation, inositol 1,4,5-trisphosphate (IP_3) and diacylglycerol (DAG), mediate the mobilization of intracellular calcium and the activation

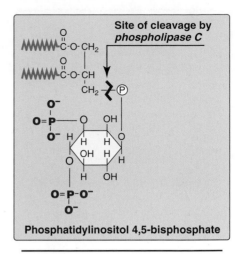

Phosphatidylinositol 4,5-bisphosphate

Figure 17.7
Structure of phosphatidylinositol 4,5-bisphosphate (PIP_2). Cleavage by *phospholipase C* produces IP_3 and DAG.

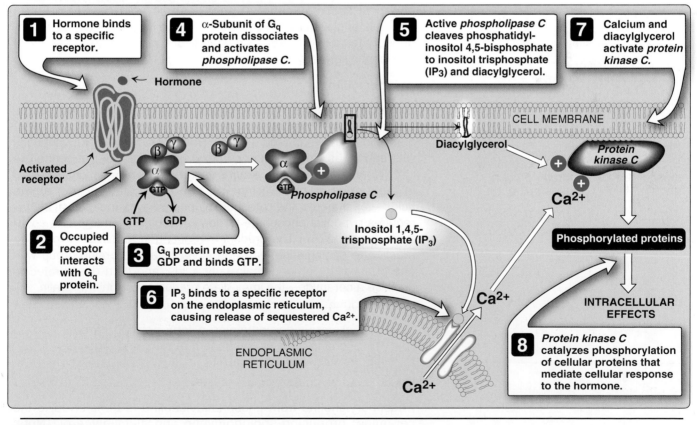

Figure 17.8
Role of inositol trisphosphate and diacylglycerol in intracellular signaling.

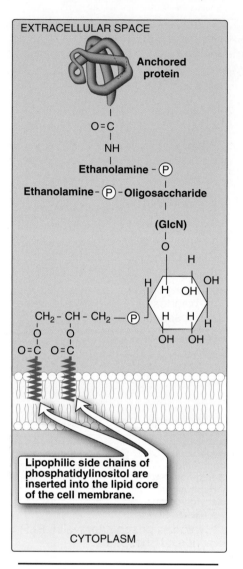

Figure 17.9
Example of a glycosyl phosphatidylinositol (GPI) membrane protein
anchor. GlcN = glucosamine.

of *protein kinase C*, respectively, which act synergistically to evoke specific cellular responses. Signal transmission across the membrane is thus accomplished.

2. **Role of PI in membrane protein anchoring:** Specific proteins can be covalently attached via a carbohydrate bridge to membrane-bound PI (Figure 17.9). [Note: Examples of such proteins include *alkaline phosphatase* (a digestive enzyme found on the surface of the small intestine that attacks organic phosphates), and *acetylcholine esterase* (an enzyme of the postsynaptic membrane that degrades the neurotransmitter acetylcholine). Cell surface proteins bound to glycosyl phosphatidylinositol (GPI) are also found in a variety of parasitic protozoans (for example, trypanosomes and leishmania).] Being attached to a membrane lipid (rather than being an integral part of the membrane) allows GPI-anchored proteins increased lateral mobility on the surface of the plasma membrane. The protein can be cleaved from its anchor by the action of *phospholipase C* (see Figure 17.8), releasing diacylglycerol. [Note: A deficiency in the synthesis of GPI in hematopoietic cells results in a hemolytic disease, paroxysmal nocturnal hemoglobinuria.]

E. Phosphatidylglycerol and cardiolipin

Phosphatidylglycerol occurs in relatively large amounts in mitochondrial membranes and is a precursor of cardiolipin. It is synthesized by a two-step reaction from CDP-diacylglycerol and glycerol 3-phosphate. Cardiolipin (diphosphatidylglycerol, see Figure 17.2) is composed of two molecules of phosphatidic acid connected by a molecule of glycerol. It is synthesized by the transfer of diacylglycerophosphate from CDP-diacylglycerol to a preexisting molecule of phosphatidylglycerol.

F. Sphingomyelin

Sphingomyelin, a sphingosine-based phospholipid, is a major structural lipid in the membranes of nerve tissue. The synthesis of sphingomyelin is shown in Figure 17.10. Briefly, palmitoyl CoA condenses with serine, as CoA and the carboxyl group (as CO_2) of serine are lost. [Note: This reaction, like the decarboxylation reactions involved in the synthesis of PE from PS, and of regulators from amino acids—for example, the catecholamines from tyrosine (see p. 286)—requires pyridoxal phosphate (a derivative of vitamin B_6) as a coenzyme (see p. 378).] The product is reduced in an NADPH-requiring reaction to sphinganine, which is acylated at the amino group with one of a variety of long-chain fatty acids, and then desaturated to produce a ceramide—the immediate precursor of sphingomyelin.

A ceramide containing a fatty acid 30 carbons long is a major component of skin, and regulates skin's water permeability.

Phosphorylcholine from phosphatidylcholine is transferred to the ceramide, producing sphingomyelin and diacylglycerol. [Note: Sphingomyelin of the myelin sheath contains predominantly longer-

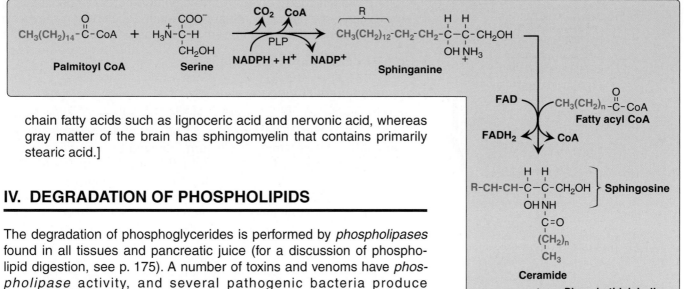

chain fatty acids such as lignoceric acid and nervonic acid, whereas gray matter of the brain has sphingomyelin that contains primarily stearic acid.]

IV. DEGRADATION OF PHOSPHOLIPIDS

The degradation of phosphoglycerides is performed by *phospholipases* found in all tissues and pancreatic juice (for a discussion of phospholipid digestion, see p. 175). A number of toxins and venoms have *phospholipase* activity, and several pathogenic bacteria produce *phospholipases* that dissolve cell membranes and allow the spread of infection. Sphingomyelin is degraded by the lysosomal *phospholipase*, *sphingomyelinase*.

A. Degradation of phosphoglycerides

Phospholipases hydrolyze the phosphodiester bonds of phosphoglycerides, with each enzyme cleaving the phospholipid at a specific site. The major enzymes responsible for degrading phosphoglycerides are shown in Figure 17.11. [Note: Removal of the fatty acid from carbon 1 or 2 of a phosphoglyceride produces a lysophosphoglyceride, which is the substrate for *lysophospholipases*.] *Phospholipases* release molecules that can serve as messengers (for example, DAG and IP$_3$), or that are the substrates for synthesis of messengers (for example, arachidonic acid). [Note: *Phospholipases* are responsible not only for degrading phospholipids, but also for "remodeling" them. For example, *phospholipases A$_1$* and *A$_2$*

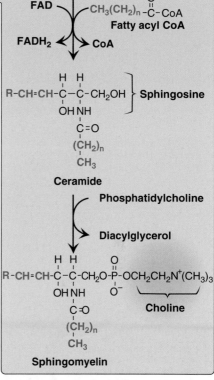

Figure 17.10
Synthesis of sphingomyelin. PLP = pyridoxal phosphate.

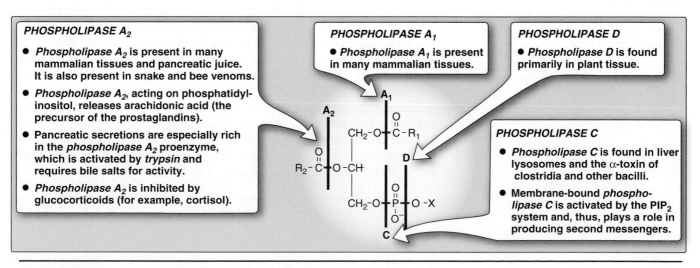

Figure 17.11
Degradation of glycerophospholipids by *phospholipases*.

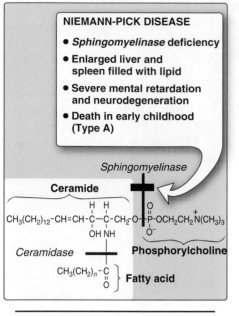

NIEMANN-PICK DISEASE

- *Sphingomyelinase* deficiency
- Enlarged liver and spleen filled with lipid
- Severe mental retardation and neurodegeneration
- Death in early childhood (Type A)

Figure 17.12
Degradation of sphingomyelin.

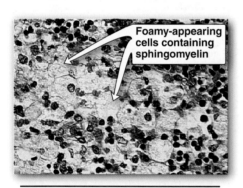

Foamy-appearing cells containing sphingomyelin

Figure 17.13
Accumulation of lipids in spleen cells from a patient with Niemann-Pick disease.

remove specific fatty acids from membrane-bound phospholipids; these can be replaced with alternative fatty acids using *fatty acyl CoA transferase*. This mechanism is used as one way to create the unique lung surfactant, DPCC (see p. 204), and to insure that carbon 2 of PI (and sometimes of PC) is bound to arachidonic acid.]

B. Degradation of sphingomyelin

Sphingomyelin is degraded by *sphingomyelinase*, a lysosomal enzyme that hydrolytically removes phosphorylcholine, leaving a ceramide. The ceramide is, in turn, cleaved by *ceramidase* into sphingosine and a free fatty acid (Figure 17.12). [Note: The ceramide and sphingosine released regulate signal transduction pathways, in part by influencing the activity of *protein kinase C* and, thus, the phosphorylation of its protein substrates. They also promote apoptosis.] Niemann-Pick disease (Types A and B) is an autosomal recessive disease caused by the inability to degrade sphingomyelin. The deficient enzyme is *sphingomyelinase*—a type of *phospholipase C*. In the severe infantile form (Type A—less than 1% normal activity), the liver and spleen are the primary sites of lipid deposits and are, therefore, tremendously enlarged. The lipid consists primarily of the sphingomyelin that cannot be degraded (Figure 17.13). Infants with this lysosomal storage disease experience rapid and progressive neurodegeneration as a result of deposition of sphingomyelin in the central nervous system, and they die in early childhood. A less severe variant (Type B—5% or more) causes little to no damage to neural tissue, but lungs, spleen, liver, and bone marrow are affected, resulting in a chronic form of the disease, with a life expectancy into adulthood. Although Niemann-Pick disease occurs in all ethnic groups, Type A occurs with greater frequency in the Ashkenazi Jewish population than in the general population.

V. OVERVIEW OF GLYCOLIPIDS

Glycolipids are molecules that contain both carbohydrate and lipid components. Like the phospholipid sphingomyelin, glycolipids are derivatives of ceramides in which a long-chain fatty acid is attached to the amino alcohol sphingosine. They are, therefore, more precisely called glycosphingolipids. [Note: Ceramides, then, are the precursors of both phosphorylated and glycosylated sphingolipids.] Like the phospholipids, glycosphingolipids are essential components of all membranes in the body, but they are found in greatest amounts in nerve tissue. They are located in the outer leaflet of the plasma membrane, where they interact with the extracellular environment. As such, they play a role in the regulation of cellular interactions, growth, and development.

When cells are transformed (that is, when their cell division and growth are dysregulated), there is a dramatic change in the glycosphingolipid composition of the plasma membrane.

Glycosphingolipids are antigenic, and they have been identified as a source of blood group antigens, various embryonic antigens specific for particular stages of fetal development, and some tumor antigens. [Note: The carbohydrate portion of a glycolipid is the antigenic determinant.] They also serve as cell surface receptors for cholera and tetanus toxins, as well as for certain viruses and microbes. Genetic disorders associated with an inability to properly degrade the glycosphingolipids result in lysosomal accumulation of these compounds.

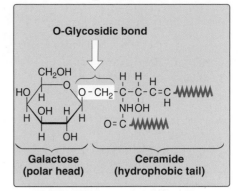

Figure 17.14
Structure of a neutral glyco-sphingolipid, galactocerebroside (▪▪▪▪▪ is a fatty acid hydrocarbon chain).

VI. STRUCTURE OF GLYCOSPHINGOLIPIDS

The glycosphingolipids differ from sphingomyelin in that they do not contain phosphate, and the polar head function is provided by a monosaccharide or oligosaccharide attached directly to the ceramide by an O-glycosidic bond (Figure 17.14). The number and type of carbohydrate moieties present help determine the type of glycosphingolipid.

A. Neutral glycosphingolipids

The simplest neutral (uncharged) glycosphingolipids are the cerebrosides. These are ceramide monosaccharides that contain either a molecule of galactose (galactocerebroside—the most common cerebroside found in membranes, see Figure 17.14) or glucose (glucocerebroside, which serves primarily as an intermediate in the synthesis and degradation of the more complex glycosphingolipids). [Note: Members of a group of galactocerebrosides (or glucocerebrosides) may also differ from each other in the type of fatty acid attached to the sphingosine.] As their name implies, cerebrosides are found predominantly in the brain and peripheral nervous tissue, with high concentrations in the myelin sheath. Ceramide oligosaccharides (or globosides) are produced by attaching additional monosaccharides (including GalNAc) to a glucocerebroside. Examples of these compounds include:

Cerebroside (glucocerebroside): Cer-Glc

Globoside (lactosylceramide): Cer-Glc-Gal

Globoside (Forssman antigen): Cer-Glc-Gal-Gal-GalNac-GalNac

(Cer = ceramide, Glc = glucose, Gal = galactose, GalNac = N-acetylgalactosamine)

B. Acidic glycosphingolipids

Acidic glycosphingolipids are negatively charged at physiologic pH. The negative charge is provided by N-acetylneuraminic acid (NANA, a sialic acid, see Figure 17.15) in gangliosides, or by sulfate groups in sulfatides.

1. **Gangliosides:** These are the most complex glycosphingolipids, and are found primarily in the ganglion cells of the central nervous system, particularly at the nerve endings. They are derivatives of ceramide oligosaccharides, and contain one or more molecules of NANA. The notation for these compounds is G (for ganglioside),

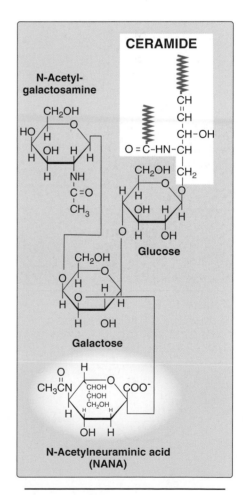

Figure 17.15
Structure of the ganglioside G_{M2}.

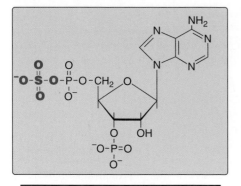

Figure 17.16
Structure of 3'-phosphoadenosine-
5'-phosphosulfate (PAPS).

plus a subscript M, D, T, or Q to indicate whether there is one (mono), two (di), three (tri), or four (quatro) molecules of NANA in the ganglioside, respectively. Additional numbers and letters in the subscript designate the monomeric sequence of the carbohydrate attached to the ceramide. (See Figure 17.15 for the structure of G_{M2}.) Gangliosides are of medical interest because several lipid storage disorders involve the accumulation of NANA-containing glycosphingolipids in cells (see Figure 17.20, p. 212).

2. **Sulfatides:** Sulfoglycosphingolipids (sulfatides) are cerebrosides that contain sulfated galactosyl residues, and are therefore negatively charged at physiologic pH. Sulfatides are found predominantly in nerve tissue and kidney.

VII. SYNTHESIS AND DEGRADATION OF GLYCOSPHINGOLIPIDS

Synthesis of glycosphingolipids occurs primarily in the Golgi by sequential addition of glycosyl monomers transferred from UDP–sugar donors to the acceptor molecule. The mechanism is similar to that used in glycoprotein synthesis (see p. 166).

A. Enzymes involved in synthesis

The enzymes involved in the synthesis of glycosphingolipids are *glycosyl transferases*, each specific for a particular sugar nucleotide and acceptor. [Note: These enzymes may recognize both glycosphingolipids and glycoproteins as substrates.]

B. Addition of sulfate groups

A sulfate group from the sulfate carrier, 3'-phosphoadenosine-5'-phosphosulfate (PAPS, Figure 17.16), is added by a *sulfotransferase* to the 3'-hydroxyl group of the galactose in a galactocerebroside. Galactocerebroside 3-sulfate is the major sulfatide in the brain (Figure 17.17). [Note: PAPS is also the sulfur donor in glycosaminoglycan synthesis (see p. 162), and steroid hormone catabolism (see p. 240).] An overview of the synthesis of sphingolipids is shown in Figure 17.18.

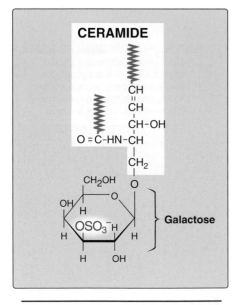

Figure 17.17
Structure of galactocerebroside 3-
sulfate.

C. Degradation of glycosphingolipids

Glycosphingolipids are internalized by endocytosis as described for the glycosaminoglycans. All of the enzymes required for the degradative process are present in lysosomes, which fuse with the endocytotic vesicles. The lysosomal enzymes hydrolytically and irreversibly cleave specific bonds in the glycosphingolipid. As seen with the glycosaminoglycans (see p. 163) and glycoproteins (see p. 170), degradation is a sequential process following the rule "last on, first off," in which the last group added during synthesis is the first group removed in degradation. [Note: Defects in the degradation of the polysaccharide chains in these three glycoconjugates also result in lysosomal storage diseases.]

D. Sphingolipidoses

In a normal individual, synthesis and degradation of glycosphingolipids are balanced, so that the amount of these compounds pre-

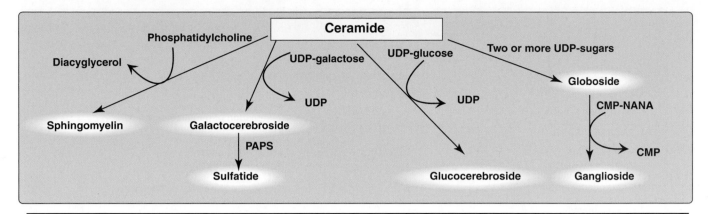

Figure 17.18
Overview of sphingolipid synthesis.

sent in membranes is constant. If a specific lysosomal *hydrolase* required for degradation is partially or totally missing, a sphingolipid accumulates. Lysosomal lipid storage diseases caused by these deficiencies are called sphingolipidoses. The result of a specific *hydrolase* deficiency may be seen dramatically in nerve tissue, where neurologic deterioration can lead to early death. [Note: Ganglioside turnover in the central nervous system is extensive during neonatal development.] Figure 17.20 provides an outline of the pathway of sphingolipid degradation and descriptions of some sphingolipidoses.

1. **Common properties:** A specific lysosomal hydrolytic enzyme is deficient in each disorder. Therefore, usually only a single sphingolipid (the substrate for the deficient enzyme) accumulates in the involved organs in each disease. [Note: The rate of biosynthesis of the accumulating lipid is normal.] The disorders are progressive and, although many are fatal in childhood, extensive phenotypic variability is seen leading to the designation of different clinical types, such as Types A and B in Niemann-Pick disease. Genetic variability is also seen because a given disorder can be caused by any one of a variety of mutations within a single gene. The sphingolipidoses are autosomal recessive diseases, except for Fabry disease, which is X-linked. The incidence of the sphingolipidoses is low in most populations, except for Gaucher and Tay-Sachs diseases, which, like Niemann-Pick disease, show a high frequency in the Ashkenazi Jewish population.

2. **Diagnosis and treatment:** A specific sphingolipidosis can be diagnosed by measuring enzyme activity in cultured fibroblasts or peripheral leukocytes, or by analysis of DNA (see p. 473). Histologic examination of the affected tissue is also useful. [Note: Shell-like inclusion bodies are seen in Tay-Sachs, and a wrinkled tissue paper appearance of the cytosol is seen in Gaucher disease (Figure 17.19).] Prenatal diagnosis, using cultured amniocytes or chorionic villi, is available. Gaucher disease, in which macrophages become engorged with glucocerebroside, and Fabry disease, in which globosides accumulate in the vascular endothelial lysosomes of the brain, heart, kidneys, and skin, are treated by recombinant human enzyme replacement therapy, but the mone-

The "crumpled tissue paper" appearance of the cytoplasm of Gaucher cells is caused by enlarged, elongated lysosomes filled with glucocerebroside.

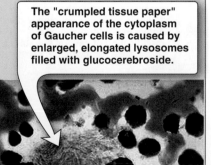

Figure 17.19
Aspirated bone marrow cells from patient with Gaucher disease.

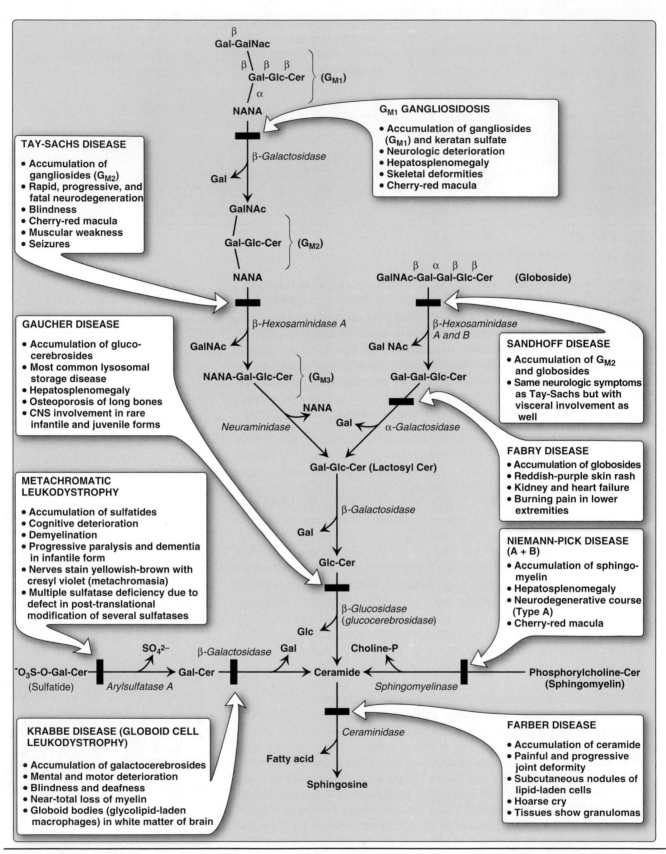

Figure 17.20
Degradation of sphingolipids showing the lysosomal enzymes affected in related genetic diseases, the sphingolipidoses. All of the diseases are autosomal recessive except Fabry disease, which is X-linked, and all can be fatal in early life. (Cer = ceramide).

tary cost is extremely high. Gaucher has also been treated by bone marrow transplantation (because macrophages are derived from hematopoietic stem cells), and by substrate reduction therapy through pharmacological reduction of glucosylceramide, the substrate for the deficient enzyme.

VIII. PROSTAGLANDINS AND RELATED COMPOUNDS

Prostaglandins, and the related compounds thromboxanes and leukotrienes, are collectively known as eicosanoids to reflect their origin from polyunsaturated fatty acids with 20 carbons. They are extremely potent compounds that elicit a wide range of responses, both physiologic (inflammatory response) and pathologic (hypersensitivity). They ensure gastric integrity and renal function, regulate smooth muscle contraction (intestine and uterus are key sites) and blood vessel diameter, and maintain platelet homeostasis. Although they have been compared to hormones in terms of their actions, eicosanoids differ from the true hormones in that they are produced in very small amounts in almost all tissues rather than in specialized glands. They also act locally rather than after transport in the blood to distant sites, as occurs with true hormones such as insulin. Eicosanoids are not stored, and they have an extremely short half-life, being rapidly metabolized to inactive products. Their biologic actions are mediated by plasma membrane G protein–coupled receptors (see p. 94), which are different in different organ systems. Examples of prostaglandins and related structures are shown in Figure 17.21.

A. Synthesis of prostaglandins and thromboxanes

The dietary precursor of the prostaglandins is the essential fatty acid, linoleic acid, an ω-6 fatty acid. It is desaturated and elongated to arachidonic acid (also an ω-6), the immediate precursor of the predominant class of prostaglandins (those with two double bonds) in humans (Figure 17.22). [Note: Arachidonic acid is incorporated into membrane-bound phospholipids. It is released by *phospholipase A_2* in response to a variety of signals (Figure 17.23).]

1. **Synthesis of PGH$_2$:** The first step in prostaglandin synthesis is the oxidative cyclization of free arachidonic acid to yield PGH$_2$ by *prostaglandin endoperoxide synthase* (*PGH synthase*). This enzyme is an endoplasmic reticulum membrane-bound protein that has two catalytic activities: *fatty acid cyclooxygenase* (*COX*), which requires two molecules of O_2, and *peroxidase*, which is dependent on reduced glutathione (see p. 148). PGH$_2$ is converted to a variety of prostaglandins and thromboxanes, as shown in Figure 17.23, by cell-specific *synthases*.

    a. **Isozymes of PGH synthase:** Two isozymes, usually denoted as *COX-1* and *COX-2*, of *PGH synthase* are known. *COX-1* is made constitutively in most tissues, and is required for maintenance of healthy gastric tissue, renal homeostasis, and platelet aggregation. *COX-2* is inducible in a limited number of tissues in response to products of activated immune and inflammatory cells. [Note: The increase in prostaglandin synthesis subsequent to the induction of *COX-2* mediates the pain, heat, redness, and swelling of inflammation, and the fever of infection.]

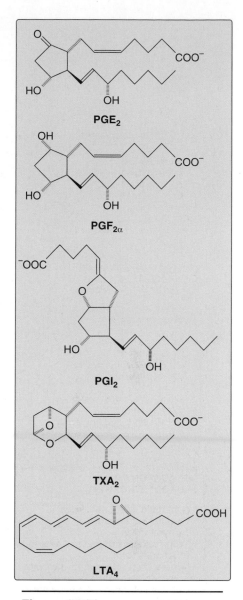

Figure 17.21
Examples of prostaglandin structures. Prostaglandins are named as follows: PG plus a third letter (for example, A, D, E, F), which designates the type and arrangement of functional groups in the molecule. The subscript number indicates the number of double bonds in the molecule. PGI$_2$ is known as prostacyclin. Thromboxanes are designated by TX and leukotrienes by LT.

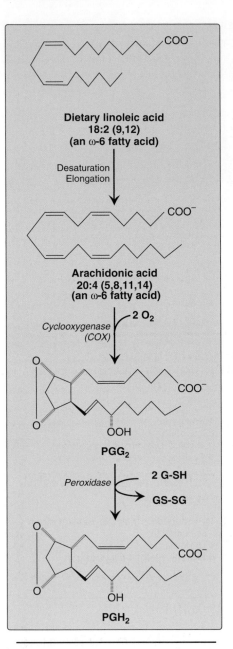

Figure 17.22
Oxidation and cyclization of arachidonic acid by the two catalytic activities of prostaglandin endoperoxide synthase. G-SH = reduced glutathione; GS-SG = oxidized glutathione.

2. Inhibition of prostaglandin synthesis: The synthesis of prostaglandins can be inhibited by a number of unrelated compounds. For example, cortisol (a steroidal anti-inflammatory agent) inhibits *phospholipase A2* activity (see Figure 17.23) and, therefore, the precursor of the prostaglandins, arachidonic acid, is not made available from membrane phospholipids. Aspirin, indomethacin, and phenylbutazone (all nonsteroidal anti-inflammatory agents [NSAIDS]) inhibit both *COX-1* and *COX-2* and, thus, prevent the synthesis of the parent prostaglandin, PGH$_2$. [Note: Systemic inhibition of *COX-1*, with subsequent damage to the stomach and the kidneys, and impaired clotting of blood, is the basis of aspirin's toxicity.] Inhibitors specific for *COX-2* (for example, celecoxib[1]) were designed to reduce pathologic inflammatory processes while maintaining the physiologic functions of *COX-1*; however, their use has been associated with increased risk of heart attacks.

B. Synthesis of leukotrienes

Arachidonic acid is converted to a variety of linear hydroperoxy acids by a separate pathway involving a family of *lipoxygenases* (LOXs). For example, *5-lipoxygenase* converts arachidonic acid to 5-hydroxy-6,8,11,14 eicosatetraenoic acid (5-HPETE, see Figure 17.23). 5-HPETE is converted to a series of leukotrienes, the nature of the final products varying according to the tissue. Leukotrienes are mediators of allergic response and inflammation. Their synthesis is not affected by NSAIDs. [Note: Aspirin-induced asthma is a response to overproduction of leukotrienes with NSAID use. NSAIDs, however, also favor synthesis of lipoxins (LXs), lipid mediators with anti-inflammatory effects.] Inhibitors of *5-lipoxygenase* and leukotriene receptor antagonists are used in the treatment of asthma.[2]

C. Role of prostaglandins in platelet homeostasis

Thromboxane A$_2$ (TXA$_2$) is produced by *COX-1* in activated platelets. It promotes adherence and aggregation of circulating platelets, and contraction of vascular smooth muscle, thus promoting formation of blood clots (thrombi). Prostacyclin (PGI$_2$), produced by *COX-2* in vascular endothelial cells, inhibits platelet aggregation and stimulates vasodilation, and so impedes thrombogenesis. The opposing effects of TXA$_2$ and PGI$_2$ limit thrombi formation to sites of vascular injury. [Note: Aspirin has an antithrombogenic effect. It inhibits *COX-1* (and TXA$_2$ synthesis) in platelets, and *COX-2* (and PGI$_2$ synthesis) in endothelial cells by irreversible acetylation of these isozymes (Figure 17.24). The inhibition of *COX-1* cannot be overcome in platelets, which lack nuclei. However, the inhibition of *COX-2* can be overcome in endothelial cells, because they have a nucleus and, therefore, can generate more of the enzyme. This difference is the basis of low-dose aspirin therapy used to lower the risk of stroke and heart attacks by decreasing formation of thrombi.]

[1]See Chapter 41 in *Lippincott's Illustrated Reviews: Pharmacology* for a discussion of anti-inflammatory drugs.
[2]See Chapter 27 in *Lippincott's Illustrated Reviews: Pharmacology* for a discussion of the treatment of asthma.

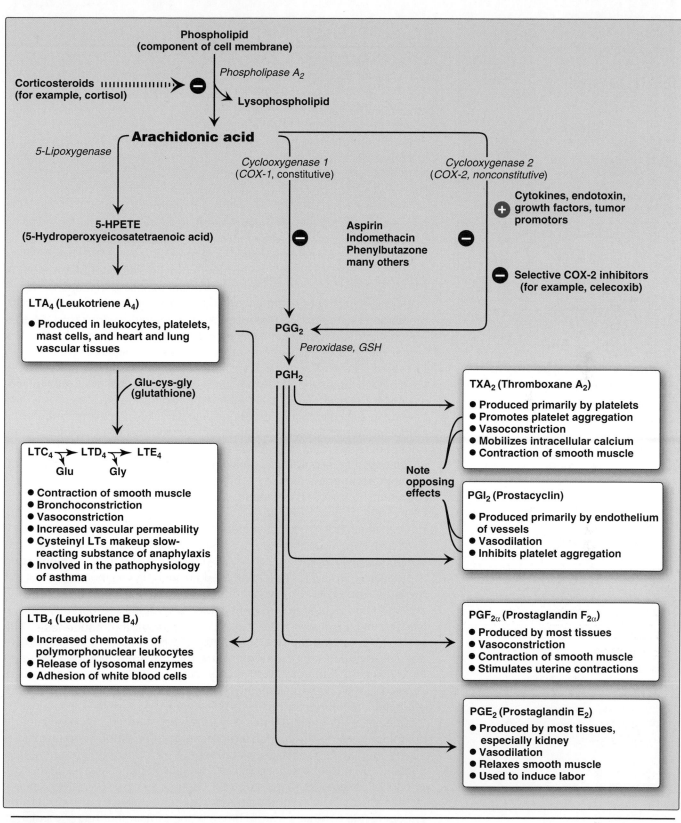

Figure 17.23
Overview of the biosynthesis and function of some important prostaglandins, leukotrienes, and a thromboxane from arachidonic acid.

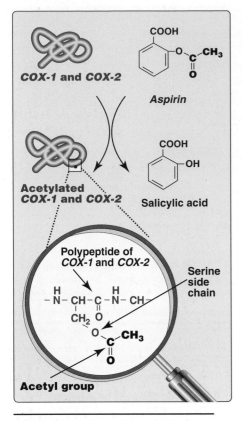

Figure 17.24
Irreversible acetylation of *COX-1 and COX-2* by aspirin.

IX. CHAPTER SUMMARY

Phospholipids are **polar**, **ionic** compounds composed of an **alcohol** (for example, **choline** or **ethanolamine**) attached by a phosphodiester bridge to either **diacylglycerol** (producing **phosphatidylcholine** or **phosphatidyl-ethanolamine**) or to **sphingosine** (Figure 17.25). The alcohol **sphingosine** attached to a long-chain fatty acid produces a **ceramide**. Addition of a **phosphorylcholine** produces the phospholipid **sphingomyelin**, which is the only significant sphingophospholipid in humans. Phospholipids are the predominant lipids of **cell membranes**. Nonmembrane-bound phospho-lipids serve as components of **lung surfactant** and **bile**. **Dipalmitoylphos-phatidylcholine** (**DPPC**, also called **dipalmitoyl lecithin**, **DPPL**) is the major lipid component of **lung surfactant**. Insufficient surfactant production causes **respiratory distress syndrome**. **Phosphatidylinositol** (**PI**) serves as a reservoir for **arachidonic acid** in membranes. The phosphorylation of membrane-bound PI produces **phosphatidylinositol 4,5-bisphosphate** (**PIP$_2$**). This compound is degraded by **phospholipase C** in response to the binding of a variety of neurotransmitters, hormones, and growth factors to membrane receptors. The products of this degradation, **inositol 1,4,5-tris-phosphate** (**IP$_3$**) and **diacylglycerol** mediate the mobilization of intracellu-lar **calcium** and the activation of **protein kinase C**, which act synergistically to evoke cellular responses. Specific proteins can be covalently attached via a carbohydrate bridge to membrane-bound phosphatidylinositol (**glyco-syl phosphatidylinositol**, or **GPI**). A deficiency in the synthesis of GPI in hematopoietic cells results in a hemolytic disease, **paroxysmal nocturnal hemoglobinuria**. The **degradation** of phosphoglycerides is performed by **phospholipases** found in all tissues and pancreatic juice. **Sphingomyelin** is degraded to a ceramide plus phosphorylcholine by the lysosomal enzyme **sphingomyelinase**. A deficiency in sphingomyelinase causes **Niemann-Pick (A + B) disease**. **Glycolipids** (glycosphingolipids) are derivatives of **ceramides** to which carbohydrates have been attached. When one sugar molecule is added to the ceramide, a **cerebroside** is pro-duced. If an oligosaccharide is added, a **globoside** is produced. If an acidic N-acetylneuraminic acid (NANA) molecule is added, a **ganglioside** is produced. Glycolipids are found predominantly in cell membranes of the **brain** and **peripheral nervous tissue**, with high concentrations in the **myelin sheath**. They are very **antigenic**. Glycolipids are degraded in the **lysosomes** by hydrolytic enzymes. A deficiency of one of these enzymes produces a **sphingolipidosis**, in each of which a characteristic sphin-golipid accumulates. **Prostaglandins** (**PG**), **thromboxanes** (**TX**), and **leukotrienes** (**LT**) are produced in very small amounts in almost all tissues, act locally and have an extremely short half-life. **They serve as mediators of the inflammatory response.** The dietary precursor of the eicosanoids is the essential fatty acid, **linoleic acid**. It is desaturated and elongated to **arachidonic acid**—the immediate precursor of prostaglandins—which is stored in the membrane as a component of a phospholipid, generally phosphatidylinositol. Arachidonic acid is released from the phospholipid by **phospholipase A$_2$**. Synthesis of the **PG** and **TX** begins with the oxidative cyclization of free arachidonic acid to yield PGH$_2$ by **prostaglandin endoperoxide synthase**—an ER membrane protein that has two catalytic activities: **fatty acid cyclooxygenase** (**COX**) and **peroxidase**. Opposing effects of PGI$_2$ and TXA$_2$ limit clot formation. There are two isozymes of the synthase: **COX-1** (constitutive) and **COX-2**. NSAIDs inhibit both. **LT** are linear molecules produced by the **5-lipoxygenase** pathway. They mediate allergic response and are unaffected by NSAIDs.

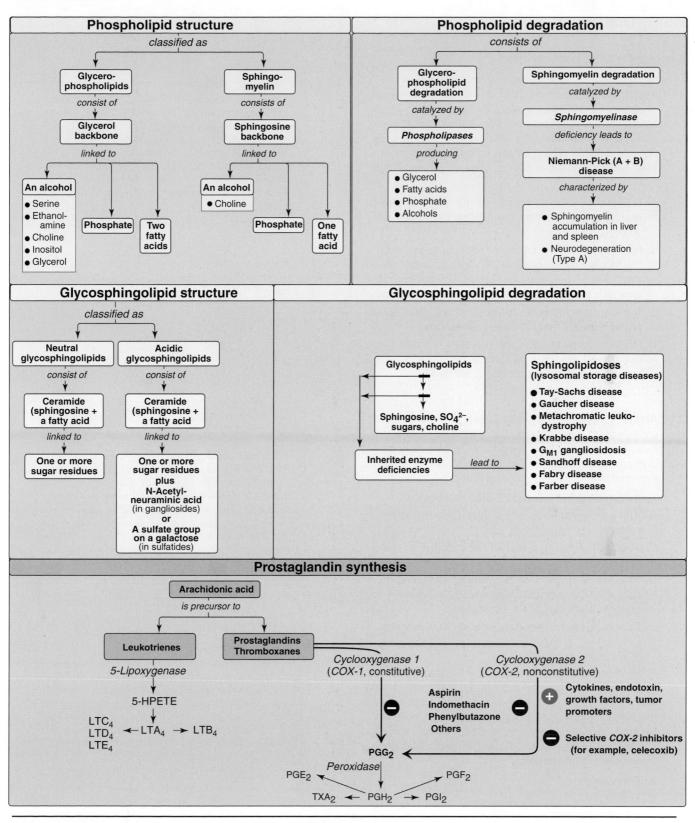

Figure 17.25
Key concept map for complex lipids.

Study Questions

Choose the ONE correct answer.

17.1 Aspirin-induced asthma (AIA) is a severe reaction to nonsteroidal anti-inflammatory drugs (NSAIDs) characterized by bronchoconstriction 30 minutes to several hours after ingestion. It is seen in as many as 20% of adults. Which of the following statements best explains the symptoms seen in patients with AIA?

A. NSAIDs inhibit the activity of the CFTR protein, resulting in thickened secretions that block airways.

B. NSAIDs inhibit COX but not lipoxygenase, resulting in the flow of arachidonic acid to leukotriene synthesis.

C. NSAIDs activate the COX activity of PGH synthase, resulting in increased synthesis of prostaglandins that promote vasodilation.

D. NSAIDs activate phospholipases, resulting in decreased amounts of dipalmytoylphosphatidylcholine and alveolar collapse (atelectasis).

Correct answer = B. NSAIDs inhibit COX but not lipoxygenase, so any arachidonic acid available is used for the synthesis of bronchoconstricting-leukotrienes. NSAIDs have no effect on the CFTR protein, defects in which are the cause of cystic fibrosis. Steroids, not NSAIDs, inhibit phospholipase A_2. COX is inhibited by NSAIDs, not activated. NSAIDs have no effect on phospholipases.

17.2 An infant, born at 28 weeks of gestation, rapidly gave evidence of respiratory distress. Lab and x-ray results supported the diagnosis of infant respiratory distress syndrome (RDS). Which of the following statements about this syndrome is true?

A. It is unrelated to the baby's premature birth.

B. It is a consequence of too few Type II pneumocytes.

C. The lecithin/sphingomyelin ratio in the amniotic fluid is likely to be greater than two.

D. The concentration of dipalmitoylphosphatidylcholine in the amniotic fluid would be expected to be lower than that of a full-term baby.

E. RDS is an easily treated disorder with low mortality.

Correct answer = D. Dipalmitoylphosphatidylcholine (DPPC, or dipalmitoyl lecithin) is the lung surfactant found in mature, healthy lungs. RDS can occur in lungs that make too little of this compound. If the lecithin/sphingomyelin ratio in amniotic is greater than two, a newborn's lungs are considered to be sufficiently mature—premature lungs would be expected to have a ratio lower than two. The RDS would not be due to too few Type II pneumocytes—these cells would simply be secreting sphingomyelin rather than DPPC at 28 weeks of gestation.

17.3 A 25-year-old woman with a history that included hepatosplenomegaly with eventual removal of the spleen, bone and joint pain with several fractures of the femur, and a liver biopsy that showed wrinkled-looking cells with accumulations of glucosylceramides was presented at Grand Rounds. The likely diagnosis for this patient is:

A. Fabry disease.

B. Farber disease.

C. Gaucher disease.

D. Krabbe disease.

E. Niemann-Pick disease.

Correct answer = C. The adult form of Gaucher disease causes hepatosplenomegaly, osteoporosis of the long bones, and the characteristic wrinkled appearance of the cytosol of cells. This is also the sphingolipidosis in which glucosylceramides accumulate. The deficient enzyme is β-glucosidase (a glucocerebrosidase).

Cholesterol and Steroid Metabolism

18

I. OVERVIEW

Cholesterol, the characteristic steroid alcohol of animal tissues, performs a number of essential functions in the body. For example, cholesterol is a structural component of all cell membranes, modulating their fluidity, and, in specialized tissues, cholesterol is a precursor of bile acids, steroid hormones, and vitamin D. It is therefore of critical importance that the cells of the body be assured an appropriate supply of cholesterol. To meet this need, a complex series of transport, biosynthetic, and regulatory mechanisms has evolved. The liver plays a central role in the regulation of the body's cholesterol homeostasis. For example, cholesterol enters the liver's cholesterol pool from a number of sources including dietary cholesterol, as well as cholesterol synthesized de novo by extrahepatic tissues and by the liver itself. Cholesterol is eliminated from the liver as unmodified cholesterol in the bile, or it can be converted to bile salts that are secreted into the intestinal lumen. It can also serve as a component of plasma lipoproteins sent to the peripheral tissues. In humans, the balance between cholesterol influx and efflux is not precise, resulting in a gradual deposition of cholesterol in the tissues, particularly in the endothelial linings of blood vessels. This is a potentially life-threatening occurrence when the lipid deposition leads to plaque formation, causing the narrowing of blood vessels (atherosclerosis) and increased risk of cardio-, cerebro- and peripheral vascular disease. Figure 18.1 summarizes the major sources of liver cholesterol and the routes by which cholesterol leaves the liver.

II. STRUCTURE OF CHOLESTEROL

Cholesterol is a very hydrophobic compound. It consists of four fused hydrocarbon rings (A-D) called the "steroid nucleus"), and it has an eight-carbon, branched hydrocarbon chain attached to carbon 17 of the D ring. Ring A has a hydroxyl group at carbon 3, and ring B has a double bond between carbon 5 and carbon 6 (Figure 18.2).

A. Sterols

Steroids with eight to ten carbon atoms in the side chain at carbon 17 and a hydroxyl group at carbon 3 are classified as sterols.

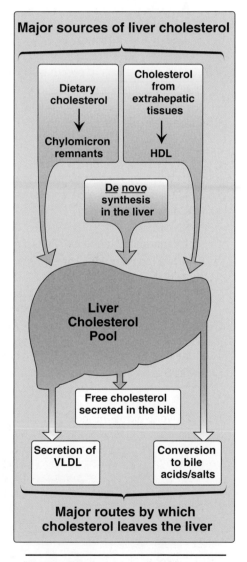

Major sources of liver cholesterol

Dietary cholesterol → Chylomicron remnants

Cholesterol from extrahepatic tissues → HDL

De novo synthesis in the liver

Liver Cholesterol Pool

Free cholesterol secreted in the bile

Secretion of VLDL

Conversion to bile acids/salts

Major routes by which cholesterol leaves the liver

Figure 18.1
Sources of liver cholesterol (influx) and routes by which cholesterol leaves the liver (efflux).

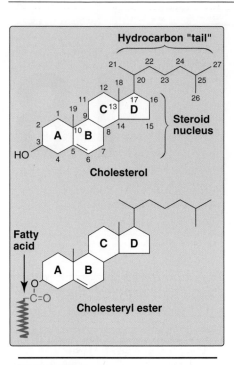

Figure 18.2
Structure of cholesterol and its ester.

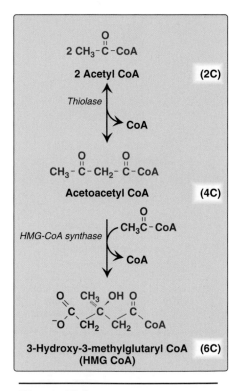

Figure 18.3
Synthesis of HMG CoA.

Cholesterol is the major sterol in animal tissues. [Note: Plant sterols, such as β-sitosterol are poorly absorbed by humans. After entering the enterocytes, they are actively transported back into the intestinal lumen. Because some cholesterol is transported as well, plant sterols appear to reduce the absorption of dietary cholesterol. This has led to clinically useful dietary treatment of hypercholesteremia. Daily ingestion of plant steroid esters (in the form of commercially available trans fatty acid–free margarine) is one of a number of dietary strategies leading to the reduction of plasma cholesterol levels (see p. 363).]

B. Cholesteryl esters

Most plasma cholesterol is in an esterified form (with a fatty acid attached at carbon 3, see Figure 18.2), which makes the structure even more hydrophobic than free (unesterified) cholesterol. Cholesteryl esters are not found in membranes, and are normally present only in low levels in most cells. Because of their hydrophobicity, cholesterol and its esters must be transported in association with protein as a component of a lipoprotein particle (see p. 227) or be solubilized by phospholipids and bile salts in the bile (see p. 226).

III. SYNTHESIS OF CHOLESTEROL

Cholesterol is synthesized by virtually all tissues in humans, although liver, intestine, adrenal cortex, and reproductive tissues, including ovaries, testes, and placenta, make the largest contributions to the body's cholesterol pool. As with fatty acids, all the carbon atoms in cholesterol are provided by acetate, and NADPH provides the reducing equivalents. The pathway is endergonic, being driven by hydrolysis of the high-energy thioester bond of acetyl coenzyme A (CoA) and the terminal phosphate bond of adenosine triphosphate (ATP). Synthesis requires enzymes in both the cytosol and the membrane of the smooth endoplasmic reticulum (ER). The pathway is responsive to changes in cholesterol concentration, and regulatory mechanisms exist to balance the rate of cholesterol synthesis within the body against the rate of cholesterol excretion. An imbalance in this regulation can lead to an elevation in circulating levels of plasma cholesterol, with the potential for vascular disease.

A. Synthesis of 3-hydroxy-3-methylglutaryl (HMG) CoA

The first two reactions in the cholesterol synthetic pathway are similar to those in the pathway that produces ketone bodies (see Figure 16.22, p. 196). They result in the production of HMG CoA (Figure 18.3). First, two acetyl CoA molecules condense to form acetoacetyl CoA. Next, a third molecule of acetyl CoA is added, producing HMG CoA, a six-carbon compound. [Note: Liver parenchymal cells contain two isoenzymes of *HMG CoA synthase*. The cytosolic enzyme participates in cholesterol synthesis, whereas the mitochondrial enzyme functions in the pathway for ketone body synthesis.]

B. Synthesis of mevalonate

The next step, the reduction of HMG CoA to mevalonate, is catalyzed by *HMG CoA reductase*, and is the rate-limiting and key regulated step in cholesterol synthesis. It occurs in the cytosol, uses two molecules of NADPH as the reducing agent, and releases CoA, making the reaction irreversible (Figure 18.4). [Note: *HMG CoA reductase* is an intrinsic membrane protein of the ER, with the enzyme's catalytic domain projecting into the cytosol. Regulation of *HMG CoA reductase* activity is discussed below.]

C. Synthesis of cholesterol

The reactions and enzymes involved in the synthesis of cholesterol from mevalonate are illustrated in Figure 18.5. [Note: The numbers shown in brackets below correspond to numbered reactions shown in this figure.]

[1] Mevalonate is converted to 5-pyrophosphomevalonate in two steps, each of which transfers a phosphate group from ATP.

[2] A five-carbon isoprene unit—isopentenyl pyrophosphate (IPP)—is formed by the decarboxylation of 5-pyrophosphomevalonate. The reaction requires ATP. [Note: IPP is the precursor of a family of molecules with diverse functions, the isoprenoids. Cholesterol is a sterol isoprenoid. Nonsterol isoprenoids include dolichol (see p. 167) and ubiquinone (Coenzyme Q) (see p. 75).]

[3] IPP is isomerized to 3,3-dimethylallyl pyrophosphate (DPP).

[4] IPP and DPP condense to form ten-carbon geranyl pyrophosphate (GPP).

[5] A second molecule of IPP then condenses with GPP to form 15-carbon farnesyl pyrophosphate (FPP). [Note: Covalent attachment of farnesyl to proteins, a process known as "prenylation," is one mechanism for anchoring proteins to plasma membranes.]

[6] Two molecules of FPP combine, releasing pyrophosphate, and are reduced, forming the 30-carbon compound squalene. [Note: Squalene is formed from six isoprenoid units. Because three ATP are hydrolyzed per mevalonate residue converted to IPP, a total of 18 ATP are required to make the polyisoprenoid squalene.]

[7] Squalene is converted to the sterol lanosterol by a sequence of reactions catalyzed by ER-associated enzymes that use molecular oxygen and NADPH. The hydroxylation of squalene triggers the cyclization of the structure to lanosterol.

[8] The conversion of lanosterol to cholesterol is a multistep process, resulting in the shortening of the carbon chain from 30 to 27 carbons, removal of the two methyl groups at carbon 4, migration of the double bond from carbon 8 to carbon 5, and reduction of the double bond between carbon 24 and carbon 25. [Note: This ER-associated pathway includes several different enzymatic reactions. Smith-Lemli-Opitz syndrome (SLOS), a relatively common autosomal recessive disorder of cholesterol biosynthesis, is caused by a partial deficiency in *7-dehydrocholesterol-7-reductase*—an enzyme involved in the migration of the double bond. SLOS is one of several multisystem, embryonic malformation syndromes associated with impaired cholesterol synthesis.]

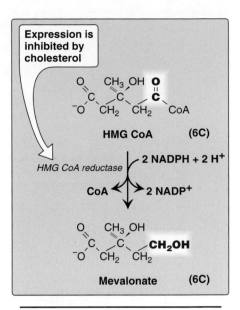

Figure 18.4
Synthesis of mevalonate.

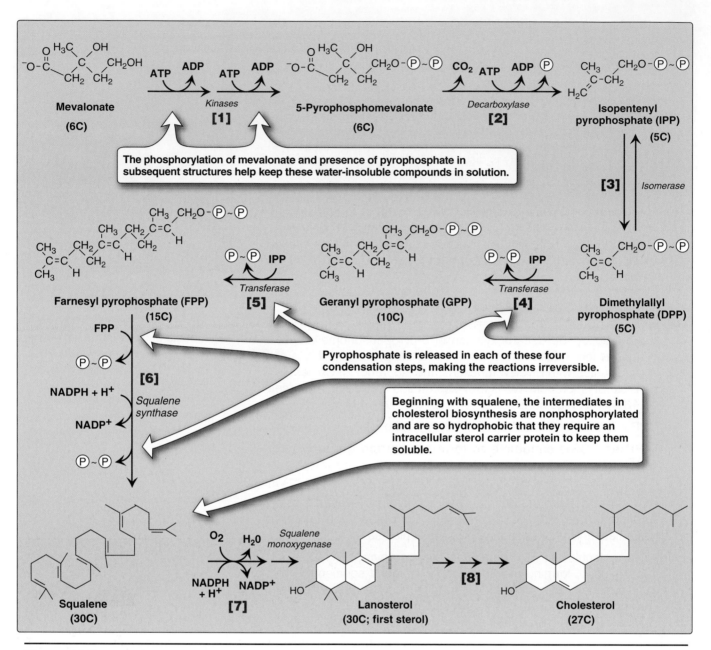

Figure 18.5
Synthesis of cholesterol from mevalonate.

D. Regulation of cholesterol synthesis

HMG CoA reductase, the rate-limiting enzyme, is the major control point for cholesterol biosynthesis, and is subject to different kinds of metabolic control.

1. **Sterol-dependent regulation of gene expression:** Expression of the gene for *HMG CoA reductase* is controlled by the transcription factor, SREBP-2 (sterol regulatory element–binding protein-2) that binds DNA at the cis-acting sterol regulatory element (SRE) of the *reductase* gene. SREBP is an integral protein of the ER membrane, and associates with a second ER membrane protein, SCAP (SREBP cleavage–activating protein). When sterol levels in

the cell are low, the SREBP-SCAP complex is sent out of the ER to the Golgi. In the Golgi, SREBP is sequentially acted upon by two *proteases*, which generate a soluble fragment that enters the nucleus, binds the SRE, and functions as a transcription factor. This results in increased synthesis of *HMG CoA reductase* and, therefore, increased cholesterol synthesis (Figure 18.6). If sterols are abundant, however, they bind SCAP at its sterol-sensing domain and induce the binding of SCAP to yet other ER membrane proteins (insigs). This results in the retention of the SCAP-SREBP complex in the ER, thus preventing the activation of SREBP, and leading to down-regulation of cholesterol synthesis.

2. **Sterol-accelerated enzyme degradation:** The *reductase* itself is a sterol-sensing integral protein of the ER membrane. When sterol levels in the cell are high, the *reductase* binds to insig proteins. Binding leads to ubiquitination and proteasomal degradation of the *reductase* (see p. 247).

3. **Sterol-independent phosphorylation/dephosphorylation:** *HMG CoA reductase* activity is controlled covalently through the actions of *adenosine monophosphate (AMP)–activated protein kinase (AMPK,* see p. 183) and a *phosphoprotein phosphatase* (see Figure 18.6). The phosphorylated form of the enzyme is inactive, whereas the dephosphorylated form is active. [Note: *AMPK* is activated by AMP, so cholesterol synthesis, like fatty acid synthesis, is decreased when ATP availability is decreased.]

4. **Hormonal regulation:** The amount (and, therefore, the activity) of *HMG CoA reductase* is controlled hormonally. An increase in insulin and thyroxine favors up-regulation of the expression of the gene for *HMG CoA reductase*. Glucagon and the glucocorticoids have the opposite effect.

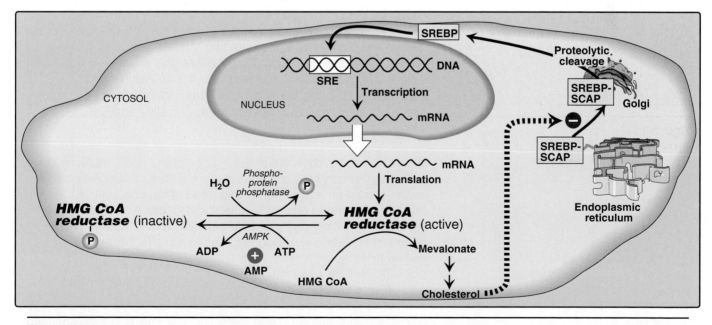

Figure 18.6
Regulation of *HMG CoA reductase*. SRE = sterol regulatory element; SREBP = sterol regulatory element-binding protein; SCAP = SREBP cleavage–activating protein.

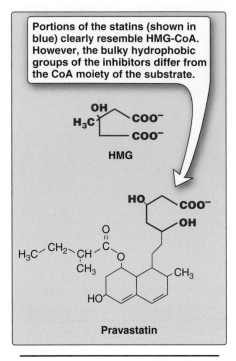

Portions of the statins (shown in blue) clearly resemble HMG-CoA. However, the bulky hydrophobic groups of the inhibitors differ from the CoA moiety of the substrate.

HMG

Pravastatin

Figure 18.7
Structural similarity of HMG and pravastatin, a clinically useful cholesterol-lowering drug of the "statin" family.

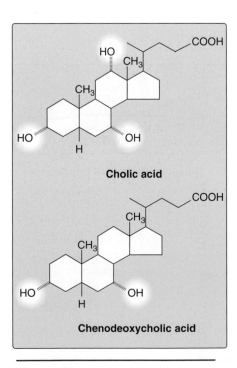

Cholic acid

Chenodeoxycholic acid

Figure 18.8
Bile acids.

5. Inhibition by drugs: The statin drugs (atorvastatin, fluvastatin, lovastatin, pravastatin, rosuvastatin, and simvastatin) are structural analogs of HMG CoA, and are (or are metabolized to) reversible, competitive inhibitors of *HMG CoA reductase* (Figure 18.7). They are used to decrease plasma cholesterol levels in patients with hypercholesterolemia.[1]

IV. DEGRADATION OF CHOLESTEROL

The ring structure of cholesterol cannot be metabolized to CO_2 and H_2O in humans. Rather, the intact sterol nucleus is eliminated from the body by conversion to bile acids and bile salts, which are excreted in the feces, and by secretion of cholesterol into the bile, which transports it to the intestine for elimination. Some of the cholesterol in the intestine is modified by bacteria before excretion. The primary compounds made are the isomers coprostanol and cholestanol, which are reduced derivatives of cholesterol. Together with cholesterol, these compounds make up the bulk of neutral fecal sterols.

V. BILE ACIDS AND BILE SALTS

Bile consists of a watery mixture of organic and inorganic compounds. Phosphatidylcholine (lecithin, see p. 202) and bile salts (conjugated bile acids) are quantitatively the most important organic components of bile. Bile can either pass directly from the liver where it is synthesized into the duodenum through the common bile duct, or be stored in the gallbladder when not immediately needed for digestion.

A. Structure of the bile acids

The bile acids contain 24 carbons, with two or three hydroxyl groups and a side chain that terminates in a carboxyl group. The carboxyl group has a pK_a of about six and, therefore, is not fully ionized at physiologic pH—hence, the term "bile acid." The bile acids are amphipathic in that the hydroxyl groups are α in orientation (they lie "below" the plane of the rings) and the methyl groups are β (they lie "above" the plane of the rings). Therefore, the molecules have both a polar and a nonpolar face, and can act as emulsifying agents in the intestine, helping prepare dietary triacylglycerol and other complex lipids for degradation by pancreatic digestive enzymes.

B. Synthesis of bile acids

Bile acids are synthesized in the liver by a multistep, multiorganelle pathway in which hydroxyl groups are inserted at specific positions on the steroid structure, the double bond of the cholesterol B ring is reduced, and the hydrocarbon chain is shortened by three carbons, introducing a carboxyl group at the end of the chain. The most common resulting compounds, cholic acid (a triol) and chenodeoxycholic acid (a diol, Figure 18.8), are called "primary" bile acids. [Note: The rate-limiting step in bile acid synthesis is the introduction of a hydroxyl group at carbon 7 of the steroid nucleus by *cholesterol-7-α-hydroxylase*, an ER-associated cytochrome P450 (CYP) enzyme found only in liver. The enzyme is down-regulated by cholic acid (Figure 18.9)]

[1]See Chapter 21 in *Lippincott's Illustrated Reviews: Pharmacology* for a discussion of the statins and other drugs to treat hyperlipidemia.

C. Synthesis of bile salts

Before the bile acids leave the liver, they are conjugated to a molecule of either glycine or taurine (an endproduct of cysteine metabolism) by an amide bond between the carboxyl group of the bile acid and the amino group of the added compound. These new structures include glycocholic and glycochenodeoxycholic acids, and taurocholic and taurochenodeoxycholic acids (Figure 18.10). The ratio of glycine to taurine forms in the bile is approximately 3:1. Addition of glycine or taurine results in the presence of a carboxyl group with a lower pK$_a$ (from glycine) or a sulfonate group (from taurine), both of which are fully ionized (negatively charged) at physiologic pH; thus, the conjugated forms are called bile salts. Bile salts are more effective detergents than bile acids because of their enhanced amphipathic nature. Therefore, only the conjugated forms—that is, the bile salts—are found in the bile. Individuals with genetic deficiencies in the conversion of cholesterol to bile acids are treated with exogenously supplied chenodeoxycholic acid.

> Bile salts provide the only significant mechanism for cholesterol excretion, both as a metabolic product of cholesterol and as a solubilizer of cholesterol in bile.

D. Action of intestinal flora on bile salts

Bacteria in the intestine can remove glycine and taurine from bile salts, regenerating bile acids. They can also convert some of the primary bile acids into "secondary" bile acids by removing a hydroxyl group, producing deoxycholic acid from cholic acid and lithocholic acid from chenodeoxycholic acid (Figure 18.11).

E. Enterohepatic circulation

Bile salts secreted into the intestine are efficiently reabsorbed (greater than 95%) and reused. The liver converts both primary and secondary bile acids into bile salts by conjugation with glycine or taurine, and secretes them into the bile. The mixture of bile acids and bile salts is absorbed primarily in the ileum via a Na$^+$-bile salt cotransporter. They are actively transported out of the ileal mucosal cells into the portal blood, and are efficiently taken up by the hepatocytes via an isoform of the cotransporter. [Note: Bile acids are hydrophobic and require a carrier in the portal blood. Albumin carries them in a noncovalent complex, just as it transports fatty acids in blood (see p. 181).] The continuous process of secretion of bile salts into the bile, their passage through the duodenum where some are converted to bile acids, their uptake in the ileum, and subsequent return to the liver as a mixture of bile acids and salts is termed the enterohepatic circulation (see Figure 18.11). Between 15 and 30 g of bile salts are secreted from the liver into the duodenum each day, yet only about 0.5 g (less than 3%) is lost daily in the feces. Approximately 0.5 g/day is synthesized from cholesterol in the liver to replace the lost bile acids. Bile acid sequestrants, such as cholestyramine, bind bile acids in the gut, prevent their reabsorption,

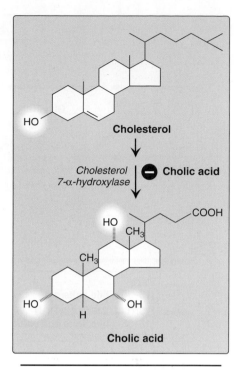

Figure 18.9
Synthesis of cholic acid, a bile acid.

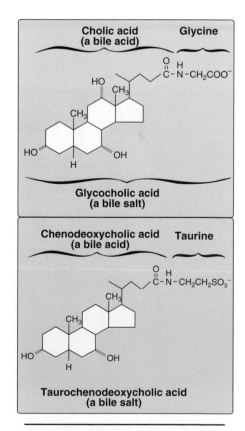

Figure 18.10
Bile salts. [Note "cholic" in the names.]

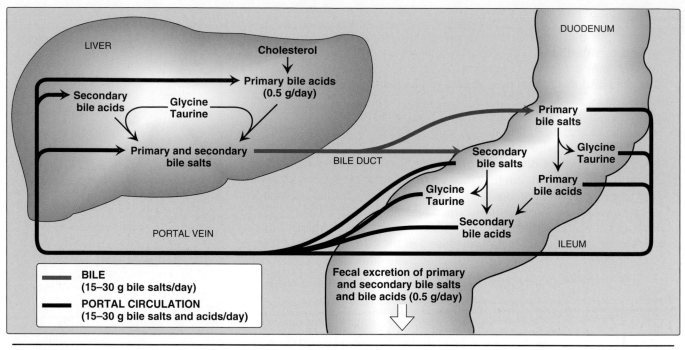

Figure 18.11
Enterohepatic circulation of bile salts and bile acids.

and so promote their excretion. They are used in the treatment of hypercholesterolemia because the removal of bile acids relieves the inhibition on bile acid synthesis in the liver, thereby diverting additional cholesterol into that pathway. [Note: Dietary fiber also binds bile acids and increases their excretion (see p. 366).]

F. Bile salt deficiency: cholelithiasis

The movement of cholesterol from the liver into the bile must be accompanied by the simultaneous secretion of phospholipid and bile salts. If this dual process is disrupted and more cholesterol enters the bile than can be solubilized by the bile salts and phosphatidyl choline present, the cholesterol may precipitate in the gallbladder, leading to cholesterol gallstone disease—cholelithiasis (Figure 18.12). This disorder is typically caused by a decrease of bile acids in the bile, which may result from: 1) gross malabsorption of bile acids from the intestine, as seen in patients with severe ileal disease; 2) obstruction of the biliary tract, interrupting the enterohepatic circulation; 3) severe hepatic dysfunction, leading to decreased synthesis of bile salts, or other abnormalities in bile production; or 4) excessive feedback suppression of bile acid synthesis as a result of an accelerated rate of recycling of bile acids. Cholelithiasis also may result from increased biliary cholesterol excretion, as seen with the use of fibrates. [Note: Fibrates, such as gemfibrozil, are derivatives of fibric acid. They are used to reduce triacylglycerol levels in blood through up-regulation of fatty acid β-oxidation.] Laparoscopic cholecystectomy (surgical removal of the gallbladder through a small incision) is currently the treatment of choice. However, for patients who are unable to undergo surgery, oral administration of chenodeoxycholic acid to supplement the body's supply of bile acids results in a gradual (months to years) dissolution of the gallstones.

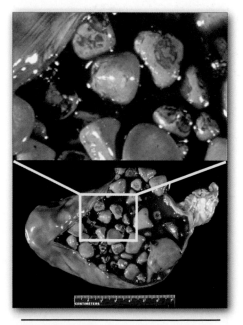

Figure 18.12
Gallbladder with gallstones.

VI. PLASMA LIPOPROTEINS

The plasma lipoproteins are spherical macromolecular complexes of lipids and specific proteins (apolipoproteins or apoproteins). The lipoprotein particles include chylomicrons (CM), very-low-density lipoproteins (VLDL), low-density lipoproteins (LDL), and high-density lipoproteins (HDL). They differ in lipid and protein composition, size, density (Figure 18.13), and site of origin. Lipoproteins function both to keep their component lipids soluble as they transport them in the plasma and to provide an efficient mechanism for transporting their lipid contents to (and from) the tissues. In humans, the transport system is less perfect than in other animals and, as a result, humans experience a gradual deposition of lipid—especially cholesterol—in tissues. This is a potentially life-threatening occurrence when the lipid deposition contributes to plaque formation, causing the narrowing of blood vessels (atherosclerosis).

A. Composition of plasma lipoproteins

Lipoproteins are composed of a neutral lipid core (containing triacylglycerol and cholesteryl esters) surrounded by a shell of amphipathic apolipoproteins, phospholipid, and nonesterified (free) cholesterol (Figure 18.14). These amphipathic compounds are oriented so that their polar portions are exposed on the surface of the lipoprotein, thus making the particle soluble in aqueous solution. The triacylglycerol and cholesterol carried by the lipoproteins are obtained either from the diet (exogenous source) or from de novo synthesis (endogenous source). [Note: Lipoprotein particles constantly interchange lipids and apolipoproteins with each other; therefore, the actual apolipoprotein and lipid content of each class of particles can be somewhat variable.]

1. **Size and density of lipoprotein particles:** Chylomicrons are the lipoprotein particles lowest in density and largest in size, and contain the highest percentage of lipid and the lowest percentage of protein. VLDLs and LDLs are successively denser, having higher ratios of protein to lipid. HDL particles are the densest. Plasma lipoproteins can be separated on the basis of their electrophoretic mobility, as shown in Figure 18.15, or on the basis of their density by ultracentrifugation.

2. **Apolipoproteins:** The apolipoproteins associated with lipoprotein particles have a number of diverse functions, such as providing recognition sites for cell-surface receptors, and serving as activators or coenzymes for enzymes involved in lipoprotein metabolism. Some of the apolipoproteins are required as essential structural components of the particles and cannot be removed (in fact, the particles cannot be produced without them), whereas others are transferred freely between lipoproteins. Apolipoproteins are divided by structure and function into five major classes, A through E, with most classes having subclasses, for example, apolipoprotein (or apo) A-I and apo C-II. [Note: Functions of all of the apolipoproteins are not yet known.]

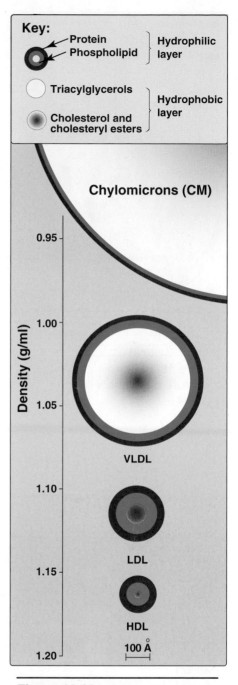

Figure 18.13
Approximate size and density of serum lipoproteins. Each family of lipoproteins exhibits a range of sizes and densities; this figure shows typical values. The width of the rings approximates the amount of each component. [Note: Although cholesterol and its esters are shown as one component in the center of each particle, physically cholesterol is a surface component whereas cholesteryl esters are located in the interior of the lipoproteins.]

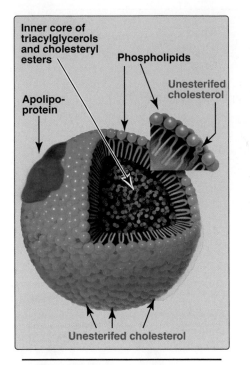

Figure 18.14
Structure of a typical lipoprotein particle.

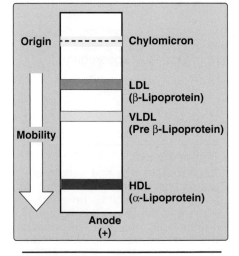

Figure 18.15
Electrophoretic mobility of plasma lipoproteins. The order of LDL and VLDL is reversed if ultra-centrifugation is used as the separation technique.

B. Metabolism of chylomicrons

Chylomicrons are assembled in intestinal mucosal cells and carry dietary triacylglycerol, cholesterol, fat-soluble vitamins, and cholesteryl esters (plus additional lipids made in these cells) to the peripheral tissues (Figure 18.16). [Note: TAGs account for close to 90% of the lipids in a chylomicron.]

1. **Synthesis of apolipoproteins:** Apolipoprotein B-48 is unique to chylomicrons. Its synthesis begins on the rough ER; it is glycosylated as it moves through the RER and Golgi. [Note: Apo B-48 is so named because it constitutes the N-terminal, 48% of the protein coded for by the gene for apo B. Apo B-100, which is synthesized by the liver and found in VLDL and LDL, represents the entire protein coded for by the apo B gene. Posttranscriptional editing (see p. 457) of a cytosine to a uracil in intestinal apo B-100 mRNA creates a nonsense codon (see p. 433), allowing translation of only 48% of the mRNA.]

2. **Assembly of chylomicrons:** The enzymes involved in triacylglycerol, cholesterol, and phospholipid synthesis are located in the smooth ER. Assembly of the apolipoproteins and lipid into chylomicrons requires microsomal triacylglycerol transfer protein (MTP, see p. 178), which loads apo B-48 with lipid. This occurs before transition from the ER to the Golgi, where the particles are packaged in secretory vesicles. These fuse with the plasma membrane releasing the lipoproteins, which then enter the lymphatic system and, ultimately, the blood.

3. **Modification of nascent chylomicron particles:** The particle released by the intestinal mucosal cell is called a "nascent" chylomicron because it is functionally incomplete. When it reaches the plasma, the particle is rapidly modified, receiving apolipoprotein E (which is recognized by hepatic receptors) and C. The latter includes apo C-II, which is necessary for the activation of *lipoprotein lipase*, the enzyme that degrades the triacylglycerol contained in the chylomicron (see below). The source of these apolipoproteins is circulating HDL (see Figure 18.16).

4. **Degradation of triacylglycerol by lipoprotein lipase:** *Lipoprotein lipase* is an extracellular enzyme that is anchored by heparan sulfate to the capillary walls of most tissues, but predominantly those of adipose tissue and cardiac and skeletal muscle. Adult liver does not have this enzyme. [Note: A *hepatic lipase* is found on the surface of endothelial cells of the liver. It plays some role in triacylglycerol degradation in CM and VLDL, and is particularly important in HDL metabolism (see p. 236).] *Lipoprotein lipase*, activated by apo C-II on circulating lipoprotein particles, hydrolyzes the triacylglycerol contained in these particles to yield fatty acids and glycerol. The fatty acids are stored (by the adipose) or used for energy (by the muscle). If they are not immediately taken up by a cell, the long-chain fatty acids are transported by serum albumin until their uptake does occur. Glycerol is used by the liver, for example, in lipid synthesis, glycolysis, or gluconeogenesis. [Note: Patients with a deficiency of *lipoprotein lipase* or

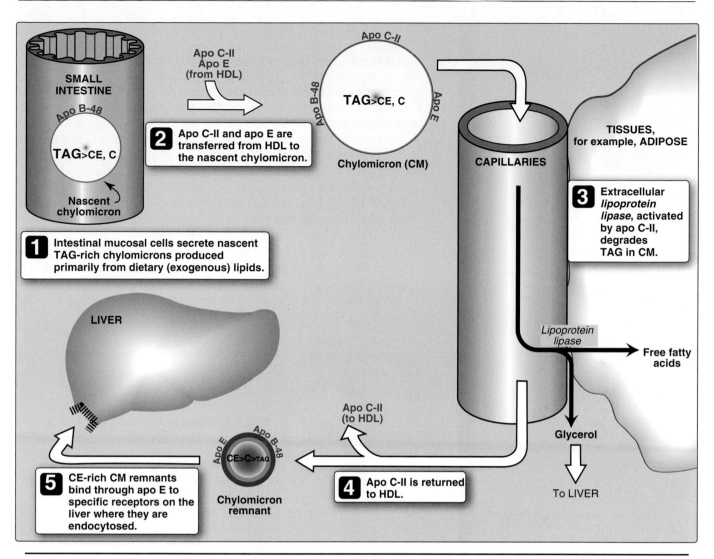

Figure 18.16
Metabolism of chylomicrons. CM = chylomicron; TAG = triacylglycerol; C = cholesterol; CE = cholesteryl esters.
Apo B-48, apo C-II, and apo E are apolipoproteins found as specific components of plasma lipoproteins.
The lipoproteins are not drawn to scale (see Figure 18.13 for details of the size and density of lipoproteins).

apo C-II (Type 1 hyperlipoproteinemia, or familial *lipoprotein lipase* deficiency) show a dramatic accumulation—1000 mg/dl or greater—of chylomicron-triacylglycerol in the plasma (hypertri-acylglycerolemia) even in the fasted state.]

5. **Regulation of lipoprotein lipase activity:** *Lipoprotein lipase* synthesis and transfer to the luminal surface of the capillary is stimulated by insulin (signifying a fed state, see p. 321). Furthermore, isomers of *lipoprotein lipase* have different K_m values for triacylglycerol (reminiscent of the *hexokinase/glucokinase* story, see p. 98). For example, the adipose enzyme has a large K_m (see p. 59), allowing the removal of fatty acids from circulating lipoprotein particles and their storage as triacylglycerols only when plasma lipoprotein concentrations are elevated. Conversely, heart muscle *lipoprotein lipase* has a small K_m, allowing the heart continuing access to the circulating fuel, even when plasma lipoprotein con-

centrations are low. [Note: The highest concentration of *lipoprotein lipase* is in cardiac muscle, reflecting the use of fatty acids to provide much of the energy needed for cardiac function.]

6. **Formation of chylomicron remnants:** As the chylomicron circulates and more than 90% of the triacylglycerol in its core is degraded by *lipoprotein lipase*, the particle decreases in size and increases in density. In addition, the C apoproteins (but not apo E) are returned to HDL. The remaining particle, called a "remnant," is rapidly removed from the circulation by the liver, whose cell membranes contain lipoprotein receptors that recognize apo E (see Figure 18.16). Chylomicron remnants bind to these receptors and are taken into the hepatocytes by endocytosis. The endocytosed vesicle then fuses with a lysosome, and the apolipoproteins, cholesteryl esters, and other components of the remnant are hydrolytically degraded, releasing amino acids, free cholesterol, and fatty acids. The receptor is recycled. (A more detailed discussion of the mechanism of receptor-mediated endocytosis is illustrated for LDL in Figure 18.20.)

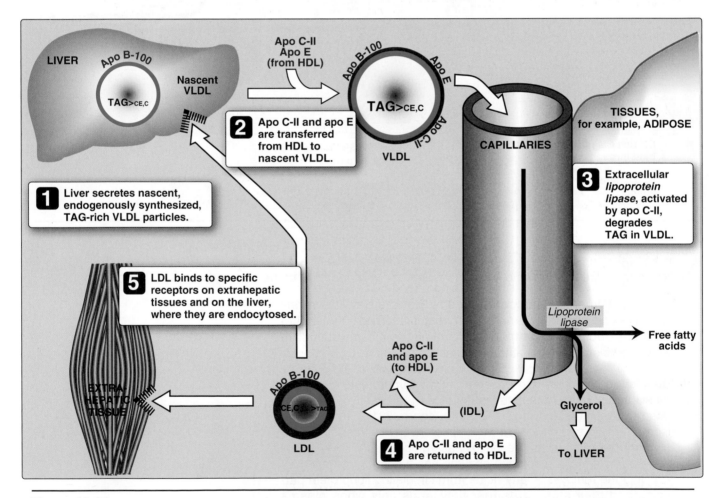

Figure 18.17
Metabolism of VLDL and LDL. TAG = triacylglycerol; VLDL = very-low-density lipoprotein; LDL = low-density-lipoprotein; IDL = intermediate-density lipoprotein; C = cholesterol; CE = cholesteryl esters. Apo B-100, apo C-II, and apo E are apolipoproteins found as specific components of plasma lipoproteins. Lipoproteins are not drawn to scale (see Figure 18.13 for details of the size and density of lipoproteins).

C. Metabolism of VLDL

VLDLs are produced in the liver (Figure 18.17). They are composed predominantly of endogenous triacylglycerol (approximately 60%), and their function is to carry this lipid from the liver (site of synthesis) to the peripheral tissues. There, the triacylglycerol is degraded by *lipoprotein lipase*, as discussed for chylomicrons (see p. 228). [Note: "Fatty liver" (hepatic steatosis) occurs in conditions in which there is an imbalance between hepatic triacylglycerol synthesis and the secretion of VLDL. Such conditions include obesity, uncontrolled diabetes mellitus, and chronic ethanol ingestion.]

1. Release of VLDL: VLDL are secreted directly into the blood by the liver as nascent VLDL particles containing apo B-100. They must obtain apo C-II and apo E from circulating HDL (see Figure 18.17). As with chylomicrons, apo C-II is required for activation of *lipoprotein lipase*. [Note: Abetalipoproteinemia is a rare hypolipoproteinemia caused by a defect in microsomal triacylglycerol transfer protein (MTP), leading to an inability to load apo B with lipid. As a consequence, no VLDL or chylomicrons are formed, and triacylglycerols accumulate in the liver and intestine.]

2. Modification of circulating VLDL: As VLDL pass through the circulation, triacylglycerol is degraded by *lipoprotein lipase*, causing the VLDL to decrease in size and become denser. Surface components, including the C and E apoproteins, are returned to HDL, but the particles retain apo B-100. Finally, some triacylglycerols are transferred from VLDL to HDL in an exchange reaction that concomitantly transfers some cholesteryl esters from HDL to VLDL. This exchange is accomplished by *cholesteryl ester transfer protein* (*CETP*, Figure 18.18).

3. Production of LDL from VLDL in the plasma: With these modifications, the VLDL is converted in the plasma to LDL. Intermediate-sized particles, the intermediate-density lipoproteins (IDL) or VLDL remnants, are observed during this transition. IDLs can also be taken up by cells through receptor-mediated endocytosis that uses apo E as the ligand. [Note: Apo E is normally present in three isoforms, E-2, E-3, and E-4. Apo E-2 binds poorly to receptors, and patients who are homozygotic for apo E-2 are deficient in the clearance of chylomicron remnants and IDL. These individuals have familial Type III hyperlipoproteinemia (familial dysbetalipoproteinemia, or broad beta disease), with hypercholesterolemia and premature atherosclerosis. Not yet understood is the fact that the E-4 isoform confers increased susceptibility to and decreased age of onset of late-onset Alzheimer disease, doubling the lifetime risk.]

D. Metabolism of LDL

LDL particles contain much less triacylglycerol than their VLDL predecessors, and have a high concentration of cholesterol and cholesteryl esters (Figure 18.19).

1. Receptor-mediated endocytosis: The primary function of LDL particles is to provide cholesterol to the peripheral tissues (or return it to the liver). They do so by binding to cell surface mem-

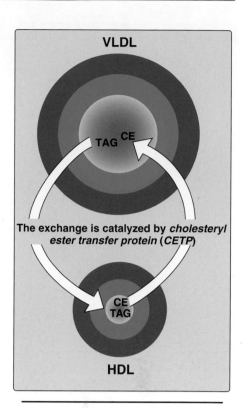

Figure 18.18
Transfer of cholesteryl esters (CE) from HDL to VLDL in exchange for triacylglycerol (TAG).

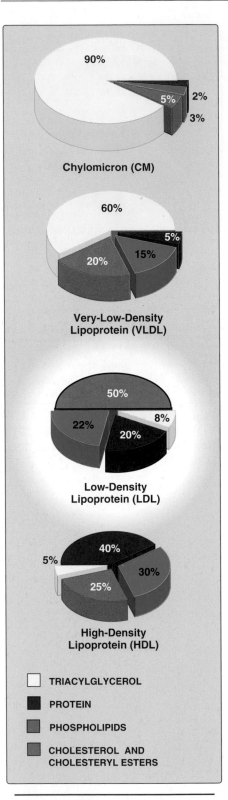

Figure 18.19
Composition of the plasma lipoproteins. Note the high concentration of cholesterol and cholesteryl esters in LDL.

brane LDL receptors that recognize apo B-100 (but not apo B-48). Because these LDL receptors can also bind apo E, they are known as apo B-100/apo E receptors. A summary of the uptake and degradation of LDL particles is presented in Figure 18.20. [Note: The numbers in brackets below refer to corresponding numbers on that figure.] A similar mechanism of receptor-mediated endocytosis is used for the cellular uptake and degradation of chylomicron remnants and IDLs by the liver.

[1] LDL receptors are negatively charged glycoproteins that are clustered in pits on cell membranes. The cytosolic side of the pit is coated with the protein clathrin, which stabilizes the shape of the pit.

[2] After binding, the LDL-receptor complex is internalized by endocytosis. [Note: A deficiency of functional LDL receptors causes a significant elevation in plasma LDL and, therefore, of plasma cholesterol. Patients with such deficiencies have Type II hyperlipidemia (familial hypercholesterolemia, FH) and premature atherosclerosis. FH can also be caused by increased activity of a *protease* that degrades the receptor and by defects in apo B-100 that reduce its binding to the receptor.]

[3] The vesicle containing LDL loses its clathrin coat and fuses with other similar vesicles, forming larger vesicles called endosomes.

[4] The pH of the endosome falls (due to the proton-pumping activity of endosomal *ATPase*), which allows separation of the LDL from its receptor. The receptors then migrate to one side of the endosome, whereas the LDLs stay free within the lumen of the vesicle. [Note: This structure is called CURL—the Compartment for Uncoupling of Receptor and Ligand.]

[5] The receptors can be recycled, whereas the lipoprotein remnants in the vesicle are transferred to lysosomes and degraded by lysosomal *acid hydrolases*, releasing free cholesterol, amino acids, fatty acids, and phospholipids. These compounds can be reutilized by the cell. [Note: Storage diseases caused by rare autosomal recessive deficiencies in the ability to hydrolyze lysosomal cholesteryl esters (Wolman disease), or to transport unesterified cholesterol out of the lysosome (Niemann-Pick disease, Type C) have been identified.]

2. **Effect of endocytosed cholesterol on cellular cholesterol homeostasis:** The chylomicron remnant-, IDL-, and LDL-derived cholesterol affects cellular cholesterol content in several ways (see Figure 18.20). First, *HMG CoA reductase* is inhibited by high cholesterol, as a result of which, de novo cholesterol synthesis decreases. Second, synthesis of new LDL receptor protein is reduced by decreasing the expression of the LDL receptor gene, thus limiting further entry of LDL cholesterol into cells. [Note: Regulation of the LDL receptor gene involves a SRE and a SREBP (SREBP-2), as was seen in the regulation of the gene for *HMG CoA reductase* (see p. 222).] Third, if the cholesterol is not required immediately for some structural or synthetic purpose, it is esterified by *acyl CoA:cholesterol acyltransferase* (*ACAT*). *ACAT*

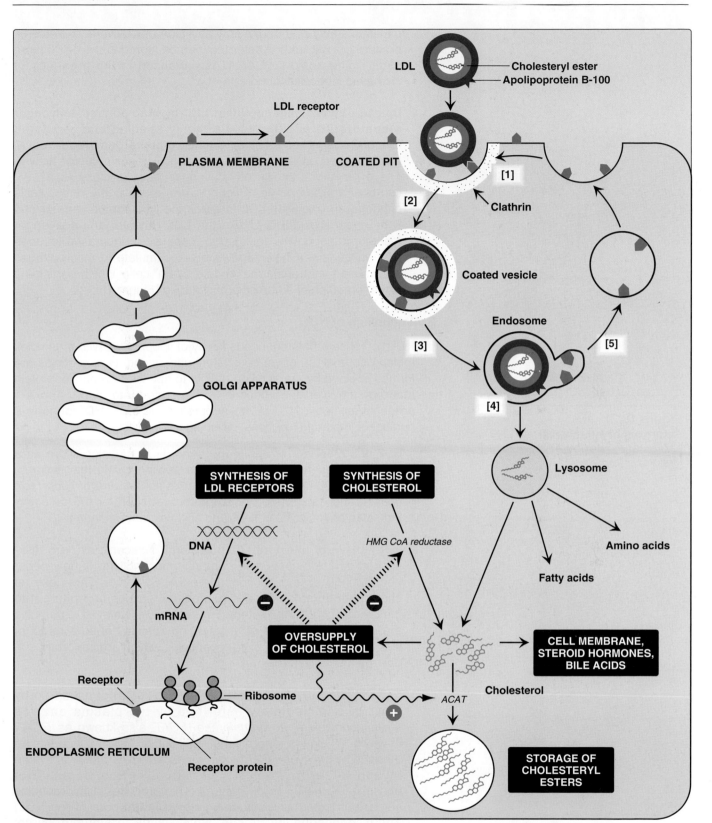

Figure 18.20
Cellular uptake and degradation of LDL. *ACAT = acyl CoA:cholesterol acyltransferase.*

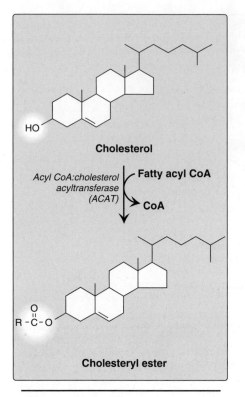

Cholesterol

Acyl CoA:cholesterol acyltransferase (ACAT)

Fatty acyl CoA

CoA

O
‖
R -C- O

Cholesteryl ester

Figure 18.21
Synthesis of intracellular cholesteryl ester by *ACAT*.

transfers a fatty acid from a fatty acyl CoA derivative to cholesterol, producing a cholesteryl ester that can be stored in the cell (Figure 18.21). The activity of *ACAT* is enhanced in the presence of increased intracellular cholesterol.

3. **Uptake of chemically modified LDL by macrophage scavenger receptors:** In addition to the highly specific and regulated receptor-mediated pathway for LDL uptake described above, macrophages possess high levels of scavenger receptor activity. These receptors, known as scavenger receptor class A (SR-A), can bind a broad range of ligands, and mediate the endocytosis of chemically modified LDL in which the lipid components or apo B have been oxidized. Unlike the LDL receptor, the scavenger receptor is not down-regulated in response to increased intracellular cholesterol. Cholesteryl esters accumulate in macrophages and cause their transformation into "foam" cells, which participate in the formation of atherosclerotic plaque (Figure 18.22).

E. Metabolism of HDL

HDL comprise a heterogeneous family of lipoproteins with a complex metabolism that is not yet completely understood. HDL particles are formed in blood by the addition of lipid to apo A-1, an apolipoprotein made by the liver and intestine and secreted into blood. Apo A-1 accounts for about 70% of the apoproteins in HDL. HDL perform a number of important functions, including the following:

1. **HDL is a reservoir of apolipoproteins:** HDL particles serve as a circulating reservoir of apo C-II (the apolipoprotein that is transferred to VLDL and chylomicrons, and is an activator of *lipoprotein lipase*), and apo E (the apolipoprotein required for the receptor-mediated endocytosis of IDLs and chylomicron remnants).

2. **HDL uptake of unesterified cholesterol:** Nascent HDL are disk-shaped particles containing primarily phospholipid (largely phosphatidylcholine) and apolipoproteins A, C, and E. They take up cholesterol from non-hepatic (peripheral) tissues and return it to the liver as cholesteryl esters (Figure 18.23). [Note: HDL particles are excellent acceptors of unesterified cholesterol as a result of their high concentration of phospholipids, which are important solubilizers of cholesterol.]

3. **Esterification of cholesterol:** When cholesterol is taken up by HDL, it is immediately esterified by the plasma enzyme *lecithin:cholesterol acyltransferase* (*LCAT*, also known as *PCAT*, in which "P" stands for phosphatidylcholine). This enzyme is synthesized by the liver. *LCAT* binds to nascent HDL, and is activated by apo A-I. *LCAT* transfers the fatty acid from carbon 2 of phosphatidylcholine to cholesterol. This produces a hydrophobic cholesteryl ester, which is sequestered in the core of the HDL, and lysophosphatidylcholine, which binds to albumin. [Note: Esterification maintains the cholesterol concentration gradient, allowing continued efflux of cholesterol to HDL.] As the discoidal nascent HDL accumulates cholesteryl esters, it first becomes a

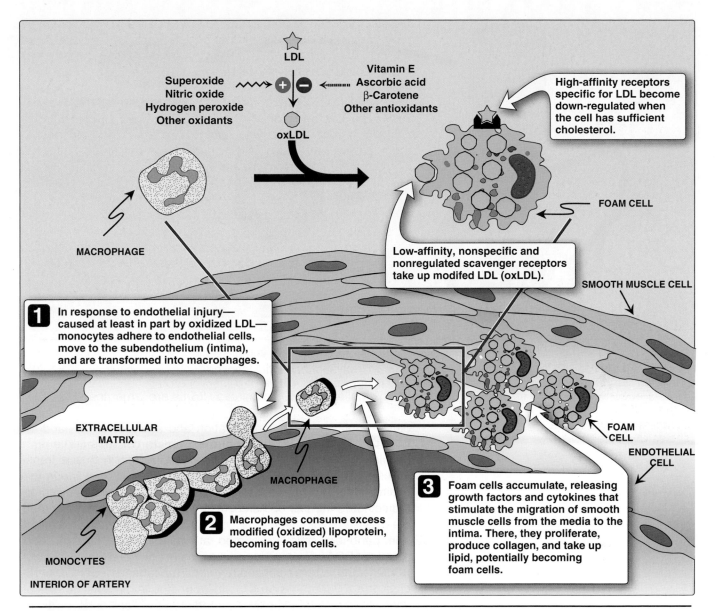

Figure 18.22
Role of oxidized lipoproteins in plaque formation in arterial wall.

spherical, relatively cholesteryl ester–poor HDL3 and, eventually, a cholesteryl ester–rich HDL2 particle that carries these esters to the liver. *Cholesterol ester transfer protein* (*CETP*, see p. 231) moves some of the cholesteryl esters from HDL to VLDL in exchange for triacylglycerol, relieving product inhibition of *LCAT*. Because VLDL are catabolized to LDL, the cholesteryl esters are ultimately taken up by the liver.

4. **Reverse cholesterol transport:** The selective transfer of cholesterol from peripheral cells to HDL, and from HDL to the liver for bile acid synthesis or disposal via the bile, and to steroidogenic cells for hormone synthesis, is a key component of cholesterol homeostasis. This is, in part, the basis for the inverse relationship seen

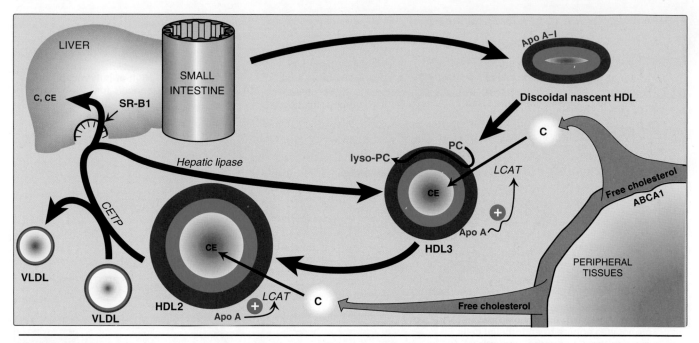

Figure 18.23
Metabolism of HDL. PC = phosphatidylcholine; lyso-PC = lysophosphatidylcholine. *LCAT* = *Lecithin cholesterol transferase*. CETP = cholesteryl ester transfer protein. ABCA1 = transport protein.
[Note: For convenience the size of VLDLs are shown smaller than HDL, whereas VLDLs are larger than HDL.]

between plasma HDL concentration and atherosclerosis, and for HDL's designation as the "good" cholesterol carrier. Reverse cholesterol transport involves efflux of cholesterol from peripheral cells to HDL, esterification of cholesterol by *LCAT*, binding of the cholesteryl ester–rich HDL (HDL2) to liver and steroidogenic cells, the selective transfer of the cholesteryl esters into these cells, and the release of lipid-depleted HDL (HDL3). The efflux of cholesterol from peripheral cells is mediated, at least in part, by the transport protein, ABCA1. [Note: Tangier disease is a very rare deficiency of ABCA1, and is characterized by the virtual absence of HDL particles due to degradation of lipid-poor apo A-1.] The uptake of cholesteryl esters by the liver is mediated by a cell-surface receptor, SR-B1 (scavenger receptor class B type 1) that binds HDL (see p, 234 for SR-A). It is not yet clear as to whether the HDL particle itself is taken up, the cholesteryl esters extracted, and the lipid-poor HDL released back into the blood, or if there is selective uptake of the cholesteryl ester alone. [Note: *Hepatic lipase*, with its ability to degrade both TAG and phospholipids, also participates in the conversion of HDL2 to HDL3.]

ABCA1 is an ATP-binding cassette (ABC) protein. ABC proteins use energy from ATP hydrolysis to transport materials, including lipids, in and out of cells and across intracellular compartments. In addition to Tangier disease, defects in specific ABC proteins result in X-linked adrenoleukodystrophy, respiratory distress syndrome due to decreased surfactant secretion, and cystic fibrosis.

F. Role of lipoprotein (a) in heart disease

Lipoprotein (a), or Lp(a), is a particle that, when present in large quantities in the plasma, is associated with an increased risk of coronary heart disease. Lp(a) is nearly identical in structure to an LDL particle. Its distinguishing feature is the presence of an additional apolipoprotein molecule, apo(a), that is covalently linked at a single site to apo B-100. Circulating levels of Lp(a) are determined primarily by genetics. However, factors such as diet may play some role, as trans fatty acids have been shown to increase Lp(a), and estrogen decreases both LDL and Lp(a). [Note: Apo(a) is structurally homologous to plasminogen—the precursor of a blood *protease* whose target is fibrin, the main protein component of blood clots. It is hypothesized that elevated Lp(a) slows the breakdown of blood clots that trigger heart attacks because it competes with plasminogen for binding to fibrin. Niacin reduces Lp(a) and raises HDL.]

VII. STEROID HORMONES

Cholesterol is the precursor of all classes of steroid hormones: glucocorticoids (for example, cortisol), mineralocorticoids (for example, aldosterone), and sex hormones—androgens, estrogens, and progestins (Figure 18.24). [Note: Glucocorticoids and mineralocorticoids are collectively called corticosteroids.] Synthesis and secretion occur in the adrenal cortex (cortisol, aldosterone, and androgens), ovaries and placenta (estrogens and progestins), and testes (testosterone). Steroid hormones are transported by the blood from their sites of synthesis to their target organs. Because of their hydrophobicity, they must be complexed with a plasma protein. Plasma albumin can act as a nonspecific carrier, and does carry aldosterone. However, specific steroid-carrier plasma proteins bind the steroid hormones more tightly than does albumin, for example, corticosteroid-binding globulin (transcortin) is responsible for transporting cortisol. A number of genetic diseases are caused by deficiencies in specific steps in the biosynthesis of steroid hormones. Some representative diseases are described in Figure 18.25.

A. Synthesis of steroid hormones

Synthesis involves shortening the hydrocarbon chain of cholesterol, and hydroxylation of the steroid nucleus. The initial and rate-limiting reaction converts cholesterol to the 21-carbon pregnenolone. It is catalyzed by the *cholesterol side-chain cleavage enzyme complex* (*desmolase, P450scc*)— a cytochrome P450 (CYP) mixed function *oxidase* of the inner mitochondrial membrane (see p. 149). NADPH and molecular oxygen are required for the reaction. The cholesterol substrate can be newly synthesized, taken up from lipoproteins, or released from cholesteryl esters stored in the cytosol of steroidogenic tissues. An important control point is the movement of cholesterol into mito-

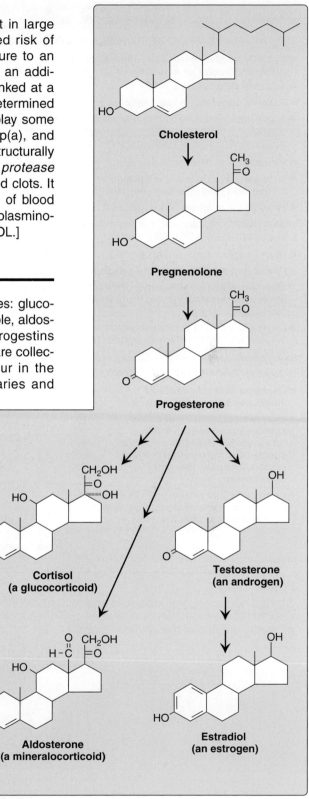

Figure 18.24
Key steroid hormones.

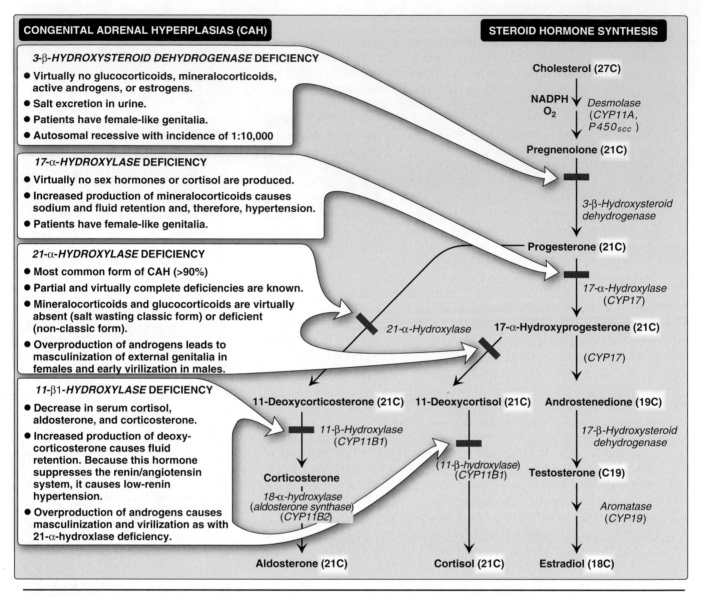

CONGENITAL ADRENAL HYPERPLASIAS (CAH)

STEROID HORMONE SYNTHESIS

3-β-HYDROXYSTEROID DEHYDROGENASE **DEFICIENCY**
- Virtually no glucocorticoids, mineralocorticoids, active androgens, or estrogens.
- Salt excretion in urine.
- Patients have female-like genitalia.
- Autosomal recessive with incidence of 1:10,000

17-α-HYDROXYLASE **DEFICIENCY**
- Virtually no sex hormones or cortisol are produced.
- Increased production of mineralocorticoids causes sodium and fluid retention and, therefore, hypertension.
- Patients have female-like genitalia.

21-α-HYDROXYLASE **DEFICIENCY**
- Most common form of CAH (>90%)
- Partial and virtually complete deficiencies are known.
- Mineralocorticoids and glucocorticoids are virtually absent (salt wasting classic form) or deficient (non-classic form).
- Overproduction of androgens leads to masculinization of external genitalia in females and early virilization in males.

11-β1-HYDROXYLASE **DEFICIENCY**
- Decrease in serum cortisol, aldosterone, and corticosterone.
- Increased production of deoxy-corticosterone causes fluid retention. Because this hormone suppresses the renin/angiotensin system, it causes low-renin hypertension.
- Overproduction of androgens causes masculinization and virilization as with 21-α-hydroxlase deficiency.

Cholesterol (27C)

NADPH $\downarrow$ *Desmolase*
O$_2$ (*CYP11A*, *P450$_{scc}$*)

Pregnenolone (21C)

3-β-Hydroxysteroid dehydrogenase

Progesterone (21C)

17-α-Hydroxylase (CYP17)

21-α-Hydroxylase   17-α-Hydroxyprogesterone (21C)

(*CYP17*)

11-Deoxycorticosterone (21C)   11-Deoxycortisol (21C)   Androstenedione (19C)

11-β-Hydroxylase (CYP11B1)   (*11-β-hydroxylase*) (*CYP11B1*)   *17-β-Hydroxysteroid dehydrogenase*

Corticosterone   Testosterone (C19)

18-α-hydroxylase (aldosterone synthase) (CYP11B2)   *Aromatase (CYP19)*

Aldosterone (21C)   Cortisol (21C)   Estradiol (18C)

Figure 18.25
Steroid hormone synthesis and associated diseases. [Note: 3-β-*hydroxysteroid dehydrogenase*, *CYP17*, and *CYP11B2* are bifunctional enzymes. Synthesis of testosterone and the estrogens from cholesterol occurs primarily outside of the adrenal gland.]

chondria. This process is mediated by StAR (steroidogenic acute regulatory protein). Pregnenolone is the parent compound for all steroid hormones (see Figure 18.25). Pregnenolone is oxidized and then isomerized to progesterone which is further modified to the other steroid hormones by hydroxylation reactions that occur in the ER and mitochondria. Like *desmolase*, the enzymes primarily are CYP proteins. A defect in the activity or amount of an enzyme in this pathway can lead to a deficiency in the synthesis of hormones beyond the affected step, and to an excess in the hormones or metabolites before that step. Because all members of the pathway have potent biologic activity, serious metabolic imbalances occur if enzyme deficiencies are present (see Figure 18.25). Collectively these disorders are known as the congenital adrenal hyperplasias. [Note: Addison disease, due to autoimmune destruction of the adrenal cortex, is characterized by adrenocortical insufficiency.]

B. Secretion of adrenal cortical steroid hormones

Steroid hormones are secreted on demand from their tissues of origin in response to hormonal signals. The corticosteroids and androgens are made in different regions of the adrenal cortex, and are secreted into blood in response to different signals.

1. **Cortisol:** Its production in the middle layer (zona fasciculata) of the adrenal cortex is controlled by the hypothalamus, to which the pituitary gland is attached (Figure 18.26). In response to severe stress (for example, infection), corticotropin-releasing hormone (CRH), produced by the hypothalamus, travels through capillaries to the anterior lobe of the pituitary, where it induces the production and secretion of adrenocorticotropic hormone (ACTH). The polypeptide ACTH, the "stress hormone," stimulates the adrenal cortex to synthesize and secrete the glucocorticoid cortisol. Cortisol allows the body to respond to stress through its effects on intermediary metabolism (for example, increased gluconeogenesis) and the inflammatory and immune responses. As cortisol levels rise, the release of CRH and ACTH is inhibited. [Note: ACTH binds to a membrane G-protein coupled receptor, resulting in cAMP production and activation of *protein kinase A* (see p. 94). *PKA* phosphorylates the *esterase* that converts cholesteryl ester to cholesterol and stimulates synthesis of StAR protein.]

2. **Aldosterone:** Its production in the outer layer (zona glomerulosa) of the adrenal cortex is induced by a decrease in the plasma Na^+/K^+ ratio, and by the hormone, angiotensin II. Angiotensin II (an octapeptide) is produced from angiotensin I (a decapeptide) by *angiotensin-converting enzyme* (*ACE*), an enzyme found predominantly in the lungs, but which is also distributed widely in the body. [Note: Angiotensin I is produced in the blood by cleavage of an inactive precursor, angiotensinogen, secreted by the liver. Cleavage is accomplished by the enzyme *renin*, made and secreted by the kidney.] Angiotensin II binds to cell-surface receptors. However, in contrast to ACTH, its effects are mediated through the phosphatidylinositol 4,5-bisphosphate (PIP_2) pathway (see p. 205) and not by cAMP. Aldosterone's primary effect is on the kidney tubules, where it stimulates sodium uptake and potassium excretion (Figure 18.27). [Note: An effect of aldosterone is an increase in blood pressure. Competitive inhibitors of *ACE* are used to treat *renin*-dependent hypertension.]

3. **Androgens:** Both the inner (zona reticularis) and middle layers of the adrenal cortex produce androgens, primarily dehydroepiandrosterone and androstenedione. Although adrenal androgens themselves are weak, they are converted in peripheral tissues to testosterone—a stronger androgen—and to estrogens.

> Estrogens are derived from androstenedione and testosterone by *aromatase* (*CYP19*). *Aromatase* inhibitors are used in the treatment of estrogen-responsive breast cancer in postmenopausal women.

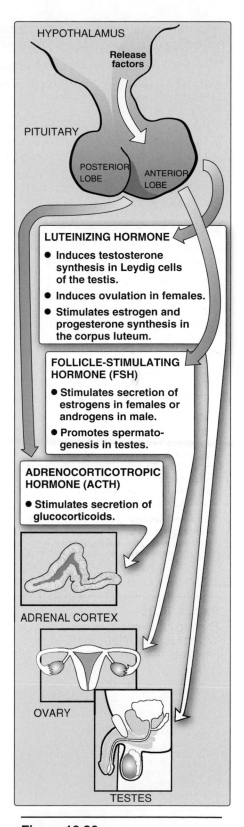

HYPOTHALAMUS

Release factors

PITUITARY

POSTERIOR LOBE

ANTERIOR LOBE

LUTEINIZING HORMONE
- Induces testosterone synthesis in Leydig cells of the testis.
- Induces ovulation in females.
- Stimulates estrogen and progesterone synthesis in the corpus luteum.

FOLLICLE-STIMULATING HORMONE (FSH)
- Stimulates secretion of estrogens in females or androgens in male.
- Promotes spermatogenesis in testes.

ADRENOCORTICOTROPIC HORMONE (ACTH)
- Stimulates secretion of glucocorticoids.

ADRENAL CORTEX

OVARY

TESTES

Figure 18.26
Pituitary hormone stimulation of steroid hormone synthesis and secretion.

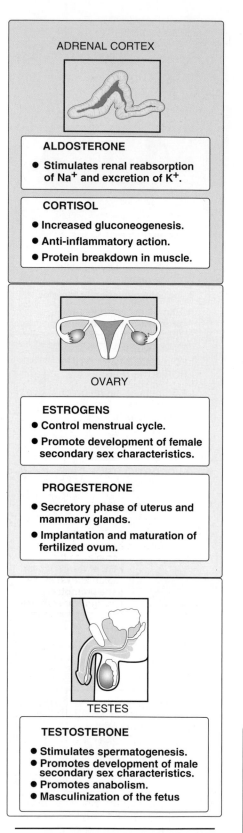

ADRENAL CORTEX

ALDOSTERONE
- Stimulates renal reabsorption of Na$^+$ and excretion of K$^+$.

CORTISOL
- Increased gluconeogenesis.
- Anti-inflammatory action.
- Protein breakdown in muscle.

OVARY

ESTROGENS
- Control menstrual cycle.
- Promote development of female secondary sex characteristics.

PROGESTERONE
- Secretory phase of uterus and mammary glands.
- Implantation and maturation of fertilized ovum.

TESTES

TESTOSTERONE
- Stimulates spermatogenesis.
- Promotes development of male secondary sex characteristics.
- Promotes anabolism.
- Masculinization of the fetus.

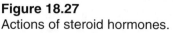

Figure 18.27
Actions of steroid hormones.

C. Secretion of steroid hormones from gonads

The testes and ovaries synthesize hormones necessary for sexual differentiation and reproduction. A single hypothalamic-releasing factor, gonadotropin-releasing hormone, stimulates the anterior pituitary to release the glycoproteins, luteinizing hormone (LH) and follicle-stimulating hormone (FSH). Like ACTH, LH and FSH bind to surface receptors and cause an increase in cAMP. LH stimulates the testes to produce testosterone and the ovaries to produce estrogens and progesterone (see Figure 18.27). FSH regulates the growth of ovarian follicles and stimulates testicular spermatogenesis.

D. Mechanism of steroid hormone action

Each steroid hormone diffuses across the plasma membrane of its target cell and binds to a specific cytosolic or nuclear receptor. These receptor–ligand complexes accumulate in the nucleus, dimerize, and bind to specific regulatory DNA sequences (hormone-response elements, HRE) in association with coactivator proteins, thereby causing promoter activation and increased transcription of targeted genes (Figure 18.28). An HRE is found in the promoter (or an enhancer element, see p. 424) for genes that respond to a specific steroid hormone, thus ensuring coordinated regulation of these genes. Hormone–receptor complexes can also inhibit transcription in association with corepressors. [Note: The binding of a hormone to its receptor causes a conformational change in the receptor that uncovers its DNA-binding domain, allowing the complex to interact through a zinc-finger motif with the appropriate sequence on the DNA. Receptors for the steroid hormones, plus those for thyroid hormone, retinoic acid (see p. 382), and 1,25-dihydroxycholecalciferol (Vitamin D, see p. 386), are members of a "superfamily" of structurally related gene regulators that function in a similar way.]

E. Further metabolism of steroid hormones

Steroid hormones are generally converted into inactive metabolic excretion products in the liver. Reactions include reduction of unsaturated bonds and the introduction of additional hydroxyl groups. The resulting structures are made more soluble by conjugation with glucuronic acid or sulfate (from 3'-phosphoadenosyl-5'-phosphosulfate, see p. 162). Approximately 20–30% of these metabolites are secreted into the bile and then excreted in the feces, whereas the remainder are released into the blood and filtered from the plasma in the kidney, passing into the urine. These conjugated metabolites are fairly water-soluble and do not need protein carriers.

VIII. CHAPTER SUMMARY

Cholesterol is a **hydrophobic** compound, with a single hydroxyl group—located at carbon 3 of the A ring—to which a fatty acid can be attached, producing an even more hydrophobic **cholesteryl ester**. Cholesterol is synthesized by virtually all human tissues, although primarily by **liver**, **intestine**, **adrenal cortex**, and **reproductive tissues** (Figure 18.29). All the carbon atoms in cholesterol are provided by **acetate**, and **NADPH** provides the reducing equivalents. The pathway is driven by hydrolysis of the high-energy thioester bond of acetyl CoA and the terminal phosphate bond of ATP. Cholesterol is synthesized in the **cytoplasm**. The **rate-limiting and regulated step** in cholesterol synthesis is catalyzed by the SER—membrane protein, hydroxymethylglutaryl (**HMG**) **CoA reductase**, which produces **mevalonate** from HMG CoA. The enzyme is regulated by a number of mechanisms: 1) **Expression of the gene for HMG CoA reductase** is activated when cholesterol levels are low, via the transcription factor, SREBP-2, bound to a sterol response element (SRE), resulting in increased enzyme and, therefore, more cholesterol synthesis; 2) HMG CoA reductase activity is controlled by **adenosine monophosphate** (**AMP**)–**activated protein kinase** (**AMPK**, which phosphorylates and **inactivates** HMG CoA reductase) and an **insulin-activated protein phosphatase** (which **activates** HMG CoA reductase); 3) Expression of the gene for the reductase is upregulated by insulin and downregulated by glucagon. Statins are **competitive inhibitors** of HMG CoA reductase. These drugs are used to decrease plasma cholesterol in patients with **hypercholesterolemia**. The ring structure of cholesterol can not be degraded in humans.

Cholesterol can be eliminated from the body either by **conversion to bile salts** or by **secretion into the bile**. **Bile salts** and **phosphatidylcholine** are quantitatively the most important organic components of bile. Bile salts are **conjugated bile acids** produced by the **liver** and **stored in the gallbladder**. The **primary bile acids**, **cholic** or **chenodeoxycholic acids**, are **amphipathic**, and can serve as **emulsifying agents**. The rate-limiting step in bile acid synthesis is catalyzed by **cholesterol-7-α-hydroxylase**, which is **inhibited** by **bile acids**. Before the bile acids leave the liver, they are conjugated to a molecule of either **glycine** or **taurine**, producing the **primary bile salts**: **glycocholic** or **taurocholic acid**, and **glycochenodeoxycholic** or **taurochenodeoxycholic acid**. Bile salts are more amphipathic than bile acids and, therefore, are more effective emulsifiers. In the intestine, bacteria can remove the glycine and taurine, and can remove a hydroxyl group from the steroid nucleus, producing the **secondary bile acids—deoxycholic** and **lithocholic acids**. More than 95% of the bile acids and salts are efficiently reabsorbed from the intestine by a sodium-bile salt cotransporter. They are then actively transported out of the ileal mucosal cells into the portal blood, where they are carried by albumin back to the liver (**enterohepatic circulation; bile acid sequestrants reduce this**) and are taken up by the hepatic form of the cotransporter. In the liver, the primary and secondary bile acids are reconverted to bile salts, and secreted into the bile. If more cholesterol enters the bile than can be solubilized by the available bile salts and phosphatidylcholine, **cholesterol gallstone disease** (**cholelithiasis**) can occur.

The plasma lipoproteins include **chylomicrons (CM)**, **very-low-density lipoproteins (VLDL)**, **low-density lipoproteins (LDL)**, and **high-density lipoproteins (HDL)**. They function to keep lipids (primarily **triacylglycerol (TAG)** and **cholesteryl esters**) soluble as they transport them between tissues. Lipoproteins are composed of a **neutral lipid** (**TAG, cholesteryl esters**, or both) surrounded by a shell of amphipathic **apolipoproteins**, **phospholipid**, and **nonesterified cholesterol**. **CM** are assembled in **intestinal mucosal cells** from **dietary lipids** (primarily, **TAG**). Each nascent CM particle has one molecule of **apolipoprotein (apo) B-48**. They are released from the cells into the lymphatic system

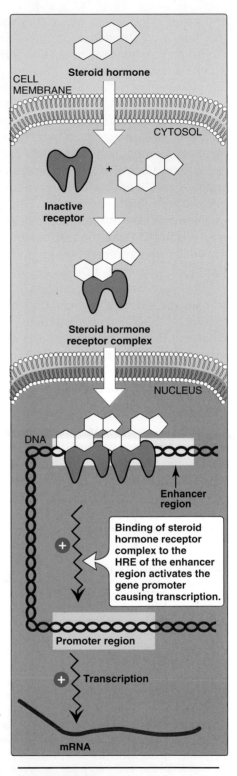

Figure 18.28
Activation of transcription by interaction of steroid hormone-receptor complex with hormone response element (HRE).

and travel to the blood, where they receive **apo C-II** and **apo E** from **HDLs**. Apo C-II activates endothelial **lipoprotein lipase**, which degrades the TAG in CM to fatty acids and glycerol. The **fatty acids** that are released are **stored** (in the **adipose**) or used for **energy** (by the **muscle**). The **glycerol** is metabolized by the **liver**. Patients with a **deficiency** of **lipoprotein lipase** or **apo C-II** show a dramatic accumulation of CM in the plasma (**Type I hyperlipoproteinemia or familial lipoprotein lipase deficiency**). After most of the TAG is removed, apo C-II is returned to the HDL, and the **CM remnant**—carrying most of the **dietary cholesterol**—binds to a **receptor** on the **liver** that recognizes **apo E**. The particle is **endocytosed** and its contents degraded by **lysosomal enzymes**. Defective uptake of CM remnants causes Type III hyperlipoproteinemia. **Nascent VLDL** are produced in the **liver**, and are composed predominantly of **TAG**. They contain a single molecule of **apo B-100**. Like nascent CM, VLDL receive **apo C-II** and **apo E** from **HDL** in the plasma. The **function** of VLDL is to **carry hepatic TAG** to the **peripheral tissues** where **lipoprotein lipase** degrades the lipid. As TAG is removed from the VLDL, the particle receives **cholesteryl esters** from **HDL**. This process is accomplished by **cholesteryl ester transfer protein (CETP)**. Eventually, VLDL in the **plasma** is **converted to LDL**—a much smaller, denser particle. Apo C-II and apo E are returned to HDL, but the LDL retains **apo B-100**, which is recognized by **receptors** on **peripheral tissues** and the **liver**. LDL undergo **receptor-mediated endocytosis**, and their contents are degraded in the **lysosomes**. A **deficiency of functional LDL receptors** causes **Type II hyperlipoproteinemia (familial hypercholesterolemia)**. The endocytosed cholesterol **inhibits HMG CoA reductase** and **decreases synthesis of LDL receptors**. Some of it can also be esterified by **acyl CoA:cholesterol acyltransferase** (**ACAT**) and stored. **HDL** are created by **lipidation of apo A-1** synthesized in the **liver** and **intestine**. They have a number of functions, including: 1) serving as a **circulating reservoir of apo C-II** and **apo E** for chylomicrons and VLDL; 2) removing **unesterified cholesterol** from from peripheral tissues via ABCA1and **esterifying it** using **lecithin:cholesterol acyl transferase (LCAT)**, a liver-synthesized plasma enzyme that is activated by **apo A-1**; and 3) delivering these cholesteryl esters to the liver (**reverse cholesterol transport**) for uptake via SR-B1.

Cholesterol is the precursor of all classes of steroid hormones (**glucocorticoids, mineralocorticoids**, and **sex hormones—androgens, estrogens**, and **progestins**). **Synthesis**, using primarily **cytochrome P450 (CYP) mixed-function oxidases**, occurs in the **adrenal cortex** (**cortisol, aldosterone**, and **androgens**), **ovaries** and **placenta** (**estrogens** and **progestins**), and **testes** (**testosterone**). Each steroid hormone diffuses across the plasma membrane of its target cell and binds to a specific **cytosolic** or **nuclear receptor**. These **receptor–ligand complexes** accumulate in the nucleus, dimerize, and **bind** to specific regulatory DNA sequences (**hormone-response elements**) in association with coactivator proteins, thereby causing **promoter activation** and **increased transcription** of targeted genes. In association with corepressors, **transcription is decreased**.

Study Questions

Choose the ONE correct answer.

18.1 A 35-year-old woman was seen in the emergency room because of recurrent abdominal pain. The history revealed a 2-year pattern of pain in the upper right quadrant, beginning several hours after the ingestion of a meal rich in fried/fatty food. Ultrasonographic examination demonstrated the presence of numerous stones in the gallbladder. The patient initially elected treatment consisting of exogenously supplied chenodeoxycholic acid, but eventually underwent surgery for the removal of the gallbladder, and had a full recovery. The rationale for the initial treatment of this patient with chenodeoxycholic acid is that this compound:

A. interferes with the enterohepatic circulation.

B. inhibits cholesterol synthesis.

C. increases <u>de novo</u> bile acid production.

D. increases cholesterol solubility in bile.

Correct answer = D. Chenodeoxycholic acid is a bile acid used in the treatment of gallstones. It is an amphipathic molecule that can act like an emulsifying agent and help solubilize cholesterol. The compound will not affect the enterohepatic circulation, interfere with cholesterol synthesis, increase bile acid production, or stimulate VLDL production.

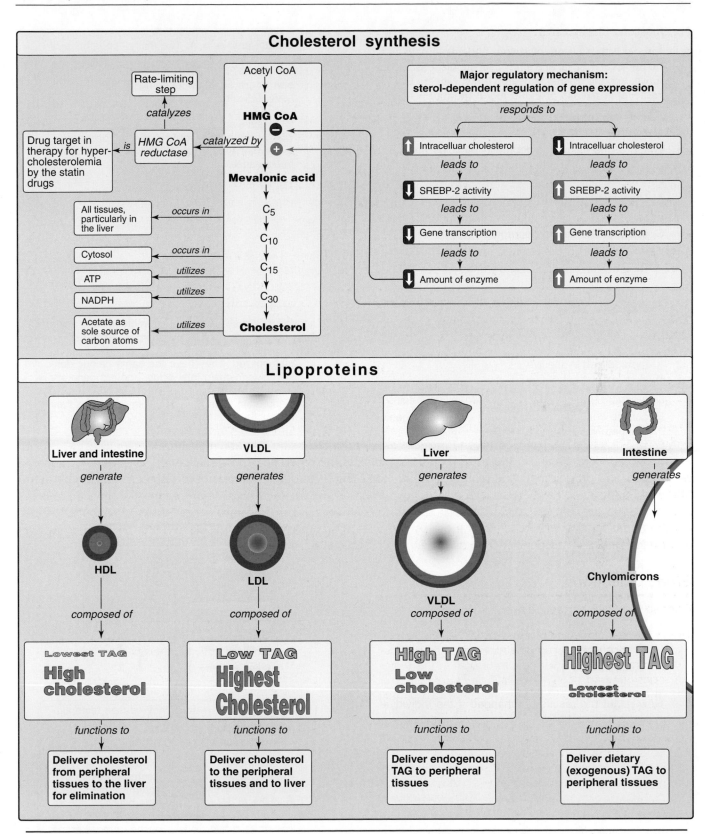

Figure 18.29
Concept map for cholesterol and the lipoproteins.

For Questions 18.2 and 18.3:

A young girl with a history of severe abdominal pain was taken to her local hospital at 5 a.m. in severe distress. Blood was drawn, and the plasma appeared milky, with the triacylglycerol level in excess of 2,000 mg/dl (normal = 4–150 mg/dl). The patient was placed on a diet severely limited in fat, but supplemented with medium-chain fatty acids.

18.2 Which of the following lipoprotein particles are most likely responsible for the appearance of the patient's plasma?

A. Chylomicrons.

B. Very-low-density lipoproteins.

C. Intermediate-density lipoproteins.

D. Low-density-lipoproteins.

E. High-density-lipoproteins.

> Correct answer = A. The milky appearance of her blood was a result of triacylglycerol-rich chylomicrons. Because 5 a.m. is presumably several hours after her evening meal, she must have difficulty clearing these lipoprotein particles. IDL, LDL, or HDL contain primarily cholesteryl esters and, if one or more of these particles was elevated, it would cause hypercholesterolemia. VLDL do not cause the described "milky appearance" in plasma.

18.3 Medium-chain fatty acids are given because they:

A. are more calorically dense than long-chain fatty acids.

B. enter directly into the portal blood, and can be metabolized by the liver.

C. are activators of lipoprotein lipase.

D. are more efficiently packed into serum lipoproteins.

E. can be converted into a variety of gluconeogenic precursors.

E. stimulates VLDL production by the liver.

> Correct answer = B. Medium-chain fatty acids are not packaged in chylomicrons, but rather are carried by albumin to the liver where they can be metabolized. They have the same caloric density as long-chain fatty acids, and are generally much more ketogenic than glycogenic. Lipoprotein lipase does not play a role in their metabolism.

18.4 Complete the following table for an individual with classic 21-α-hydroxylase deficiency relative to a normal individual.

Measured	Increased	Decreased
Aldosterone		
Cortisol		
Androstenedione		
ACTH		
Blood glucose		
Blood pressure		

How might the results be changed if the individual was deficient in 17-α-hydroxylase, rather than 21-α-hydroxylase?

Measured	Increased	Decreased
Aldosterone		X
Cortisol		X
Androstenedione	X	
ACTH	X	
Blood glucose		X
Blood pressure		X

> 21-α-Hydroxylase deficiency causes mineralocorticoids (aldosterone) and glucocorticoids (cortisol) to be virtually absent. Because aldosterone increases blood pressure, and cortisol increases blood glucose, their deficiencies result in a decrease in blood pressure and blood glucose, respectively. Cortisol normally feeds back to inhibit ACTH release by the pituitary, and so its absence results in an elevation in ACTH. The loss of 21-α-hydroxylase pushes progesterone and pregnenolone to androgen synthesis, thus, androstenedione levels rise. With 17-α-hydroxylase deficiency, sex hormone synthesis would be inhibited. Mineralocorticoid production would be increased, leading to hypertension.

Amino Acids: Disposal of Nitrogen

19

I. OVERVIEW

Unlike fats and carbohydrates, amino acids are not stored by the body, that is, no protein exists whose sole function is to maintain a supply of amino acids for future use. Therefore, amino acids must be obtained from the diet, synthesized de novo, or produced from normal protein degradation. Any amino acids in excess of the biosynthetic needs of the cell are rapidly degraded. The first phase of catabolism involves the removal of the α-amino groups (usually by transamination and subsequent oxidative deamination), forming ammonia and the corresponding α-keto acid—the "carbon skeletons" of amino acids. A portion of the free ammonia is excreted in the urine, but most is used in the synthesis of urea (Figure 19.1), which is quantitatively the most important route for disposing of nitrogen from the body. In the second phase of amino acid catabolism, described in Chapter 20, the carbon skeletons of the α-ketoacids are converted to common intermediates of energy producing, metabolic pathways. These compounds can be metabolized to CO_2 and water, glucose, fatty acids, or ketone bodies by the central pathways of metabolism described in Chapters 8–13, and 16.

II. OVERALL NITROGEN METABOLISM

Amino acid catabolism is part of the larger process of the metabolism of nitrogen-containing molecules. Nitrogen enters the body in a variety of compounds present in food, the most important being amino acids contained in dietary protein. Nitrogen leaves the body as urea, ammonia, and other products derived from amino acid metabolism. The role of body proteins in these transformations involves two important concepts: the amino acid pool and protein turnover.

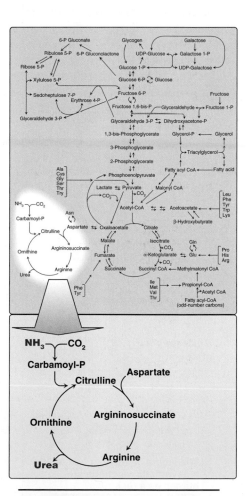

Figure 19.1
Urea cycle shown as part of the essential reactions of energy metabolism. (See Figure 8.2, p. 92, for a more detailed view of the metabolic pathway.)

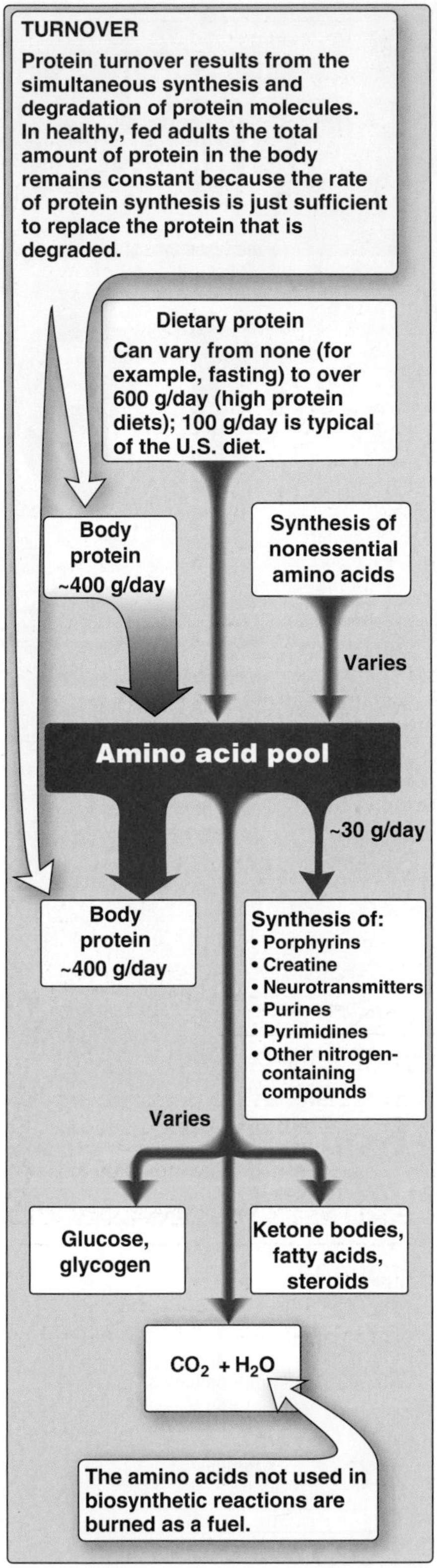
TURNOVER
Protein turnover results from the simultaneous synthesis and degradation of protein molecules. In healthy, fed adults the total amount of protein in the body remains constant because the rate of protein synthesis is just sufficient to replace the protein that is degraded.
Dietary protein
Can vary from none (for example, fasting) to over 600 g/day (high protein diets); 100 g/day is typical of the U.S. diet.
Body protein ~400 g/day
Synthesis of nonessential amino acids
Varies
Amino acid pool
~30 g/day
Body protein ~400 g/day
Synthesis of:
• Porphyrins
• Creatine
• Neurotransmitters
• Purines
• Pyrimidines
• Other nitrogen-containing compounds
Varies
Glucose, glycogen
Ketone bodies, fatty acids, steroids
CO2 + H2O
The amino acids not used in biosynthetic reactions are burned as a fuel.

Figure 19.2
Sources and fates of amino acids.

A. Amino acid pool

Free amino acids are present throughout the body, for example, in cells, blood, and the extracellular fluids. For the purpose of this discussion, envision all these amino acids as if they belonged to a single entity, called the amino acid pool. This pool is supplied by three sources: 1) amino acids provided by the degradation of body proteins, 2) amino acids derived from dietary protein, and 3) synthesis of nonessential amino acids from simple intermediates of metabolism (Figure 19.2). Conversely, the amino pool is depleted by three routes: 1) synthesis of body protein, 2) amino acids consumed as precursors of essential nitrogen-containing small molecules, and 3) conversion of amino acids to glucose, glycogen, fatty acids, ketone bodies, or CO_2 + H_2O (Figure 19.2). Although the amino acid pool is small (comprised of about 90–100 g of amino acids) in comparison with the amount of protein in the body (about 12 kg in a 70-kg man), it is conceptually at the center of whole-body nitrogen metabolism.

> In healthy, well-fed individuals, the input to the amino acid pool is balanced by the output, that is, the amount of amino acids contained in the pool is constant. The amino acid pool is said to be in a steady state, and the individual is said to be in nitrogen balance.

B. Protein turnover

Most proteins in the body are constantly being synthesized and then degraded, permitting the removal of abnormal or unneeded proteins. For many proteins, regulation of synthesis determines the concentration of protein in the cell, with protein degradation assuming a minor role. For other proteins, the rate of synthesis is constitutive, that is, relatively constant, and cellular levels of the protein are controlled by selective degradation.

1. **Rate of turnover:** In healthy adults, the total amount of protein in the body remains constant, because the rate of protein synthesis is just sufficient to replace the protein that is degraded. This process, called protein turnover, leads to the hydrolysis and resynthesis of 300–400 g of body protein each day. The rate of protein turnover varies widely for individual proteins. Short-lived proteins (for example, many regulatory proteins and misfolded proteins) are rapidly degraded, having half-lives measured in minutes or hours. Long-lived proteins, with half-lives of days to weeks, constitute the majority of proteins in the cell. Structural proteins, such as collagen, are metabolically stable, and have half-lives measured in months or years.

2. **Protein degradation:** There are two major enzyme systems responsible for degrading damaged or unneeded proteins: the ATP-dependent ubiquitin-proteasome system of the cytosol, and the ATP-independent degradative enzyme system of the lyso-

somes. Proteasomes degrade mainly endogenous proteins, that is, proteins that were synthesized within the cell. Lysosomal enzymes (*acid hydrolases*, see p. 162) degrade primarily extracellular proteins, such as plasma proteins that are taken into the cell by endocytosis, and cell-surface membrane proteins that are used in receptor-mediated endocytosis.

a. **Ubiquitin-proteasome proteolytic pathway:** Proteins selected for degradation by the ubiquitin-proteasome system are first covalently attached to ubiquitin, a small, globular, non-enzymic protein. Ubiquitination of the target substrate occurs through linkage of the α-carboxyl group of the C-terminal glycine of ubiquitin to the ε-amino group of a lysine on the protein substrate by a three-step, enzyme-catalyzed, ATP-dependent process. The consecutive addition of ubiquitin moieties generates a polyubiquitin chain. Proteins tagged with ubiquitin are then recognized by a large, barrel-shaped, macromolecular, proteolytic complex called a proteasome, which functions like a garbage disposal (Figure 19.3). The proteasome unfolds, deubiquitinates, and cuts the target protein into fragments that are then further degraded to amino acids, which enter the amino acid pool. [Note: The ubiquitins are recycled.] It is noteworthy that the selective degradation of proteins by the ubiquitin-proteosome complex (unlike simple hydrolysis by proteolytic enzymes) requires energy in the form of ATP.

b. **Chemical signals for protein degradation:** Because proteins have different half-lives, it is clear that protein degradation cannot be random, but rather is influenced by some structural aspect of the protein. For example, some proteins that have been chemically altered by oxidation or tagged with ubiquitin are preferentially degraded. The half-life of a protein is influenced by the nature of the N-terminal residue. For example, proteins that have serine as the N-terminal amino acid are long-lived, with a half-life of more than 20 hours. In contrast, proteins with aspartate as the N-terminal amino acid have a half-life of only 3 minutes. Additionally, proteins rich in sequences containing proline, glutamate, serine, and threonine (called PEST sequences after the one-letter designations for these amino acids) are rapidly degraded and, therefore, exhibit short intracellular half-lives.

III. DIGESTION OF DIETARY PROTEINS

Most of the nitrogen in the diet is consumed in the form of protein, typically amounting to 70–100 g/day in the American diet (see Figure 19.2). Proteins are generally too large to be absorbed by the intestine. [Note: An example of an exception to this rule is that newborns can take up maternal antibodies in breast milk.] They must, therefore, be hydrolyzed to yield di- and tripeptides as well as individual amino acids, which can be absorbed. Proteolytic enzymes responsible for degrading proteins are produced by three different organs: the stomach, the pancreas, and the small intestine (Figure 19.4).

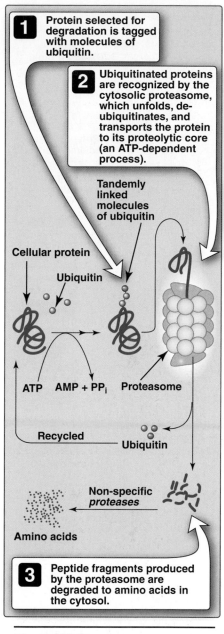

1 Protein selected for degradation is tagged with molecules of ubiquitin.

2 Ubiquitinated proteins are recognized by the cytosolic proteasome, which unfolds, de-ubiquitinates, and transports the protein to its proteolytic core (an ATP-dependent process).

Tandemly linked molecules of ubiquitin

Cellular protein

Ubiquitin

ATP   AMP + PP$_i$ Proteasome

Recycled   Ubiquitin

Non-specific *proteases*

Amino acids

3 Peptide fragments produced by the proteasome are degraded to amino acids in the cytosol.

Figure 19.3
The ubiquitin-proteasome degradation pathway of proteins.

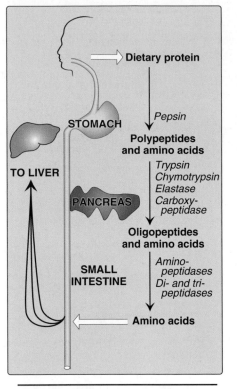

Figure 19.4
Digestion of dietary proteins by the proteolytic enzymes of the gastrointestinal tract.

A. Digestion of proteins by gastric secretion

The digestion of proteins begins in the stomach, which secretes gastric juice—a unique solution containing hydrochloric acid and the proenzyme, pepsinogen.

1. **Hydrochloric acid:** Stomach acid is too dilute (pH 2–3) to hydrolyze proteins. The acid, secreted by the parietal cells, functions instead to kill some bacteria and to denature proteins, thus making them more susceptible to subsequent hydrolysis by *proteases*.

2. **Pepsin:** This acid-stable *endopeptidase* is secreted by the chief cells of the stomach as an inactive zymogen (or proenzyme), pepsinogen. In general, zymogens contain extra amino acids in their sequences that prevent them from being catalytically active. [Note: Removal of these amino acids permits the proper folding required for an active enzyme.] Pepsinogen is activated to *pepsin*, either by HCl, or autocatalytically by other *pepsin* molecules that have already been activated. *Pepsin* releases peptides and a few free amino acids from dietary proteins.

B. Digestion of proteins by pancreatic enzymes

On entering the small intestine, large polypeptides produced in the stomach by the action of *pepsin* are further cleaved to oligopeptides and amino acids by a group of pancreatic *proteases*.

1. **Specificity:** Each of these enzymes has a different specificity for the amino acid R-groups adjacent to the susceptible peptide bond (Figure 19.5). For example, *trypsin* cleaves only when the carbonyl group of the peptide bond is contributed by arginine or lysine. These enzymes, like *pepsin* described above, are synthesized and secreted as inactive zymogens.

2. **Release of zymogens:** The release and activation of the pancreatic zymogens is mediated by the secretion of cholecystokinin and secretin, two polypeptide hormones of the digestive tract (see p. 176).

3. **Activation of zymogens:** *Enteropeptidase* (formerly called *enterokinase*)—an enzyme synthesized by and present on the luminal surface of intestinal mucosal cells of the brush border membrane—converts the pancreatic zymogen trypsinogen to *trypsin* by removal of a hexapeptide from the N-terminus of trypsinogen. *Trypsin* subsequently converts other trypsinogen molecules to *trypsin* by cleaving a limited number of specific peptide bonds in the zymogen. *Enteropeptidase* thus unleashes a cascade of proteolytic activity, because *trypsin* is the common activator of all the pancreatic zymogens (see Figure 19.5).

4. **Abnormalities in protein digestion:** In individuals with a deficiency in pancreatic secretion (for example, due to chronic pancreatitis, cystic fibrosis, or surgical removal of the pancreas), the digestion and absorption of fat and protein are incomplete. This results in the abnormal appearance of lipids (called steatorrhea, see p. 177) and undigested protein in the feces.

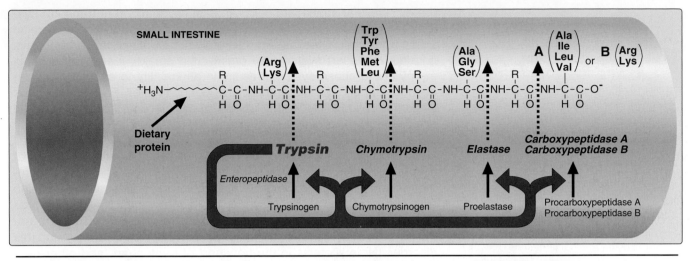

Figure 19.5
Cleavage of dietary protein by *proteases* from the pancreas. The peptide bonds susceptible to hydrolysis are shown for each of the five major pancreatic *proteases*. [Note: The first three are serine *endopeptidases*, whereas the last two are *exopeptidases*.]

> Celiac disease (celiac sprue) is a disease of mal-absorption resulting from immune-mediated damage to the small intestine in response to ingestion of gluten (or gliadin produced from gluten), a protein found in wheat, barley and rye.

C. Digestion of oligopeptides by enzymes of the small intestine

The luminal surface of the intestine contains *aminopeptidase*—an *exopeptidase* that repeatedly cleaves the N-terminal residue from oligopeptides to produce even smaller peptides and free amino acids.

D. Absorption of amino acids and small peptides

Free amino acids are taken into the enterocytes by a Na⁺-linked secondary transport system of the apical membrane. Di- and tri-peptides, however, are taken up by a H⁺-linked transport system. The peptides are hydrolyzed in the cytosol to amino acids that are released into the portal system by facilitated diffusion. Thus, only free amino acids are found in the portal vein after a meal containing protein. These amino acids are either metabolized by the liver or released into the general circulation. [Note: Branched-chain amino acids are important examples of amino acids that are not metabolized by the liver, but instead are sent from the liver primarily to muscle via the blood.]

IV. TRANSPORT OF AMINO ACIDS INTO CELLS

The concentration of free amino acids in the extracellular fluids is significantly lower than that within the cells of the body. This concentration gradient is maintained because active transport systems, driven by the hydrolysis of ATP, are required for movement of amino acids from

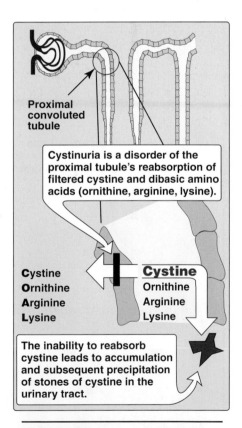

Cystinuria is a disorder of the proximal tubule's reabsorption of filtered cystine and dibasic amino acids (ornithine, arginine, lysine).

Cystine	Cystine
Ornithine	Ornithine
Arginine	Arginine
Lysine	Lysine

The inability to reabsorb cystine leads to accumulation and subsequent precipitation of stones of cystine in the urinary tract.

Figure 19.6
Genetic defect seen in cystinuria. [Note: Cystinura is distinct from cystinosis, a rare defect in the transport of cystine out of lysosomes that results in the formation of cystine crystals within the lysosome, and tissue damage.]

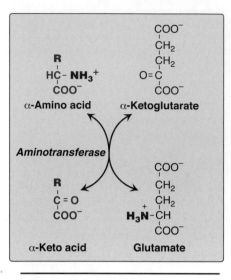

Figure 19.7
Aminotransferase reaction using α-ketoglutarate as the amino-group acceptor.

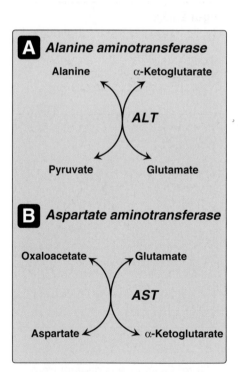

Figure 19.8
Reactions catalyzed during amino acid catabolism. A. *Alanine aminotransferase (ALT)*. B. *Aspartate aminotransferase (AST)*.

the extracellular space into cells. At least seven different transport systems are known that have overlapping specificities for different amino acids. The small intestine and the proximal tubule of the kidney have common transport systems for amino acid uptake; therefore, a defect in any one of these systems results in an inability to absorb particular amino acids into the gut and into the kidney tubules. For example, one system is responsible for the uptake of cystine and the dibasic amino acids, ornithine, arginine, and lysine (represented as "COAL"). In the inherited disorder cystinuria, this carrier system is defective, and all four amino acids appear in the urine (Figure 19.6). Cystinuria occurs at a frequency of 1 in 7,000 individuals, making it one of the most common inherited diseases, and the most common genetic error of amino acid transport. The disease expresses itself clinically by the precipitation of cystine to form kidney stones (calculi), which can block the urinary tract. Oral hydration is an important part of treatment for this disorder. [Note: Defects in the transport of tryptophan (and other neutral amino acids) can result in Hartnup disorder and pellagra-like (see p. 380) dermatologic and neurologic symptoms.]

V. REMOVAL OF NITROGEN FROM AMINO ACIDS

The presence of the α-amino group keeps amino acids safely locked away from oxidative breakdown. Removing the α-amino group is essential for producing energy from any amino acid, and is an obligatory step in the catabolism of all amino acids. Once removed, this nitrogen can be incorporated into other compounds or excreted, with the carbon skeletons being metabolized. This section describes transamination and oxidative deamination—reactions that ultimately provide ammonia and aspartate, the two sources of urea nitrogen (see p. 253).

A. Transamination: the funneling of amino groups to glutamate

The first step in the catabolism of most amino acids is the transfer of their α-amino group to α-ketoglutarate (Figure 19.7). The products are an α-keto acid (derived from the original amino acid) and glutamate. α-Ketoglutarate plays a pivotal role in amino acid metabolism by accepting the amino groups from most amino acids, thus becoming glutamate. Glutamate produced by transamination can be oxidatively deaminated (see below), or used as an amino group donor in the synthesis of nonessential amino acids. This transfer of amino groups from one carbon skeleton to another is catalyzed by a family of enzymes called *aminotransferases* (formerly called *transaminases*). These enzymes are found in the cytosol and mitochondria of cells throughout the body—especially those of the liver, kidney, intestine, and muscle. All amino acids, with the exception of lysine and threonine, participate in transamination at some point in their catabolism. [Note: These two amino acids lose their α-amino groups by deamination (see pp. 265–266).]

1. **Substrate specificity of aminotransferases:** Each *aminotransferase* is specific for one or, at most, a few amino group donors. *Aminotransferases* are named after the specific amino group donor, because the acceptor of the amino group is almost always α-ketoglutarate. The two most important *aminotransferase* reactions are catalyzed by *alanine aminotransferase (ALT) and aspartate aminotransferase (AST)*, Figure 19.8).

a. **Alanine aminotransferase (ALT)**: *ALT* is present in many tissues. The enzyme catalyzes the transfer of the amino group of alanine to α-ketoglutarate, resulting in the formation of pyruvate and glutamate. The reaction is readily reversible. However, during amino acid catabolism, this enzyme (like most *aminotransferases*) functions in the direction of glutamate synthesis. Thus, glutamate, in effect, acts as a "collector" of nitrogen from alanine.

b. **Aspartate aminotransferase (AST)**: *AST* is an exception to the rule that *aminotransferases* funnel amino groups to form glutamate. During amino acid catabolism, *AST* transfers amino groups from glutamate to oxaloacetate, forming aspartate, which is used as a source of nitrogen in the urea cycle (see p. 253). [Note: The *AST* reaction is also reversible.]

2. **Mechanism of action of aminotransferases**: All *aminotransferases* require the coenzyme pyridoxal phosphate (a derivative of vitamin B_6, see p. 378), which is covalently linked to the ε-amino group of a specific lysine residue at the active site of the enzyme. *Aminotransferases* act by transferring the amino group of an amino acid to the pyridoxal part of the coenzyme to generate pyridoxamine phosphate. The pyridoxamine form of the coenzyme then reacts with an α-keto acid to form an amino acid, at the same time regenerating the original aldehyde form of the coenzyme. Figure 19.9 shows these two component reactions for the reaction catalyzed by *AST*.

3. **Equilibrium of transamination reactions**: For most transamination reactions, the equilibrium constant is near one. This allows the reaction to function in both amino acid degradation through removal of α-amino groups (for example, after consumption of a protein-rich meal) and biosynthesis through addition of amino groups to the carbon skeletons of α-keto acids (for example, when the supply of amino acids from the diet is not adequate to meet the synthetic needs of cells).

4. **Diagnostic value of plasma aminotransferases**: *Aminotransferases* are normally intracellular enzymes, with the low levels found in the plasma representing the release of cellular contents during normal cell turnover. The presence of elevated plasma levels of *aminotransferases* indicates damage to cells rich in these enzymes. For example, physical trauma or a disease process can cause cell lysis, resulting in release of intracellular enzymes into the blood. Two *aminotransferases*—*AST* and *ALT*—are of particular diagnostic value when they are found in the plasma.

a. **Liver disease**: Plasma *AST* and *ALT* are elevated in nearly all liver diseases, but are particularly high in conditions that cause extensive cell necrosis, such as severe viral hepatitis, toxic injury, and prolonged circulatory collapse. *ALT* is more specific than *AST* for liver disease, but the latter is more sensitive because the liver contains larger amounts of *AST*. Serial enzyme measurements are often useful in determining the course of liver damage. Figure 19.10 shows the early release of *ALT* into the serum, following ingestion of a liver

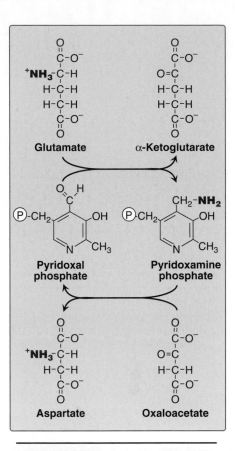

Figure 19.9
Cyclic interconversion of pyridoxal phosphate and pyridoxamine phosphate during the *aspartate aminotransferase* reaction. [Note: ℗ = phosphate group.]

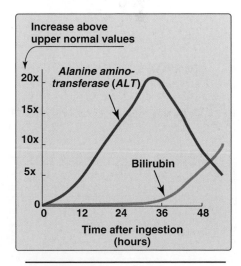

Figure 19.10
Pattern of serum *alanine aminotransferase (ALT)* and bilirubin in the plasma, following poisoning with the toxic mushroom Amanita phalloides.

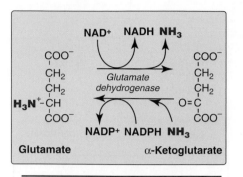

Figure 19.11
Oxidative deamination by
glutamate dehydrogenase.

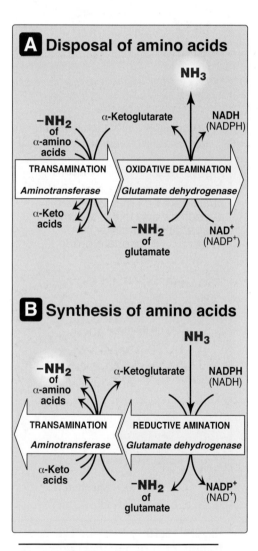

Figure 19.12
Combined actions of *aminotransferase*
and *glutamate dehydrogenase* reactions.

toxin. [Note: Elevated serum bilirubin results from hepatocellular damage that decreases the hepatic conjugation and excretion of bilirubin (see p. 284).]

b. **Nonhepatic disease:** *Aminotransferases* may be elevated in nonhepatic disease, such as myocardial infarction and muscle disorders. However, these disorders can usually be distinguished clinically from liver disease.

B. Glutamate dehydrogenase: the oxidative deamination of amino acids

In contrast to transamination reactions that transfer amino groups, oxidative deamination by *glutamate dehydrogenase* results in the liberation of the amino group as free ammonia (NH_3) (Figure 19.11). These reactions occur primarily in the liver and kidney. They provide α-keto acids that can enter the central pathway of energy metabolism, and ammonia, which is a source of nitrogen in urea synthesis.

1. **Glutamate dehydrogenase:** As described above, the amino groups of most amino acids are ultimately funneled to glutamate by means of transamination with α-ketoglutarate. Glutamate is unique in that it is the only amino acid that undergoes rapid oxidative deamination—a reaction catalyzed by *glutamate dehydrogenase* (see Figure 19.11). Therefore, the sequential action of transamination (resulting in the collection of amino groups from most amino acids onto α-ketoglutarate to produce glutamate) and the oxidative deamination of that glutamate (regenerating α-ketoglutarate) provide a pathway whereby the amino groups of most amino acids can be released as ammonia.

   a. **Coenzymes:** *Glutamate dehydrogenase* is unusual in that it can use either NAD^+ or $NADP^+$ as a coenzyme (see Figure 19.11). NAD^+ is used primarily in oxidative deamination (the simultaneous loss of ammonia coupled with the oxidation of the carbon skeleton (Figure 19.12A), and NADPH is used in reductive amination (the simultaneous gain of ammonia coupled with the reduction of the carbon skeleton, Figure 19.12B).

   b. **Direction of reactions:** The direction of the reaction depends on the relative concentrations of glutamate, α-ketoglutarate, and ammonia, and the ratio of oxidized to reduced coenzymes. For example, after ingestion of a meal containing protein, glutamate levels in the liver are elevated, and the reaction proceeds in the direction of amino acid degradation and the formation of ammonia (see Figure 19.12A). [Note: the reaction can also be used to synthesize amino acids from the corresponding α-keto acids (see Figure 19.12B).]

   c. **Allosteric regulators:** Guanosine triphosphate (GTP) is an allosteric inhibitor of *glutamate dehydrogenase*, whereas adenosine diphosphate (ADP) is an activator. Thus, when energy levels are low in the cell, amino acid degradation by *glutamate dehydrogenase* is high, facilitating energy production from the carbon skeletons derived from amino acids.

2. D-Amino acid oxidase: D-Amino acids (see p. 5) are found in plants and in the cell walls of microorganisms, but are not used in the synthesis of mammalian proteins. D-Amino acids are, however, present in the diet, and are efficiently metabolized by the kidney and liver. *D-Amino acid oxidase* (*DAO*) is an FAD-dependent peroxisomal enzyme that catalyzes the oxidative deamination of these amino acid isomers, producing α-keto acids, ammonia, and hydrogen peroxide. The α-keto acids can enter the general pathways of amino acid metabolism, and be reaminated to L-isomers, or catabolized for energy. [Note: *DAO* degrades D-serine, the isomeric form of serine that modulates NMDA-type glutamate receptors. Increased *DAO* activity has been linked to increased susceptibility to schizophrenia.] *L-amino acid oxidases* are components of several snake venoms.

C. Transport of ammonia to the liver

Two mechanisms are available in humans for the transport of ammonia from the peripheral tissues to the liver for its ultimate conversion to urea. The first, found in most tissues, uses *glutamine synthetase* to combine ammonia (NH_3) with glutamate to form glutamine—a nontoxic transport form of ammonia (Figure 19.13). The glutamine is transported in the blood to the liver where it is cleaved by *glutaminase* to produce glutamate and free ammonia (see p. 256). The second transport mechanism, used primarily by muscle, involves transamination of pyruvate (the end product of aerobic glycolysis) to form alanine (see Figure 19.8). Alanine is transported by the blood to the liver, where it is converted to pyruvate, again by transamination. In the liver, the pathway of gluconeogenesis can use the pyruvate to synthesize glucose, which can enter the blood and be used by muscle—a pathway called the glucose-alanine cycle.

VI. UREA CYCLE

Urea is the major disposal form of amino groups derived from amino acids, and accounts for about 90% of the nitrogen-containing components of urine. One nitrogen of the urea molecule is supplied by free ammonia, and the other nitrogen by aspartate. [Note: Glutamate is the immediate precursor of both ammonia (through oxidative deamination by *glutamate dehydrogenase*) and aspartate nitrogen (through transamination of oxaloacetate by *AST*).] The carbon and oxygen of urea are derived from CO_2. Urea is produced by the liver, and then is transported in the blood to the kidneys for excretion in the urine.

A. Reactions of the cycle

The first two reactions leading to the synthesis of urea occur in the mitochondria, whereas the remaining cycle enzymes are located in the cytosol (Figure 19.14). [Note: Gluconeogenesis (see p. 117) and heme synthesis (see p. 278) also involve both the mitochondrial matrix and the cytosol.]

1. Formation of carbamoyl phosphate: Formation of carbamoyl phosphate by *carbamoyl phosphate synthetase I* is driven by cleavage of two molecules of ATP. Ammonia incorporated into carbamoyl phosphate is provided primarily by the oxidative deamina-

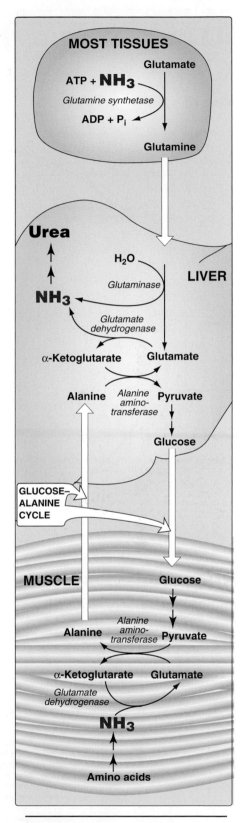

Figure 19.13
Transport of ammonia from peripheral tissues to the liver.

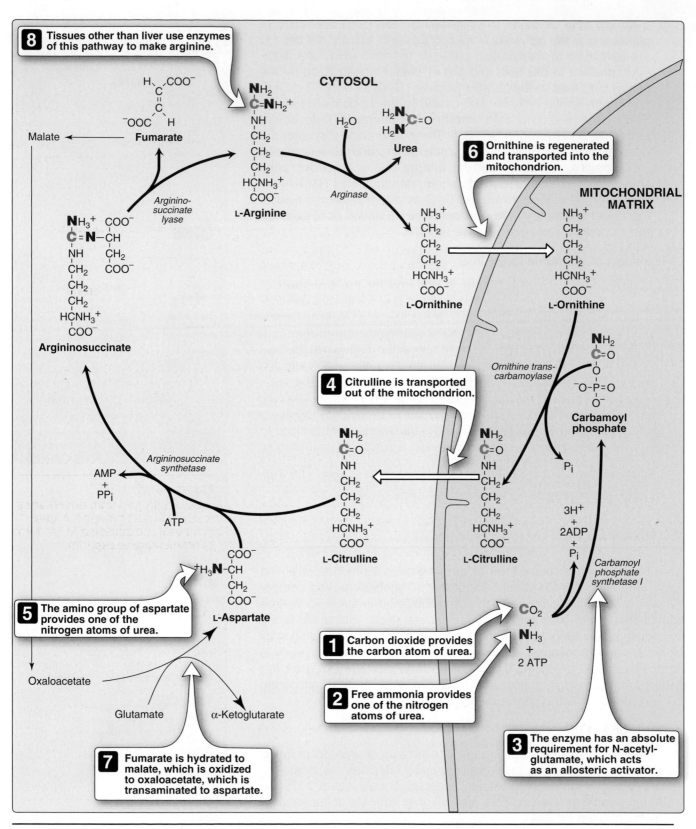

Figure 19.14
Reactions of the urea cycle.

tion of glutamate by mitochondrial *glutamate dehydrogenase* (see Figure 19.11). Ultimately, the nitrogen atom derived from this ammonia becomes one of the nitrogens of urea. *Carbamoyl phosphate synthetase I* requires N-acetylglutamate as a positive allosteric activator (see Figure 19.14). [Note: *Carbamoyl phosphate synthetase II* participates in the biosynthesis of pyrimidines (see p. 302). It does not require N-acetylglutamate, uses glutamine as the nitrogen source, and occurs in the cytosol.]

2. **Formation of citrulline:** The carbamoyl portion of carbamoyl phosphate is transferred to ornithine by *ornithine transcarbamoylase* (*OTC*) as the high-energy phosphate is released as P_i. The reaction product, citrulline, is transported to the cytosol. [Note: Ornithine and citrulline are basic amino acids that participate in the urea cycle, moving across the inner mitochondrial membrane via a cotransporter. They are not incorporated into cellular proteins because there are no codons for these amino acids (see p. 432).] Ornithine is regenerated with each turn of the urea cycle, much in the same way that oxaloacetate is regenerated by the reactions of the citric acid cycle (see p. 109).

3. **Synthesis of argininosuccinate:** *Argininosuccinate synthetase* combines citrulline with aspartate to form argininosuccinate. The α-amino group of aspartate provides the second nitrogen that is ultimately incorporated into urea. The formation of argininosuccinate is driven by the cleavage of ATP to adenosine monophosphate (AMP) and pyrophosphate. This is the third and final molecule of ATP consumed in the formation of urea.

4. **Cleavage of argininosuccinate:** Argininosuccinate is cleaved by *argininosuccinate lyase* to yield arginine and fumarate. The arginine formed by this reaction serves as the immediate precursor of urea. Fumarate produced in the urea cycle is hydrated to malate, providing a link with several metabolic pathways. For example, the malate can be transported into the mitochondria via the malate shuttle, reenter the tricarboxylic acid cycle, and get oxidized to oxaloacetate (OAA), which can be used for gluconeogenesis (see p. 120). Alternatively, the OAA can be converted to aspartate via transamination (see Figure 19.8), and can enter the urea cycle (see Figure 19.14).

5. **Cleavage of arginine to ornithine and urea:** *Arginase* cleaves arginine to ornithine and urea, and occurs almost exclusively in the liver. Thus, whereas other tissues, such as the kidney, can synthesize arginine by these reactions, only the liver can cleave arginine and, thereby, synthesize urea.

6. **Fate of urea:** Urea diffuses from the liver, and is transported in the blood to the kidneys, where it is filtered and excreted in the urine. A portion of the urea diffuses from the blood into the intestine, and is cleaved to CO_2 and NH_3 by bacterial *urease*. This ammonia is partly lost in the feces, and is partly reabsorbed into the blood. In patients with kidney failure, plasma urea levels are elevated, promoting a greater transfer of urea from blood into the gut. The intestinal action of *urease* on this urea becomes a clinically important source of ammonia, contributing to the hyperammonemia often seen in these patients. Oral administration of neomycin reduces the number of intestinal bacteria responsible for this NH_3 production.

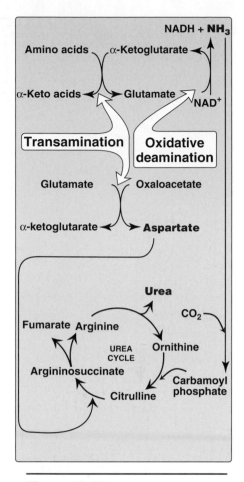

Figure 19.15
Flow of nitrogen from amino acids to urea. Amino groups for urea synthesis are collected in the form of ammonia and aspartate.

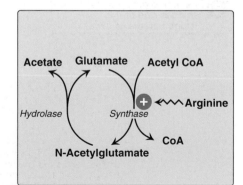

Figure 19.16
Formation and degradation of N-acetylglutamate, an allosteric activator of *carbamoyl phosphate synthetase I*.

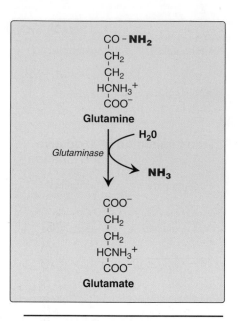

Figure 19.17
Hydrolysis of glutamine to form ammonia.

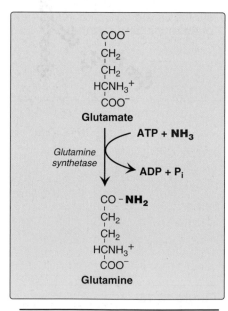

Figure 19.18
Synthesis of glutamine.

B. Overall stoichiometry of the urea cycle

$$\text{Aspartate} + NH_3 + CO_2 + 3\,ATP + H_2O \longrightarrow$$

$$\text{urea} + \text{fumarate} + 2\,ADP + AMP + 2\,P_i + PP_i$$

Four high-energy phosphate bonds are consumed in the synthesis of each molecule of urea; therefore, the synthesis of urea is irreversible, with a large, negative ΔG (see p. 70). [Note: The ATP is replenished by oxidative phosphorylation.] One nitrogen of the urea molecule is supplied by free NH_3, and the other nitrogen by aspartate. Glutamate is the immediate precursor of both ammonia (through oxidative deamination by *glutamate dehydrogenase*) and aspartate nitrogen (through transamination of oxaloacetate by *AST*). In effect, both nitrogen atoms of urea arise from glutamate, which, in turn, gathers nitrogen from other amino acids (Figure 19.15).

C. Regulation of the urea cycle

N-Acetylglutamate is an essential activator for *carbamoyl phosphate synthetase I*—the rate-limiting step in the urea cycle (see Figure 19.14). N-Acetylglutamate is synthesized from acetyl coenzyme A and glutamate by *N-acetylglutamate synthase* (Figure 19.16), in a reaction for which arginine is an activator. Therefore, the intrahepatic concentration of N-acetylglutamate increases after ingestion of a protein-rich meal, which provides both a substrate (glutamate) and the regulator of N-acetylglutamate synthesis. This leads to an increased rate of urea synthesis.

VII. METABOLISM OF AMMONIA

Ammonia is produced by all tissues during the metabolism of a variety of compounds, and it is disposed of primarily by formation of urea in the liver. However, the level of ammonia in the blood must be kept very low, because even slightly elevated concentrations (hyperammonemia) are toxic to the central nervous system (CNS). There must, therefore, be a metabolic mechanism by which nitrogen is moved from peripheral tissues to the liver for ultimate disposal as urea, while at the same time maintaining low levels of circulating ammonia.

A. Sources of ammonia

Amino acids are quantitatively the most important source of ammonia, because most Western diets are high in protein and provide excess amino acids, which travel to the liver and undergo transdeamination— the linking of *aminotransferase* and *glutamate dehydrogenase* reactions—producing ammonia. However, substantial amounts of ammonia can be obtained from other sources.

1. **From glutamine:** The kidneys generate ammonia from glutamine by the actions of renal *glutaminase* (Figure 19.17) and *glutamate dehydrogenase*. Most of this ammonia is excreted into the urine as NH_4^+, which provides an important mechanism for maintaining the body's acid-base balance through the excretion of protons. Ammonia is also obtained from the hydrolysis of glutamine by intestinal *glutaminase*. The intestinal mucosal cells obtain

glutamine either from the blood or from digestion of dietary protein. [Note: Intestinal glutamine metabolism produces citrulline, which travels to the kidney and is used to synthesize arginine.]

2. **From bacterial action in the intestine:** Ammonia is formed from urea by the action of bacterial *urease* in the lumen of the intestine. This ammonia is absorbed from the intestine by way of the portal vein and is almost quantitatively removed by the liver via conversion to urea.

3. **From amines:** Amines obtained from the diet, and monoamines that serve as hormones or neurotransmitters, give rise to ammonia by the action of *amine oxidase* (see p. 286).

4. **From purines and pyrimidines:** In the catabolism of purines and pyrimidines, amino groups attached to the rings are released as ammonia (see Figure 22.15 and p. 304).

B. Transport of ammonia in the circulation

Although ammonia is constantly produced in the tissues, it is present at very low levels in blood. This is due both to the rapid removal of blood ammonia by the liver, and the fact that many tissues, particularly muscle, release amino acid nitrogen in the form of glutamine or alanine, rather than as free ammonia (see Figure 19.13).

1. **Urea:** Formation of urea in the liver is quantitatively the most important disposal route for ammonia. Urea travels in the blood from the liver to the kidneys, where it passes into the glomerular filtrate.

2. **Glutamine:** This amide of glutamic acid provides a nontoxic storage and transport form of ammonia (Figure 19.18). The ATP-requiring formation of glutamine from glutamate and ammonia by *glutamine synthetase* occurs primarily in the muscle and liver, but is also important in the CNS where it is the major mechanism for the removal of ammonia in the brain. Glutamine is found in plasma at concentrations higher than other amino acids—a finding consistent with its transport function. Circulating glutamine is removed by the liver and the kidneys and deaminated by *glutaminase*. In the liver, the NH_3 produced is detoxified through conversion to urea, and in the kidney it can be used in the excretion of protons. The metabolism of ammonia is summarized in Figure 19.19.

C. Hyperammonemia

The capacity of the hepatic urea cycle exceeds the normal rates of ammonia generation, and the levels of serum ammonia are normally low (5–35 µmol/L). However, when liver function is compromised, due either to genetic defects of the urea cycle or liver disease, blood levels can rise above 1,000 µmol/L. Such hyperammonemia is a medical emergency, because ammonia has a direct neurotoxic effect on the CNS. For example, elevated concentrations of ammonia in the blood cause the symptoms of ammonia intoxication, which include tremors, slurring of speech, somnolence, vomiting, cerebral edema, and blurring of vision. At high concentrations, ammonia can cause coma and death. The two major types of hyperammonemia are:

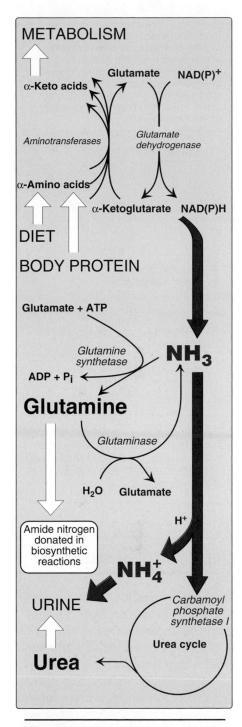

Figure 19.19
Metabolism of ammonia. Urea content in the urine is reported as urinary urea nitrogen or UUN. Urea in blood is reported as BUN (blood urea nitrogen). The enzymes *glutamate dehydrogenase*, *glutamine synthetase*, and *carbamoyl phosphate synthetase I* fix ammonia (NH_3) into organic molecules.

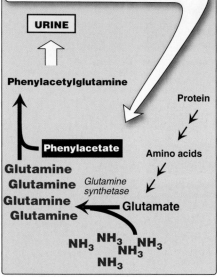

Phenylbutyrate is a prodrug that is rapidly converted to phenylacetate, which combines with glutamine to form phenylacetylglutamine. The phenylacetyglutamine, containing two atoms of nitrogen, is excreted in the urine, thus assisting in clearance of nitrogenous waste.

Figure 19.20
Treatment of patients with urea cycle defects by administration of phenylbutyrate to aid in excretion of ammonia.

1. **Acquired hyperammonemia:** Liver disease is a common cause of hyperammonemia in adults, and may be due, for example, to viral hepatitis or to hepatotoxins such as alcohol. Cirrhosis of the liver may result in formation of collateral circulation around the liver. As a result, portal blood is shunted directly into the systemic circulation and does not have access to the liver. The conversion of ammonia to urea is, therefore, severely impaired, leading to elevated levels of ammonia.

2. **Congenital hyperammonemia:** Genetic deficiencies of each of the five enzymes of the urea cycle have been described, with an overall prevalence estimated to be 1:25,000 live births. *Ornithine transcarbamoylase* deficiency, which is X-linked, is the most common of these disorders, predominantly affecting males, although female carriers may become symptomatic. All of the other urea cycle disorders follow an autosomal recessive inheritance pattern. In each case, the failure to synthesize urea leads to hyperammonemia during the first weeks following birth. [Note: The hyperammonemia seen with *arginase* deficiency is less severe because arginine contains two waste nitrogens and can be excreted in the urine.] Historically, urea cycle defects had high morbidity (neurological manifestations) and mortality. Treatment included restriction of dietary protein in the presence of sufficient calories to prevent catabolism. Administration of compounds that bind covalently to amino acids, producing nitrogen-containing molecules that are excreted in the urine, has improved survival. For example, phenylbutyrate given orally is converted to phenylacetate. This condenses with glutamine to form phenylacetylglutamine, which is excreted (Figure 19.20).

VIII. CHAPTER SUMMARY

Nitrogen enters the body in a variety of compounds present in food, the most important being amino acids contained in **dietary protein. Nitrogen leaves** the body as **urea**, **ammonia**, and other products derived from amino acid metabolism (Figure 19.21). Free amino acids in the body are produced by hydrolysis of dietary protein by proteases in the stomach and intestine, degradation of tissue proteins, and de novo synthesis. This **amino acid pool** is consumed in the synthesis of body protein, metabolized for energy, or its members serve as precursors for other nitrogen-containing compounds. Note that body protein is simultaneously degraded and resynthesized— a process known as **protein turnover**. For many proteins, **regulation of synthesis** determines the concentration of the protein in the cell, whereas the amounts of other proteins are controlled by **selective degradation**. The ATP-dependent **ubiquitin/proteasome** and ATP-independent **lysosomal acid hydrolases** are the two major enzyme systems that are responsible for **degrading damaged or unneeded proteins**. Nitrogen cannot be stored, and amino acids in excess of the biosynthetic needs of the cell are immediately degraded. The first phase of **catabolism** involves the transfer of the α-amino groups by PLP-dependent **transamination**, followed by **oxidative deamination of glutamate**, forming **ammonia** and the corresponding α-keto acids. A portion of the **free ammonia** is excreted in the **urine**, some is used in converting glutamate to glutamine, but most is used in the synthesis of **urea**, which is quantitatively the most important route for disposing of nitrogen from the body. The two major causes of **hyperammonemia** (with its CNS effects) are liver disease and inherited deficiencies of enzymes (such as ornithine transcarbamolyase) in the urea cycle.

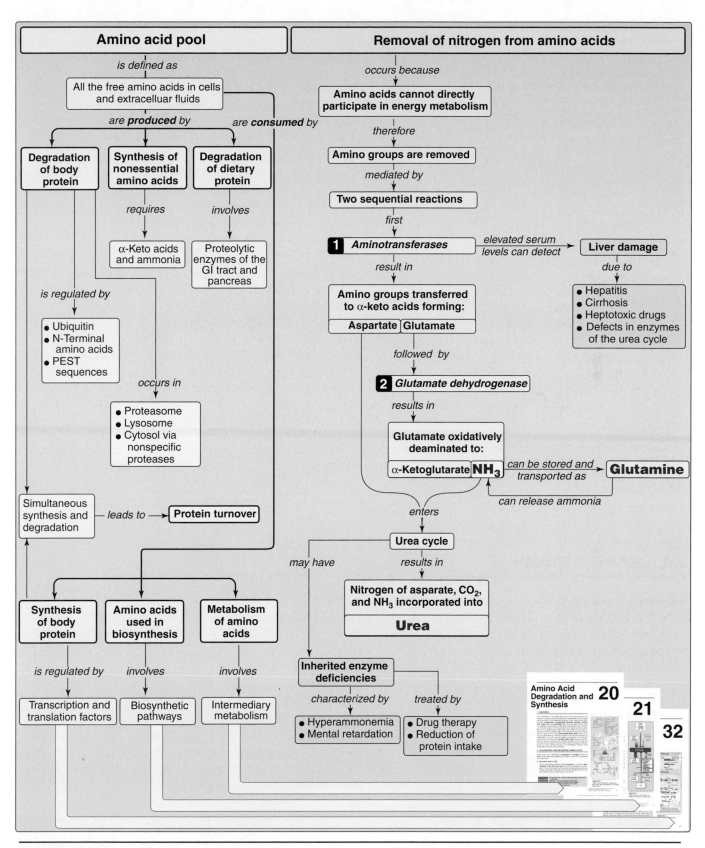

Figure 19.21
Key concept map for nitrogen metabolism.

Study Questions:

Choose the ONE best answer.

19.1 In the transamination reaction shown below, which of the following are the products, X and Y?

Oxaloacetate X

Glutamate Y

A. Alanine, α-ketoglutarate.
B. Glutamate, α-ketoglutarate.
C. Asparate, α-ketoglutarate.
D. Pyruvate, aspartate.
E. Pyruvate, alanine.

19.2 Which one of the following statements about the urea cycle is correct?

A. The two nitrogen atoms that are incorporated into urea enter the cycle as ammonia and alanine.
B. Urea is produced directly by the hydrolysis of ornithine.
C. ATP is required for the reaction in which argininosuccinate is cleaved to form arginine.
D. Urinary urea is increased by a diet rich in protein.
E. The urea cycle occurs exclusively in the cytosol.

For Questions 19.3 and 19.4:

A female neonate did well until approximately 24 hours of age when she became lethargic. A sepsis workup proved negative. At 56 hours, she started showing focal seizure activity. The plasma ammonia level was found to be 1,100 μmol/L (normal 5–35 μmol/L). Quantitative plasma amino acid levels revealed a marked elevation of argininosuccinate.

19.3 Which one of the following enzymic activities is most likely to be deficient in this patient?

A. Arginase.
B. Argininosuccinate lyase.
C. Argininosuccinate synthase.
D. Carbamoyl phosphate synthetase I.
E. Ornithine transcarbamoylase.

19.4 Which one of the following would also be elevated in the blood of this patient?

A. Asparagine.
B. Glutamine.
C. Lysine.
D. Urea.
E. Uric acid.

Correct answer = C. Transaminase reactions always have an amino acid and an α-keto acid as substrates. The products of the reaction are also an amino acid (corresponding to the α-keto substrate) and an α-keto acid (corresponding to the amino acid substrate). Three amino acid α-keto acid pairs commonly encountered in metabolism are:

alanine/pyruvate
aspartate/oxaloacetate
glutamate/α-ketoglutarate

In this question, glutamate is deaminated to form α-ketoglutarate, and oxaloacetate is aminated to form aspartate.

Correct answer = D. The amino nitrogen of dietary protein is excreted as urea. The two nitrogens enter the urea cycle as ammonia and aspartate. Urea is produced by the hydrolysis of arginine. The cleavage of argininosuccinate does not require ATP. The urea cycle occurs partly in the mitochondria.

Correct answer = B. Genetic deficiencies of each of the five enzymes of the urea cycle, as well as deficiencies in N-acetyglutamate synthase, have been described. The accumulation of argininosuccinate in the plasma of this patient means that the enzymes required for its synthesis are functional, but the enzyme (argininosuccinate lyase or argininosuccinase) required for its cleavage to arginine plus fumarate is not.

Correct answer = B. With the exception of arginase, deficiencies of the enzymes of the urea cycle result in the failure to synthesize urea and lead to hyperammonemia in the first few weeks after birth. Glutamine will also be elevated because it acts as a nontoxic storage and transport form of ammonia. Thus, elevated glutamine always accompanies hyperammonemia. Asparagine does not serve this sequestering role. Urea would be decreased due to impaired activity of the urea cycle. Lysine and uric acid would not be elevated. Treatment of this patient includes limiting protein in the diet and administering compounds that bind covalently to amino acids, producing nitrogen-containing molecules that are excreted in the urine. For example, phenylbutyrate given orally is converted to phenylacetate. This compound condenses with glutamine to form phenylacetylglutamine, which is excreted.

Amino Acid Degradation and Synthesis

20

I. OVERVIEW

The catabolism of the amino acids involves the removal of α-amino groups, followed by the breakdown of the resulting carbon skeletons. These pathways converge to form seven intermediate products: oxaloacetate, pyruvate, α-ketoglutarate, fumarate, succinyl coenzyme A (CoA), acetyl CoA, and acetoacetate. These products directly enter the pathways of intermediary metabolism, resulting either in the synthesis of glucose or lipid or in the production of energy through their oxidation to CO_2 by the citric acid cycle. Figure 20.1 provides an overview of these pathways, with a more detailed summary presented later in Figure 20.14 (see p. 269). Nonessential amino acids (Figure 20.2) can be synthesized in sufficient amounts from the intermediates of metabolism or, as in the case of cysteine and tyrosine, from essential amino acids. In contrast, the essential amino acids cannot be synthesized (or produced in sufficient amounts) by the body and, therefore, must be obtained from the diet in order for normal protein synthesis to occur. Genetic defects in the pathways of amino acid metabolism can cause serious disease.

II. GLUCOGENIC AND KETOGENIC AMINO ACIDS

Amino acids can be classified as glucogenic, ketogenic, or both based on which of the seven intermediates are produced during their catabolism (see Figure 20.2).

A. Glucogenic amino acids

Amino acids whose catabolism yields pyruvate or one of the intermediates of the citric acid cycle are termed glucogenic. These intermediates are substrates for gluconeogenesis (see p. 117) and, therefore, can give rise to the net formation of glucose in the liver and kidney.

Color-coding used in this chapter:	• **BLUE CAPS TEXT** = names of seven products of amino acid metabolism
	• Red text = names of glucogenic amino acids
	• Brown text = names of glucogenic and ketogenic amino acids
	• Green text = names of ketogenic amino acids
	• Cyan text = one-carbon compounds

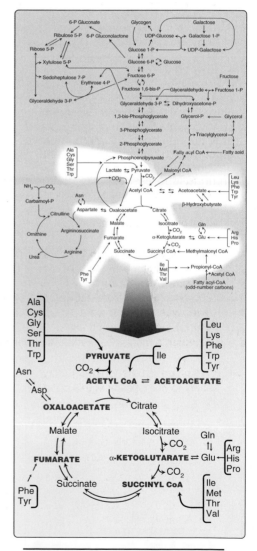

Figure 20.1
Amino acid metabolism shown as a part of the central pathways of energy metabolism. (See figure 8.2, p. 92, for a more detailed view of these processes.

Glucogenic	Glucogenic and Ketogenic	Ketogenic
Nonessential		
Alanine Arginine Asparagine Aspartate Cysteine Glutamate Glutamine Glycine Proline Serine	Tyrosine	
Essential		
Histidine Methionine Threonine Valine	Isoleucine Phenyl-alanine Tryptophan	Leucine Lysine

Figure 20.2
Classification of amino acids. [Note: Some amino acids can become conditionally essential. For example, supplementation with glutamine and arginine has been shown to improve outcomes in patients with trauma, post-operative infections, and immunosuppression.]

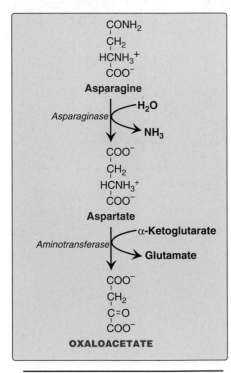

Figure 20.3
Metabolism of asparagine and aspartate. [Note: Recall that carbons from aspartate can form fumarate in the urea cycle (see p. 254).]

B. Ketogenic amino acids

Amino acids whose catabolism yields either acetoacetate or one of its precursors (acetyl CoA or acetoacetyl CoA) are termed ketogenic (see Figure 20.2). Acetoacetate is one of the ketone bodies, which also include 3-hydroxybutyrate and acetone (see p. 195). Leucine and lysine are the only exclusively ketogenic amino acids found in proteins. Their carbon skeletons are not substrates for gluconeogenesis and, therefore, cannot give rise to the net formation of glucose.

III. CATABOLISM OF THE CARBON SKELETONS OF AMINO ACIDS

The pathways by which amino acids are catabolized are conveniently organized according to which one (or more) of the seven intermediates listed above is produced from a particular amino acid.

A. Amino acids that form oxaloacetate

Asparagine is hydrolyzed by *asparaginase*, liberating ammonia and aspartate (Figure 20.3). Aspartate loses its amino group by transamination to form oxaloacetate (see Figure 20.3). [Note: Some rapidly dividing leukemic cells are unable to synthesize sufficient asparagine to support their growth. This makes asparagine an essential amino acid for these cells, which therefore require asparagine from the blood. *Asparaginase*, which hydrolyzes asparagine to aspartate, can be administered systemically to treat leukemic patients.[1] *Asparaginase* lowers the level of asparagine in the plasma and, therefore, deprives cancer cells of a required nutrient.]

B. Amino acids that form α-ketoglutarate via glutamate

1. **Glutamine:** This amino acid is converted to glutamate and ammonia by the enzyme *glutaminase* (see p. 256). Glutamate is converted to α-ketoglutarate by transamination, or through oxidative deamination by *glutamate dehydrogenase* (see p. 252).

2. **Proline:** This amino acid is oxidized to glutamate. Glutamate is transaminated or oxidatively deaminated to form α-ketoglutarate.

3. **Arginine:** This amino acid is cleaved by *arginase* to produce ornithine. [Note: This reaction occurs primarily in the liver as part of the urea cycle (see p. 255).] Ornithine is subsequently converted to α-ketoglutarate; glutamate semi-aldehyde is an intermediate.

4. **Histidine:** This amino acid is oxidatively deaminated by *histidase* to urocanic acid, which subsequently forms N-formiminoglutamate (FIGlu, Figure 20.4). FIGlu donates its formimino group to tetrahydrofolate (THF), leaving glutamate, which is degraded as described above. [Note: Individuals deficient in folic acid excrete increased amounts of FIGlu in the urine, particularly after ingestion of a large dose of histidine. The FIGlu excretion test has been used in diagnosing a deficiency of folic acid.] (See p. 267 for a discussion of folic acid, THF, and one-carbon metabolism.)

[1]See Chapter 39 in *Lippincott's Illustrated Reviews: Pharmacology* for a discussion of the use of asparaginase as an antileukemic drug.

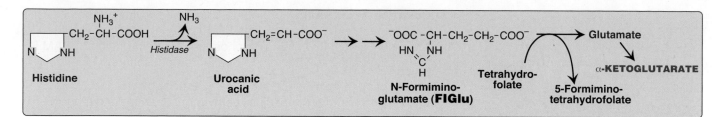

Figure 20.4
Degradation of histidine.

C. Amino acids that form pyruvate

1. **Alanine:** This amino acid loses its amino group by reversible transamination to form pyruvate (Figure 20.5). [Note: Alanine is the major gluconeogenic amino acid.]

2. **Serine:** This amino acid can be converted to glycine and N^5,N^{10}-methylenetetrahydrofolate (Figure 20.6A). Serine can also be converted to pyruvate by *serine dehydratase* (Figure 20.6B).

3. **Glycine:** This amino acid can be converted to serine by the reversible addition of a methylene group from N^5,N^{10}-methylene-tetrahydrofolic acid (see Figure 20.6A) or oxidized to CO_2 and NH_3. [Note: Glycine can be converted to glyoxylate. Glyoxylate can be oxidized to oxalate, or transaminated to glycine. Deficiency of the *transaminase* causes overproduction of oxalate and kidney damage (primary oxaluria Type 1).]

4. **Cystine:** This amino acid is reduced to cysteine, using NADH + H+ as a reductant. **Cysteine** undergoes desulfuration to yield pyruvate. [Note: The sulfate released can be used to synthesize 3'-phosphoadenosine-5'-phosphosulfate (PAPS), an activated sulfur donor to acceptors such as glycosaminoglycans (see p. 162).]

5. **Threonine:** This amino acid is converted to pyruvate or to α-ketobutyrate, which forms succinyl CoA.

D. Amino acids that form fumarate

1. **Phenylalanine and tyrosine:** Hydroxylation of phenylalanine produces tyrosine (Figure 20.7). This reaction, catalyzed by tetrahydrobiopterin-requiring *phenylalanine hydroxylase*, initiates the catabolism of phenylalanine. Thus, the metabolism of phenylalanine and tyrosine merge, leading ultimately to the formation of fumarate and acetoacetate. Phenylalanine and tyrosine are, therefore, both glucogenic and ketogenic.

2. **Inherited deficiencies:** Inherited deficiencies in the enzymes of phenylalanine and tyrosine metabolism lead to the diseases phenylketonuria (see p. 270) and alkaptonuria (see p. 274), and the condition of albinism (see p. 273).

E. Amino acids that form succinyl CoA: methionine

Methionine is one of four amino acids that form succinyl CoA. This sulfur-containing amino acid deserves special attention because it is converted to S-adenosylmethionine (SAM), the major methyl-group donor in one-carbon metabolism (Figure 20.8). Methionine is also the source of homocysteine—a metabolite associated with atherosclerotic vascular disease (see p. 265).

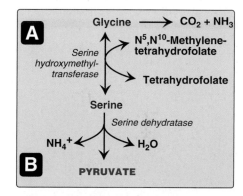

Figure 20.5
Transamination of alanine to form pyruvate.

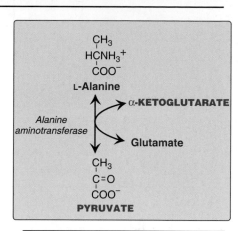

Figure 20.6
A. Interconversion of serine and glycine, and oxidation of glycine. B. Dehydration of serine to form pyruvate.

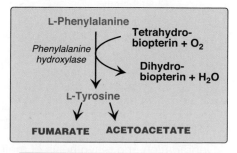

Figure 20.7
Degradation of phenylalanine.

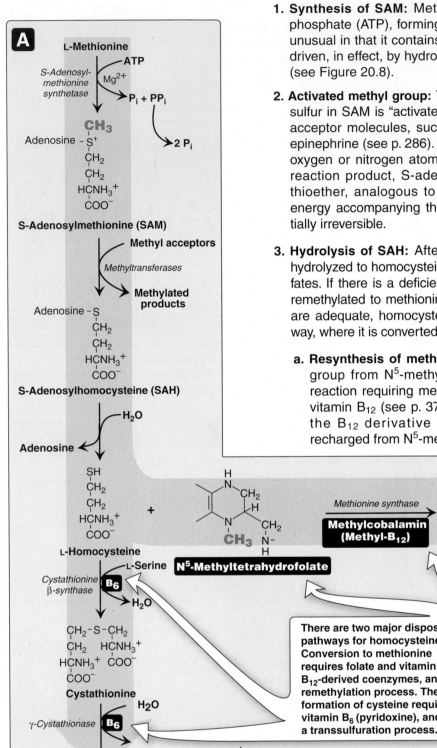

1. **Synthesis of SAM:** Methionine condenses with adenosine triphosphate (ATP), forming SAM—a high-energy compound that is unusual in that it contains no phosphate. The formation of SAM is driven, in effect, by hydrolysis of all three phosphate bonds in ATP (see Figure 20.8).

2. **Activated methyl group:** The methyl group attached to the tertiary sulfur in SAM is "activated," and can be transferred to a variety of acceptor molecules, such as norepinephrine in the synthesis of epinephrine (see p. 286). The methyl group is usually transferred to oxygen or nitrogen atoms, but sometimes to carbon atoms. The reaction product, S-adenosylhomocysteine (SAH), is a simple thioether, analogous to methionine. The resulting loss of free energy accompanying the reaction makes methyl transfer essentially irreversible.

3. **Hydrolysis of SAH:** After donation of the methyl group, SAH is hydrolyzed to homocysteine and adenosine. Homocysteine has two fates. If there is a deficiency of methionine, homocysteine may be remethylated to methionine (see Figure 20.8). If methionine stores are adequate, homocysteine may enter the transsulfuration pathway, where it is converted to cysteine.

   a. **Resynthesis of methionine:** Homocysteine accepts a methyl group from N^5-methyltetrahydrofolate (N^5-methyl-THF) in a reaction requiring methylcobalamin, a coenzyme derived from vitamin B_{12} (see p. 375). The methyl group is transferred from the B_{12} derivative to homocysteine, and cobalamin is recharged from N^5-methyl-THF.

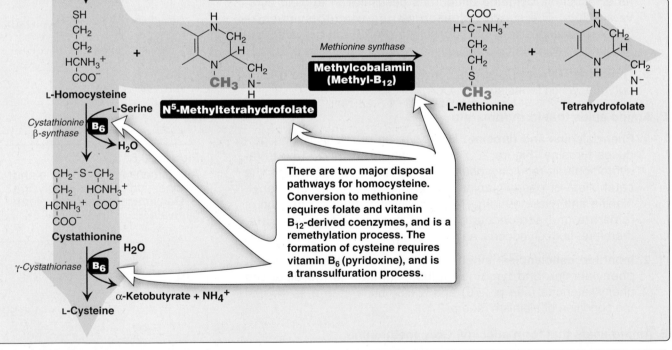

There are two major disposal pathways for homocysteine. Conversion to methionine requires folate and vitamin B_{12}-derived coenzymes, and is a remethylation process. The formation of cysteine requires vitamin B_6 (pyridoxine), and is a transsulfuration process.

Figure 20.8
Degradation and resynthesis of methionine. [Note: The resynthesis of methionine from homocysteine is the only reaction in which THF both carries and donates a methyl group. In all other reactions, SAM is the methyl group carrier and donor.]

b. Synthesis of cysteine: Homocysteine condenses with serine, forming cystathionine, which is hydrolyzed to α-ketobutyrate and cysteine (see Figure 20.8). This vitamin B$_6$–requiring sequence has the net effect of converting serine to cysteine, and homocysteine to α-ketobutyrate, which is oxidatively decarboxylated to form propionyl CoA. Propionyl CoA is converted to succinyl CoA (see p. 194). Because homocysteine is synthesized from the essential amino acid methionine, cysteine is not an essential amino acid as long as sufficient methionine is available.

4. **Relationship of homocysteine to vascular disease:** Elevations in plasma homocysteine levels promote oxidative damage, inflammation, and endothelial dysfunction, and are an independent risk factor for occlusive vascular disease (Figure 20.9). Mild elevations are seen in about 7% of the population. Epidemiologic studies have shown that plasma homocysteine levels are inversely related to plasma levels of folate, B$_{12}$, and B$_6$—the three vitamins involved in the conversion of homocysteine to methionine or cysteine. Supplementation with these vitamins has been shown to reduce circulating levels of homocysteine. However, in patients with established cardiovascular disease, vitamin therapy does not decrease cardiovascular events or death. This raises the question as to whether homocysteine is a cause of the vascular damage or merely a marker of such damage. [Note: Large elevations in plasma homocysteine as a result of rare deficiencies in *cystathionine β-synthase* are seen in patients with classic homocystinuria. These individuals experience premature vascular disease, with about 25% dying from thrombotic complications before 30 years of age.]

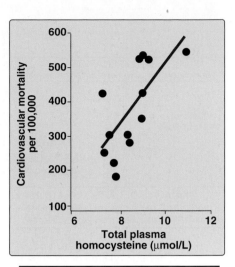

Figure 20.9
Association between cardio-vascular disease mortality and total plasma homocysteine.

> Elevated homocysteine or decreased folic acid levels in pregnant women are associated with increased incidence of neural tube defects (improper closure, as in spina bifida) in the fetus. Periconceptual supplementation with folate reduces the risk of such defects.

F. Other amino acids that form succinyl CoA

Degradation of valine, isoleucine, and threonine also results in the production of succinyl CoA—a tricarboxylic acid (TCA) cycle intermediate and glucogenic compound.

1. **Valine and isoleucine:** These amino acids are branched-chain amino acids that generate propionyl CoA, which is converted to succinyl CoA by biotin- and vitamin B$_{12}$–requiring reactions (Figure 20.10).

2. **Threonine:** This amino acid is dehydrated to α-ketobutyrate, which is converted to propionyl CoA and then to succinyl CoA. Threonine can also be converted to pyruvate. [Note: Propionyl CoA, then, is generated by the catabolism of certain amino acids and odd-numbered fatty acids (see p. 193).]

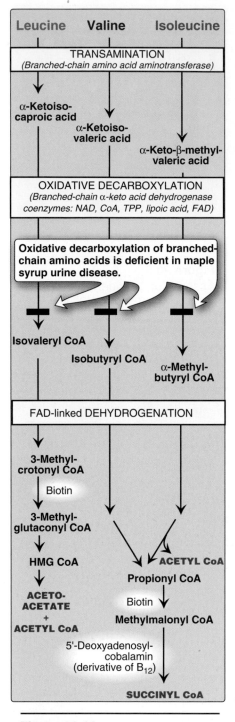

Figure 20.10
Degradation of leucine, valine, and isoleucine. TPP = thiamine pyrophosphate. [Note: *3-Methylcrotonyl CoA carboxylase* is one of four biotin-requiring carboxylases we have encountered. The other three are *pyruvate carboxylase*, *acetyl CoA carboxylase*, and *propionyl CoA carboxylase*.]

G. Amino acids that form acetyl CoA or acetoacetyl CoA

Leucine, isoleucine, lysine, and tryptophan form acetyl CoA or acetoacetyl CoA directly, without pyruvate serving as an intermediate (through the *pyruvate dehydrogenase* reaction, see p. 109). As mentioned previously, phenylalanine and tyrosine also give rise to acetoacetate during their catabolism (see Figure 20.7). Therefore, there are a total of six ketogenic amino acids.

1. **Leucine:** This amino acid is exclusively ketogenic in its catabolism, forming acetyl CoA and acetoacetate (see Figure 20.10). The initial steps in the catabolism of leucine are similar to those of the other branched-chain amino acids, isoleucine and valine (see below).

2. **Isoleucine:** This amino acid is both ketogenic and glucogenic, because its metabolism yields acetyl CoA and propionyl CoA. The first three steps in the metabolism of isoleucine are similar to the initial steps in the degradation of the other branched-chain amino acids, valine and leucine (see Figure 20.10).

3. **Lysine:** An exclusively ketogenic amino acid, this amino acid is unusual in that neither of its amino groups undergoes transamination as the first step in catabolism. Lysine is ultimately converted to acetoacetyl CoA.

4. **Tryptophan:** This amino acid is both glucogenic and ketogenic because its metabolism yields alanine and acetoacetyl CoA.

H. Catabolism of the branched-chain amino acids

The branched-chain amino acids, isoleucine, leucine, and valine, are essential amino acids. In contrast to other amino acids, they are metabolized primarily by the peripheral tissues (particularly muscle), rather than by the liver. Because these three amino acids have a similar route of catabolism, it is convenient to describe them as a group (see Figure 20.10).

1. **Transamination:** Removal of the amino groups of all three amino acids is catalyzed by a single, vitamin B_6–requiring enzyme, *branched-chain amino acid aminotransferase*.

2. **Oxidative decarboxylation:** Removal of the carboxyl group of the α-keto acids derived from leucine, valine, and isoleucine is catalyzed by a single multienzyme complex, *branched-chain α-keto acid dehydrogenase complex.* This complex uses thiamine pyrophosphate, lipoic acid, FAD, NAD^+, and CoA as its coenzymes. [Note: This reaction is similar to the conversion of pyruvate to acetyl CoA by *pyruvate dehydrogenase* (see p. 110) and the oxidation of α-ketoglutarate to succinyl CoA by *α-ketoglutarate dehydrogenase* (see p. 112).] An inherited deficiency of *branched-chain α-keto acid dehydrogenase* results in accumulation of the branched-chain α-keto acid substrates in the urine. Their sweet odor prompted the name maple syrup urine disease (see p. 272).

3. **Dehydrogenation:** Oxidation of the products formed in the above reaction yields α-β-unsaturated acyl CoA derivatives. This reaction is analogous to the FAD-linked dehydrogenation described in the β-oxidation scheme of fatty acid degradation (see p. 192). [Note: Deficiency in the *dehydrogenase* specific for isovaleryl CoA

causes neurological problems, and is associated with a "sweaty feet" odor in body fluids.]

4. **End products:** The catabolism of isoleucine ultimately yields acetyl CoA and succinyl CoA, rendering it both ketogenic and glucogenic. Valine yields succinyl CoA and is glucogenic. Leucine is ketogenic, being metabolized to acetoacetate and acetyl CoA. [Note: Branched-chain amino acid catabolism also results in glutamine and alanine being sent out into the blood from muscle.]

IV. ROLE OF FOLIC ACID IN AMINO ACID METABOLISM

Some synthetic pathways require the addition of single carbon groups that exist in a variety of oxidation states, including formyl, methenyl, methylene, and methyl. These single carbon groups can be transferred from carrier compounds such as THF and SAM to specific structures that are being synthesized or modified. The "one-carbon pool" refers to single carbon units attached to this group of carriers. [Note: CO_2, the dehydrated form of carbonic acid, is carried by the vitamin biotin, which is a prosthetic group for most carboxylation reactions, but is not considered a member of the one-carbon pool. Defects in the ability to add or remove biotin from *carboxylases* result in multiple *carboxylase* deficiency; treatment is supplementation with biotin.]

A. Folic acid: a carrier of one-carbon units

The active form of folic acid, tetrahydrofolic acid (THF), is produced from folate by *dihydrofolate reductase* in a two-step reaction requiring two NADPH. The carbon unit carried by THF is bound to nitrogen N^5 or N^{10}, or to both N^5 and N^{10}. THF allows one-carbon compounds to be recognized and manipulated by biosynthetic enzymes. Figure 20.11 shows the structures of the various members of the THF family and their interconversions, and indicates the sources of the one-carbon units and the synthetic reactions in which the specific members participate. [Note: Folate deficiency presents as a megaloblastic anemia due to decreased availability of the purines and of the TMP needed for DNA synthesis (see p. 303).]

V. BIOSYNTHESIS OF NONESSENTIAL AMINO ACIDS

Nonessential amino acids are synthesized from intermediates of metabolism or, as in the case of tyrosine and cysteine, from the essential amino acids phenylalanine and methionine, respectively. The synthetic reactions for the nonessential amino acids are described below, and are summarized later in Figure 20.14. [Note: Some amino acids found in proteins, such as hydroxyproline and hydroxylysine (see p. 45), are modified after their incorporation into the protein (posttranslational modification, see p. 443).]

A. Synthesis from α-keto acids

Alanine, aspartate, and glutamate are synthesized by transfer of an amino group to the α-keto acids pyruvate, oxaloacetate, and α-keto-glutarate, respectively. These transamination reactions (Figure 20.12, and see p. 250) are the most direct of the biosynthetic pathways.

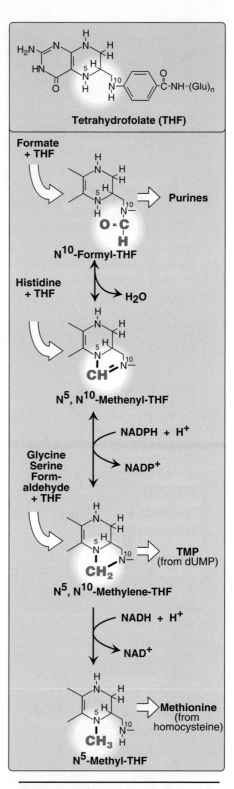

Figure 20.11

Summary of the interconversions and uses of the carrier, tetrahydrofolate. [Note: N^5, N^{10}-Methenyl-THF arises from 5-formimino-THF (see Figure 20.4).]

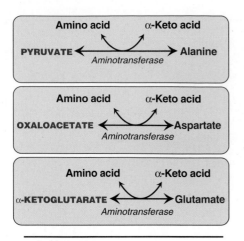

Figure 20.12
Formation of alanine, aspartate, and glutamate from the corresponding α-keto acids.

Glutamate is unusual in that it can also be synthesized by the reverse of oxidative deamination, catalyzed by *glutamate dehydrogenase* (see p. 252).

B. Synthesis by amidation

1. **Glutamine:** This amino acid, which contains an amide linkage with ammonia at the γ-carboxyl, is formed from glutamate by *glutamine synthetase* (see Figure 19.18, p. 256). The reaction is driven by the hydrolysis of ATP. In addition to producing glutamine for protein synthesis, the reaction also serves as a major mechanism for the transport of ammonia in a nontoxic form (see p. 256 for a discussion of ammonia metabolism).

2. **Asparagine:** This amino acid, which contains an amide linkage with ammonia at the β-carboxyl, is formed from aspartate by *asparagine synthetase,* using glutamine as the amide donor. The reaction requires ATP, and, like the synthesis of glutamine, has an equilibrium far in the direction of asparagine synthesis.

C. Proline

Glutamate is converted to proline by cyclization and reduction reactions.

D. Serine, glycine, and cysteine

1. **Serine:** This amino acid arises from 3-phosphoglycerate, an intermediate in glycolysis (see Figure 8.18, p. 101), which is first oxidized to 3-phosphopyruvate, and then transaminated to 3-phosphoserine. Serine is formed by hydrolysis of the phosphate ester. Serine can also be formed from glycine through transfer of a hydroxymethyl group by *serine hydroxymethyl transferase* using N^5,N^{10}-methylene-THF as the one carbon donor (see Figure 20.6A).

2. **Glycine:** This amino acid is synthesized from serine by removal of a hydroxymethyl group, also by *serine hydroxymethyl transferase* (see Figure 20.6A). THF is the one carbon acceptor.

3. **Cysteine:** This amino acid is synthesized by two consecutive reactions in which homocysteine combines with serine, forming cystathionine that, in turn, is hydrolyzed to α-ketobutyrate and cysteine (see Figure 20.8). Homocysteine is derived from methionine as described on p. 264. Because methionine is an essential amino acid, cysteine synthesis can be sustained only if the dietary intake of methionine is adequate.

E. Tyrosine

Tyrosine is formed from phenylalanine by *phenylalanine hydroxylase.* The reaction requires molecular oxygen and the coenzyme tetrahydrobiopterin (BH_4), which can be synthesized from guanosine triphosphate (GTP) by the body. One atom of molecular oxygen becomes the hydroxyl group of tyrosine, and the other atom is reduced to water. During the reaction, BH_4 is oxidized to dihydrobiopterin (BH_2). BH_4 is regenerated from BH_2 by NADH-requiring *dihydropteridine reductase.* Tyrosine, like cysteine, is formed from an essential amino acid and is, therefore, nonessential only in the presence of adequate dietary phenylalanine.

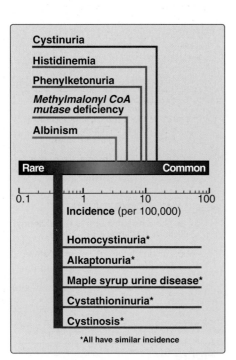

Figure 20.13
Incidence of inherited diseases of amino acid metabolism. [Note: Cystinuria is the most common genetic error of amino acid transport.]

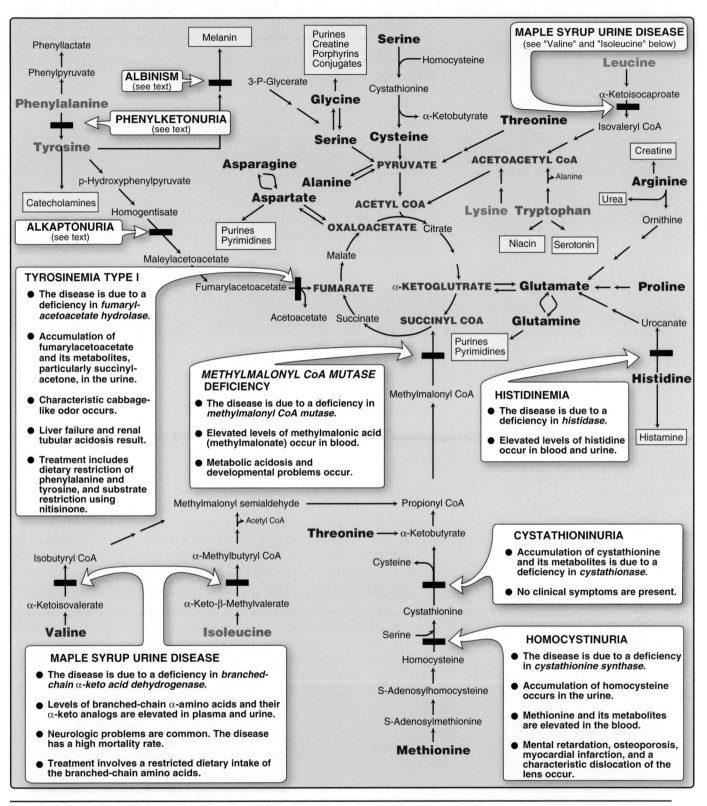

Figure 20.14

Summary of the metabolism of amino acids in humans. Genetically determined enzyme deficiencies are summarized in white boxes. Nitrogen-containing compounds derived from amino acids are shown in small, yellow boxes. Classification of amino acids is color coded: **Red** = glucogenic; **brown** = glucogenic and ketogenic; **green** = ketogenic. Compounds in **BLUE ALL CAPS** are the seven metabolites to which all amino acid metabolism converges.

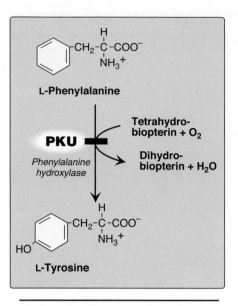

Figure 20.15
A deficiency in *phenylalanine hydroxylase* results in the disease phenylketonuria (PKU).

VI. METABOLIC DEFECTS IN AMINO ACID METABOLISM

Inborn errors of metabolism are commonly caused by mutant genes that generally result in abnormal proteins, most often enzymes. The inherited defects may be expressed as a total loss of enzyme activity or, more frequently, as a partial deficiency in catalytic activity. Without treatment, the inherited defects of amino acid metabolism almost invariably result in mental retardation or other developmental abnormalities as a consequence of harmful accumulation of metabolites. Although more than 50 of these disorders have been described, many are rare, occurring in less than 1 per 250,000 in most populations (Figure 20.13). Collectively, however, they constitute a very significant portion of pediatric genetic diseases (Figure 20.14). Phenylketonuria is the most important disease of amino acid metabolism because it is relatively common and responds to dietary treatment.

> Screening of newborns for a number of the amino acid disorders by tandem mass spectrometry of blood obtained from a heel prick is possible; however, exactly which disorders are screened for currently varies from state to state, and only phenylketonuria screening is mandated by all states.

A. Phenylketonuria

Phenylketonuria (PKU), caused by a deficiency of *phenylalanine hydroxylase* (Figure 20.15), is the most common clinically encountered inborn error of amino acid metabolism (prevalence 1:15,000). Biochemically, it is characterized by accumulation of phenylalanine (and a deficiency of tyrosine). Hyperphenylalaninemia may also be caused by deficiencies in any of the several enzymes required to synthesize BH_4, or in *dihydropteridine reductase*, which regenerates BH_4 from BH_2 (Figure 20.16). Such deficiencies indirectly raise phenylalanine concentrations, because *phenylalanine hydroxylase*

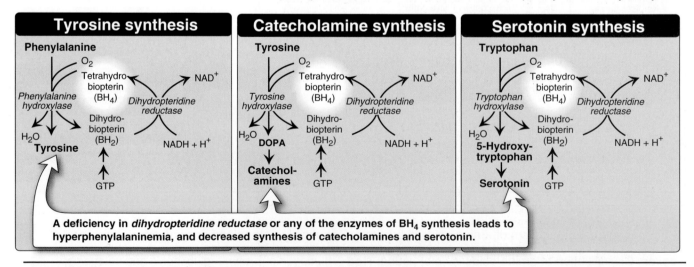

Figure 20.16
Biosynthetic reactions involving amino acids and tetrahydrobiopterin.

requires BH$_4$ as a coenzyme. BH$_4$ is also required for *tyrosine hydroxylase* and *tryptophan hydroxylase*, which catalyze reactions leading to the synthesis of neurotransmitters, such as serotonin and the catecholamines. Simply restricting dietary phenylalanine does not reverse the central nervous system (CNS) effects due to deficiencies in neurotransmitters. Replacement therapy with BH$_4$ or L-DOPA and 5-hydroxytryptophan (products of the affected *tyrosine hydroxylase–* and *tryptophan hydroxylase–*catalyzed reactions) improves the clinical outcome in these variant forms of hyperphenylalaninemia, although the response is unpredictable.

1. Characteristics of classic PKU:

a. Elevated phenylalanine: Phenylalanine is present in elevated concentrations in tissues, plasma, and urine. Phenyllactate, phenylacetate, and phenylpyruvate, which are not normally produced in significant amounts in the presence of functional *phenylalanine hydroxylase*, are also elevated in PKU (Figure 20.17). These metabolites give urine a characteristic musty ("mousey") odor. [Note: The disease acquired its name from the presence of a phenylketone (now known to be phenylpyruvate) in the urine.]

b. CNS symptoms: Mental retardation, failure to walk or talk, seizures, hyperactivity, tremor, microcephaly, and failure to grow are characteristic findings in PKU. The patient with untreated PKU typically shows symptoms of mental retardation by the age of 1 year, and rarely achieves an IQ greater than 50 (Figure 20.18). [Note: These clinical manifestations are now rarely seen as a result of neonatal screening programs.]

c. Hypopigmentation: Patients with phenylketonuria often show a deficiency of pigmentation (fair hair, light skin color, and blue eyes). The hydroxylation of tyrosine by *tyrosinase*, which is the first step in the formation of the pigment melanin, is competitively inhibited by the high levels of phenylalanine present in PKU.

2. Neonatal screening and diagnosis of PKU:
Early diagnosis of phenylketonuria is important because the disease is treatable by dietary means. Because of the lack of neonatal symptoms, laboratory testing for elevated blood levels of phenylalanine is mandatory for detection. However, the infant with PKU frequently has normal blood levels of phenylalanine at birth because the mother clears increased blood phenylalanine in her affected fetus through the placenta. Normal levels of phenylalanine may persist until the newborn is exposed to 24–48 hours of protein feeding. Thus, screening tests are typically done after this time to avoid false negatives. For newborns with a positive screening test, diagnosis is confirmed through quantitative determination of phenylalanine levels.

3. Prenatal diagnosis of PKU:
Classic PKU is a family of diseases caused by any of 100 or more different mutations in the gene that codes for *phenylalanine hydroxylase* (*PAH*). The frequency of any given mutation varies among populations, and the disease is often doubly heterozygous, that is, the *PAH* gene has a different mutation in each allele. Despite this complexity, prenatal diagnosis is possible (see p. 477).

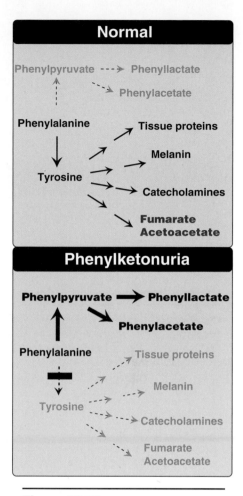

Figure 20.17
Pathways of phenylalanine metabolism in normal individuals and in patients with phenylketonuria.

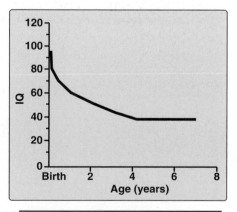

Figure 20.18
Typical intellectual ability in untreated PKU patients of different ages.

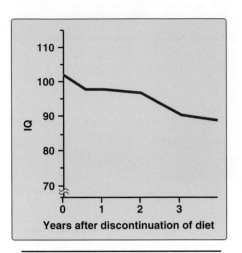

Figure 20.19
Changes in IQ scores after discontinuation of low-phenylalanine diet in patients with phenylketonuria.

4. Treatment of PKU: Most natural protein contains phenylalanine, and it is impossible to satisfy the body's protein requirement when ingesting a normal diet without exceeding the phenylalanine limit. Therefore, in PKU, blood phenylalanine is maintained close to the normal range by feeding synthetic amino acid preparations low in phenylalanine, supplemented with some natural foods (such as fruits, vegetables, and certain cereals) selected for their low phenylalanine content. The amount is adjusted according to the tolerance of the individual as measured by blood phenylalanine levels. The earlier treatment is started, the more completely neurologic damage can be prevented. [Note: Treatment must begin during the first 7–10 days of life to prevent mental retardation.] Because phenylalanine is an essential amino acid, overzealous treatment that results in blood phenylalanine levels below normal is avoided because this can lead to poor growth and neurologic symptoms. In patients with PKU, tyrosine cannot be synthesized from phenylalanine and, therefore, it becomes an essential amino acid and so must be supplied in the diet. Discontinuance of the phenylalanine-restricted diet before 8 years of age is associated with poor performance on IQ tests. Adult PKU patients show deterioration of IQ scores after discontinuation of the diet (Figure 20.19). Lifelong restriction of dietary phenylalanine is, therefore, recommended. [Note: Individuals with PKU are advised to avoid aspartame, an artificial sweetener that contains phenylalanine.]

5. Maternal PKU: If women with PKU who are not on a low-phenylalanine diet become pregnant, the offspring are affected with "maternal PKU syndrome." High blood phenylalanine levels in the mother cause microcephaly, mental retardation, and congenital heart abnormalities in the fetus—phenlyalanine is a teratogen. Some of these developmental responses to high phenylalanine occur during the first months of pregnancy. Thus, dietary control of blood phenylalanine must begin prior to conception, and must be maintained throughout the pregnancy.

B. Maple syrup urine disease

Maple syrup urine disease (MSUD) is a rare (1:185,000), autosomal recessive disorder in which there is a partial or complete deficiency in *branched-chain α-keto acid dehydrogenase*, an enzyme complex that decarboxylates leucine, isoleucine, and valine (see Figure 20.10). These amino acids and their corresponding α-keto acids accumulate in the blood, causing a toxic effect that interferes with brain functions. The disease is characterized by feeding problems, vomiting, dehydration, severe metabolic acidosis, and a characteristic maple syrup odor to the urine. If untreated, the disease leads to mental retardation, physical disabilities, and even death.

1. Classification: The term "maple syrup urine disease" includes a classic type and several variant forms of the disorder. The classic form is the most common type of MSUD. Leukocytes or cultured skin fibroblasts from these patients show little or no *branched-chain α-keto acid dehydrogenase* activity. Infants with classic MSUD show symptoms within the first several days of life. If not diagnosed and treated, classic MSUD is lethal in the first weeks of life. Patients with intermediate forms have a higher level of enzyme activity (approximately 3–15% of normal). The symptoms are milder and show an onset from infancy to adulthood. Patients with the rare thiamine-dependent variant of MSUD achieve increased activity of branched-chain *α-keto acid dehydrogenase* if given large doses of this vitamin.

2. **Screening and diagnosis:** As with PKU, prenatal diagnosis and neonatal screening are available, and most affected individuals are compound heterozygotes.

3. **Treatment:** The disease is treated with a synthetic formula that contains limited amounts of leucine, isoleucine, and valine—sufficient to provide the branched-chain amino acids necessary for normal growth and development without producing toxic levels. Early diagnosis and lifelong dietary treatment is essential if the child with MSUD is to develop normally. [Note: Branched-chain amino acids are an important energy source in times of metabolic need, and individuals with MSUD are at risk of decompensation during periods of increased protein catabolism.]

C. Albinism

Albinism refers to a group of conditions in which a defect in tyrosine metabolism results in a deficiency in the production of melanin. These defects result in the partial or full absence of pigment from the skin, hair, and eyes. Albinism appears in different forms, and it may be inherited by one of several modes: autosomal recessive (primary mode), autosomal dominant, or X-linked. Complete albinism (also called *tyrosinase*-negative oculocutaneous albinism) results from a deficiency of copper-requiring *tyrosinase*, causing a total absence of pigment from the hair, eyes, and skin (Figure 20.20). It is the most severe form of the condition. In addition to hypopigmentation, affected individuals have vision defects and photophobia (sunlight hurts their eyes). They are at increased risk for skin cancer.

D. Homocystinuria

The homocystinurias are a group of disorders involving defects in the metabolism of homocysteine. The diseases are inherited as autosomal recessive illnesses, characterized by high plasma and urinary levels of homocysteine and methionine and low levels of cysteine. The most common cause of homocystinuria is a defect in the enzyme *cystathionine β-synthase*, which converts homocysteine to cystathionine (Figure 20.21). Individuals who are homozygous for *cystathionine β-synthase* deficiency exhibit ectopia lentis (displacement of the lens of the eye), skeletal abnormalities, a tendency to form thrombi (blood clots), osteoporosis, and neurological deficits. Patients can be responsive or nonresponsive to oral administration of pyridoxine (vitamin B_6)—a coenzyme of *cystathionine β-synthase*. Vitamin B_6–responsive patients usually have a milder and later onset of clinical symptoms compared with B_6-nonresponsive patients. Treatment includes restriction of methionine intake and supplementation with vitamins B_6, B_{12}, and folate.

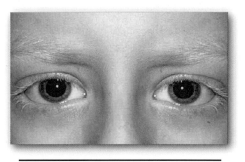

Figure 20.20
Patient with oculocutaneous albinism, showing white eyebrows and lashes.

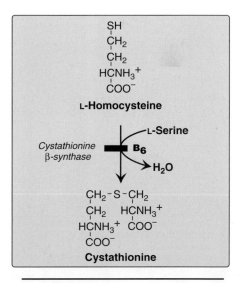

Figure 20.21
Enzyme deficiency in homocystinuria.

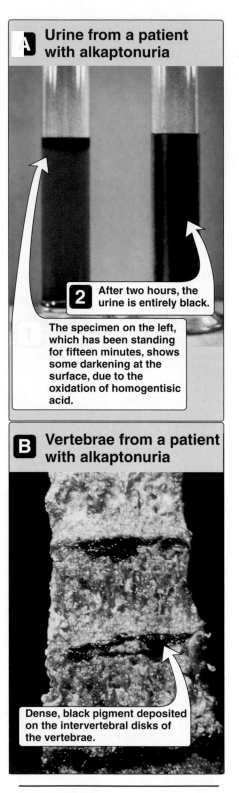

A Urine from a patient with alkaptonuria

2 After two hours, the urine is entirely black.

The specimen on the left, which has been standing for fifteen minutes, shows some darkening at the surface, due to the oxidation of homogentisic acid.

B Vertebrae from a patient with alkaptonuria

Dense, black pigment deposited on the intervertebral disks of the vertebrae.

Figure 20.22
A patient with alkaptonuria.
A. Urine. B. Vertebrae.

E. Alkaptonuria (Alcaptonuria)

Alkaptonuria is a rare metabolic condition involving a deficiency in *homogentisic acid oxidase*, resulting in the accumulation of homogentisic acid. [Note: This reaction occurs in the degradative pathway of tyrosine, p. 269.] The condition has three characteristic symptoms: homogentisic aciduria (the patient's urine contains elevated levels of homogentisic acid, which is oxidized to a dark pigment on standing, Figure 20.22A), large joint arthritis, and black ochronotic pigmentation of cartilage and collagenous tissue (Figure 20.22B). Patients with alkaptonuria are usually asymptomatic until about age 40. Dark staining of the diapers sometimes can indicate the disease in infants, but usually no symptoms are present until later in life. Diets low in protein—especially in phenylalanine and tyrosine—help reduce the levels of homogentisic acid, and decrease the amount of pigment deposited in body tissues. Although alkaptonuria is not life-threatening, the associated arthritis may be severely crippling.

VII. CHAPTER SUMMARY

Amino acids whose catabolism yields **pyruvate** or one of the **intermediates of the tricarboxylic acid cycle** are termed **glucogenic**. (Figure 20.23).They can give rise to the net formation of **glucose** in the **liver** and the **kidney**. The solely glucogenic amino acids are glutamine, glutamate, proline, arginine, histidine, alanine, serine, glycine, cysteine, methionine, valine, threonine, aspartate, and asparagine. Amino acids whose catabolism yields either **acetoacetate** or one of its precursors, **acetyl coenzyme A (CoA)** or **acetoacetyl CoA**, are termed **ketogenic**. Leucine and lysine are solely ketogenic. Tyrosine, phenylalanine, tryptophan, and isoleucine are both ketogenic and glucogenic. **Nonessential** amino acids can be synthesized from metabolic intermediates, or from the carbon skeletons of essential amino acids. **Essential amino acids** need to be obtained from the **diet**. They include histidine, methionine, threonine, valine, isoleucine, phenylalanine, tryptophan, leucine and lysine. **Phenylketonuria (PKU)** is caused by a **deficiency** of **phenylalanine hydroxylase**—the enzyme that converts phenylalanine to tyrosine. **Hyperphenylalaninemia** may also be caused by deficiencies in the enzymes that synthesize or reduce the hydroxylase's coenzyme, **tetrahydrobiopterin**. Untreated patients with PKU suffer from **mental retardation**, failure to walk or talk, seizures, hyperactivity, tremor, microcephaly, failure to grow and a characteristic smell of the urine. Treatment involves controlling dietary phenylalanine. Note that tyrosine becomes an essential dietary component for people with PKU. **Maple syrup urine disease (MSUD)** is a recessive disorder in which there is a partial or complete **deficiency** in **branched-chain α-keto acid dehydrogenase**—an enzyme that decarboxylates **leucine**, **isoleucine**, and **valine**. Symptoms include feeding problems, vomiting, dehydration, severe metabolic acidosis, and a characteristic smell of the urine. If untreated, the disease leads to **mental retardation**, physical disabilities, and death. Treatment of MSUD involves a synthetic formula that contains limited amounts of leucine, isoleucine, and valine. Other important genetic diseases associated with amino acid metabolism include **albinism**, **homocystinuria**, **methylmalonyl CoA mutase deficiency**, **alkaptonuria**, **histidinemia**, **tyrosinemia**, and **cystathioninuria**.

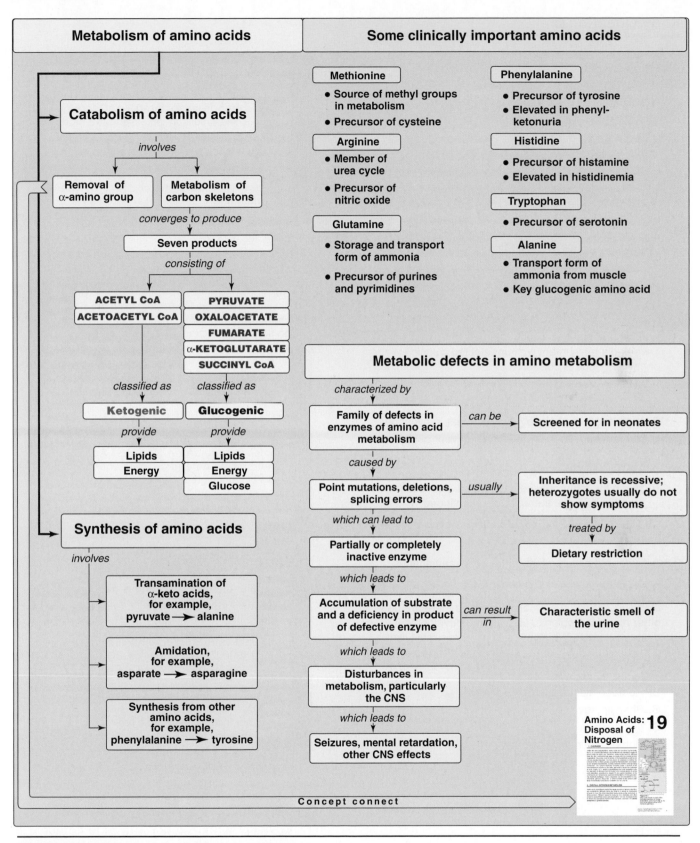

Figure 20.23
Key concept map for amino acid metabolism.

The concept map reads as follows:

Metabolism of amino acids

Catabolism of amino acids — *involves*:
- Removal of α-amino group
- Metabolism of carbon skeletons

converges to produce **Seven products** *consisting of*:
- ACETYL CoA / ACETOACETYL CoA — *classified as* **Ketogenic** — *provide* Lipids, Energy
- PYRUVATE, OXALOACETATE, FUMARATE, α-KETOGLUTARATE, SUCCINYL CoA — *classified as* **Glucogenic** — *provide* Lipids, Energy, Glucose

Synthesis of amino acids — *involves*:
- Transamination of α-keto acids, for example, pyruvate → alanine
- Amidation, for example, asparate → asparagine
- Synthesis from other amino acids, for example, phenylalanine → tyrosine

Some clinically important amino acids

Methionine
- Source of methyl groups in metabolism
- Precursor of cysteine

Arginine
- Member of urea cycle
- Precursor of nitric oxide

Glutamine
- Storage and transport form of ammonia
- Precursor of purines and pyrimidines

Phenylalanine
- Precursor of tyrosine
- Elevated in phenyl-ketonuria

Histidine
- Precursor of histamine
- Elevated in histidinemia

Tryptophan
- Precursor of serotonin

Alanine
- Transport form of ammonia from muscle
- Key glucogenic amino acid

Metabolic defects in amino metabolism — *characterized by*:
- Family of defects in enzymes of amino acid metabolism — *can be* Screened for in neonates
- *caused by* Point mutations, deletions, splicing errors — *usually* Inheritance is recessive; heterozygotes usually do not show symptoms — *treated by* Dietary restriction
- *which can lead to* Partially or completely inactive enzyme
- *which leads to* Accumulation of substrate and a deficiency in product of defective enzyme — *can result in* Characteristic smell of the urine
- *which leads to* Disturbances in metabolism, particularly the CNS
- *which leads to* Seizures, mental retardation, other CNS effects

Concept connect

Amino Acids: 19 Disposal of Nitrogen

Study Questions:

Choose the ONE correct answer.

20.1 Which one of the following statements concerning amino acids is correct?

  A. An increase in gluconeogenesis from amino acids results in a decrease in urea formation.
  B. All essential amino acids are glycogenic.
  C. Ornithine and citrulline are found in tissue proteins.
  D. Cysteine is an essential amino acid in individuals consuming a diet severely limited in methionine.
  E. In the presence of adequate dietary sources of tyrosine, phenylalanine is not an essential amino acid.

Correct answer = D. Methionine is the precursor of cysteine. An increase in the availability of gluconeogenic amino acids from the catabolism of body protein is associated with increased ammonia and results in increased urea production. The essential amino acids leucine and lysine are ketogenic. Ornithine and citrulline are amino acids that are intermediates in the urea cycle, but are not found in tissue proteins because there are no codons for them. Phenylalanine is essential regardless of the level of tyrosine.

20.2 Which one of the following statements concerning a 1-week-old male infant with undetected classic phenylketonuria is correct?

  A. Tyrosine is a nonessential amino acid for the infant.
  B. High levels of phenylpyruvate appear in his urine.
  C. Therapy must begin within the first year of life.
  D. A diet devoid of phenylalanine should be initiated immediately.
  E. When the infant reaches adulthood, it is recommended that diet therapy be discontinued.

Correct answer = B. Phenyllactate, phenylacetate, and phenylpyruvate, which are not normally produced in significant amounts in the presence of functional phenylalanine hydroxylase, are elevated in PKU, and appear in the urine. In patients with PKU, tyrosine cannot be synthesized from phenylalanine and, hence, becomes essential and must be supplied in the diet. Treatment must begin during the first 7–10 days of life to prevent mental retardation. Discontinuance of the phenylalanine-restricted diet before 8 years of age is associated with poor performance on IQ tests. Adult PKU patients show deterioration of attention and speed of mental processing after discontinuation of the diet. Elevated levels of phenylalanine are teratogenic. Lifelong restriction of dietary phenylalanine is, therefore, recommended.

20.3 A 4-year-old boy of a first-degree consanguineous couple was noted by the parents to have darkening of the urine to an almost black color when it was left standing. He has a normal sibling, and there are no other medical problems. Growth and development to date are normal. Which of the following is most likely to be elevated in this patient?

  A. Methylmalonate.
  B. Homogentisate.
  C. Phenylpyruvate.
  D. α-Ketoisovalerate.
  E. Homocysteine.

Correct answer = B. Alkaptonuria is a rare metabolic disease involving a deficiency in homogentisic acid oxidase, and the subsequent accumulation of homogentisic acid in the urine, which turns dark upon standing. The elevation of methylmalonate (due to methylmalonyl CoA mutase deficiency), phenylpyruvate (due to phenylalanine hydroxylase deficiency), α-ketoisovalerate (due to branched-chain α-keto acid dehydrogenase deficiency), and homocysteine (due to cystathionine β-synthase deficiency) are inconsistent with a healthy child with darkening of the urine.

20.4 What enzyme is deficient in: homocystinuria, methylmalonic acidemia, MSUD, oculocutaneous albinism, PKU?

Answer: Cystathionine β-synthase, methylmalonyl CoA mutase, branched-chain α-keto acid dehydrogenase, tyrosinase, phenylanine hydroxylase. [Note:Deficiency of dihydropteridine reductase or any of the enzymes needed for BH4 synthesis can also result in hyperphenylalaninemia.]

Conversion of Amino Acids to Specialized Products

21

I. OVERVIEW

In addition to serving as building blocks for proteins, amino acids are precursors of many nitrogen-containing compounds that have important physiologic functions (Figure 21.1). These molecules include porphyrins, neurotransmitters, hormones, purines, and pyrimidines.

II. PORPHYRIN METABOLISM

Porphyrins are cyclic compounds that readily bind metal ions—usually Fe^{2+} or Fe^{3+}. The most prevalent metalloporphyrin in humans is heme, which consists of one ferrous (Fe^{2+}) iron ion coordinated in the center of the tetrapyrrole ring of protoporphyrin IX (see p. 280). Heme is the prosthetic group for hemoglobin, myoglobin, the cytochromes, *catalase, nitric oxide synthase*, and *peroxidase*. These hemeproteins are rapidly synthesized and degraded. For example, 6–7 g of hemoglobin are synthesized each day to replace heme lost through the normal turnover of erythrocytes. Coordinated with the turnover of hemeproteins is the simultaneous synthesis and degradation of the associated porphyrins, and recycling of the bound iron ions.

A. Structure of porphyrins

Porphyrins are cyclic molecules formed by the linkage of four pyrrole rings through methenyl bridges (Figure 21.2). Three structural features of these molecules are relevant to understanding their medical significance.

1. **Side chains:** Different porphyrins vary in the nature of the side chains that are attached to each of the four pyrrole rings. Uroporphyrin contains acetate ($-CH_2-COO^-$) and propionate ($-CH_2-CH_2-COO^-$) side chains, coproporphyrin contains methyl ($-CH_3$) and propionate groups, and protoporphyrin IX (and heme) contains vinyl ($-CH=CH_2$), methyl, and propionate groups. [Note: The methyl and vinyl groups are produced by decarboxylation of acetate and propionate side chains, respectively.]

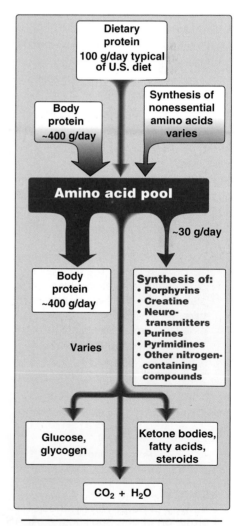

Figure 21.1
Amino acids as precursors of nitrogen-containing compounds.

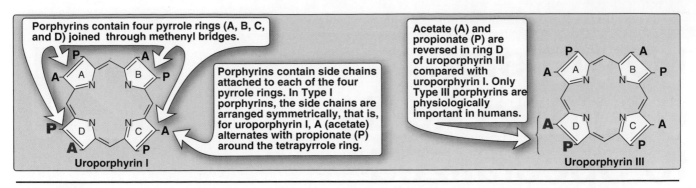

Figure 21.2
Structures of uroporphyrin I and uroporphyrin III. A = acetate and P = propionate.

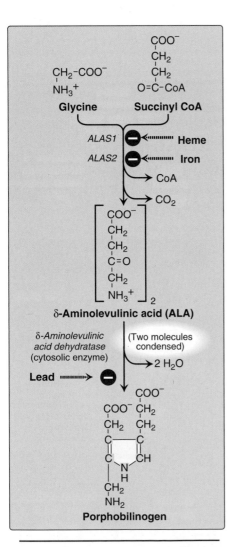

Figure 21.3
Pathway of porphyrin synthesis: Formation of porphobilinogen. *ALAS = δ-aminolevulinic acid synthase.* (Continued in Figures 21.4 and 21.5.)

2. Distribution of side chains: The side chains of porphyrins can be ordered around the tetrapyrrole nucleus in four different ways, designated by Roman numerals I to IV. Only Type III porphyrins, which contain an asymmetric substitution on ring D (see Figure 21.2), are physiologically important in humans. [Note: Protoporphyrin IX is a member of the Type III series.]

3. Porphyrinogens: These porphyrin precursors (for example, uroporphyrinogen) exist in a chemically reduced, colorless form, and serve as intermediates between porphobilinogen and the oxidized, colored protoporphyrins in heme biosynthesis.

B. Biosynthesis of heme

The major sites of heme biosynthesis are the liver, which synthesizes a number of heme proteins (particularly cytochrome P450 proteins), and the erythrocyte-producing cells of the bone marrow, which are active in hemoglobin synthesis. [Note: Over 85% of all heme synthesis occurs in erythroid tissue.] In the liver, the rate of heme synthesis is highly variable, responding to alterations in the cellular heme pool caused by fluctuating demands for heme proteins. In contrast, heme synthesis in erythroid cells is relatively constant, and is matched to the rate of globin synthesis. The initial reaction and the last three steps in the formation of porphyrins occur in mitochondria, whereas the intermediate steps of the biosynthetic pathway occur in the cytosol (see Figure 21.8). [Note: Mature red blood cells lack mitochondria and are unable to synthesize heme.]

1. Formation of δ-aminolevulinic acid (ALA): All the carbon and nitrogen atoms of the porphyrin molecule are provided by glycine (a nonessential amino acid) and succinyl coenzyme A (an intermediate in the citric acid cycle) that condense to form ALA in a reaction catalyzed by *ALA synthase* (*ALAS*) (Figure 21.3) This reaction requires pyridoxal phosphate (PLP) as a coenzyme, and is the committed and rate-limiting step in porphyrin biosynthesis. [Note: There are two isoforms of *ALAS*, 1 and 2, each controlled by different mechanisms. Erythroid tissue produces only *ALAS2*, the gene for which is located on the X-chromosome. Loss of function mutations in *ALAS2* result in X-linked sideroblastic anemia.]

a. End-product inhibition of ALAS1 by hemin: When porphyrin production exceeds the availability of the apoproteins that require it, heme accumulates and is converted to hemin by the oxidation of Fe^{2+} to Fe^{3+}. Hemin decreases the activity of hepatic *ALAS1* by causing decreased synthesis of the enzyme, through inhibition of mRNA synthesis and use (heme decreases stability of the mRNA), and by inhibiting mitochondrial import of the enzyme. [Note: In erythroid cells, *ALAS2* is controlled by the availability of intracellular iron.]

b. Effect of drugs on ALA synthase activity: Administration of any of a large number of drugs results in a significant increase in hepatic *ALAS1* activity. These drugs are metabolized by the *microsomal cytochrome P450 monooxygenase* system—a hemeprotein *oxidase* system found in the liver (see p. 149). In response to these drugs, the synthesis of cytochrome P450 proteins increases, leading to an enhanced consumption of heme—a component of cytochrome P450 proteins. This, in turn, causes a decrease in the concentration of heme in liver cells. The lower intracellular heme concentration leads to an increase in the synthesis of *ALAS1* (derepression), and prompts a corresponding increase in ALA synthesis.

2. Formation of porphobilinogen: The condensation of two molecules of ALA to form porphobilinogen by Zn-containing *ALA dehydratase* (*porphobilinogen synthase*) is extremely sensitive to inhibition by heavy metal ions, for example, lead that replace the zinc (see Figure 21.3). This inhibition is, in part, responsible for the elevation in ALA and the anemia seen in lead poisoning.

3. Formation of uroporphyrinogen: The condensation of four porphobilinogens produces the linear tetrapyrrole, hydroxymethylbilane, which is isomerized and cyclized by *uroporphyrinogen III synthase* to produce the asymmetric uroporphyrinogen III. This cyclic tetrapyrrole undergoes decarboxylation of its acetate groups, generating coproporphyrinogen III (Figure 21.4). These reactions occur in the cytosol.

4. Formation of heme: Coproporphyrinogen III enters the mitochondrion, and two propionate side chains are decarboxylated to vinyl groups generating protoporphyrinogen IX, which is oxidized to protoporphyrin IX. The introduction of iron (as Fe^{2+}) into protoporphyrin IX occurs spontaneously, but the rate is enhanced by *ferrochelatase*, an enzyme that, like *ALA dehydratase*, is inhibited by lead (Figure 21.5).

C. Porphyrias

Porphyrias are rare, inherited (or occasionally acquired) defects in heme synthesis, resulting in the accumulation and increased excretion of porphyrins or porphyrin precursors (see Figure 21.8). [Note: With few exceptions, porphyrias are inherited as autosomal dominant disorders.] The mutations that cause the porphyrias are heterogenous (not all are at the same DNA locus), and nearly every affected family has its own mutation. Each porphyria results in the accumulation of a unique pattern of intermediates caused by the deficiency of an enzyme in the heme synthetic pathway. [Note: "Porphyria" refers to the purple color caused by pigment-like porphyrins in the urine of some patients with defects in heme synthesis.]

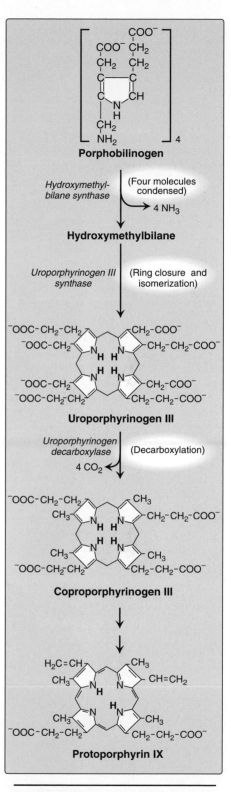

Figure 21.4
Pathway of porphyrin synthesis: Formation of protoporphyrin IX. (Continued from Figure 21.3.)

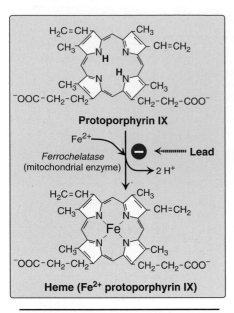

Figure 21.5
Pathway of porphyrin synthesis: Formation of heme. (Continued from Figures 21.3 and 21.4)

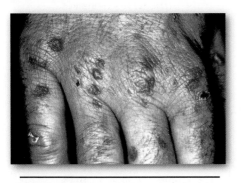

Figure 21.6
Skin eruptions in a patient with porphyria cutanea tarda.

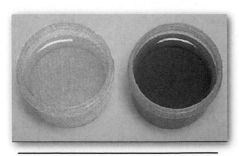

Figure 21.7
Urine from a patient with porphyria cutanea tarda (right) and from a patient with normal porphyrin excretion (left).

1. **Clinical manifestations:** The porphyrias are classified as erythropoietic or hepatic, depending on whether the enzyme deficiency occurs in the erythropoietic cells of the bone marrow or in the liver. Hepatic porphyrias can be further classified as chronic or acute. In general, individuals with an enzyme defect prior to the synthesis of the tetrapyrroles manifest abdominal and neuropsychiatric signs, whereas those with enzyme defects leading to the accumulation of tetrapyrrole intermediates show photosensitivity—that is, their skin itches and burns (pruritus) when exposed to visible light. [Note: Photosenstivity is a result of the oxidation of colorless porphyrinogens to colored porphyrins, which are photosensitizing molecules that are thought to participate in the formation of superoxide radicals from oxygen. These reactive oxygen species can oxidatively damage membranes, and cause the release of destructive enzymes from lysosomes.]

   a. **Chronic hepatic porphyria:** Porphyria cutanea tarda, the most common porphyria, is a chronic disease of the liver. The disease is associated with a deficiency in *uroporphyrinogen decarboxylase,* but clinical expression of the enzyme deficiency is influenced by various factors, such as hepatic iron overload, exposure to sunlight, alcohol ingestion, and the presence of hepatitis B or C, or HIV infections. Clinical onset is typically during the fourth or fifth decade of life. Porphyrin accumulation leads to cutaneous symptoms (Figure 21.6), and urine that is red to brown in natural light (Figure 21.7), and pink to red in fluorescent light.

   b. **Acute hepatic porphyrias:** Acute hepatic porphyrias (*ALA dehydratase* deficiency, acute intermittent porphyria, hereditary coproporphyria, and variegate porphyria) are characterized by acute attacks of gastrointestinal, neuropsychiatric, and motor symptoms that may be accompanied by photosensitivity. Porphyrias leading to accumulation of ALA and porphobilinogen, such as acute intermittent porphyria, cause abdominal pain and neuropsychiatric disturbances, ranging from anxiety to delirium. Symptoms of the acute hepatic porphyrias are often precipitated by administration of drugs such as barbiturates and ethanol, which induce the synthesis of the heme-containing cytochrome P450 microsomal drug oxidation system. This further decreases the amount of available heme, which, in turn, promotes the increased synthesis of *ALAS1*.

   c. **Erythropoietic porphyrias:** The erythropoietic porphyrias (congenital erythropoietic porphyria and erythropoietic protoporphyria) are characterized by skin rashes and blisters that appear in early childhood. The diseases are complicated by cholestatic liver cirrhosis and progressive hepatic failure.

2. **Increased ALA synthase activity:** One common feature of the porphyrias is a decreased synthesis of heme. In the liver, heme normally functions as a repressor of the gene for *ALAS1*. Therefore, the absence of this end product results in an increase in the synthesis of *ALA synthase1* (derepression). This causes an increased synthesis of intermediates that occur prior to the genetic block. The accumulation of these toxic intermediates is the major pathophysiology of the porphyrias.

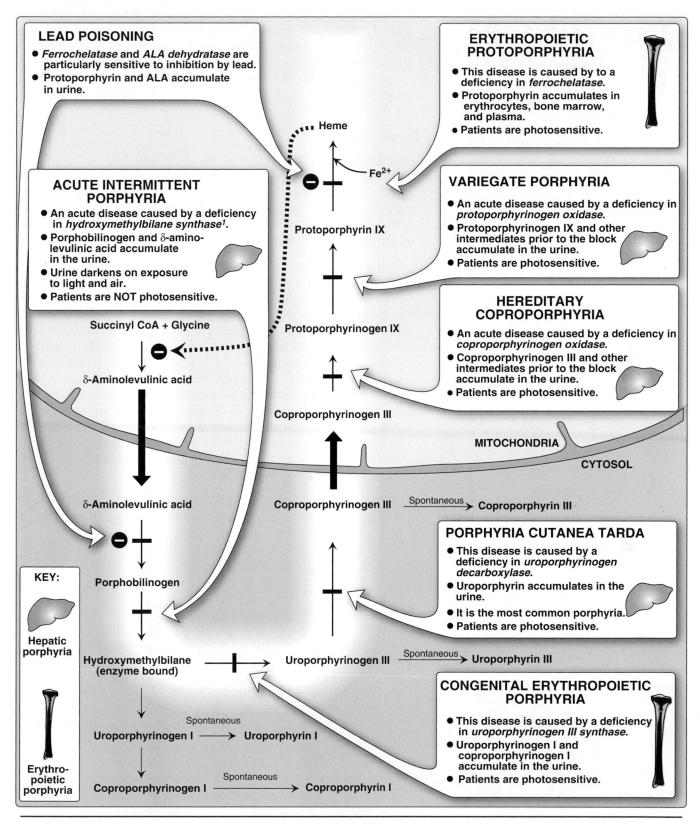

LEAD POISONING
- *Ferrochelatase* and *ALA dehydratase* are particularly sensitive to inhibition by lead.
- Protoporphyrin and ALA accumulate in urine.

ERYTHROPOIETIC PROTOPORPHYRIA
- This disease is caused by to a deficiency in *ferrochelatase*.
- Protoporphyrin accumulates in erythrocytes, bone marrow, and plasma.
- Patients are photosensitive.

ACUTE INTERMITTENT PORPHYRIA
- An acute disease caused by a deficiency in *hydroxymethylbilane synthase*[1].
- Porphobilinogen and δ-amino-levulinic acid accumulate in the urine.
- Urine darkens on exposure to light and air.
- Patients are NOT photosensitive.

VARIEGATE PORPHYRIA
- An acute disease caused by a deficiency in *protoporphyrinogen oxidase*.
- Protoporphyrinogen IX and other intermediates prior to the block accumulate in the urine.
- Patients are photosensitive.

HEREDITARY COPROPORPHYRIA
- An acute disease caused by a deficiency in *coproporphyrinogen oxidase*.
- Coproporphyrinogen III and other intermediates prior to the block accumulate in the urine.
- Patients are photosensitive.

Heme

Fe^{2+}

Protoporphyrin IX

Protoporphyrinogen IX

Coproporphyrinogen III

Succinyl CoA + Glycine

δ-Aminolevulinic acid

MITOCHONDRIA

CYTOSOL

δ-Aminolevulinic acid

Coproporphyrinogen III ──Spontaneous──> Coproporphyrin III

PORPHYRIA CUTANEA TARDA
- This disease is caused by a deficiency in *uroporphyrinogen decarboxylase*.
- Uroporphyrin accumulates in the urine.
- It is the most common porphyria.
- Patients are photosensitive.

KEY:

Hepatic porphyria

Porphobilinogen

Hydroxymethylbilane (enzyme bound)

Uroporphyrinogen III ──Spontaneous──> Uroporphyrin III

Erythro-poietic porphyria

Uroporphyrinogen I ──Spontaneous──> Uroporphyrin I

Coproporphyrinogen I ──Spontaneous──> Coproporphyrin I

CONGENITAL ERYTHROPOIETIC PORPHYRIA
- This disease is caused by a deficiency in *uroporphyrinogen III synthase*.
- Uroporphyrinogen I and coproporphyrinogen I accumulate in the urine.
- Patients are photosensitive.

Figure 21.8
Summary of heme synthesis. [1]Also referred to as *porphobilinogen deaminase*.

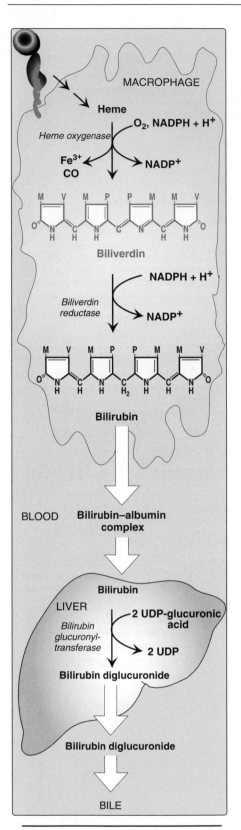

Figure 21.9
Formation of bilirubin from heme.
UDP = uridine diphosphate.

3. Treatment: During acute porphyria attacks, patients require medical support, particularly treatment for pain and vomiting. The severity of symptoms of the porphyrias can be diminished by intravenous injection of hemin and glucose, which decreases the synthesis of *ALAS1*. Avoidance of sunlight and ingestion of β-carotene (a free-radical scavenger) are helpful in porphyrias with photosensitivity.

D. Degradation of heme

After approximately 120 days in the circulation, red blood cells are taken up and degraded by the reticuloendothelial system, particularly in the liver and spleen (Figure 21.9). Approximately 85% of heme destined for degradation comes from senescent red blood cells, and 15% is from turnover of immature red blood cells and cytochromes from nonerythroid tissues.

1. Formation of bilirubin: The first step in the degradation of heme is catalyzed by the microsomal *heme oxygenase* system of the reticuloendothelial cells. In the presence of NADPH and O_2, the enzyme adds a hydroxyl group to the methenyl bridge between two pyrrole rings, with a concomitant oxidation of ferrous iron to Fe^{3+}. A second oxidation by the same enzyme system results in cleavage of the porphyrin ring. The green pigment biliverdin is produced as ferric iron and CO are released (see Figure 21.9). [Note: The CO has biologic function, acting as a signaling molecule and vasodilator.] Biliverdin is reduced, forming the red-orange bilirubin. Bilirubin and its derivatives are collectively termed bile pigments. [Note: The changing colors of a bruise reflect the varying pattern of intermediates that occurs during heme degradation.]

> Bilirubin, unique to mammals, appears to function as an antioxidant. In this role, it is oxidized to biliverdin, which is then reduced by *biliverdin reductase*, regenerating bilirubin.

2. Uptake of bilirubin by the liver: Bilirubin is only slightly soluble in plasma and, therefore, is transported to the liver by binding noncovalently to albumin. [Note: Certain anionic drugs, such as salicylates and sulfonamides, can displace bilirubin from albumin, permitting bilirubin to enter the central nervous system. This causes the potential for neural damage in infants.] Bilirubin dissociates from the carrier albumin molecule, enters a hepatocyte via facilitated diffusion, and binds to intracellular proteins, particularly the protein ligandin.

3. Formation of bilirubin diglucuronide: In the hepatocyte, the solubility of bilirubin is increased by the addition of two molecules of glucuronic acid. [Note: This process is referred to as conjugation.] The reaction is catalyzed by microsomal *bilirubin glucuronyltransferase* using uridine diphosphate-glucuronic acid as the glucuronate donor. [Note: Varying degrees of deficiency of this enzyme result in Crigler-Najjar I and II and Gilbert syndrome, with Crigler-Najjar I being the most severe deficiency.]

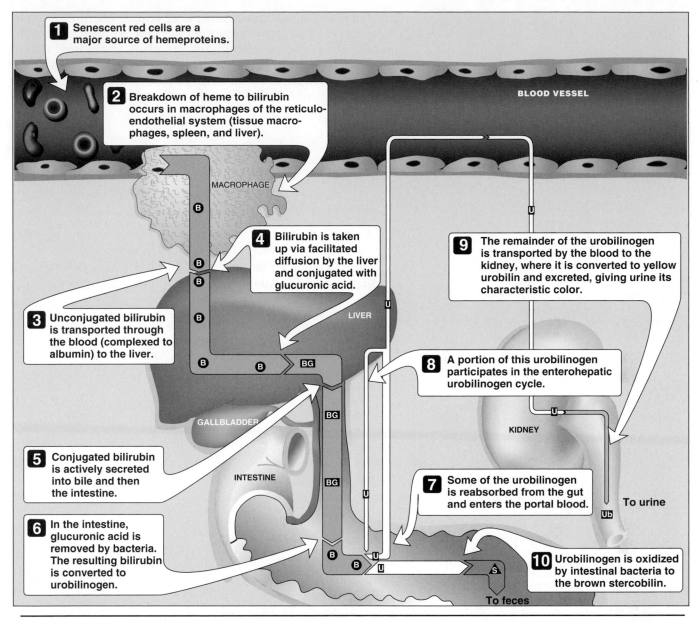

Figure 21.10
Catabolism of heme **B** = bilirubin; **BG** = bilirubin diglucuronide; **U** = urobilinogen; **Ub** = urobilin; **S** = stercobilin.

4. Secretion of bilirubin into bile: Bilirubin diglucuronide (conjugated bilirubin) is actively transported against a concentration gradient into the bile canaliculi and then into the bile. This energy-dependent, rate-limiting step is susceptible to impairment in liver disease. [Note: A deficiency in the protein required for transport of conjugated bilirubin out of the liver results in Dubin-Johnson syndrome.] Unconjugated bilirubin is normally not secreted.

5. Formation of urobilins in the intestine: Bilirubin diglucuronide is hydrolyzed and reduced by bacteria in the gut to yield urobilinogen, a colorless compound. Most of the urobilinogen is oxidized by intestinal bacteria to stercobilin, which gives feces the characteristic brown color. However, some of the urobilinogen is reabsorbed from the gut and enters the portal blood. A portion of

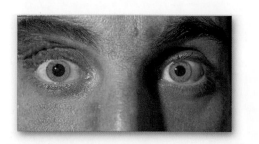

Figure 21.11
Jaundiced patient, with the sclerae of his eyes appearing yellow.

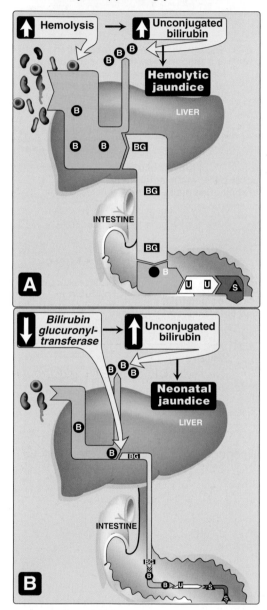

Figure 21.12
Alterations in the metabolism of heme.
A. Hemolytic jaundice. B. Neonatal jaundice.
BG = bilirubin glucuronide; B = bilirubin;
U = urobilinogen; S = stercobilin.

this urobilinogen participates in the enterohepatic urobilinogen cycle in which it is taken up by the liver, and then resecreted into the bile. The remainder of the urobilinogen is transported by the blood to the kidney, where it is converted to yellow urobilin and excreted, giving urine its characteristic color. The metabolism of bilirubin is summarized in Figure 21.10.

E. Jaundice

Jaundice (also called icterus) refers to the yellow color of skin, nail beds, and sclerae (whites of the eyes) caused by deposition of bilirubin, secondary to increased bilirubin levels in the blood (hyperbilirubinemia, Figure 21.11). Although not a disease, jaundice is usually a symptom of an underlying disorder.

1. **Types of jaundice:** Jaundice can be classified into three major forms described below. However, in clinical practice, jaundice is often more complex than indicated in this simple classification. For example, the accumulation of bilirubin may be a result of defects at more than one step in its metabolism.

   a. **Hemolytic jaundice:** The liver has the capacity to conjugate and excrete over 3,000 mg of bilirubin per day, whereas the normal production of bilirubin is only 300 mg/day. This excess capacity allows the liver to respond to increased heme degradation with a corresponding increase in conjugation and secretion of bilirubin diglucuronide. However, massive lysis of red blood cells (for example, in patients with sickle cell anemia, *pyruvate kinase* or *glucose 6-phosphate dehydrogenase* deficiency) may produce bilirubin faster than it can be conjugated. Unconjugated bilirubin levels in the blood become elevated, causing jaundice (Figure 21.12A). [Note: More conjugated bilirubin is excreted into the bile, the amount of urobilinogen entering the enterohepatic circulation is increased, and urinary urobilinogen is increased.]

   b. **Hepatocellular jaundice:** Damage to liver cells (for example, in patients with cirrhosis or hepatitis) can cause unconjugated bilirubin levels in the blood to increase as a result of decreased conjugation. Urobilinogen is increased in the urine because hepatic damage decreases the enterohepatic circulation of this compound, allowing more to enter the blood, from which it is filtered into the urine. The urine thus darkens, whereas stools may be a pale, clay color. Plasma levels of *AST* and *ALT* (see p. 251) are elevated. [Note: If conjugated bilirubin is not efficiently secreted from the liver into bile (intrahepatic cholestasis), it can diffuse ("leak") into the blood, causing a conjugated hyperbilirubinemia.]

   c. **Obstructive jaundice:** In this instance, jaundice is not caused by overproduction of bilirubin or decreased conjugation, but instead results from obstruction of the bile duct (extrahepatic cholestasis). For example, the presence of a tumor or bile stones may block the bile ducts, preventing passage of bilirubin into the intestine. Patients with obstructive jaundice experience gastrointestinal pain and nausea, and produce stools that are a pale, clay color, and urine that darkens upon standing. The liver "regurgitates" conjugated bilirubin into the blood (hyperbilirubinemia). The compound is eventually excreted in the urine. Urinary urobiloinogen is absent. [Note: Prolonged obstruction of the bile duct can lead to liver damage and a subsequent rise in unconjugated bilirubin.]

2. **Jaundice in newborns:** Newborn infants, particularly if premature, often accumulate bilirubin, because the activity of hepatic *bilirubin glucuronyltransferase* is low at birth—it reaches adult levels in about 4 weeks (Figures 21.12B and 21.13). Elevated bilirubin, in excess of the binding capacity of albumin, can diffuse into the basal ganglia and cause toxic encephalopathy (kernicterus). Thus, newborns with significantly elevated bilirubin levels are treated with blue fluorescent light (Figure 21.14), which converts bilirubin to more polar and, hence, water-soluble isomers. These photoisomers can be excreted into the bile without conjugation to glucuronic acid.

3. **Determination of bilirubin concentration:** Bilirubin is most commonly determined by the van den Bergh reaction, in which diazotized sulfanilic acid reacts with bilirubin to form red azodipyrroles that are measured colorimetrically. In aqueous solution, the water-soluble, conjugated bilirubin reacts rapidly with the reagent (within one minute), and is said to be "direct-reacting." The unconjugated bilirubin, which is much less soluble in aqueous solution, reacts more slowly. However, when the reaction is carried out in methanol, both conjugated and unconjugated bilirubin are soluble and react with the reagent, providing the total bilirubin value. The "indirect-reacting" bilirubin, which corresponds to the unconjugated bilirubin, is obtained by subtracting the direct-reacting bilirubin from the total bilirubin. [Note: In normal plasma, only about 4% of the total bilirubin is conjugated or direct-reacting, because most is secreted into bile.]

III. OTHER NITROGEN-CONTAINING COMPOUNDS

A. Catecholamines

Dopamine, norepinephrine, and epinephrine are biologically active (biogenic) amines that are collectively termed catecholamines. Dopamine and norepinephrine are synthesized in the brain and function as neurotransmitters. Norepinephrine is also synthesized in the adrenal medulla, as is epinephrine.

1. **Function:** Outside the nervous system, norepinephrine and its methylated derivative, epinephrine, are hormone regulators of carbohydrate and lipid metabolism. Norepinephrine and epinephrine are released from storage vesicles in the adrenal medulla in response to fright, exercise, cold, and low levels of blood glucose. They increase the degradation of glycogen and triacylglycerol, as well as increase blood pressure and the output of the heart. These effects are part of a coordinated response to prepare the individual for stress, and are often called the "fight-or-flight" reactions.

2. **Synthesis of catecholamines:** The catecholamines are synthesized from tyrosine, as shown in Figure 21.15. Tyrosine is first hydroxylated by *tyrosine hydroxylase* to form 3,4-dihydroxyphenyl-

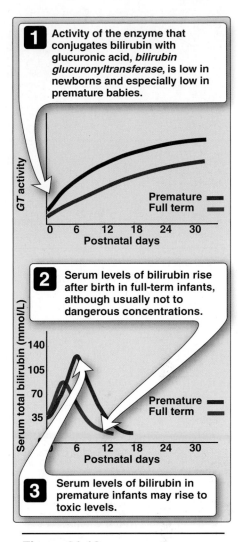

1 Activity of the enzyme that conjugates bilirubin with glucuronic acid, *bilirubin glucuronyltransferase*, is low in newborns and especially low in premature babies.

GT activity

Premature
Full term

0   6   12   18   24   30
Postnatal days

2 Serum levels of bilirubin rise after birth in full-term infants, although usually not to dangerous concentrations.

Serum total bilirubin (mmol/L)

140
105
70
35

6   12   18   24   30
Postnatal days

Premature
Full term

3 Serum levels of bilirubin in premature infants may rise to toxic levels.

Figure 21.13
Neonatal jaundice. *GT* = *glucuronyltransferase.*

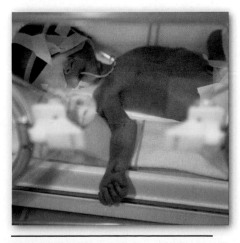

Figure 21.14
Phototherapy in neonatal jaudice

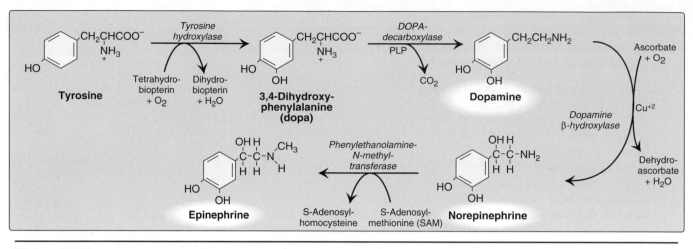

Figure 21.15
Synthesis of catecholamines. PLP = pyridoxal phosphate.

alanine (DOPA) in a reaction analogous to that described for the hydroxylation of phenylalanine (see p. 268). The tetrahydro-biopterin (BH$_4$)-requiring enzyme is abundant in the central nervous system, the sympathetic ganglia, and the adrenal medulla, and is the rate-limiting step of the pathway. DOPA is decarboxylated in a reaction requiring pyridoxal phosphate (PLP, see p. 378) to form dopamine, which is hydroxylated by *dopamine β-hydroxylase* to yield norepinephrine in a reaction that requires ascorbate (vitamin C) and copper. Epinephrine is formed from norepinephrine by an N-methylation reaction using S-adenosylmethionine (SAM) as the methyl donor (see p. 264).

> Parkinson disease, a neurodegenerative movement disorder, is due to insufficient dopamine production as a result of the idiopathic loss of dopamine-producing cells in the brain. Administration of L-DOPA (levodopa) is the most common treatment.

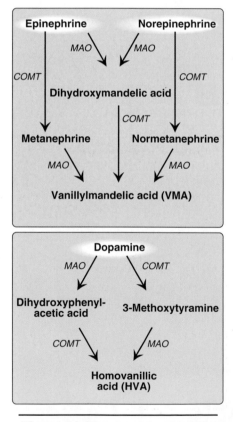

Figure 21.16
Metabolism of the catecholamines by *catechol-O-methyltranferase* (*COMT*) and *monoamine oxidase* (*MAO*).

3. **Degradation of catecholamines:** The catecholamines are inactivated by oxidative deamination catalyzed by *monoamine oxidase* (*MAO*), and by O-methylation carried out by *catechol-O-methyltransferase* using SAM as the methyl donor (Figure 21.16). The two reactions can occur in either order. The aldehyde products of the *MAO* reaction are oxidized to the corresponding acids. The metabolic products of these reactions are excreted in the urine as vanillylmandelic acid (VMA) from epinephrine and norepinephrine, and homovanillic acid from dopamine. [Note: VMA is increased with pheochromocytomas, tumors of the adrenal characterized by excessive production of catecholamines.]

4. **MAO inhibitors:** *MAO* is found in neural and other tissues, such as the intestine and liver. In the neuron, this enzyme oxidatively deaminates and inactivates any excess neurotransmitter molecules (norepinephrine, dopamine, or serotonin) that may

leak out of synaptic vesicles when the neuron is at rest. *MAO* inhibitors may irreversibly or reversibly inactivate the enzyme, permitting neurotransmitter molecules to escape degradation and, therefore, to both accumulate within the presynaptic neuron and to leak into the synaptic space. This causes activation of norepinephrine and serotonin receptors, and may be responsible for the antidepressant action of these drugs.

B. Histamine

Histamine is a chemical messenger that mediates a wide range of cellular responses, including allergic and inflammatory reactions, gastric acid secretion, and possibly neurotransmission in parts of the brain. A powerful vasodilator, histamine is formed by decarboxylation of histidine in a reaction requiring PLP (Figure 21.17). It is secreted by mast cells as a result of allergic reactions or trauma. Histamine has no clinical applications, but agents that interfere with the action of histamine have important therapeutic applications.

C. Serotonin

Serotonin, also called 5-hydroxytryptamine (5HT), is synthesized and stored at several sites in the body (Figure 21.18). By far the largest amount of serotonin is found in cells of the intestinal mucosa. Smaller amounts occur in the central nervous system, where it functions as a neurotransmitter, and in platelets. Serotonin is synthesized from tryptophan, which is hydroxylated in a BH_4-requiring reaction analogous to that catalyzed by *phenylalanine hydroxylase*. The product, 5-hydroxytryptophan, is decarboxylated to serotonin, which is also degraded by *MAO*. Serotonin has multiple physiologic roles, including pain perception, regulation of sleep, appetite, temperature, blood pressure, cognitive functions, and mood (causes a feeling of well-being). [Note: Serotonin is converted to melatonin in the pineal gland via acetylation and methylation.]

D. Creatine

Creatine phosphate (also called phosphocreatine), the phosphorylated derivative of creatine found in muscle, is a high-energy compound that provides a small but rapidly mobilized reserve of high-energy phosphates that can be reversibly transferred to ADP (Figure 21.9) to maintain the intracellular level of ATP during the first few minutes of intense muscular contraction. [Note: The amount of creatine phosphate in the body is proportional to the muscle mass.]

1. **Synthesis:** Creatine is synthesized from glycine and the guanidino group of arginine, plus a methyl group from SAM (see Figure 21.19). Creatine is reversibly phosphorylated to creatine phosphate by *creatine kinase*, using ATP as the phosphate donor. [Note: The presence of *creatine kinase* (MB isozyme) in the plasma is indicative of heart damage, and is used in the diagnosis of myocardial infarction (see p. 65).]

2. **Degradation:** Creatine and creatine phosphate spontaneously cyclize at a slow but constant rate to form creatinine, which is excreted in the urine. The amount of creatinine excreted is propor-

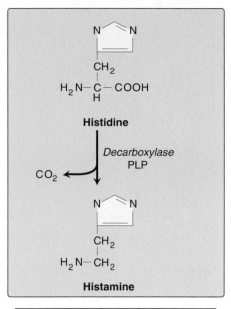

Figure 21.17
Biosynthesis of histamine. PLP = pyridoxal phosphate.

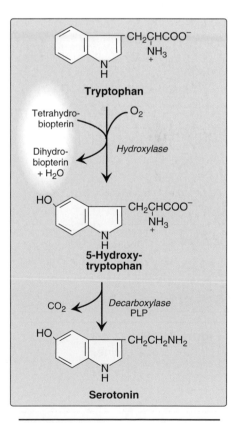

Figure 21.18
Synthesis of serotonin. PLP = pyridoxal phosphate.

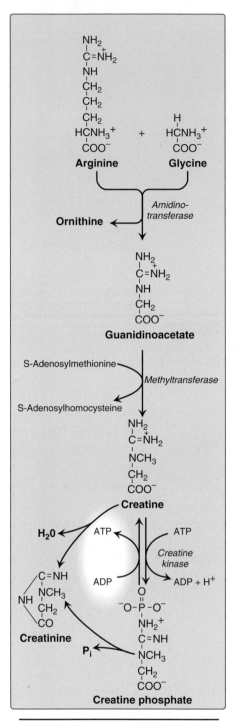

Figure 21.19
Synthesis of creatine.

tional to the total creatine phosphate content of the body, and thus can be used to estimate muscle mass. When muscle mass decreases for any reason (for example, from paralysis or muscular dystrophy), the creatinine content of the urine falls. In addition, any rise in blood creatinine is a sensitive indicator of kidney malfunction, because creatinine normally is rapidly removed from the blood and excreted. A typical adult male excretes about 15 mmol of creatinine per day.

E. Melanin

Melanin is a pigment that occurs in several tissues, particularly the eye, hair, and skin. It is synthesized from tyrosine in the epidermis by pigment-forming cells called melanocytes. Its function is to protect underlying cells from the harmful effects of sunlight. [Note: A defect in melanin production results in albinism, the most common form being due to defects in copper-containing *tyrosinase* (see p. 273).]

IV. CHAPTER SUMMARY

Amino acids are precursors of many nitrogen-containing compounds including **porphyrins**, which, in combination with ferrous (Fe^{2+}) iron, form **heme** (Figure 21.20). The major sites of **heme biosynthesis** are the **liver**, which synthesizes a number of heme proteins (particularly cytochrome P450), and the **erythrocyte-producing cells** of the bone marrow, which are active in hemoglobin synthesis. In the liver, the rate of heme synthesis is highly variable, responding to alterations in the cellular heme pool caused by fluctuating demands for hemeproteins. In contrast, heme synthesis in erythroid cells is relatively constant, and is matched to the rate of globin synthesis. **Porphyrin synthesis** start with **glycine** and **succinyl CoA**. The **committed step** in heme synthesis is the formation of δ-aminolevulinic acid (ALA). This reaction is catalyzed by **ALA synthase-1** in liver (inhibited by hemin, the oxidized form of heme that accumulates in the cell when heme is being underutilized) and ALA synthase-2 in erythroid tissues (regulated by iron). **Porphyrias** are caused by inherited or acquired defects in heme synthesis, resulting in the accumulation and increased excretion of porphyrins or porphyrin precursors. With few exceptions, **porphyrias** are inherited as **autosomal dominant** disorders. **Degradation** of hemeproteins occurs in the **reticuloendothelial system**, particularly in the **liver** and **spleen**. The first step in the degradation of heme is the production of the green pigment **biliverdin**, which is subsequently reduced to **bilirubin**. Bilirubin is transported to the liver, where its solubility is increased by the addition of two molecules of **glucuronic acid**. Bilirubin diglucuronide is transported into the **bile canaliculi**, where it is first hydrolyzed and reduced by bacteria in the gut to yield **urobilinogen**, then oxidized by intestinal bacteria to **stercobilin**. **Jaundice** refers to the yellow color of the skin and sclera that is caused by deposition of bilirubin, secondary to increased bilirubin levels in the blood. Three commonly encountered type of jaundice are **hemolytic jaundice**, **obstructive jaundice**, and **hepatocellular jaundice**. Other important N-containing compounds derived from amino acids include the **catecholamines** (dopamine, norepinephrine, and epinephrine), **creatine**, **histamine**, **serotonin**, and **melanin**.

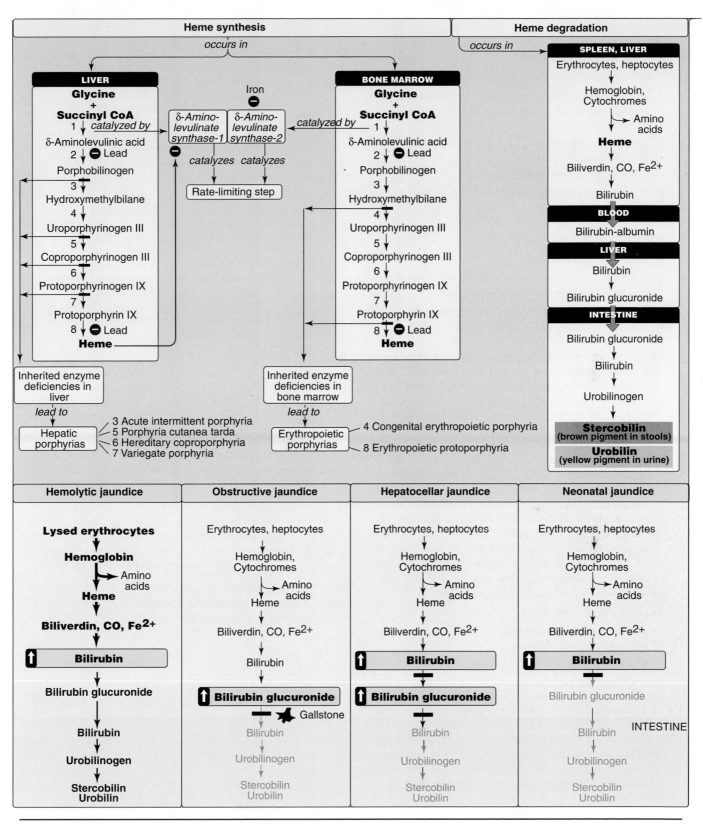

Figure 21.20
Key concept map for heme metabolism. ▬ = Block in the pathway.

Study Questions

Choose the ONE best answer.

21.1 δ-Aminolevulinic acid synthase activity:

    A. in liver is frequently decreased in individuals treated with drugs, such as the barbiturate phenobarbital.

    B. catalyzes a rate-limiting reaction in porphyrin biosynthesis.

    C. requires the coenzyme biotin.

    D. is strongly inhibited by heavy metal ions such as lead.

    E. occurs in the cytosol.

> Correct answer = B. The activity of δ-aminolevulinic acid synthase controls the rate of porphyrin synthesis. The hepatic form of the enzyme is increased in patients treated with certain drugs, and requires pyridoxal phosphate as a coenzyme. Another enzyme in the pathway (δ-aminolevulinic acid dehydrase) is extremely sensitive to the presence of heavy metals.

21.2 The catabolism of hemoglobin:

    A. occurs in red blood cells.

    B. involves the oxidative cleavage of the porphyrin ring.

    C. results in the liberation of carbon dioxide.

    D. results in the formation of protoporphyrinogen.

    E. is the sole source of bilirubin.

> Correct answer = B. The cyclic heme molecule is oxidatively cleaved to form biliverdin. The catabolism occurs in the cells of the reticuloendothelial system, particularly the spleen, and results in the liberation of carbon monoxide. Protoporphyrinogen is an intermediate in the synthesis, not degradation, of heme. Cytochromes and other non-hemoglobin hemeproteins are also precursors of bilirubin.

21.3 A 50-year-old man presented with painful blisters on the backs of his hands. He was a golf instructor, and indicated that the blisters had erupted shortly after the golfing season began. He did not have recent exposure to poison ivy or sumac, new soaps or detergents, or new medications. He denied having previous episodes of blistering. He had partial complex seizure disorder that had begun about three years earlier after a head injury. The patient had been taking phenytoin—his only medication—since the onset of the seizure disorder. He admitted to an average weekly ethanol intake of about eighteen 12-oz cans of beer. The patient's urine was reddish orange. Cultures obtained from skin lesions failed to grow organisms. A 24-hour urine collection showed elevated uroporphyrin (1,000 mg; normal, <27mg). The most likely presumptive diagnosis is:

    A. porphyria cutanea tarda.

    B. acute intermittent porphyria.

    C. hereditary coproporphyria.

    D. congenital erythropoietic porphyria.

    E. erythropoietic protoporphyria.

> Correct answer = A. The disease is associated with a deficiency in uroporphyrinogen decarboxylase, but clinical expression of the enzyme deficiency is influenced by hepatic injury caused by iron overload, chronic ethanol consumption, and the presence of hepatitis B or C and HIV infections. Exposure to sunlight can also be a precipitating factor. Clinical onset is typically during the fourth or fifth decade of life. Porphyrin accumulation leads to cutaneous symptoms and urine that is red to brown. Treatment of the patient's seizure disorder with phenytoin caused increased synthesis of ALA synthase, and, therefore, of uroporphyrinogen, the substrate of the deficient enzyme. The laboratory and clinical findings are inconsistent with other porphyrias.

21.4 A 10-year-old boy is referred to a specialist because of skin that blisters easily, urine that darkens on standing, and stained teeth. Lab studies are remarkable for high levels of uroporphyrin I and coproporphyrin I in plasma, with uroporphyrin I being present in the urine. The most likely biochemical pathology in this case is:

    A. deficiency of ALA synthase.

    B. deficiency of bilirubin glucuronyltransferase.

    C. deficiency of uroporphyrinogen III synthase.

    D. down-regulation of tyrosinase.

    E. inhibition of ALA dehydratase by lead.

> Correct answer = C. A deficiency of uroporphyrinogen III synthase results in accumulation of hydroxymethylbilane and the spontaneous conversion of this substrate to porphyrins of the Type I series. A deficiency of ALA synthase or inhibition of ALA dehydratase by lead would not allow the synthesis of porphobilinogen, the first pyrrole product in the heme biosynthetic pathway, and thus would not result in uro- or coproporphyrin synthesis. Deficiency of the glucuronyltransferase would not present with the systems described, and lab studies would be remarkable for an elevation of unconjugated bilirubin. Down-regulation of tyrosinase would result in decreased pigmentation.

Nucleotide Metabolism

22

I. OVERVIEW

Ribonucleoside and deoxyribonucleoside phosphates (nucleotides) are essential for all cells. Without them, neither RNA nor DNA can be produced and, therefore, proteins cannot be synthesized or cells proliferate. Nucleotides also serve as carriers of activated intermediates in the synthesis of some carbohydrates, lipids, and conjugated proteins, for example, UDP-glucose and CDP-choline, and are structural components of several essential coenzymes, such as coenzyme A, FAD, NAD$^+$, and NADP$^+$. Nucleotides, such as cyclic adenosine monophosphate (cAMP) and cyclic guanosine monophosphate (cGMP), serve as second messengers in signal transduction pathways. In addition, nucleotides play an important role as "energy currency" in the cell. Finally, nucleotides are important regulatory compounds for many of the pathways of intermediary metabolism, inhibiting or activating key enzymes. The purine and pyrimidine bases found in nucleotides can be synthesized <u>de novo</u>, or can be obtained through salvage pathways that allow the reuse of the preformed bases resulting from normal cell turnover. [Note: Little of the purines and pyrimidines supplied by diet are utilized, and are degraded instead.]

II. NUCLEOTIDE STRUCTURE

Nucleotides are composed of a nitrogenous base, a pentose monosaccharide, and one, two, or three phosphate groups. The nitrogen-containing bases belong to two families of compounds: the purines and the pyrimidines.

A. Purine and pyrimidine structures

Both DNA and RNA contain the same purine bases: adenine (A) and guanine (G). Both DNA and RNA contain the pyrimidine cytosine (C), but they differ in their second pyrimidine base: DNA contains thymine (T), whereas RNA contains uracil (U). T and U differ in that only T has a methyl group (Figure 22.1). [Note: Unusual (modified) bases are

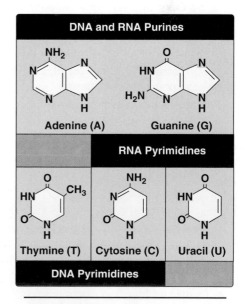

Figure 22.1
Purines and pyrimidines commonly found in DNA and RNA.

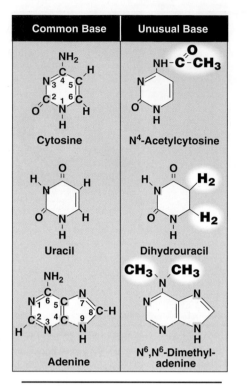

Figure 22.2
Examples of unusual bases.

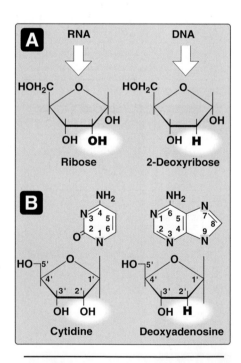

Figure 22.3
A. Pentoses found in nucleic acids.
B. Examples of the numbering systems for purine- and pyrimidine-containing nucleosides.

occasionally found in some species of DNA and RNA, for example, in some viral DNA, and in transfer RNA. Base modifications include methylation, glycosylation, acetylation, or reduction. Some examples of unusual bases are shown in Figure 22.2. The presence of an unusual base in a nucleotide sequence may aid in its recognition by specific enzymes, or protect it from being degraded by *nucleases*.]

B. Nucleosides

The addition of a pentose sugar to a base produces a nucleoside. If the sugar is ribose, a ribonucleoside is produced; if the sugar is 2-deoxyribose, a deoxyribonucleoside is produced (Figure 22.3A). The ribonucleosides of A, G, C, and U are named adenosine, guanosine, cytidine, and uridine, respectively. The deoxyribonucleosides of A, G, C, and T have the added prefix, "deoxy-," for example, deoxyadenosine. [Note: The compound deoxythymidine is often simply called thymidine, with the "deoxy-" prefix being understood.] The carbon and nitrogen atoms in the rings of the base and the sugar are numbered separately (Figure 22.3B). Note that the carbons in the pentose are numbered 1' to 5'. Thus, when the 5'-carbon of a nucleoside (or nucleotide) is referred to, a carbon atom in the pentose, rather than an atom in the base, is being specified.

C. Nucleotides

The addition of one or more phosphate groups to a nucleoside produces a nucleotide. The first phosphate group is attached by an ester linkage to the 5'-OH of the pentose. Such a compound is called a nucleoside 5'-phosphate or a 5'-nucleotide. The type of pentose is denoted by the prefix in the names "5'-ribonucleotide" and "5'-deoxyribonucleotide." If one phosphate group is attached to the 5'-carbon of the pentose, the structure is a nucleoside monophosphate, like adenosine monophosphate (AMP) (also called adenylate). If a second or third phosphate is added to the nucleoside, a nucleoside diphosphate (for example, adenosine diphosphate or ADP) or triphosphate (for example, adenosine triphosphate or ATP) results (Figure 22.4). The second and third phosphates are each connected to the nucleotide by a "high-energy" bond. [Note: The phosphate groups are responsible for the negative charges associated with nucleotides, and cause DNA and RNA to be referred to as "nucleic acids."]

III. SYNTHESIS OF PURINE NUCLEOTIDES

The atoms of the purine ring are contributed by a number of compounds, including amino acids (aspartic acid, glycine, and glutamine), CO_2, and N^{10}–formyltetrahydrofolate (Figure 22.5). The purine ring is constructed primarily in the liver by a series of reactions that add the donated carbons and nitrogens to a preformed ribose 5-phosphate. (See p. 147 for the synthesis of ribose 5-phosphate by the pentose phosphate pathway).

A. Synthesis of 5-phosphoribosyl-1-pyrophosphate (PRPP)

PRPP is an "activated pentose" that participates in the synthesis and salvage of purines and pyrimidines. Synthesis of PRPP from ATP and ribose 5-phosphate is catalyzed by *PRPP synthetase (ribose phosphate pyrophosphokinase,* Figure 22.6). This X-linked enzyme is activated by inorganic phosphate and inhibited by purine nucleotides (end-product inhibition). [Note: The sugar moiety of PRPP is ribose, and, therefore, ribonucleotides are the end products of <u>de novo</u> purine synthesis. When deoxyribonucleotides are required for DNA synthesis, the ribose sugar moiety is reduced (see p. 297).]

B. Synthesis of 5'-phosphoribosylamine

Synthesis of 5'-phosphoribosylamine from PRPP and glutamine is shown in Figure 22.7. The amide group of glutamine replaces the pyrophosphate group attached to carbon 1 of PRPP. The enzyme, *glutamine:phosphoribosylpyrophosphate amidotransferase,* is inhibited by the purine 5'-nucleotides AMP and GMP—the end products of the pathway. This is the committed step in purine nucleotide biosynthesis. The rate of the reaction is also controlled by the intracellular concentration of PRPP. [Note: The intracellular concentration of PRPP is normally far below the K_m for the *amidotransferase.* Therefore, any small change in the PRPP concentration causes a proportional change in the rate of the reaction (see p. 59).]

C. Synthesis of inosine monophosphate, the "parent" purine nucleotide

The next nine steps in purine nucleotide biosynthesis leading to the synthesis of inosine monophosphate (IMP, whose base is hypoxanthine) are illustrated in Figure 22.7. This pathway requires ATP as an energy source. Two steps in the pathway require N^{10}-formyltetrahydrofolate (see p. 267).

D. Synthetic inhibitors of purine synthesis

Some synthetic inhibitors of purine synthesis (for example, the sulfonamides[1]), are designed to inhibit the growth of rapidly dividing microorganisms without interfering with human cell functions (see Figure 22.7). Other purine synthesis inhibitors, such as structural analogs of folic acid (for example, methotrexate[2]), are used pharmacologically to control the spread of cancer by interfering with the synthesis of nucleotides and, therefore, of DNA and RNA (see Figure 22.7).

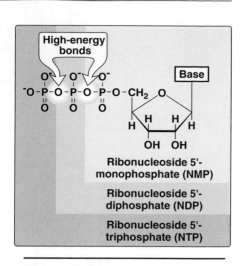

Figure 22.4
Ribonucleoside monophosphate, diphosphate, and triphosphate.

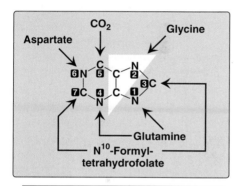

Figure 22.5
Sources of the individual atoms in the purine ring. The order in which the atoms are added is shown by the numbers in the black boxes (see Figure 22.7).

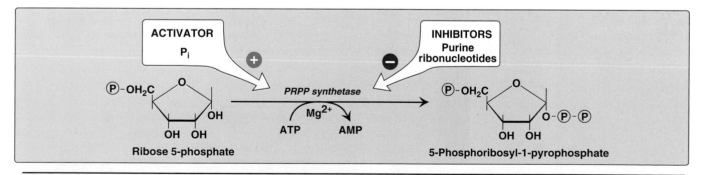

Figure 22.6
Synthesis of 5-phosphoribosyl-1-pyrophosphate (PRPP), showing the activator and inhibitors of the reaction.

[1,2]See Chapter 33 in ***Lippincott's Illustrated Reviews: Pharmacology*** for a discussion of sulfonamides and methotrexate.

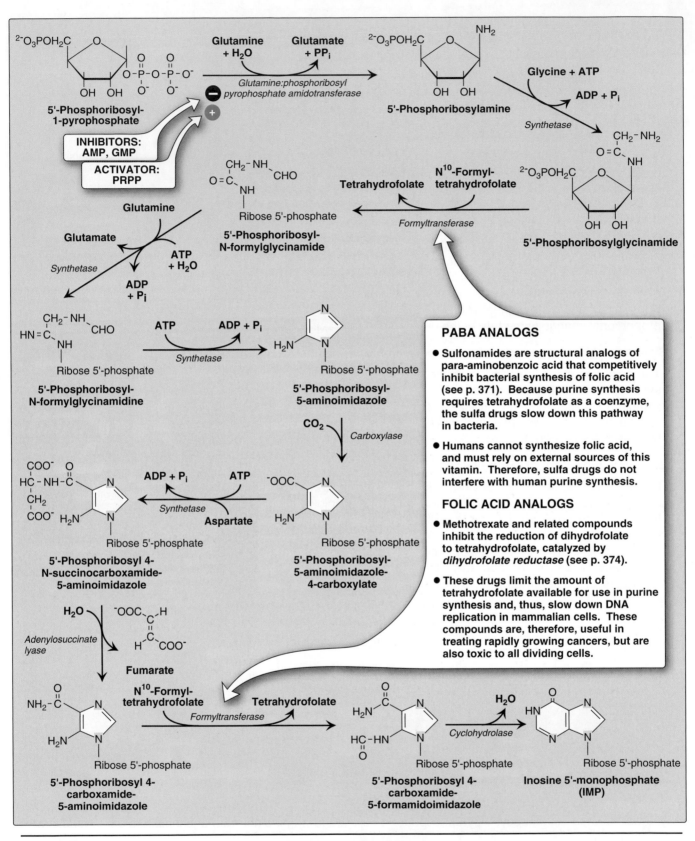

Figure 22.7
Synthesis of purine nucleotides, showing the inhibitory effect of some structural analogs.

Inhibitors of human purine synthesis are extremely toxic to tissues, especially to developing structures such as in a fetus, or to cell types that normally replicate rapidly, including those of bone marrow, skin, gastrointestinal (GI) tract, immune system, or hair follicles. As a result, individuals taking such anticancer drugs can experience adverse effects, including anemia, scaly skin, GI tract disturbance, immunodeficiencies, and hair loss.

E. Conversion of IMP to AMP and GMP

The conversion of IMP to either AMP or GMP uses a two-step, energy-requiring pathway (Figure 22.8). Note that the synthesis of AMP requires guanosine triphosphate (GTP) as an energy source, whereas the synthesis of GMP requires ATP. Also, the first reaction in each pathway is inhibited by the end product of that pathway. This provides a mechanism for diverting IMP to the synthesis of the species of purine present in lesser amounts. If both AMP and GMP are present in adequate amounts, the de novo pathway of purine synthesis is turned off at the *amidotransferase* step.

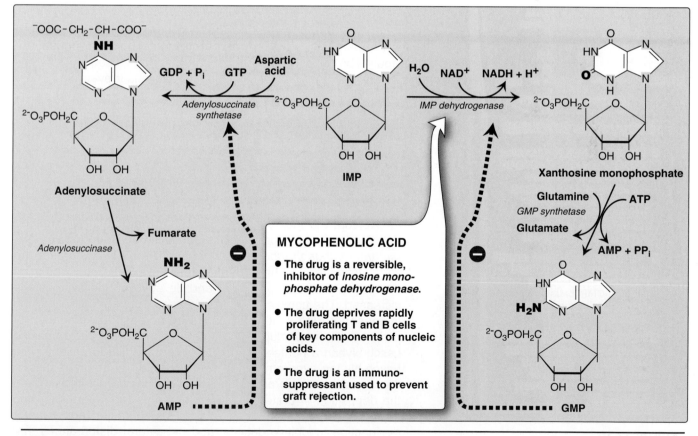

Figure 22.8
Conversion of IMP to AMP and GMP showing feedback inhibition.

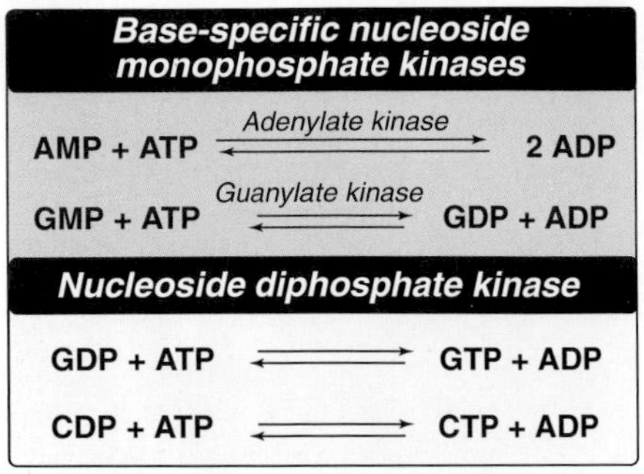

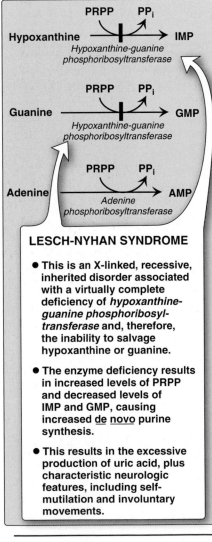

Figure 22.9
Conversion of nucleoside monophosphates to nucleoside
diphosphates and triphosphates.

LESCH-NYHAN SYNDROME

● This is an X-linked, recessive,
inherited disorder associated
with a virtually complete
deficiency of *hypoxanthine-
guanine phosphoribosyl-
transferase* and, therefore,
the inability to salvage
hypoxanthine or guanine.

● The enzyme deficiency results
in increased levels of PRPP
and decreased levels of
IMP and GMP, causing
increased <u>de novo</u> purine
synthesis.

● This results in the excessive
production of uric acid, plus
characteristic neurologic
features, including self-
mutilation and involuntary
movements.

Figure 22.10
Salvage pathways of purine
nucleotide synthesis.

F. Conversion of nucleoside monophosphates to nucleoside diphosphates and triphosphates

Nucleoside diphosphates are synthesized from the corresponding
nucleoside monophosphates by base-specific *nucleoside monophosphate kinases* (Figure 22.9). [Note: These *kinases* do not discriminate between ribose or deoxyribose in the substrate.] ATP is
generally the source of the transferred phosphate, because it is present in higher concentrations than the other nucleoside triphosphates. *Adenylate kinase* is particularly active in liver and muscle,
where the turnover of energy from ATP is high. Its function is to
maintain an equilibrium among AMP, ADP, and ATP. Nucleoside
diphosphates and triphosphates are interconverted by *nucleoside
diphosphate kinase*—an enzyme that, unlike the *monophosphate
kinases*, has broad specificity.

G. Salvage pathway for purines

Purines that result from the normal turnover of cellular nucleic acids,
or the small amount that is obtained from the diet and not degraded,
can be converted to nucleoside triphosphates and used by the body.
This is referred to as the "salvage pathway" for purines.

1. **Conversion of purine bases to nucleotides:** Two enzymes are
   involved: *adenine phosphoribosyltransferase* (*APRT*) and *hypoxanthine-guanine phosphoribosyltransferase* (*HGPRT*). Both
   enzymes use PRPP as the source of the ribose 5-phosphate
   group. The release of pyrophosphate and its subsequent hydrolysis by *pyrophosphatase* makes these reactions irreversible (Figure
   22.10). [Note: Adenosine is the only purine nucleoside to be salvaged. It is phosphorylated to AMP by *adenosine kinase*.]

2. **Lesch-Nyhan syndrome:** This syndrome is a rare, X-linked, recessive disorder associated with a virtually complete deficiency of
   HGPRT. This deficiency results in an inability to salvage hypoxanthine or guanine, from which excessive amounts of uric acid,
   the end product of purine degradation, are produced (see p. 298).
   In addition, the lack of this salvage pathway causes increased
   PRPP levels and decreased IMP and GMP levels. As a result,
   glutamine:phosphoribosylpyrophosphate amidotransferase (the
   committed step in purine synthesis) has excess substrate and
   decreased inhibitors available, and <u>de novo</u> purine synthesis is
   increased. The combination of decreased purine reutilization and
   increased purine synthesis results in increased degradation of
   purines and the production of large amounts of uric acid, making
   Lesch-Nyhan a heritable cause of hyperuricemia. In patients with
   Lesch-Nyhan syndrome, the hyperuricemia frequently results in
   the formation of uric acid stones in the kidneys (urolithiasis) and
   the deposition of urate crystals in the joints (gouty arthritis) and
   soft tissues. In addition, the syndrome is characterized by motor
   dysfunction, cognitive deficits, and behavioral disturbances that
   include self-mutilation (biting of lips and fingers, Figure 22.11).

IV. SYNTHESIS OF DEOXYRIBONUCLEOTIDES

The nucleotides described thus far all contain ribose (ribonucleotides). The nucleotides required for DNA synthesis, however, are 2'-deoxyribonucleotides, which are produced from ribonucleoside diphosphates by the enzyme *ribonucleotide reductase* during the S-phase of the cell cycle (see p. 407). [Note: The same enzyme acts on pyrimidine ribonucleotides.]

A. Ribonucleotide reductase

Ribonucleotide reductase (*ribonucleoside diphosphate reductase*) is composed of two nonidentical dimeric subunits, R1 and R2, and is specific for the reduction of purine nucleoside diphosphates (ADP and GDP), and pyrimidine nucleoside diphosphates, cytidine diphosphate (CDP) and uridine diphosphate (UDP) to their deoxyforms (dADP, dGDP, dCDP, and dUDP). The immediate donors of the hydrogen atoms needed for the reduction of the 2'-hydroxyl group are two sulfhydryl groups on the enzyme itself, which, during the reaction, form a disulfide bond (Figure 22.12).

1. **Regeneration of reduced enzyme:** In order for *ribonucleotide reductase* to continue to produce deoxyribonucleotides, the disulfide bond created during the production of the 2'-deoxy carbon must be reduced. The source of the reducing equivalents for this purpose is thioredoxin—a peptide coenzyme of *ribonucleotide reductase*. Thioredoxin contains two cysteine residues separated by two amino acids in the peptide chain. The two sulfhydryl groups of thioredoxin donate their hydrogen atoms to *ribonucleotide reductase*, in the process forming a disulfide bond (see p. 19).

2. **Regeneration of reduced thioredoxin:** Thioredoxin must be converted back to its reduced form in order to continue to perform its function. The necessary reducing equivalents are provided by NADPH + H⁺, and the reaction is catalyzed by *thioredoxin reductase* (see Figure 22.12).

B. Regulation of deoxyribonucleotide synthesis

Ribonucleotide reductase is responsible for maintaining a balanced supply of the deoxyribonucleotides required for DNA synthesis. To achieve this, the regulation of the enzyme is complex. In addition to the catalytic (active) site, there are allosteric sites on the enzyme involved in regulating its activity (Figure 22.13).

1. **Activity sites:** The binding of dATP to allosteric sites (known as the activity sites) on the enzyme inhibits the overall catalytic activity of the enzyme and, therefore, prevents the reduction of any of the four nucleoside diphosphates. This effectively prevents DNA synthesis, and explains the toxicity of increased levels of dATP seen in conditions such as *adenosine deaminase* deficiency (see p. 301). In contrast, ATP bound to these sites activates the enzyme.

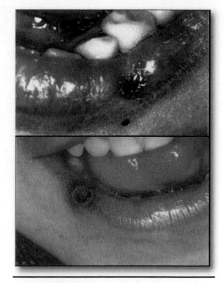

Figure 22.11
Lesions on the lips of Lesch-Nyhan patients caused by self-mutilation.

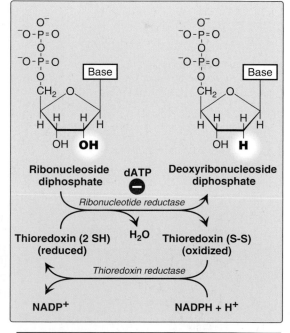

Figure 22.12
Conversion of ribonucleotides to deoxyribonucleotides.

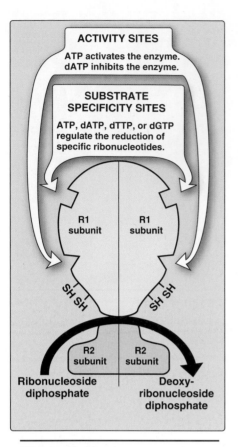

Figure 22.13
Regulation of *ribonucleotide reductase*.

2. Substrate specificity sites: The binding of nucleoside tri-phosphates to additional allosteric sites (known as the substrate specificity sites) on the enzyme regulates substrate specificity, causing an increase in the conversion of different species of ribonucleotides to deoxyribonucleotides as they are required for DNA synthesis. For example, deoxythymidine triphosphate (dTTP) binding at the specificity sites causes a conformational change that allows reduction of GDP to dGDP at the catalytic site.

> The drug hydroxyurea destroys the free radical required for enzymic activity of *ribonucleotide reductase*, and thus inhibits the generation of substrates for DNA synthesis. Hydroxyurea has been used in the treatment of cancers such as chronic myelogenous leukemia. Hydroxyurea is also used in the treatment of sickle cell disease (see p. 36); however, the increase in fetal hemoglobin seen with hydroxyurea has not been linked to its effect on *ribonucleotide reductase*.

V. DEGRADATION OF PURINE NUCLEOTIDES

Degradation of dietary nucleic acids occurs in the small intestine, where a family of pancreatic enzymes hydrolyzes the nucleic acids to nucleotides. Inside the intestinal mucosal cells, purine nucleotides are sequentially degraded by specific enzymes to nucleosides and free bases, with uric acid as the end product of this pathway. [Note: Purine nucleotides from de novo synthesis are degraded in the liver primarily. The free bases are sent out from liver and salvaged by peripheral tissues.]

A. Degradation of dietary nucleic acids in the small intestine

Ribonucleases and *deoxyribonucleases*, secreted by the pancreas, hydrolyze dietary RNA and DNA primarily to oligonucleotides. Oligonucleotides are further hydrolyzed by pancreatic *phosphodiesterases*, producing a mixture of 3'- and 5'-mononucleotides. In the intestinal mucosal cells, a family of *nucleotidases* removes the phosphate groups hydrolytically, releasing nucleosides that are further degraded to free bases. Dietary purine bases are not used to any appreciable extent for the synthesis of tissue nucleic acids. Instead, they are generally converted to uric acid in intestinal mucosal cells. Most of the uric acid enters the blood, and is eventually excreted in the urine. A summary of this pathway is shown in Figure 22.14. [Note: Mammals other than primates express *urate oxidase* which cleaves the purine ring, generating allantoin. Use of recombinant *urate oxidase* is a potential therapeutic strategy to lower urate levels.]

B. Formation of uric acid

A summary of the steps in the production of uric acid and genetic diseases associated with deficiencies of specific degradative enzymes are shown in Figure 22.15. [Note: The bracketed numbers refer to specific reactions in the figure.]

[1] An amino group is removed from AMP to produce IMP by *AMP deaminase*, or from adenosine to produce inosine (hypoxanthine-ribose) by *adenosine deaminase*.

[2] IMP and GMP are converted into their nucleoside forms—inosine and guanosine—by the action of *5'-nucleotidase*.

[3] *Purine nucleoside phosphorylase* converts inosine and guanosine into their respective purine bases, hypoxanthine and guanine. [Note: A *mutase* interconverts ribose 1- and ribose 5-phosphate.]

[4] Guanine is deaminated to form xanthine.

[5] Hypoxanthine is oxidized by *xanthine oxidase* to xanthine, which is further oxidized by *xanthine oxidase* to uric acid, the final product of human purine degradation. Uric acid is excreted primarily in the urine.

C. Diseases associated with purine degradation

1. Gout: Gout is a disorder characterized by high levels of uric acid— the end product of purine catabolism—in blood (hyperuricemia), as a result of either the overproduction or underexcretion of uric acid. The hyperuricemia can lead to the deposition of mono-sodium urate crystals in the joints, and an inflammatory response to the crystals, causing first acute and then progressing to chronic gouty arthritis. Nodular masses of monosodium urate crystals (tophi) may be deposited in the soft tissues, resulting in chronic tophaceous gout (Figure 22.16). Formation of uric acid stones in the kidney (urolithiasis) may also be seen. [Note: Hyperuricemia is typically asymptomatic and does not lead to gout, but gout is preceded by hyperuricemia.] The definitive diagnosis of gout requires aspiration and examination of synovial fluid (Figure 22.17) from an affected joint (or material from a tophus) using polarized light microscopy to confirm the presence of needle-shaped mono-sodium urate crystals (Figure 22.18).

a. Underexcretion of uric acid: In the vast majority of patients, the hyperuricemia leading to gout is caused by underexcretion of uric acid. Underexcretion can be primary, due to as-yet-unidentified inherent excretory defects, or secondary to known disease processes that affect how the kidney handles urate, for example lactic acidosis (lactate and urate compete for the same renal transporter), and to environmental factors such as the use of drugs, for example, thiazide diuretics, or exposure to lead (saturnine gout).

b. Overproduction of uric acid: A less common cause of gout is hyperuricemia from the overproduction of uric acid. Primary hyperuricemia is, for the most part, idiopathic (having no known cause). However, several identified mutations in the gene for X-linked *PRPP synthetase* result in the enzyme having an increased V_{max} (see p. 58) for the production of PRPP, a lower K_m (see p. 59) for ribose 5-phosphate, or a decreased sensitivity to purine nucleotides—its allosteric inhibitors (see p. 62). In each case, increased availability of PRPP increases purine production, resulting in elevated levels of plasma uric acid. Lesch-Nyhan syndrome (see p. 296) also causes hyperuricemia as a

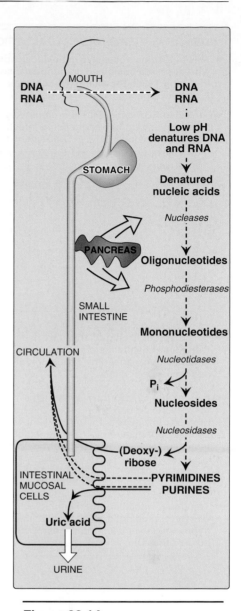

Figure 22.14
Digestion of dietary nucleic acids. [Note: Much of the metabolism of the mononucleotides occurs within the intestinal mucosal cells.]

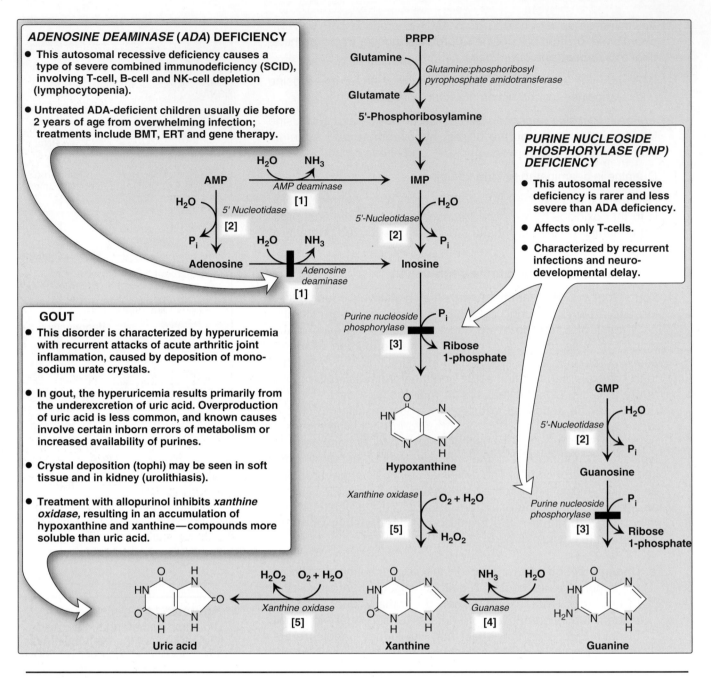

Figure 22.15
The degradation of purine nucleotides to uric acid, illustrating some of the genetic diseases associated with this pathway. [Note: The numbers in brackets refer to the corresponding numbered citations in the text.]

result of the decreased salvage of hypoxanthine and guanine, and the subsequent increased availability of PRPP. Secondary hyperuricemia is typically the consequence of increased availability of purines, for example, in patients with myeloproliferative disorders or who are undergoing chemotherapy and so have a high rate of cell turnover. Hyperuricemia leading to gout can also be the result of seemingly unrelated metabolic diseases, such as von Gierke disease (see Figure 11.8 on p. 129) or fructose intolerance (see p. 138).

A diet rich in meat and seafood (particularly shellfish) is associated with increased risk of gout. In addition, a diet rich in low-fat dairy products was shown to be associated with a decreased risk.

c. **Treatment of gout:** Acute attacks of gout are treated with anti-inflammatory agents. Colchicine, steroidal drugs such as prednisone, and nonsteroidal drugs such as indomethacin are used. [Note: Colchicine prevents formation of microtubules, thus decreasing the movement of neutrophils into the affected area. Like the other anti-inflammatory drugs, it has no effect on uric acid levels.] Long-term therapeutic strategies for gout involve lowering the uric acid level below its saturation point, thereby preventing the deposition of urate crystals. Uricosuric agents, such as probenecid or sulfinpyrazone, that increase renal excretion of uric acid, are used in patients who are "underexcretors" of uric acid. Allopurinol, a structural analog of hypoxanthine, inhibits uric acid synthesis and is used in patients who are "overproducers" of uric acid. Allopurinol is converted in the body to oxypurinol, which inhibits *xanthine oxidase* (*XO*), resulting in an accumulation of hypoxanthine and xanthine (see Figure 22.15)—compounds more soluble than uric acid and, therefore, less likely to initiate an inflammatory response. In patients with normal levels of *HGPRT*, the hypoxanthine can be salvaged, thus reducing the levels of PRPP and, therefore, <u>de novo</u> purine synthesis. Febuxostat, a non-purine inhibitor of *XO*, is now available. [Note: Uric acid levels in the blood normally are close to the saturation point. One reason for this may be the strong antioxidant effects of uric acid.]

2. **Adenosine deaminase (ADA) deficiency:** *ADA* is expressed in a variety of tissues, but, in humans, lymphocytes have the highest activity of this cytoplasmic enzyme. A deficiency of *ADA* results in an accumulation of adenosine, which is converted to its ribonucleotide or deoxyribonucleotide forms by cellular *kinases*. As dATP levels rise, *ribonucleotide reductase* is inhibited, thus preventing the production of all deoxyribose-containing nucleotides (see p. 297). Consequently, cells cannot make DNA and divide. [Note: The dATP and adenosine that accumulate in ADA deficiency lead to developmental arrest and apoptosis of lymphocytes.] In its most severe form, this autosomal recessive disorder causes a type of severe combined immunodeficiency disease (SCID), involving a decrease in T cells, B cells, and natural killer (NK) cells. It is estimated that in the United States, *ADA* deficiency accounts for approximately 14% of all cases of SCID. Treatment requires either bone marrow transplantation (BMT) or enzyme replacement therapy (ERT). Without appropriate treatment, children with this disorder usually die by the age of two. [Note: *Purine nucleoside phosphorylase* (*PNP*) deficiency results in a less severe immunodeficiency involving T-cells primarily.]

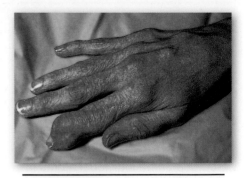

Figure 22.16
Tophaceous gout.

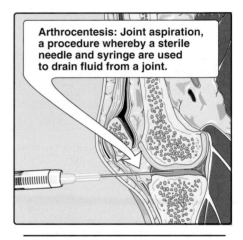

Arthrocentesis: Joint aspiration, a procedure whereby a sterile needle and syringe are used to drain fluid from a joint.

Figure 22.17
Analysis of joint fluid can help to define causes of joint swelling or arthritis, such as infection, gout, and rheumatoid disease.

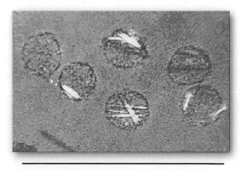

Figure 22.18
Gout can be diagnosed by the presence of negatively birefringent monosodium urate crystals in aspirated synovial fluid examined by polarized-light microscopy. Here, crystals are within polymorphonuclear leukocytes.

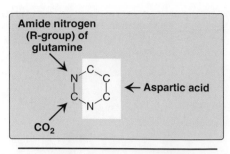

Figure 22.19
Sources of the individual atoms in the pyrimidine ring.

	CPS I	**CPS II**
Cellular location	Mitochondria	Cytosol
Pathway involved	Urea cycle	Pyrimidine synthesis
Source of nitrogen	Ammonia	γ-Amide group of glutamine
Regulators	Activator: N–acetyl-glutamate	Activator: PRPP Inhibitor: UTP

Figure 22.20
Summary of the differences between *carbamoyl phosphate synthetase (CPS) I* and *II*.

VI. PYRIMIDINE SYNTHESIS AND DEGRADATION

Unlike the synthesis of the purine ring, which is constructed on a preexisting ribose 5-phosphate, the pyrimidine ring is synthesized before being attached to ribose 5-phosphate, which is donated by PRPP. The sources of the atoms in the pyrimidine ring are glutamine, CO_2, and aspartic acid (Figure 22.19). [Note: Glutamine and aspartic acid are thus required for both purine and pyrimidine synthesis.]

A. Synthesis of carbamoyl phosphate

The regulated step of this pathway in mammalian cells is the synthesis of carbamoyl phosphate from glutamine and CO_2, catalyzed by *carbamoyl phosphate synthetase (CPS) II*. *CPS II* is inhibited by UTP (the end product of this pathway, which can be converted into the other pyrimidine nucleotides), and is activated by PRPP. [Note: Carbamoyl phosphate, synthesized by *CPS I*, is also a precursor of urea (see p. 253). Defects in *ornithine transcarbamylase* of the urea cycle promote pyrimidine synthesis due to increased availability of carbamoyl phosphate. A comparison of the two enzymes is presented in Figure 22.20.]

B. Synthesis of orotic acid

The second step in pyrimidine synthesis is the formation of carbamoylaspartate, catalyzed by *aspartate transcarbamoylase*. The pyrimidine ring is then closed hydrolytically by *dihydroorotase*. The resulting dihydroorotate is oxidized to produce orotic acid (orotate, Figure 22.21). The enzyme that produces orotate, *dihydroorotate dehydrogenase*, is associated with the inner mitochondrial membrane. All other enzymes in pyrimidine biosynthesis are cytosolic. [Note: The first three enzymic activities in this pathway (*CPS II, aspartate transcarbamoylase*, and *dihydroorotase*) are actually three different catalytic domains of a single polypeptide chain known as CAD from the first letter in the name of each domain. (See p. 19 for a discussion of domains). This is an example of a multfunctional or multicatalytic polypeptide that facilitates the ordered synthesis of an important compound. Synthesis of the purine nucleotide IMP also involves multifunctional proteins.]

C. Formation of a pyrimidine nucleotide

The completed pyrimidine ring is converted to the nucleotide orotidine 5'-monophosphate (OMP) in the second stage of pyrimidine nucleotide synthesis (see Figure 22.21). PRPP is again the ribose 5-phosphate donor. The enzyme *orotate phosphoribosyltransferase* produces OMP and releases pyrophosphate, thereby making the reaction biologically irreversible. [Note: Both purine and pyrimidine synthesis thus require glutamine, aspartic acid, and PRPP as essential precursors.] OMP, the parent pyrimidine mononucleotide, is converted to uridine monophosphate (UMP) by *orotidylate decarboxylase*, which removes the acidic carboxyl group. *Orotate phosphoribosyltransferase* and *orotidylate decarboxylase* are also catalytic domains of a single polypeptide chain called *UMP synthase*. Orotic aciduria—a rare genetic defect—may be caused by a deficiency of one or both activities of this bifunctional enzyme, resulting in orotic acid in the urine (see Figure 22.21). UMP is

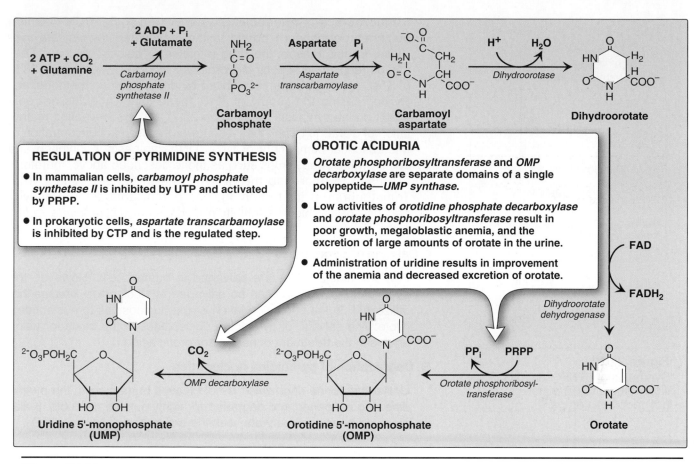

REGULATION OF PYRIMIDINE SYNTHESIS

- In mammalian cells, *carbamoyl phosphate synthetase II* is inhibited by UTP and activated by PRPP.

- In prokaryotic cells, *aspartate transcarbamoylase* is inhibited by CTP and is the regulated step.

OROTIC ACIDURIA

- *Orotate phosphoribosyltransferase* and *OMP decarboxylase* are separate domains of a single polypeptide—*UMP synthase*.

- Low activities of *orotidine phosphate decarboxylase* and *orotate phosphoribosyltransferase* result in poor growth, megaloblastic anemia, and the excretion of large amounts of orotate in the urine.

- Administration of uridine results in improvement of the anemia and decreased excretion of orotate.

Figure 22.21
<u>De</u> <u>novo</u> pyrimidine synthesis.

sequentially phosphorylated to UDP and UTP. [Note: The UDP is a substrate for *ribonucleotide reductase*, which generates dUDP. The dUDP is phosphorylated to dUTP, which is rapidly hydrolyzed to dUMP by *UTP diphosphatase* (*dUTPase*). *dUTPase*, then, plays an important role in reducing availability of dUTP as a substrate for DNA synthesis, thus preventing erroneous incorporation of uracil into DNA.]

D. Synthesis of UTP and cytidine triphosphate (CTP)

CTP is produced by amination of UTP by *CTP synthetase* (Figure 22.22), with glutamine providing the nitrogen. [Note: Some CTP is dephosphorylated to CDP, which is a substrate for *ribonucleotide reductase*. The dCDP generated can be phosphorylated to dCTP for DNA synthesis.]

E. Synthesis of thymidine monophosphate (TMP) from dUMP

dUMP is converted to dTMP by *thymidylate synthase*, which uses N^5,N^{10}-methylene tetrahydrofolate as the source of the methyl group (see p. 267 for a discussion of this coenzyme). This is an unusual reaction in that tetrahydrofolate (THF) contributes not only a one-carbon unit but also two hydrogen atoms from the pteridine ring, resulting in the oxidation of THF to dihydrofolate (DHF) (Figure 22.23). Inhibitors of *thymidylate synthase* include thymine analogs such as 5-fluorouracil, which serve as successful antitumor agents.

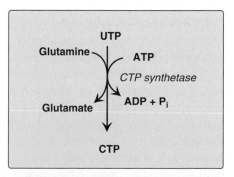

Figure 22.22
Synthesis of CTP from UTP. [Note: CTP, required for RNA synthesis, is converted to dCTP for DNA synthesis.]

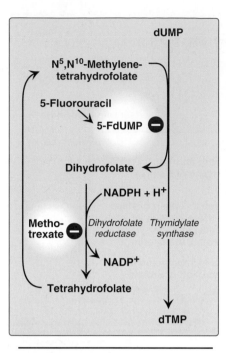

Figure 22.23
Synthesis of dTMP from dUMP, illustrating sites of action of antineoplastic drugs.

5-Fluorouracil is metabolically converted to 5-FdUMP, which becomes permanently bound to the inactivated *thymidylate synthase*; for this reason, the drug is called a "suicide" inhibitor. DHF can be reduced to THF by *dihydrofolate reductase* (see Figure 28.3, p. 374), an enzyme that is inhibited by drugs such as methotrexate. By decreasing the supply of THF, these folate analogs not only inhibit purine synthesis (see Figure 22.7), but, by preventing methylation of dUMP to dTMP, they also lower the cellular concentration of this essential component of DNA. DNA synthesis is inhibited and cell growth slowed. Drugs such as those described above, therefore, are used to decrease the growth rate of cancer cells. [Note: Trimethoprim, a folate analog, has potent antibacterial activity because of its selective inhibition of bacterial *dihydrofolate reductase*.]

F. Salvage of pyrimidines

Few pyrimidine bases are salvaged in human cells. However, the pyrimidine nucleosides can be salvaged by nucleoside *kinases* that utilize ATP in the phosphorylation of the nucleosides to nucleotides. [Note: The salvage of pyrimidine nucleosides is the basis for using uridine in the treatment of hereditary orotic aciduria.]

G. Degradation of pyrimidine nucleotides

Unlike the purine ring, which is not cleaved human cells, the pyrimidine ring is opened and degraded to highly soluble products, β-alanine and β-aminoisobutyrate, with the production of NH_3 and CO_2.

VII. CHAPTER SUMMARY

Nucleotides are composed of a **nitrogenous base** (adenine = **A**, guanine = **G**, cytosine = **C**, uracil = **U**, and thymine = **T**), a **pentose**, and one, two, or three **phosphate groups** (Figure 22.24). A and G are **purines**; C, U, and T are **pyrimidines**. If the sugar is **ribose**, the nucleotide is a **ribonucleoside phosphate** (for example, AMP), and it can have several functions in the cell, including being a component of **RNA**. If the sugar is **deoxyribose**, the nucleotide is a **deoxyribonucleoside phosphate** (for example, dAMP), and will be found almost exclusively as a component of **DNA**. The **committed step** in **purine synthesis** uses **5-phosphoribosyl-1-pyrophosphate** (**PRPP**, an "activated pentose" that provides the ribose-phosphate group for <u>de novo</u> purine and pyrimidine synthesis and purine salvage) and nitrogen from **glutamine** to produce phosphoribosyl amine. The enzyme is **glutamine:PRPP amidotransferase**, and is **inhibited** by **AMP** and **GMP** (the end products of the pathway) and activated by PRPP. Purine nucleotides can also be produced from preformed purine bases by using **salvage reactions** catalyzed by **adenine phosphoribosyltransferase (APRT)** and **hypoxanthine-guanine phosphoribosyltransferase (HGPRT)**. A near total deficiency of HGPRT causes **Lesch-Nyhan syndrome**—a severe, heritable form of hyperuricemia accompanied by compulsive self-mutilation. All deoxyribonucleotides are synthesized from ribonucleotides by the enzyme **ribonucleotide reductase**. This enzyme is highly regulated, for example, it is **strongly inhibited by dATP**—a compound that is overproduced in bone marrow cells in individuals with **adenosine deaminase deficiency**. This syndrome causes **severe combined immunodeficiency disease**. The end product of purine degradation is **uric acid**—a compound whose overproduction or undersecretion causes hyperuricemia that, if accompanied by the deposition of urate crystals in joints and soft tissues, and an inflammatory response to those crystals, results in **gout**. The first step in **pyrimidine synthesis**—the production of carbamoyl phosphate by **carbamoyl phosphate synthetase II**—is the **regulated** step in this pathway (it is **inhibited by UTP** and **activated by PRPP**). The UTP produced by this pathway can be converted to CTP. dUMP can be converted to **dTMP** using **thymidylate synthase**—an enzyme targeted by anticancer drugs such as **5-fluorouracil**. The regeneration of THF from DHF produced in the thymidylate synthase reaction requires **dihydrofolate reductase**—an enzyme targeted by the drug, **methotrexate**.

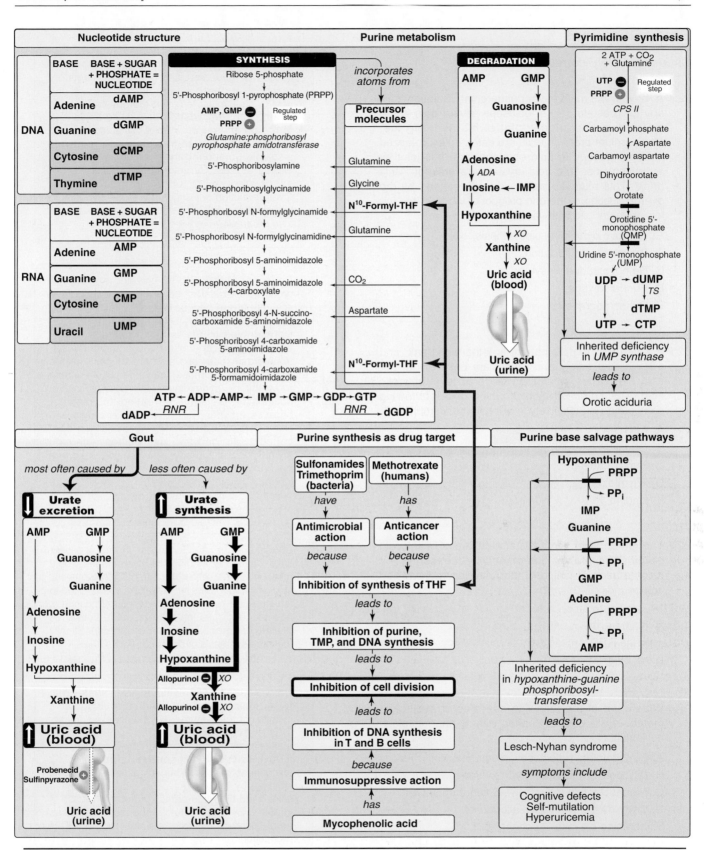

Figure 22.24
Key concept map for nucleotide metabolism. *ADA= adenosine deaminase, XO = xanthine oxidase, TS = thymidylate synthase. RNR = ribonucleotide reductase, CPS II = carbamyl phosphate synthetase II.*

Study Questions

Choose the ONE correct answer.

22.1 A 42-year-old male patient undergoing radiation therapy for prostate cancer develops severe pain in the metatarsal phalangeal joint of his right big toe. Monosodium urate crystals are detected by polarized light microscopy in fluid obtained from this joint by arthrocentesis. Uric acid crystals are present in his urine. This patient's pain is directly caused by the overproduction of the end product of which of the following metabolic pathways?

A. De novo pyrimidine biosynthesis.

B. Pyrimidine degradation.

C. De novo purine biosynthesis.

D. Purine salvage.

E. Purine degradation.

Correct answer = E. The patient's pain is caused by gout, resulting from an inflammatory response to the crystallization of excess uric acid in his joints. Radiation therapy caused cell death, with degradation of nucleic acids and their constituent purines. Uric acid, the end product of purine degradation, is a relatively insoluble compound that can cause gout and kidney stones. Pyrimidine metabolism is not associated with uric acid production. Overproduction of purines can indirectly result in hyperuricemia. Purine salvage decreases uric acid production.

22.2 A 1-year-old female patient is lethargic, weak, and anemic. Her height and weight are both low for her age. Her urine contains an elevated level of orotic acid. The administration of which of the following compounds is most likely to alleviate her symptoms?

A. Adenine.

B. Guanine.

C. Hypoxanthine.

D. Thymidine.

E. Uridine.

Correct answer = E. The elevated excretion of orotic acid indicates that the patient has orotic aciduria, a rare genetic disorder affecting the de novo pyrimidine biosynthetic pathway. Deficiencies in the enzyme activities OMP decarboxylase and/or orotate phosphoribosyltransferase (both of which are domains of the enzyme UMP synthase) leave the patient unable to synthesize pyrimidines. Uridine, a pyrimidine nucleoside, is useful in treating this disorder because it bypasses the missing enzymes and can be salvaged to UMP, which can be converted to all the other pyrimidines. Although thymidine is a pyrimidine nucleoside, it cannot be converted to other pyrimidines. Hypoxanthine, guanine, and adenine are all purine bases that have no value in helping to replace the missing pyrimidines.

22.3 The rate of DNA synthesis in a culture of cells could be most accurately determined by measuring the incorporation of which of the following radiolabeled compounds?

A. Adenine.

B. Guanine.

C. Phosphate.

D. Thymidine.

Correct answer = D. Because thymidine is essentially found only in DNA, its incorporation would most accurately reflect the rate of DNA synthesis. Uridine is found only in RNA and could be used to measure the rate of RNA synthesis. Phosphate, adenine, and guanine are present in both DNA and RNA, and could not be used to specifically measure synthesis of either one.

22.4 Which one of the following enzymes of nucleotide metabolism is correctly paired with its pharmacological inhibitor?

A. Dihydrofolate reductase—methotrexate

B. IMP dehydrogenase—hydroxyurea

C. Ribonucleotide reductase—5-fluorouracil

D. Thymidylate synthase—allopurinol

E. Xanthine oxidase—probenecid

Correct answer = A. Methotrexate interferes with folate metabolism by acting as a competitive inhibitor of the enzyme dihydrofolate reductase. This starves cells for tetrahydrofolate, and makes them unable to synthesize purines and dTMP. IMP dehydrogenase is inhibited by mycophenolic acid. Ribonucleotide reductase is inhibited by hydroxyurea. Thymidylate synthase is inhibited by 5-fluorouracil. Xanthine oxidase is inhibited by allopurinol; probenecid increases renal excretion of urate, but does not inhibit its production.

22.5 What laboratory test would help in distinguishing an orotic aciduria caused by ornithine transcarbamylase deficiency from that caused by UMP synthase deficiency?

Blood ammonia level would expected to be elevated in ornithine transcarbamylase deficiency but not in UMP synthase deficiency.

Metabolic Effects of Insulin and Glucagon

23

I. OVERVIEW

Four major organs play a dominant role in fuel metabolism: liver, adipose, muscle, and brain. These tissues contain unique sets of enzymes, such that each organ is specialized for the storage, use, or generation of specific fuels. These tissues do not function in isolation, but rather form part of a network in which one tissue may provide substrates to another, or process compounds produced by other organs. Communication between tissues is mediated by the nervous system, by the availability of circulating substrates, and by variation in the levels of plasma hormones (Figure 23.1). The integration of energy metabolism is controlled primarily by the actions of two peptide hormones: insulin and glucagon, with the catecholamines epinephrine and norepinephrine playing a supporting role. Changes in the circulating levels of these hormones allow the body to store energy when food is available in abundance, or to make stored energy available, for example, during "survival crises," such as famine, severe injury, and "fight-or-flight" situations. This chapter describes the structure, secretion, and metabolic effects of the two hormones that most profoundly affect energy metabolism.

II. INSULIN

Insulin is a polypeptide hormone produced by the β cells of the islets of Langerhans—clusters of cells that are embedded in the exocrine portion of the pancreas (Figure 23.2). The islets of Langerhans make up only about 1–2% of the total cells of the pancreas. Insulin is the most

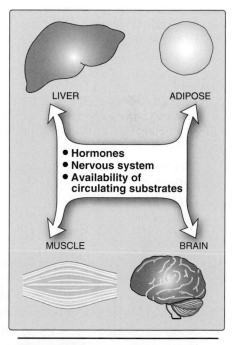

Figure 23.1
Mechanisms of communication between four major tissues.

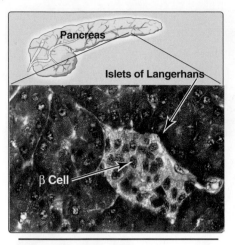

Figure 23.2
Islets of Langerhans.

important hormone coordinating the use of fuels by tissues. Its metabolic effects are anabolic, favoring, for example, synthesis of glycogen, triacylglycerols, and protein.

A. Structure of insulin

Insulin is composed of 51 amino acids arranged in two polypeptide chains, designated A and B, which are linked together by two disulfide bridges (Figure 23.3A). The insulin molecule also contains an intramolecular disulfide bridge between amino acid residues of the A chain. [Note: Pig (porcine) and beef (bovine) insulin differ from human insulin at one and three amino acid positions, respectively. When used in humans for the treatment of diabetes, antibodies to these foreign proteins develop. Use of human recombinant insulin (see p. 470) has eliminated this problem.]

B. Synthesis of insulin

The processing and transport of intermediates that occur during the synthesis of insulin are shown in Figures 23.3B and 23.4. Note that the biosynthesis involves two inactive precursors, preproinsulin and proinsulin, which are sequentially cleaved to form the active hormone plus the connecting or C-peptide (see Figure 23.4). [Note: The C-peptide is essential for proper insulin folding. Also, because of its longer half-life in the plasma, the C-peptide is a good indicator of insulin production and secretion.] Insulin is stored in the cytosol in granules that, given the proper stimulus (see below), are released by exocytosis. (See p. 166 for a discussion of the synthesis of proteins destined for secretion.) Insulin is degraded by the enzyme *insulinase* which is present in the liver and, to a lesser extent, in the kidneys. Insulin has a plasma half-life of approximately 6 minutes. This short duration of action permits rapid changes in circulating levels of the hormone.

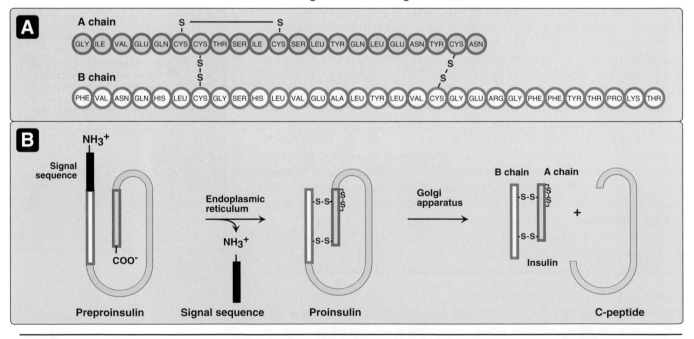

Figure 23.3
A. Structure of insulin. B. Formation of human insulin from preproinsulin.

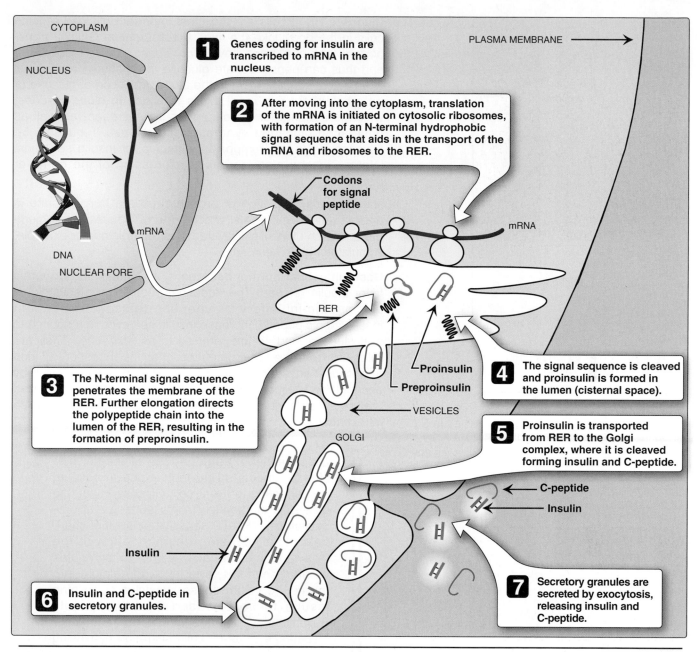

Figure 23.4
Intracellular movements of insulin and its precursors. RER = rough endoplasmic reticulum.

C. Regulation of insulin secretion

1. **Stimulation of insulin secretion:** Insulin secretion by the β cells of the islets of Langerhans of the pancreas is closely coordinated with the release of glucagon by pancreatic α cells. The relative amounts of insulin and glucagon released by the pancreas are regulated so that the rate of hepatic glucose production is kept equal to the use of glucose by peripheral tissues. In view of its coordinating role, it is not surprising that the β cell responds to a variety of stimuli. In particular, insulin secretion is increased by:

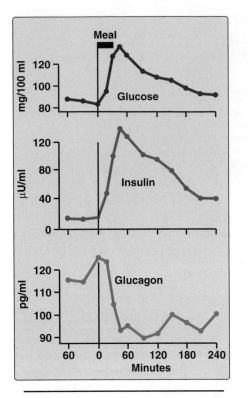

Figure 23.5
Changes in blood levels of glucose,
insulin, and glucagon after ingestion
of a carbohydrate-rich meal.

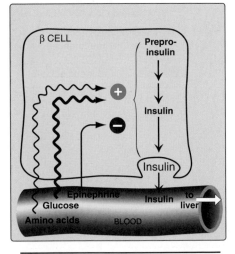

Figure 23.6
Regulation of insulin release from
pancreatic β cells.

a. Glucose: The β cells are the most important glucose-sensing cells in the body. Like the liver, β cells contain GLUT-2 transporters (see p. 97) and have *glucokinase* activity (see p. 98), and thus can phosphorylate glucose in amounts proportional to its actual concentration in the blood. Ingestion of glucose or a carbohydrate-rich meal leads to a rise in blood glucose, which is a signal for increased insulin secretion (as well as decreased glucagon synthesis and release, Figure 23.5). Glucose is the most important stimulus for insulin secretion. [Note: Glucose also increases expression of the gene for insulin.]

b. Amino acids: Ingestion of protein causes a transient rise in plasma amino acid levels, which, in turn, induces the immediate secretion of insulin. Elevated plasma arginine, for example, stimulates insulin secretion.

c. Gastrointestinal hormones: Most gastrointestinal hormones favor insulin release. The intestinal peptides cholecystokinin and gastric-inhibitory polypeptide (glucose-dependent insulinotropic peptide) increase insulin secretion in response to oral glucose, and so are referred to as "incretins." They are released from the small intestine after the ingestion of food and cause an anticipatory rise in insulin levels. This may account for the fact that the same amount of glucose given orally induces a much greater secretion of insulin than if given intravenously.

> Glucose-dependent release of insulin into blood is mediated through a rise in calcium concentration in the β cell. Glucose taken into β cells is metabolized, with subsequent production of ATP. ATP-sensitive potassium channels close, causing depolarization of the plasma membrane, activation of voltage-gated calcium channels, and influx of calcium into the cell. Calcium causes vesicles containing insulin to be released from the β cell. Sulfonylureas, oral agents used to treat type 2 diabetes, increase insulin secretion by closing ATP-sensitive potassium channels.

2. Inhibition of insulin secretion: The synthesis and release of insulin are decreased when there is a scarcity of dietary fuels, and also during periods of stress (for example, fever or infection). These effects are mediated primarily by epinephrine, which is secreted by the adrenal medulla in response to stress, trauma, or extreme exercise. Under these conditions, the release of epinephrine is controlled largely by the nervous system. Epinephrine has a direct effect on energy metabolism, causing a rapid mobilization of energy-yielding fuels, including glucose from the liver (produced by glycogenolysis or gluconeogenesis, see p. 121) and fatty acids from adipose tissue (see p. 189). In addition, epinephrine can override the normal glucose-stimulated release of insulin. Thus, in emergency situations, the sympathetic nervous

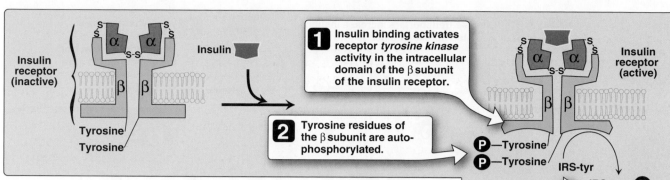

system largely replaces the plasma glucose concentration as the controlling influence over β-cell secretion. The regulation of insulin secretion is summarized in Figure 23.6.

D. Metabolic effects of insulin

1. **Effects on carbohydrate metabolism:** The effects of insulin on glucose metabolism promote its storage and are most prominent in three tissues: liver, muscle, and adipose. In the liver and muscle, insulin increases glycogen synthesis. In the muscle and adipose, insulin increases glucose uptake by increasing the number of glucose transporters (GLUT-4, see p. 97) in the cell membrane. The intravenous administration of insulin thus causes an immediate decrease in the concentration of blood glucose. In the liver, insulin decreases the production of glucose through the inhibition of glycogenolysis and gluconeogenesis.

2. **Effects on lipid metabolism:** Adipose tissue responds within minutes to administration of insulin, which causes a significant reduction in the release of fatty acids.

   a. **Decreased triacylglycerol degradation:** Insulin decreases the level of circulating free fatty acids by inhibiting the activity of *hormone-sensitive lipase* that degrades triacylglycerol in adipose tissue. Insulin acts by promoting the dephosphorylation and, hence, inactivation of the enzyme (see p. 190).

   b. **Increased triacylglycerol synthesis:** Insulin increases the transport and metabolism of glucose into adipocytes, providing the substrate glycerol 3-phosphate for triacylglycerol synthesis. Insulin also increases the *lipoprotein lipase* activity of adipose tissue by increasing the enzyme's synthesis, thus providing fatty acids for esterification. [Note: In liver, insulin promotes the conversion of glucose to triacylglycerols.]

3. **Effects on protein synthesis:** In most tissues, insulin stimulates the entry of amino acids into cells, and protein synthesis. [Note: Insulin stimulates protein synthesis through activation of factors required for translation.]

E. Mechanism of insulin action

Insulin binds to specific, high-affinity receptors in the cell membrane of most tissues, including liver, muscle, and adipose. This is the first step in a cascade of reactions ultimately leading to a diverse array of biologic actions (Figure 23.7).

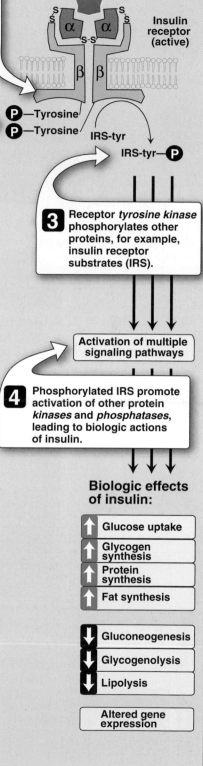

Figure 23.7
Insulin receptor. IRS = Insulin receptor substrate.

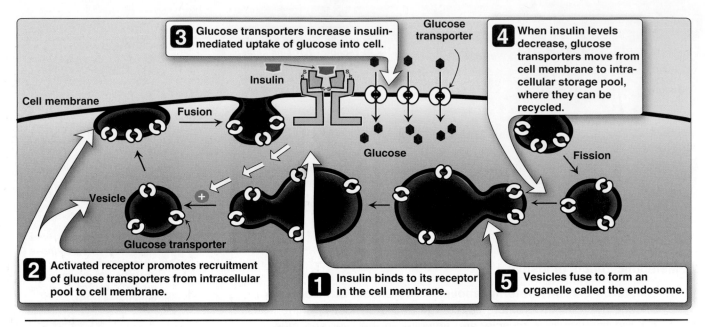

Figure 23.8
Insulin causes the recruitment of glucose transporters (GLUTs) from intracellular stores in skeletal and cardiac muscle and adipose tissue.

1. **Insulin receptor:** The insulin receptor is synthesized as a single polypeptide that is glycosylated and cleaved into α and β subunits, which are then assembled into a tetramer linked by disulfide bonds (see Figure 23.7). A hydrophobic domain in each β subunit spans the plasma membrane. The extracellular α subunit contains the insulin-binding site. The cytosolic domain of the β subunit is a *tyrosine kinase*, which is activated by insulin.

2. **Signal transduction:** The binding of insulin to the α subunits of the insulin receptor induces conformational changes that are transduced to the β subunits. This promotes a rapid autophosphorylation of specific tyrosine residues on each β subunit (see Figure 23.7). Autophosphorylation initiates a cascade of cell-signaling responses, including phosphorylation of a family of proteins called insulin receptor substrates (IRS). At least four IRS have been identified that show similar structures but different tissue distributions. Phosphorylated IRS proteins interact with other signaling molecules through specific domains, activating a number of pathways that affect gene expression, cell metabolism and growth. The actions of insulin are terminated by dephosphorylation of the receptor.

3. **Membrane effects of insulin:** Glucose transport in some tissues, such as skeletal muscle and adipocytes, increases in the presence of insulin (Figure 23.8). Insulin promotes the recruitment of insulin-sensitive glucose transporters (GLUT-4) from a pool located in intracellular vesicles. [Note: Many tissues have insulin-insensitive systems for glucose transport (Figure 23.9). For example, hepatocytes, erythrocytes, and cells of the nervous system, intestinal mucosa, renal tubules, and cornea do not require insulin for glucose uptake.]

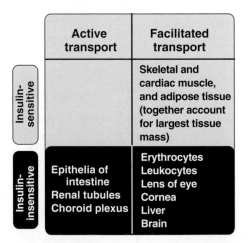

	Active transport	Facilitated transport
Insulin-sensitive		Skeletal and cardiac muscle, and adipose tissue (together account for largest tissue mass)
Insulin-insensitive	Epithelia of intestine Renal tubules Choroid plexus	Erythrocytes Leukocytes Lens of eye Cornea Liver Brain

Figure 23.9
Characteristics of glucose transport in various tissues.

4. **Receptor regulation:** Binding of insulin is followed by internalization of the hormone–receptor complex. Once inside the cell, insulin is degraded in the lysosomes. The receptors may be degraded but most are recycled to the cell surface. [Note: Elevated levels of insulin promote the degradation of receptors, thus decreasing the number of surface receptors. This is one type of "down-regulation."]

5. **Time course of insulin actions:** The binding of insulin provokes a wide range of actions. The most immediate response is an increase in glucose transport into adipocytes and skeletal muscle cells that occurs within seconds of insulin binding to its membrane receptor. Insulin-induced changes in enzymic activity in many cell types occur over minutes to hours, and reflect changes in the phosphorylation states of existing proteins. Insulin also initiates an increase in the amount of many enzymes, such as *glucokinase*, liver *pyruvate kinase, acetyl CoA carboxylase*, and *fatty acid synthase*, which requires hours to days. These changes reflect an increase in gene expression through increased transcription (mediated by SREBP-1, see p. 184) and translation.

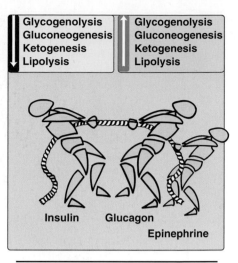

Figure 23.10
Opposing actions of insulin and glucagon plus epinephrine.

III. GLUCAGON

Glucagon is a polypeptide hormone secreted by the α cells of the pancreatic islets of Langerhans. Glucagon, along with epinephrine, cortisol, and growth hormone (the "counter-regulatory hormones"), opposes many of the actions of insulin (Figure 23.10). Most importantly, glucagon acts to maintain blood glucose levels by activation of hepatic glycogenolysis and gluconeogenesis. Glucagon is composed of 29 amino acids arranged in a single polypeptide chain. [Note: Unlike insulin, the amino acid sequence of glucagon is the same in all mammalian species examined to date.] Glucagon is synthesized as a large precursor molecule (preproglucagon) that is converted to glucagon through a series of selective proteolytic cleavages, similar to those described for insulin biosynthesis (see Figure 23.3). In contrast to insulin, preproglucagon is processed to different products in different tissues.

A. Stimulation of glucagon secretion

The α cell is responsive to a variety of stimuli that signal actual or potential hypoglycemia (Figure 23.11). Specifically, glucagon secretion is increased by:

1. **Low blood glucose:** A decrease in plasma glucose concentration is the primary stimulus for glucagon release. During an overnight or prolonged fast, elevated glucagon levels prevent hypoglycemia (see below for a discussion of hypoglycemia).

2. **Amino acids:** Amino acids derived from a meal containing protein stimulate the release of both glucagon and insulin. The glucagon effectively prevents hypoglycemia that would otherwise occur as a result of increased insulin secretion that occurs after a protein meal.

3. **Epinephrine:** Elevated levels of circulating epinephrine produced by the adrenal medulla, or norepinephrine produced by sympathetic innervation of the pancreas, or both, stimulate the release

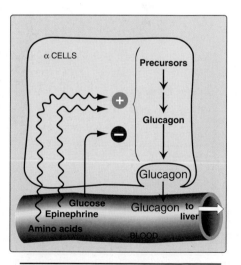

Figure 23.11
Regulation of glucagon release from pancreatic α cells. [Note: Amino acids increase release of insulin and glucagon, whereas glucose increases release of insulin only.]

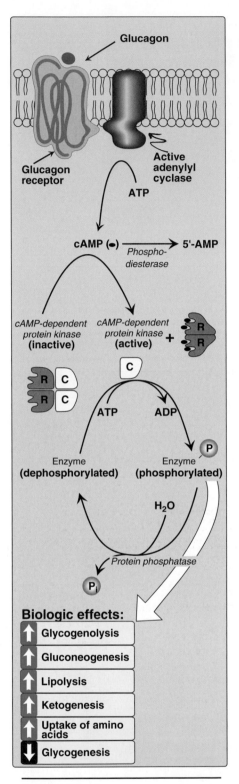

Figure 23.12
Mechanism of action of glucagon.
[Note: For clarity, G-protein
activation of *adenylyl cyclase*
has been omitted.] R = regulatory
subunit; C = catalytic subunit.

of glucagon. Thus, during periods of stress, trauma, or severe exercise, the elevated epinephrine levels can override the effect on the α cell of circulating substrates. In these situations—regardless of the concentration of blood glucose—glucagon levels are elevated in anticipation of increased glucose use. In contrast, insulin levels are depressed.

B. Inhibition of glucagon secretion

Glucagon secretion is significantly decreased by elevated blood glucose and by insulin. Both substances are increased following ingestion of glucose or a carbohydrate-rich meal (see Figure 23.5). The regulation of glucagon secretion is summarized in Figure 23.11.

C. Metabolic effects of glucagon

1. **Effects on carbohydrate metabolism:** The intravenous administration of glucagon leads to an immediate rise in blood glucose. This results from an increase in the breakdown of liver (not muscle) glycogen and an increase in gluconeogenesis.

2. **Effects on lipid metabolism:** Glucagon activates lipolysis in adipose. The free fatty acids released are taken up by liver and oxidized to acetyl coenzyme A, which is used in ketone body synthesis. [Note: The catecholamines also activate lipolysis.]

3. **Effects on protein metabolism:** Glucagon increases uptake of amino acids by the liver, resulting in increased availability of carbon skeletons for gluconeogenesis. As a consequence, plasma levels of amino acids are decreased.

D. Mechanism of action of glucagon

Glucagon binds to high-affinity G protein-coupled receptors on the cell membrane of hepatocytes. The receptors for glucagon are distinct from those that bind insulin or epinephrine. [Note: Glucagon receptors are not found on skeletal muscle.] Glucagon binding results in activation of *adenylyl cyclase* in the plasma membrane (Figure 23.12, and see p. 94). This causes a rise in cAMP (the "second messenger"), which, in turn, activates *cAMP-dependent protein kinase* and increases the phosphorylation of specific enzymes or other proteins. This cascade of increasing enzymic activities results in the phosphorylation-mediated activation or inhibition of key regulatory enzymes involved in carbohydrate and lipid metabolism. An example of such a cascade in glycogen degradation is shown on Figure 11.9, p. 131, and p. 132. [Note: Glucagon also affects gene transcription.]

IV. HYPOGLYCEMIA

Hypoglycemia is characterized by: 1) central nervous system (CNS) symptoms, including confusion, aberrant behavior, or coma; 2) a simultaneous blood glucose level equal to or less than 40 mg/dl; and 3) symptoms being resolved within minutes following the administration of glucose (Figure 23.13). Hypoglycemia is a medical emergency because the CNS has an absolute requirement for a continuous supply of bloodborne glucose to serve as fuel for energy metabolism. Transient hypoglycemia can cause cerebral dysfunction, whereas severe, prolonged hypoglycemia causes brain death. It is, therefore, not surprising that the body has multiple overlapping mechanisms to prevent or correct hypoglycemia. The most important hormone changes in combating hypoglycemia are elevated glucagon and epinephrine, combined with the diminished release of insulin.

A. Symptoms of hypoglycemia

The symptoms of hypoglycemia can be divided into two categories. Adrenergic symptoms—anxiety, palpitation, tremor, and sweating—are mediated by epinephrine release regulated by the hypothalamus in response to hypoglycemia. Usually adrenergic symptoms (that is, symptoms mediated by elevated epinephrine) occur when blood glucose levels fall abruptly. The second category of hypoglycemic symptoms is neuroglycopenic. Neuroglycopenia—the impaired delivery of glucose to the brain—results in impairment of brain function, causing headache, confusion, slurred speech, seizures, coma, and death. Neuroglycopenic symptoms often result from a gradual decline in blood glucose, often to levels below 40 mg/dl. The slow decline in glucose deprives the CNS of fuel, but fails to trigger an adequate epinephrine response.

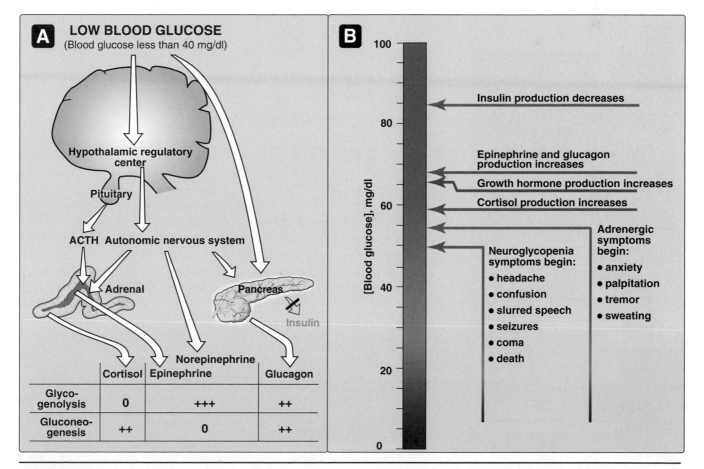

Figure 23.13
A. Actions of some of the glucoregulatory hormones in response to low blood glucose. B. Glycemic thresholds for the various responses to hypoglycemia. + = weak stimulation; ++ = moderate stimulation; +++ = strong stimulation; 0 = no effect. [Note: Normal fasted blood glucose is 70–99 mg/100 ml.]

B. Glucoregulatory systems

Humans have two overlapping glucose-regulating systems that are activated by hypoglycemia: 1) the islets of Langerhans, which release glucagon; and 2) receptors in the hypothalamus, which respond to abnormally low concentrations of blood glucose. The hypothalamic glucoreceptors can trigger both the secretion of epinephrine (mediated by the autonomic nervous system) and release of adrenocorticotropic hormone (ACTH) and growth hormone by the anterior pituitary (see Figure 23.13). [Note: ACTH increases cortisol synthesis and secretion in the adrenal cortex (see p. 239.] Glucagon, epinephrine, cortisol, and growth hormones are sometimes called the "counter-regulatory" hormones because each opposes the action of insulin on glucose use.

1. **Glucagon and epinephrine:** Hypoglycemia is combatted by decreased release of insulin and increased secretion of glucagon, epinephrine, cortisol, and growth hormone (see Figure 23.13). Glucagon and epinephrine are most important in the acute, short-term regulation of blood glucose levels. Glucagon stimulates hepatic glycogenolysis and gluconeogenesis. Epinephrine promotes glycogenolysis and lipolysis, inhibits insulin secretion, and inhibits the insulin-mediated uptake of glucose by peripheral tissues. Epinephrine is not normally essential in combating hypoglycemia, but it can assume a critical role when glucagon secretion is deficient, for example, in the late stages of type 1 (formerly called insulin-dependent) diabetes mellitus (see p. 340). The prevention or correction of hypoglycemia fails when the secretion of both glucagon and epinephrine is deficient.

2. **Cortisol and growth hormone:** These hormones are less important in the short-term maintenance of blood glucose concentrations. They do, however, play a role in the long-term management of glucose metabolism.

C. Types of hypoglycemia

Hypoglycemia may be divided into three types: 1) insulin-induced; 2) postprandial (sometimes called reactive hypoglycemia); and 3) fasting hypoglycemia. [Note: Alcohol intoxication in fasting individuals can also be associated with hypoglycemia.]

1. **Insulin-induced hypoglycemia:** Hypoglycemia occurs frequently in patients with diabetes who are receiving insulin treatment, particularly those striving to achieve tight control of blood glucose levels. Mild hypoglycemia in fully conscious patients is treated by oral administration of carbohydrate. More commonly, patients with hypoglycemia are unconscious or have lost the ability to coordinate swallowing. In these cases, glucagon, administered subcutaneously or intramuscularly, is the treatment of choice (Figure 23.14).

2. **Postprandial hypoglycemia:** This is the second most common form of hypoglycemia. It is caused by an exaggerated insulin release following a meal, prompting transient hypoglycemia with mild adrenergic symptoms. The plasma glucose level returns to normal even if the patient is not fed. The only treatment usually required is that the patient eat frequent small meals rather than the usual three large meals.

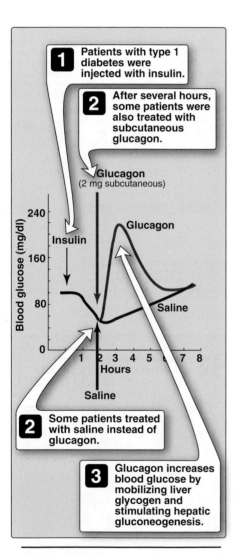

Figure 23.14
Reversal of insulin-induced hypoglycemia by administration of subcutaneous glucagon.

3. **Fasting hypoglycemia:** Low blood glucose during fasting is rare, but is more likely to present as a serious medical problem. Fasting hypoglycemia, which tends to produce neuroglycopenia symptoms, may result from a reduction in the rate of glucose production by hepatic glycogenolysis or gluconeogenesis. Thus, low blood glucose levels are often seen in patients with hepatocellular damage or adrenal insufficiency, or in fasting individuals who have consumed large quantities of ethanol (see below). Alternately, fasting hypoglycemia may be the result of an increased rate of glucose use by the peripheral tissues due to overproduction of insulin by rare pancreatic tumors. If left untreated, a patient with fasting hypoglycemia may lose consciousness and experience convulsions and coma. [Note: Defects in fatty acid oxidation also result in hypoglycemia.]

4. **Hypoglycemia and alcohol intoxication:** Alcohol is metabolized in the liver by two oxidation reactions (Figure 23.15). Ethanol is first converted to acetaldehyde by *alcohol dehydrogenase*. Acetaldehyde is subsequently oxidized to acetate by *aldehyde dehydrogenase*. [Note: This enzyme is inhibited by disulfiram, a drug that has found some use in patients desiring to stop alcohol ingestion. It causes the accumulation of acetaldehyde in the blood, which results in flushing, tachycardia, hyperventilation, and nausea.] In each reaction, electrons are transferred to NAD$^+$, resulting in a massive increase in the concentration of cytosolic NADH. The abundance of NADH favors the reduction of pyruvate to lactate, and of oxaloacetate (OAA) to malate. [Note: The rise in lactate can result in lactic acidosis and, because lactate competes with urate for excretion by the kidney, can also result in hyperuricemia.] Recall from p. 118 that pyruvate and OAA are both intermediates in the synthesis of glucose by gluconeogenesis. Thus, the ethanol-mediated increase in NADH causes the intermediates of gluconeogenesis to be diverted into alternate reaction pathways, resulting in the decreased synthesis of glucose.

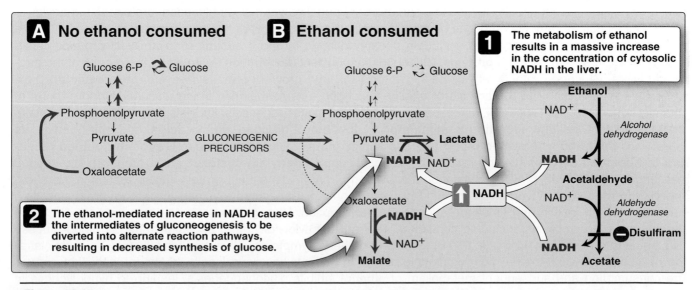

Figure 23.15
A. Normal gluconeogenesis in the absence of ethanol consumption. B. Inhibition of gluconeogenesis resulting from hepatic metabolism of ethanol.

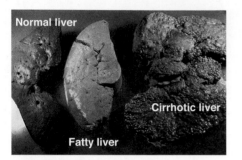

Figure 23.16
Effects of chronic alcohol consumption on liver morphology.

This can precipitate hypoglycemia, particularly in individuals who have depleted their stores of liver glycogen. [Note: Decreased availability of OAA allows acetyl CoA to be diverted to ketone body synthesis in liver (see p. 195), and can result in alcoholic ketoacidosis.] Hypoglycemia can produce many of the behaviors associated with alcohol intoxication—agitation, impaired judgement, and combativeness. Thus, alcohol consumption in vulnerable individuals—those who are fasted or have engaged in prolonged, strenuous exercise—can produce hypoglycemia that may contribute to the behavioral effects of alcohol. Alcohol consumption can also increase the risk for hypoglycemia in patients using insulin; therefore, patients in an intensive insulin treatment protocol (see p. 340) are counseled about the increased risk of hypoglycemia that generally occurs many hours after the alcohol has been consumed. [Note: Chronic alcohol consumption can also result in alcoholic fatty liver due to increased synthesis of triacylglycerols. This occurs as a result of decreased fatty acid oxidation due to a fall in the $NAD^+/NADH$ ratio, and increased lipogenesis due to the increased availability of fatty acids (decreased catabolism) and of glyceraldehyde 3-phosphate (the *dehydrogenase* is inhibited by the low $NAD^+/NADH$ ratio). With continued alcohol consumption, alcoholic fatty liver can progress first to alcoholic hepatitis, and then to alcoholic cirrhosis (Figure 23.16).]

V. CHAPTER SUMMARY

The integration of energy metabolism is controlled primarily by **insulin** and the opposing actions of **glucagon** and **epinephrine** (Figure 23.17). Changes in the circulating levels of these hormones allow the body to store energy when food is available in abundance, or to make stored energy available, for example, during "survival crises," such as famine, severe injury, and "fight-or-flight" situations. **Insulin** is a polypeptide hormone produced by the **β-cells** of the **islets of Langerhans** of the pancreas. The biosynthesis involves two inactive precursors, **preproinsulin** and **proinsulin**, which are sequentially cleaved to form the active hormone. A rise in blood glucose is the most important signal for increased insulin secretion. The synthesis and release of insulin are decreased by epinephrine, which is secreted by the adrenal cortex in response to stress, trauma, or extreme exercise. Insulin increases glucose uptake (by muscle and adipose) and the synthesis of glycogen, protein, and triacylglycerol. These actions are mediated by the binding of insulin to the α subunit of the insulin receptor, which initiates a cascade of cell-signaling responses, including phosphorylation by the β subunit of a family of proteins called **insulin receptor substrate (IRS) proteins**. Glucagon is a polypeptide hormone secreted by the α cells of the pancreatic islets. Glucagon, along with epinephrine, cortisol, and growth hormone (the "**counter-regulatory hormones**"), opposes many of the actions of insulin. Glucagon acts to maintain blood glucose during periods of potential hypoglycemia. Glucagon increases glycogenolysis, gluconeogenesis, lipolysis, ketogenesis, and uptake of amino acids. Glucagon **secretion** is **stimulated** by **low blood glucose**, **amino acids**, and **epinephrine**. Its secretion is **inhibited by elevated blood glucose** and by **insulin**. Glucagon binds to **G protein-coupled receptors** of **hepatocytes**. This binding results in the activation of **adenylate cyclase**, which produces the second messenger, **cyclic AMP (cAMP)**. Subsequent activation of cAMP-dependent protein kinase results in the phosphorylation-mediated activation or inhibition of key regulatory enzymes involved in carbohydrate and lipid metabolism. Both insulin and glucagon affect gene transcription. **Hypoglycemia** is characterized by: 1) central nervous system symptoms, including confusion, aberrant behavior, or coma; 2) a simultaneous blood glucose level equal to or less than 40 mg/dl; and 3) resolution of these symptoms within minutes following the administration of glucose. Hypoglycemia most commonly occurs in patients receiving insulin treatment with tight control. The consumption and subsequent metabolism of **ethanol** inhibits gluconeogenesis, leading to hypoglycemia in individuals with depleted stores of liver glycogen. Alcohol consumption can also increase the risk for hypoglycemia in patients using insulin. Chronic alcohol consumption can cause liver disease.

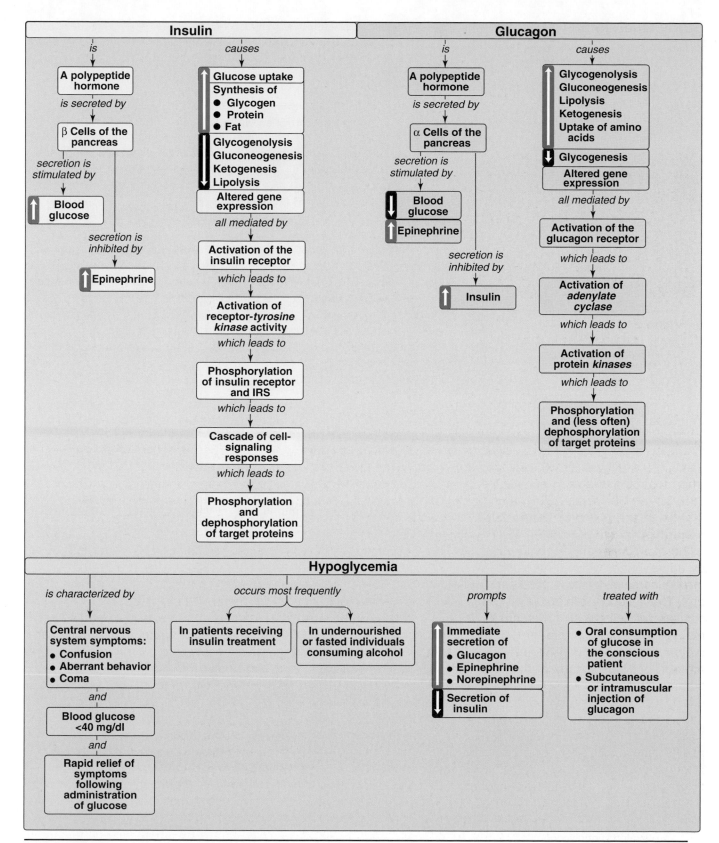

Figure 23.17
Key concept map for integration of energy metabolism.

Study Questions

Choose the ONE correct answer.

23.1 In which one of the following tissues is glucose transport into the cell insulin-sensitive?

    A. Brain.

    B. Lens of the eye.

    C. Red blood cells.

    D. Adipose tissue.

    E. Liver.

> Correct answer = D. The major tissues in which glucose transport requires insulin are muscle and adipose tissue. The metabolism of the liver responds to insulin, but hepatic glucose transport is determined by blood glucose concentration and does not require insulin. Brain, RBC, and lens of the eye have insulin-insensitive uptake of glucose.

23.2 Which one of the following is characteristic of low insulin levels?

    A. Increased glycogen synthesis.

    B. Decreased gluconeogenesis from lactate.

    C. Decreased glycogenolysis.

    D. Increased formation of 3-hydroxybutyrate.

    E. Decreased action of hormone-sensitive lipase.

> Correct answer = D. 3-Hydroxybutyrate (or β-hydroxybutyrate)—a ketone body—synthesis is enhanced in the liver by low insulin levels, which favor activation of hormone-sensitive lipase and release of fatty acids from adipose tissue. Glycogen synthesis is decreased, whereas gluconeogenesis and glycogenolysis are increased.

23.3 Which one of the following statements about glucagon is correct?

    A. High levels of blood glucose increase the release of glucagon from the α cells of the pancreas.

    B. Glucagon levels decrease following ingestion of a protein-rich meal.

    C. Glucagon increases the intracellular levels of cAMP in liver cells, causing an increase in glycogenolysis.

    D. Glucagon is the only hormone important in combating hypoglycemia.

    E. Glucagon depresses the formation of ketone bodies by the liver.

> Correct answer = C. The cAMP cascade initiated by glucagon causes the liver to degrade glycogen, releasing glucose to the blood. High levels of blood glucose decrease the release of glucagon from the α cells of the pancreas. Glucagon levels increase following ingestion of a protein-rich meal. In addition to glucagon, epinephrine and cortisol are also important in increasing glucose production in hypoglycemia. Glucagon increases the formation of ketone bodies by the liver.

23.4 A 39-year-old woman is brought to the emergency room complaining of dizziness. She recalls getting up early that morning to do as much shopping as possible and had skipped breakfast. She drank a cup of coffee for lunch and had nothing to eat during the day. She met with friends at 8 p.m. and had a drink at the bar. She soon became weak and dizzy and was transported to the hospital. Following examination, the patient was given orange juice and immediately felt better. Which one of the following best completes this sentence? "The patient has":

    A. blood glucose greater than 70 mg/dl.

    B. elevated insulin.

    C. elevated glucagon.

    D. elevated liver glycogen.

    E. presence of an insulinoma.

> Correct answer = C. The patient's glucagon level will be elevated in response to the hypoglycemia. She is most likely experiencing alcohol-induced fasting hypoglycemia. Blood glucose is expected to be 40 mg/dl or less, insulin secretion depressed because of the low blood glucose, and liver glycogen levels low because of the fast. An insulinoma, an insulin-producing tumor of the pancreas, is unlikely.

The Feed/Fast Cycle

24

I. OVERVIEW OF THE ABSORPTIVE STATE

The absorptive (fed) state is the two- to four-hour period after ingestion of a normal meal. During this interval, transient increases in plasma glucose, amino acids, and triacylglycerols (TAG) occur, the latter primarily as components of chylomicrons synthesized by the intestinal mucosal cells (see p. 228). Islet tissue of the pancreas responds to the elevated levels of glucose and amino acids with an increased secretion of insulin and a decreased release of glucagon. The elevated insulin to glucagon ratio and the ready availability of circulating substrates make the absorptive state an anabolic period characterized by increased synthesis of TAG and glycogen to replenish fuel stores, and enhanced synthesis of protein. During this absorptive period, virtually all tissues use glucose as a fuel, and the metabolic response of the body is dominated by alterations in the metabolism of liver, adipose tissue, muscle, and brain. In this chapter, an "organ map" is introduced that traces the movement of metabolites between tissues. The goal is to create an expanded and clinically useful vision of whole-body metabolism.

II. ENZYMIC CHANGES IN THE ABSORPTIVE STATE

The flow of intermediates through metabolic pathways is controlled by four mechanisms: 1) the availability of substrates; 2) allosteric regulation of enzymes; 3) covalent modification of enzymes; and 4) induction-repression of enzyme synthesis, primarily through regulation of transcription. This scheme may at first seem unnecessarily redundant; however, each mechanism operates on a different timescale (Figure 24.1), and allows the body to adapt to a wide variety of physiologic situations. In the fed state, these regulatory mechanisms ensure that available nutrients are captured as glycogen, TAG, and protein.

A. Allosteric effects

Allosteric changes usually involve rate-determining reactions. For example, glycolysis in the liver is stimulated following a meal by an increase in fructose 2,6-bisphosphate—an allosteric activator of *phosphofructokinase-1* (see p. 99). In contrast, gluconeogenesis is inhibited by fructose 2,6-bisphosphate, an allosteric inhibitor of *fructose 1,6-bisphosphatase* (see p. 121).

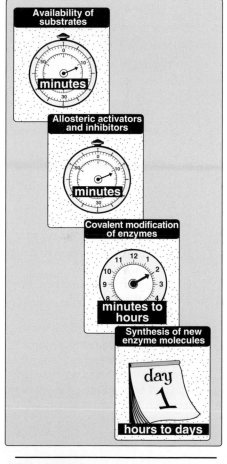

Figure 24.1
Control mechanisms of metabolism and some typical response times. [Note: Response times may vary according to the nature of the stimulus and from tissue to tissue.]

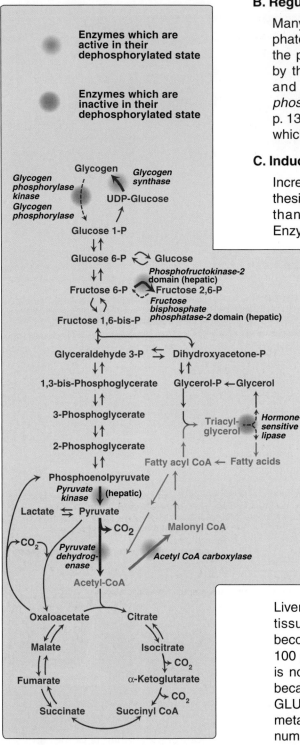

Figure 24.2
Important reactions of intermediary metabolism regulated by enzyme phosphorylation.
Blue text = intermediates of carbohydrate metabolism;
Brown text = intermediates of lipid metabolism.

B. Regulation of enzymes by covalent modification

Many enzymes are regulated by the addition or removal of phosphate groups from specific serine, threonine, or tyrosine residues of the protein. In the absorptive state, most of the enzymes regulated by these covalent modifications are in the dephosphorylated form and are active (Figure 24.2). Three exceptions are *glycogen phosphorylase kinase* (see p. 132), *glycogen phosphorylase* (see p. 132), and *hormone-sensitive lipase* of adipose tissue (see p. 190), which are inactive in their dephosphorylated form.

C. Induction and repression of enzyme synthesis

Increased (induction of) or decreased (repression of) enzyme synthesis leads to changes in the total population of active sites, rather than influencing the efficiency of existing enzyme molecules. Enzymes subject to regulation of synthesis are often those that are needed at only one stage of development or under selected physiologic conditions. For example, in the fed state, elevated insulin levels result in an increase in the synthesis of key enzymes, such as *acetyl coenzyme A (CoA) carboxylase* (see p. 184) and *3-hydroxy-3-methylglutaryl-coenzyme A (HMG-CoA) reductase* (see p. 223) involved in anabolic metabolism.

III. LIVER: NUTRIENT DISTRIBUTION CENTER

The liver is uniquely situated to process and distribute dietary nutrients because the venous drainage of the gut and pancreas passes through the hepatic portal vein before entry into the general circulation. Thus, after a meal, the liver is bathed in blood containing absorbed nutrients and elevated levels of insulin secreted by the pancreas. During the absorptive period, the liver takes up carbohydrates, lipids, and most amino acids. These nutrients are then metabolized, stored, or routed to other tissues. Thus, the liver smooths out potentially broad fluctuations in the availability of nutrients for the peripheral tissues.

A. Carbohydrate metabolism

Liver is normally a glucose-producing rather than a glucose-using tissue. However, after a meal containing carbohydrate, the liver becomes a net consumer of glucose, retaining roughly 60 of every 100 g of glucose presented by the portal system. This increased use is not a result of stimulated glucose transport into the hepatocyte, because this process is normally rapid and the glucose transporter, GLUT-2 (see p. 97), is insulin insensitive. Rather, hepatic glucose metabolism is increased by the following mechanisms. [Note: The numbers in colored circles in the text refer to Figure 24.3.]

1. **Increased phosphorylation of glucose:** Elevated levels of glucose within the hepatocyte (as a result of elevated extracellular levels) allow *glucokinase* to phosphorylate glucose to glucose 6-phosphate. (Recall that *glucokinase* is not subject to product inhibition.) This contrasts with the postabsorptive (fasted) state in which hepatic glucose levels are lower and *glucokinase* is largely dormant because of its low affinity (high K_m) for glucose (Figure 24.3, **❶**).

2. **Increased glycogen synthesis:** The conversion of glucose 6-phosphate to glycogen is favored by the activation of *glycogen synthase*—both by dephosphorylation and by increased availability of glucose 6-phosphate, its allosteric effector (see Figure 24.3, ❷).

3. **Increased activity of the hexose monophosphate pathway (HMP):** The increased availability of glucose 6-phosphate in the absorptive state, combined with the active use of NADPH in hepatic lipogenesis, stimulate the HMP (see Chapter 12, p. 145). This pathway typically accounts for 5–10% of the glucose metabolized by the liver (see Figure 24.3, ❸).

4. **Increased glycolysis:** In liver, glycolytic metabolism of glucose is significant only during the absorptive period following a carbohydrate-rich meal. The conversion of glucose to acetyl CoA is stimulated by the elevated insulin to glucagon ratio that results in increased activity (and amount) of the regulated enzymes of glycolysis, for example, *pyruvate kinase* (see p. 102). *Pyruvate dehydrogenase* (*PDH*), which converts pyruvate to acetyl CoA, is active (dephosphorylated) because pyruvate inhibits *PDH kinase* (see Figure 24.3, ❹). Acetyl CoA is used as either a building block for fatty acid synthesis, or it provides energy by oxidation in the tricarboxylic acid (TCA) cycle.

5. **Decreased gluconeogenesis:** Whereas glycolysis is stimulated in the absorptive state, gluconeogenesis is decreased. *Pyruvate carboxylase*, which catalyzes the first step in gluconeogenesis, is largely inactive due to low levels of acetyl CoA—an allosteric effector essential for enzyme activity (see p. 119). [Note: The acetyl CoA is being used for fatty acid synthesis.] The high insulin to glucagon ratio also favors inactivation of other gluconeogenic

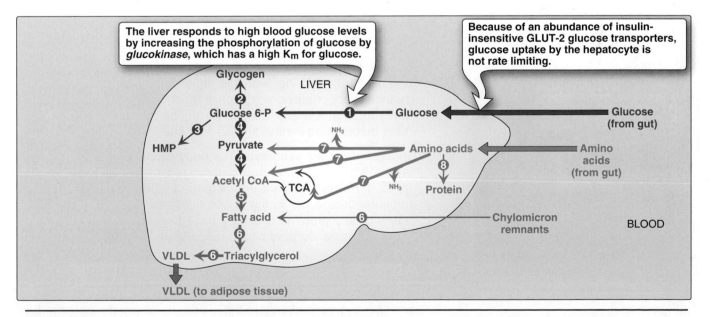

Figure 24.3
Major metabolic pathways in liver in the absorptive state. [Note: The acetyl CoA is also used for cholesterol synthesis.] The numbers in circles, which appear both in the figure and in the text, indicate important pathways for carbohydrate, fat, or protein metabolism. **Blue text** = intermediates of carbohydrate metabolism; **Brown text** = intermediates of lipid metabolism; **Green text** = intermediates of protein metabolism.

enzymes, such as *fructose 1,6-bisphosphatase* (see Figure 8.17, p. 100). [Note: Glycogenolysis is also decreased in this period.]

B. Fat metabolism

1. **Increased fatty acid synthesis:** Liver is the primary tissue for <u>de novo</u> synthesis of fatty acids (see Figure 24.3, ❺). This pathway occurs in the absorptive period, when dietary caloric intake exceeds energy expenditure by the body. Fatty acid synthesis is favored by the availability of substrates (acetyl CoA and NADPH derived from the metabolism of glucose) and by the activation of *acetyl CoA carboxylase*, both by dephosphorylation and by the presence of its allosteric activator, citrate. This enzyme catalyzes the formation of malonyl CoA from acetyl CoA—a reaction that is rate-limiting for fatty acid synthesis (see p. 183). [Note: Fatty acid oxidation is inhibited in this period by malonyl CoA.]

2. **Increased TAG synthesis:** TAG synthesis is favored because fatty acyl CoA is available both from <u>de novo</u> synthesis from acetyl CoA and from hydrolysis of the TAG component of chylomicron remnants removed from the blood by hepatocytes (see p. 178). Glycerol 3-phosphate, the backbone for TAG synthesis, is provided by the glycolytic metabolism of glucose (see p. 189). The liver packages TAG into very-low-density lipoprotein (VLDL) particles that are secreted into the blood for use by extrahepatic tissues, particularly adipose and muscle tissue (see Figure 24.3, ❻).

C. Amino acid metabolism

1. **Increased amino acid degradation:** In the absorptive period, more amino acids are present than the liver can use in the synthesis of proteins and other nitrogen-containing molecules. The surplus amino acids are not stored, but are either released into the blood for all tissues to use in protein synthesis or are deaminated, with the resulting carbon skeletons being degraded by the liver to pyruvate, acetyl CoA, or TCA cycle intermediates. These metabolites can be oxidized for energy or used in fatty acid synthesis (see Figure 24.3, ❼). The liver has limited capacity to degrade the branched-chain amino acids leucine, isoleucine, and valine. They pass through the liver essentially unchanged and are preferentially metabolized in muscle (see p. 266).

2. **Increased protein synthesis:** The body cannot store protein in the same way that it maintains glycogen or TAG reserves (see p. 327). However, a transient increase in the synthesis of hepatic proteins does occur in the absorptive state, resulting in replacement of any proteins that may have been degraded during the previous postabsorptive period (see Figure 24.3, ❽).

IV. ADIPOSE TISSUE: ENERGY STORAGE DEPOT

Adipose tissue is second only to the liver in its ability to distribute fuel molecules. In a 70-kg man, adipose tissue weighs approximately 14 kg, or about half as much as the total muscle mass. In obese individuals adipose tissue can constitute up to 70% of body weight. Nearly the entire volume of each adipocyte can be occupied by a droplet of TAG (Figure 24.4).

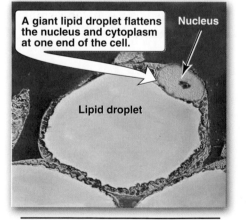

A giant lipid droplet flattens the nucleus and cytoplasm at one end of the cell.

Nucleus

Lipid droplet

Figure 24.4
Colorized transmission electron micrograph of adipocytes.

A. Carbohydrate metabolism

1. Increased glucose transport: Glucose transport by GLUT-4 into adipocytes is sensitive to the insulin concentration in the blood. Circulating insulin levels are elevated in the absorptive state, resulting in an influx of glucose into adipocytes (Figure 24.5, ❶).

2. Increased glycolysis: The increased intracellular availability of glucose results in an enhanced rate of glycolysis (see Figure 24.5, ❷). In adipose tissue, glycolysis serves a synthetic function by supplying glycerol phosphate for TAG synthesis (see p. 189).

3. Increased activity in the HMP: Adipose tissue can metabolize glucose by means of the HMP, thereby producing NADPH, which is essential for fat synthesis (see p. 186 and Figure 24.5, ❸). However in humans, <u>de novo</u> synthesis is not a major source of fatty acids in adipose tissue.

B. Fat metabolism

1. Increased synthesis of fatty acids: <u>De novo</u> synthesis of fatty acids from acetyl CoA in adipose tissue is low in humans, except when refeeding a previously fasted individual (see Figure 24.5, ❹). Instead, most of the fatty acids added to the lipid stores of adipocytes are provided by dietary fat (in the form of chylomicrons), with a lesser amount supplied by VLDL from the liver (see pp. 228 and 231).

2. Increased TAG synthesis: After consumption of a lipid-containing meal, hydrolysis of the TAG of chylomicrons (from the intestine) and VLDL (from the liver) provides adipose tissue with fatty acids (see Figure 24.5, ❺). The fatty acids are released from lipoproteins by the action of *lipoprotein lipase,* an extracellular enzyme attached to the capillary walls in many tissues—particularly adipose and muscle. Because adipocytes lack *glycerol kinase,* glycerol 3-phosphate used in TAG synthesis comes from the metabolism of glucose (see p. 189). Thus, in the fed state, elevated levels of glucose and insulin favor storage of TAG (see Figure 24.5, ❻), all the carbons of which are supplied by glucose.

3. Decreased TAG degradation: Elevated insulin favors the dephosphorylated (inactive) form of *hormone-sensitive lipase* (see p. 190). TAG degradation is thus inhibited in the fed state.

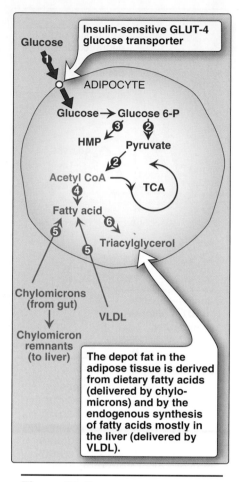

Figure 24.5
Major metabolic pathways in adipose tissue in the absorptive state. [Note: The numbers in the circles, which appear both in the figure and in the corresponding text, indicate important pathways for adipose tissue metabolism.]

V. RESTING SKELETAL MUSCLE

The energy metabolism of skeletal muscle is unique in being able to respond to substantial changes in the demand for ATP that accompanies muscle contraction. At rest, muscle accounts for approximately 30% of the oxygen consumption of the body, whereas during vigorous exercise, it is responsible for up to 90% of the total oxygen consumption. This graphically illustrates the fact that skeletal muscle, despite its potential for transient periods of anaerobic glycolysis, is an oxidative tissue. [Note: Heart muscle differs from skeletal muscle in three important ways: 1) the heart is continuously active, whereas skeletal muscle contracts intermittently on demand; 2) the heart has a completely aerobic metabolism;

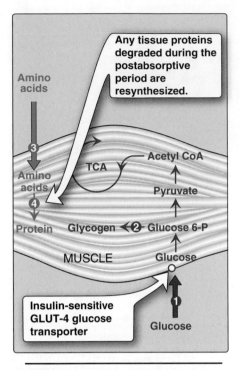

Figure 24.6
Major metabolic pathways in skeletal muscle in the absorptive state. [Note: The numbers in circles, which appear both in the figure and in the text, indicate important pathways for carbohydrate or protein metabolism.]

and 3) the heart contains negligible energy stores, such as glycogen or lipid. Thus, any interruption of the vascular supply, for example, as occurs during a myocardial infarction, results in rapid death of the myocardial cells.] Heart muscle uses fatty acids, glucose, and ketone bodies as fuels.

A. Carbohydrate metabolism

1. **Increased glucose transport:** The transient increase in plasma glucose and insulin after a carbohydrate-rich meal leads to an increase in glucose transport into muscle cells by GLUT-4 (see p. 97 and Figure 24.6, ❶). Glucose is phosphorylated to glucose 6-phosphate by *hexokinase*, and metabolized to provide the energy needs of the cells. [Note: In the fasted state fatty acids and ketone bodies are the major fuels of resting muscle.]

2. **Increased glycogen synthesis:** The increased insulin to glucagon ratio and the availability of glucose 6-phosphate favor glycogen synthesis, particularly if glycogen stores have been depleted as a result of exercise (see p. 126, and Figure 24.6, ❷).

B. Fat metabolism

Fatty acids are released from chylomicrons and VLDL by the action of *lipoprotein lipase* (see pp. 228 and 231). However, fatty acids are of secondary importance as a fuel for muscle during the fed state, in which glucose is the primary source of energy.

C. Amino acid metabolism

1. **Increased protein synthesis:** A spurt in amino acid uptake and protein synthesis occurs in the absorptive period after ingestion of a meal containing protein (see Figure 24.6, ❸ and ❹). This synthesis replaces protein degraded since the previous meal.

2. **Increased uptake of branched-chain amino acids:** Muscle is the principal site for degradation of branched-chain amino acids because it contains the required *transaminase* (see p. 266). The branched-chain amino acids, leucine, isoleucine, and valine, escape metabolism by the liver, and are taken up by muscle, where they are used for protein synthesis (see Figure 24.6, ❸) and as sources of energy.

VI. BRAIN

Although contributing only 2% of the adult weight, the brain accounts for a consistent 20% of the basal oxygen consumption of the body at rest. Because the brain is vital to the proper functioning of all organs of the body, special priority is given to its fuel needs. To provide energy, substrates must be able to cross the endothelial cells that line the blood vessels in the brain (the "blood-brain barrier"). Normally, glucose serves as the primary fuel for the brain. [Note: If blood glucose levels fall below approximately 40 mg/100 ml (normal fasted blood glucose is 70–99 mg/100 ml), cerebral function is impaired. If the hypoglycemia occurs for even a short time, severe and potentially irreversible brain damage may occur.] During a fast, however, ketone bodies play a significant role as a fuel for brain, reducing its dependence on glucose (see p. 196).

A. Carbohydrate metabolism

In the fed state, the brain uses glucose exclusively as a fuel, completely oxidizing approximately 140 g/day to CO_2 and H_2O. The brain contains no significant stores of glycogen and is, therefore, completely dependent on the availability of blood glucose (Figure 24.7, ❶).

B. Fat metabolism

The brain has no significant stores of TAG, and the fatty acids circulating in the blood make little contribution to energy production because fatty acids bound to albumin do not efficiently cross the blood-brain barrier. The intertissue exchanges characteristic of the absorptive period are summarized in Figure 24.8.

VII. OVERVIEW OF FASTING

Fasting begins if no food is ingested after the absorptive period. It may result from an inability to obtain food, the desire to lose weight rapidly, or clinical situations in which an individual cannot eat, for example, because of trauma, surgery, cancer, or burns. In the absence of food, plasma levels of glucose, amino acids, and TAG fall, triggering a decline in insulin secretion and an increase in glucagon release. The decreased insulin to glucagon ratio, and the decreased availability of circulating substrates, make the period of nutrient deprivation a catabolic period characterized by degradation of TAG, glycogen, and protein. This sets into motion an exchange of substrates among liver, adipose tissue, muscle, and brain that is guided by two priorities: 1) the need to maintain adequate plasma levels of glucose to sustain energy metabolism of the brain, red blood cells, and other glucose-requiring tissues; and 2) the need to mobilize fatty acids from adipose tissue, and the synthesis and release of ketone bodies from the liver, to supply energy to all other tissues.

A. Fuel stores

The metabolic fuels available in a normal 70–kg man at the beginning of a fast are shown in Figure 24.9. Note the enormous caloric stores available in the form of TAG compared with those contained in glycogen. [Note: Although protein is listed as an energy source, each protein also has a function, for example, as a structural component of the body, an enzyme, and so forth. Therefore, only about one third of the body's protein can be used for energy production without fatally compromising vital functions.]

B. Enzymic changes in fasting

In fasting (as in the fed state), the flow of intermediates through the pathways of energy metabolism is controlled by four mechanisms: 1) the availability of substrates; 2) allosteric regulation of enzymes; 3) covalent modification of enzymes; and 4) induction-repression of enzyme synthesis. The metabolic changes observed in fasting are generally opposite to those described for the absorptive state (see Figure 24.8). For example, most of the enzymes regulated by covalent

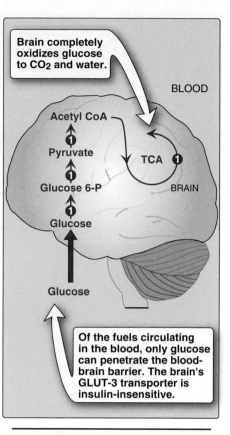

Figure 24 .7
Major metabolic pathways in brain in the absorptive state. [Note: The numbers in circles, which appear both in the figure and in the text, indicate important pathways for carbohydrate metabolism.]

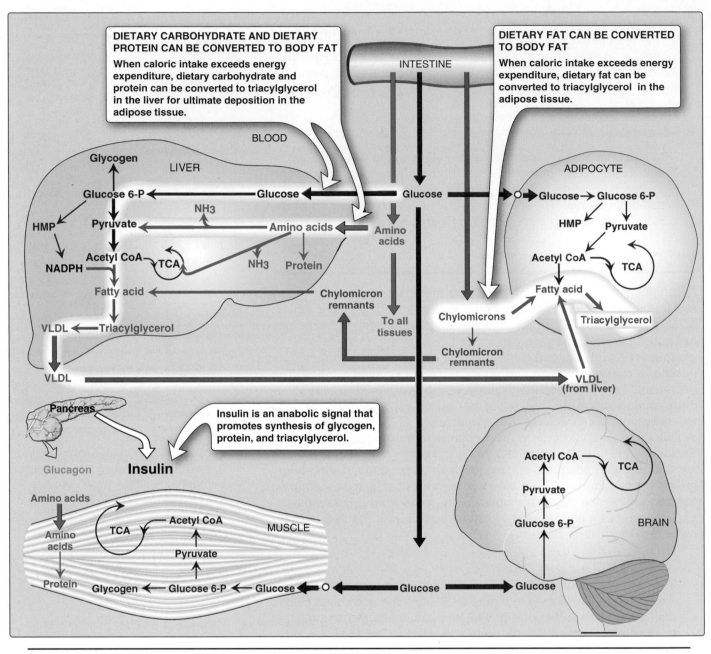

Figure 24.8
Intertissue relationships in the absorptive state. [Note: Small circles on the perimeter of tissues indicate insulin-dependent transport systems.]

modification are dephosphorylated and active in the fed state, whereas in the fasted state, they are phosphorylated and active. Three exceptions are *glycogen phosphorylase* (see p. 132), *glycogen phosphorylase kinase* (see p. 132), and *hormone-sensitive lipase* of adipose tissue (see p. 190), which are inactive in their dephosphorylated states. In fasting, substrates are not provided by the diet, but are available from the breakdown of stores and/or tissues, for example, lipolysis with release of fatty acids and glycerol from TAG in adipose tissue, and proteolysis with release of amino acids from muscle.

Recognition that the changes in fasting are the reciprocal of those in the fed state is helpful in understanding the ebb and flow of metabolism.

VIII. LIVER IN FASTING

The primary role of liver in energy metabolism during fasting is maintenance of blood glucose through the synthesis and distribution of fuel molecules for use by other organs. Thus, one speaks of "hepatic metabolism" and "extrahepatic" or "peripheral" metabolism.

A. Carbohydrate metabolism

The liver first uses glycogen degradation and then gluconeogenesis to maintain blood glucose levels to sustain energy metabolism of the brain and other glucose-requiring tissues in the fasted (postabsorptive) state. [Note: Recall the presence of *glucose 6-phosphatase* in the liver allows the production of free glucose both from glycogenolysis and from gluconeogenesis (see p. 130).]

1. **Increased glycogen degradation:** Figure 24.10 shows the sources of blood glucose after ingestion of 100 g of glucose. During the brief absorptive period, ingested glucose is the major source of blood glucose. Several hours later, blood glucose levels have declined sufficiently to cause increased secretion of glucagon and decreased release of insulin. The increased glucagon to insulin ratio causes a rapid mobilization of liver glycogen stores (which contain about 80 g of glycogen in the fed state) due to phosphorylation (activation) of *glycogen phosphorylase* (see p. 130). Note that liver glycogen is nearly exhausted after 10–18 hours of fasting; therefore, hepatic glycogenolysis is a transient response to early fasting. Figure 24.11, ❶, shows glycogen degradation as part of the overall metabolic response of the liver during fasting.

2. **Increased gluconeogenesis:** The synthesis of glucose and its release into the circulation are vital hepatic functions during fasting (see Figure 24.11, ❷). The carbon skeletons for gluconeogenesis are derived primarily from glucogenic amino acids and lactate from muscle, and glycerol from adipose. Gluconeogenesis, favored by activation of *fructose 1,6-bisphosphatase* (due to a drop in its inhibitor, fructose 2,6-bisphosphate, see p. 121) and by induction of *phosphoenolpyruvate (PEP) carboxykinase* by glucagon (see p. 122), begins 4–6 hours after the last meal and becomes fully active as stores of liver glycogen are depleted (see Figure 24.10). Gluconeogenesis plays an essential role in maintaining blood glucose during both overnight and prolonged fasting. [Note: Whereas acetyl CoA cannot be used as a substrate for gluconeogenesis, the acetyl CoA produced by hepatic oxidation of fatty acids supplied from lipolysis in adipose is an allosteric activator of *pyruvate carboxylase* (and an allosteric inhibitor of *pyruvate dehydrogenase*), and thus pushes pyruvate to gluconeogenesis (see Figure 8.24).]

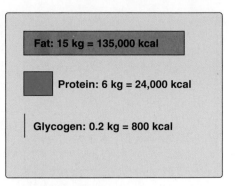

Figure 24.9
Metabolic fuels present in a 70-kg man at the beginning of a fast. Fat stores are sufficient to meet energy needs for about 3 months.

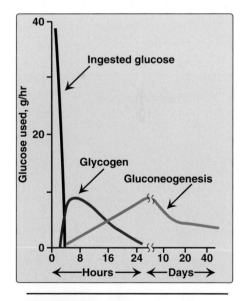

Figure 24.10
Sources of blood glucose after ingestion of 100 g of glucose.

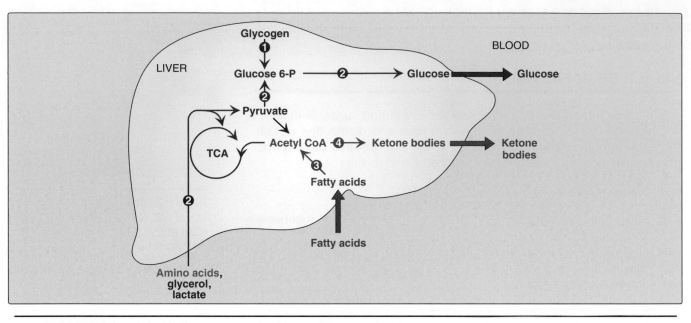

Figure 24.11
Major metabolic pathways in liver during starvation. [Note: The numbers in circles, which appear both in the figure and in the corresponding citation in the text, indicate important metabolic pathways for carbohydrate or fat.]

B. Fat metabolism

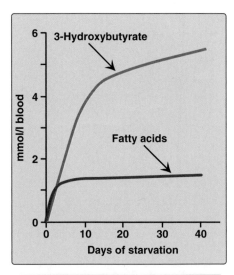

Figure 24.12
Concentrations of fatty acids and 3-hydroxybutyrate in the blood during fasting.

1. **Increased fatty acid oxidation:** The oxidation of fatty acids obtained from TAG hydrolysis in adipose tissue is the major source of energy in hepatic tissue in the postabsorptive state (see Figure 24.11, ❸). The fall in malonyl CoA due to phosphory-lation (inactivation) of *acetyl CoA carboxylase* by *AMP-activated protein kinase (AMPK)* removes the brake on *carnitine palmitoyl transferase-1 (CPT-1)*, allowing β-oxidation to occur (see p. 191). [Note: Fatty acid oxidation provides the NADH and ATP required for gluconeogenesis.]

2. **Increased synthesis of ketone bodies:** The liver is unique in being able to synthesize and release ketone bodies, primarily 3-hydroxybutyrate (formerly called β-hydroxybutyrate), for use as fuel by peripheral tissues (see p. 195), but not by the liver itself. Ketogenesis is favored when the concentration of acetyl CoA, produced from fatty acid metabolism, exceeds the oxidative capacity of the TCA cycle. [Note: Ketogenesis releases CoA, ensuring its availability for continued fatty acid oxidation.] Ketogenesis starts during the first days of fasting (Figure 24.12). The availability of circulating water-soluble ketone bodies is important in fasting because they can be used for fuel by most tissues, including brain tissue, once their level in the blood is sufficiently high. This reduces the need for gluconeogenesis from amino acid carbon skeletons, thus preserving essential protein. Ketogenesis as part of the overall hepatic response to fasting is shown in Figure 24.11, ❹. [Note: Ketone bodies are organic acids and, when present at high concentrations, can cause ketoacidosis.]

IX. ADIPOSE TISSUE IN FASTING

A. Carbohydrate metabolism

Glucose transport by insulin-sensitive GLUT-4 into the adipocyte (see p. 97) and its subsequent metabolism are depressed due to low levels of circulating insulin. This leads to a decrease in fatty acid and TAG synthesis.

B. Fat metabolism

1. **Increased degradation of TAG:** The activation of *hormone-sensitive lipase* (see p. 190) and subsequent hydrolysis of stored TAG are enhanced by the elevated catecholamines epinephrine and, particularly, norepinephrine. These compounds, which are released from the sympathetic nerve endings in adipose tissue, are physiologically important activators of *hormone-sensitive lipase* (Figure 24.13, ❶). [Note: Glucagon also activates the *lipase* (see p. 190).]

2. **Increased release of fatty acids:** Fatty acids obtained from hydrolysis of stored TAG are primarily released into the blood (see Figure 24.13, ❷). Bound to albumin, they are transported to a variety of tissues for use as fuel. The glycerol produced from TAG degradation is used as a gluconeogenic precursor by the liver. [Note: Fatty acids can also be oxidized to acetyl CoA, which can enter the TCA cycle, thus producing energy for the adipocyte. They also can be re-esterified to glycerol 3-phosphate (from glyceroneogenesis, see p. 190), generating TAG.]

3. **Decreased uptake of fatty acids:** In fasting, *lipoprotein lipase* activity of adipose tissue is low. Consequently, circulating TAG of lipoproteins is not available to adipose tissue.

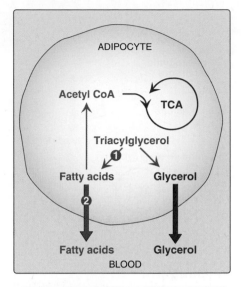

Figure 24.13
Major metabolic pathways in adipose tissue during starvation. [Note: The numbers in the circles, which appear both in the figure and in the corresponding citation in the text, indicate important pathways for fat metabolism.]

X. RESTING SKELETAL MUSCLE IN FASTING

Resting muscle uses fatty acids as its major fuel source. By contrast, exercising muscle initially uses its glycogen stores as a source of energy. During intense exercise, glucose 6-phosphate derived from glycogen is converted to lactate by anaerobic glycolysis (see p. 103). As these glycogen reserves are depleted, free fatty acids provided by the mobilization of TAG from adipose tissue become the dominant energy source.

A. Carbohydrate metabolism

Glucose transport into skeletal muscle cells via insulin-sensitive GLUT-4 proteins in the plasma membrane (see p. 97) and subsequent glucose metabolism are depressed because of low levels of circulating insulin.

B. Lipid metabolism

During the first 2 weeks of fasting, muscle uses fatty acids from adipose tissue and ketone bodies from the liver as fuels (Figure 24.14, ❶ and ❷). After about 3 weeks of fasting, muscle decreases its use of ketone bodies and oxidizes fatty acids almost exclusively. This

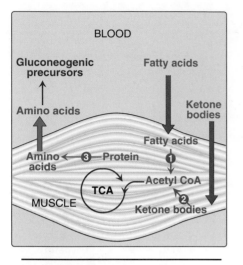

Figure 24.14
Major metabolic pathways in skeletal muscle during starvation. [Note:The numbers in the circles, which appear both in the figure and in the corresponding citation in the text, indicate important pathways for fat or protein metabolism.]

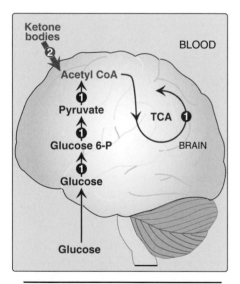

Figure 24.15
Major metabolic pathways in the brain during starvation. [Note:The numbers in the circles, which appear both in the figure and in the corresponding citation in the text, indicate important pathways for metabolism of fat or carbohydrates.]

leads to a further increase in the already elevated level of circulating ketone bodies. [Note: The increased use of ketone bodies by the brain as a result of their increased concentration in the blood is correlated with the decreased use of these compounds by the muscle.]

C. Protein metabolism

During the first few days of fasting, there is a rapid breakdown of muscle protein, providing amino acids that are used by the liver for gluconeogenesis (see Figure 24.14, ❸). Because muscle does not have glucagon receptors, muscle proteolysis likely is initiated by the fall in insulin and sustained by the rise in glucocorticoids. [Note: Alanine and glutamine are quantitatively the most important gluconeogenic amino acids released from muscle. They are produced by the catabolism of branched-chain amino acids (see p. 267).] By several weeks of fasting, the rate of muscle proteolysis decreases paralleling a decline in the need for glucose as a fuel for the brain, which has begun using ketone bodies as a source of energy.

XI. BRAIN IN FASTING

During the first days of fasting, the brain continues to use glucose exclusively as a fuel (Figure 24.15, ❶). [Note: Blood glucose is maintained by hepatic gluconeogenesis from glucogenic precursors, such as amino acids from proteolysis and glycerol from lipolysis.] In prolonged fasting (greater than 2–3 weeks), plasma ketone bodies (see Figure 24.12) reach significantly elevated levels, and replace glucose as the primary fuel for the brain (see Figure 24.15, ❷, and Figure 24.16). This reduces the need for protein catabolism for gluconeogenesis: ketone bodies spare glucose and, thus, muscle protein. The metabolic changes that occur during fasting ensure that all tissues have an adequate supply of fuel molecules. The response of the major tissues involved in energy metabolism during fasting is summarized in Figure 24.17 (see below).

XII. KIDNEY IN LONG-TERM FASTING

As fasting continues into early starvation and beyond, the kidney plays important roles. Kidney expresses the enzymes of gluconeogenesis, including *glucose 6-phosphatase*, and in late fasting about 50% of gluconeogenesis occurs here. [Note: A portion of this glucose is used by kidney itself.] Kidney also provides compensation for the acidosis that accompanies the increased production of ketone bodies (organic acids). The glutamine released from the muscle's metabolism of branched-chain amino acids is taken up by the kidney and acted upon by renal *glutaminase* and *glutamate dehydrogenase* (see p. 256), producing α-ketoglutarate that can be used as a substrate for gluconeogenesis, plus ammonia (NH_3). The NH_3 picks up H^+ from ketone body dissociation, and is excreted in the urine as NH_4^+, decreasing the acid load in the body. In long-term fasting, then, there is a switch from nitrogen disposal in the form of urea to disposal in the form of ammonia. [Note: As ketone body concentration rises, enterocytes, typically consumers of glutamine, become consumers of ketone bodies. This allows more glutamine to be available to the kidney.]

XIII. CHAPTER SUMMARY

The flow of intermediates through metabolic pathways is controlled by four mechanisms: 1) the availability of substrates; 2) allosteric activation and inhibition of enzymes; 3) covalent modification of enzymes; and 4) induction-repression of enzyme synthesis. In the absorptive state, these regulatory mechanisms ensure that available nutrients are captured as **glycogen**, **triacylglycerol**, and **protein** (Figure 24.18). The **absorptive state** is the two- to four-hour period after ingestion of a normal meal. During this interval, transient increases in plasma glucose, amino acids, and triacylglycerols occur, the last primarily as components of chylomicrons synthesized by the intestinal mucosal cells. The **pancreas** responds to the elevated levels of glucose and amino acids with an **increased secretion of insulin** and a **decrease in the release of glucagon** by the **islets of Langerhans**. The elevated insulin to glucagon ratio and the ready availability of circulating substrates make the 2–4 hours after ingestion of a meal into an **anabolic period**. During this absorptive period, virtually all tissues use **glucose** as a fuel. In addition, the **liver** replenishes its **glycogen** stores, replaces any needed **hepatic proteins**, and increases **triacylglycerol** synthesis. The latter are packaged in **very-low-density lipoproteins**, which are exported to the peripheral tissues. The **adipose** increases **triacylglycerol** synthesis and storage, whereas the **muscle** increases **protein** synthesis to replace protein degraded since the previous meal. In the fed state, the **brain** uses glucose exclusively as a fuel. In the **absence of food**, plasma levels of glucose, amino acids, and triacylglycerols fall, triggering a **decline** in **insulin secretion** and an **increase in glucagon** and **epinephrine release**. The decreased insulin to glucagon ratio, and the decreased availability of circulating substrates, makes the period of fasting a **catabolic period**. This sets into motion an **exchange of substrates** among liver, adipose tissue, muscle, and brain that is guided by two priorities: 1) the need to maintain adequate plasma levels of glucose to sustain energy metabolism of the brain and other glucose-requiring tissues; and 2) the need to mobilize fatty acids from adipose tissue and ketone bodies from liver to supply energy to all other tissues. To accomplish these goals, the **liver** degrades **glycogen** and initiates **gluconeogenesis**, using **increased fatty acid oxidation** as a source of the energy needed for gluconeogenesis, and to supply the acetyl coenzyme A building blocks for **ketone body synthesis**. The **adipose** degrades stored **triacylglycerols**, thus providing **fatty acids** and **glycerol** to the liver. The **muscle** can also use **fatty acids** as fuel, as well as **ketone bodies** supplied by the liver. Muscle **protein** is **degraded** to supply **amino acids** for the liver to use in gluconeogenesis. The **brain** can use both **glucose** and **ketone bodies** as fuels. From late fasting into starvation, the **kidneys** play important roles by **synthesizing glucose** and **excreting the protons** from ketone body dissociation as **NH₄⁺**.

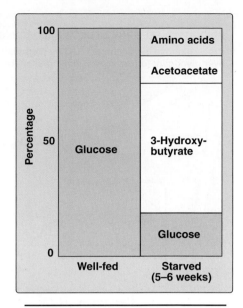

Figure 24.16
Fuel sources used by the brain to meet energy needs.

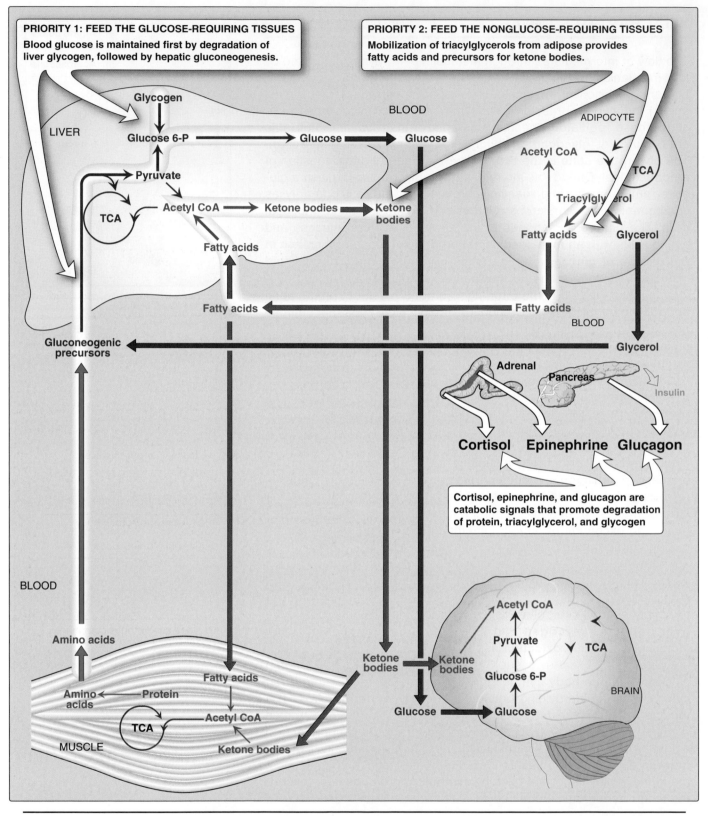

Figure 24.17
Intertissue relationships during starvation.

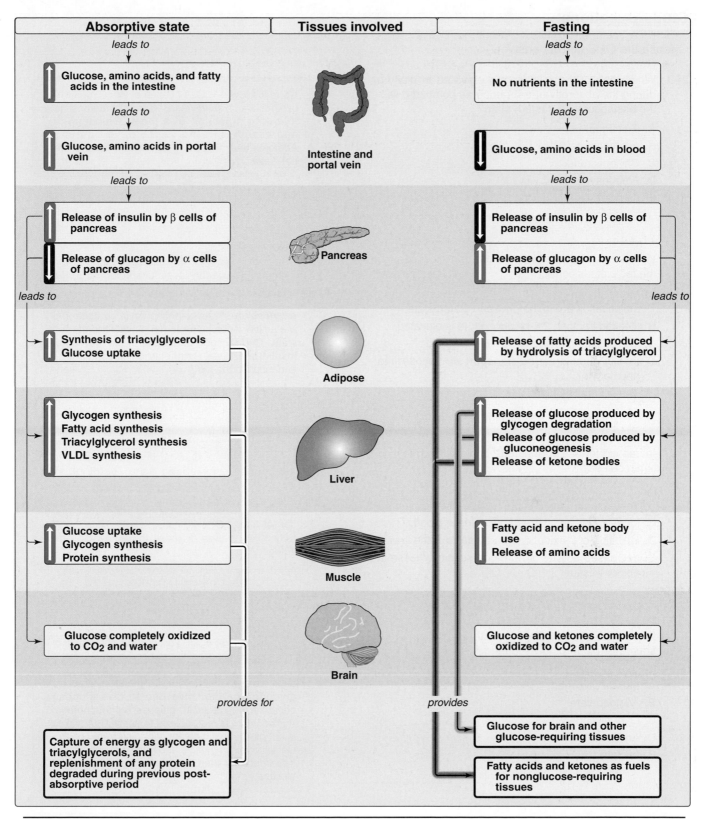

Figure 24.18
Key concept map for feed/fast cycle.

Study Questions

Choose the ONE correct answer.

24.1 Which one of the following is elevated in plasma during the absorptive (fed) period as compared with the postabsorptive (fasted) state?

A. Glucagon.

B. Acetoacetate.

C. Chylomicrons.

D. Free fatty acids.

E. Lactate.

Correct answer = C. TAG-rich chylomicrons are synthesized in (and released from) the intestine following ingestion of a meal. Glucagon is depressed in the absorptive period. Acetoacetate, free fatty acids, and lactate are not elevated.

24.2 Which one of the following statements concerning the fed state is correct?

A. Most enzymes that are regulated by covalent modification are in the phosphorylated state.

B. Hepatic fructose 2,6-bisphosphate is elevated.

C. The oxidation of acetyl CoA is increased.

D. Insulin stimulates the transport of glucose into hepatocytes.

E. The synthesis of glucokinase is repressed.

Correct answer = B. The increased insulin and decreased glucagon levels characteristic of the fed state promote the synthesis of fructose 2,6-bisphosphate. Most covalently modified enzymes are in the dephosphorylated state and are active. Acetyl CoA is not elevated in the fed state. The transport of glucose in the liver is not insulin sensitive. Synthesis of glucokinase is enhanced in the fed state.

24.3 Increased formation of ketone bodies during fasting is a result of:

A. decreased levels of circulating glucagon.

B. decreased formation of acetyl CoA in the liver.

C. increased levels of free fatty acids in blood.

D. inhibition of β-oxidation of fatty acids in the liver.

E. decreased activity of hormone-sensitive lipase in adipose tissue.

Correct answer = C. Free fatty acids bound to albumin are increased as a result of an increased activity of hormone-sensitive lipase in adipose tissue. Hepatic ketogenesis is stimulated by elevated levels of glucagon. The formation of acetyl CoA is increased. β-Oxidation of fatty acids in liver provides the acetyl CoA for ketogenesis.

24.4 Which one of the following is the most important source of blood glucose during the last hours of a 48-hour fast?

A. Muscle glycogen.

B. Acetoacetate.

C. Liver glycogen.

D. Amino acids.

E. Lactate.

Correct answer = D. The carbon skeletons of glucogenic amino acids are used by the liver for gluconeogenesis. Liver glycogen is nearly depleted by 12 hours after a meal, and muscle glycogen cannot give rise to free glucose because muscle lacks glucose 6-phosphatase. Acetoacetate is metabolized to acetyl CoA, which is not glucogenic. Lactate can arise from anaerobic glycolysis in muscle and red blood cells, but is less important than amino acids as a source of glucose.

Diabetes Mellitus

25

I. OVERVIEW OF DIABETES MELLITUS

Diabetes mellitus is not one disease, but rather is a heterogeneous group of multifactorial, polygenic syndromes characterized by an elevation of fasting blood glucose caused by a relative or absolute deficiency in insulin. Diabetes is the leading cause of adult blindness and amputation, and a major cause of renal failure, nerve damage, heart attacks, and strokes. Most cases of diabetes mellitus can be separated into two groups (Figure 25.1), type 1 (formerly called insulin-dependent diabetes mellitus) and type 2 (formerly called noninsulin-dependent diabetes). Approximately 150,000 newly diagnosed cases of type 1 and 1.3 million cases of type 2 diabetes are estimated to occur yearly in the United States. The incidence and prevalence of type 2 disease is increasing because of the aging of the United States population, and the increasing prevalence of obesity and sedentary lifestyles (see p. 349). The increase in children with type 2 diabetes is particularly disturbing.

	Type 1 Diabetes	Type 2 Diabetes
AGE OF ONSET	Usually during childhood or puberty; symptoms develop rapidly	Frequently after age 35; symptoms develop gradually
NUTRITIONAL STATUS AT TIME OF DISEASE ONSET	Frequently undernourished	Obesity usually present
PREVALENCE	10% of diagnosed diabetics	90% of diagnosed diabetics
GENETIC PREDISPOSITION	Moderate	Very strong
DEFECT OR DEFICIENCY	β Cells are destroyed, eliminating production of insulin	Insulin resistance combined with inability of β cells to produce appropriate quantities of insulin
FREQUENCY OF KETOSIS	Common	Rare
PLASMA INSULIN	Low to absent	High early in disease; low in disease of long duration
ACUTE COMPLICATIONS	Ketoacidosis	Hyperosmolar state
RESPONSE TO ORAL HYPOGLYCEMIC DRUGS	Unresponsive	Responsive
TREATMENT	Insulin is always necessary	Diet, exercise, oral hypoglycemic drugs; insulin may or may not be necessary. Reduction of risk factors (smoking cessation, blood pressure control, treatment of dyslipidemia) is essential to therapy.

Figure 25.1
Comparison of type 1 and type 2 diabetes.

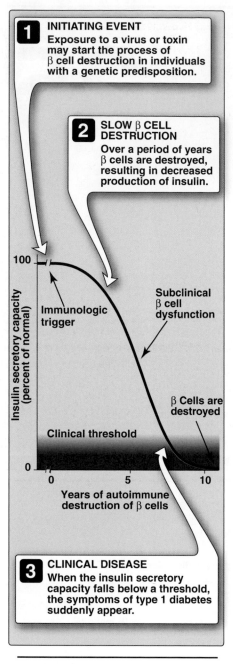

Figure 25.2
Insulin secretory capacity during onset of type 1 diabetes. [Note: Rate of autoimmune destruction of β cells may be faster or slower than shown.]

II. TYPE 1 DIABETES

Persons with type 1 diabetes constitute approximately 10% of the nearly 20 million known diabetics in the United States. The disease is characterized by an absolute deficiency of insulin caused by an auto-immune attack on the β cells of the pancreas. In type 1 diabetes, the islets of Langerhans become infiltrated with activated T lymphocytes, leading to a condition called insulitis. Over a period of years, this autoimmune attack on the β cells leads to gradual depletion of the β-cell population (Figure 25.2). However, symptoms appear abruptly when 80–90% of the β cells have been destroyed. At this point, the pancreas fails to respond adequately to ingestion of glucose, and insulin therapy is required to restore metabolic control and prevent life-threatening ketoacidosis. β Cell destruction requires both a stimulus from the environment (such as a viral infection) and a genetic determinant that allows the β cells to be recognized as "nonself." [Note: Among monozygotic (identical) twins, if one sibling develops type 1 diabetes mellitus, the other twin has only a 30–50% chance of developing the disease. This contrasts with type 2 disease (see p. 341), in which the genetic influence is stronger, and in virtually all monozygotic twinships, the disease eventually develops in both individuals.]

> Patients with type 1 diabetes have virtually no functional β cells, and can neither respond to variations in circulating fuels nor maintain a basal secretion of insulin.

A. Diagnosis of type 1 diabetes

The onset of type 1 diabetes is typically during childhood or puberty, and symptoms develop suddenly. Patients with type 1 diabetes can usually be recognized by the abrupt appearance of polyuria (frequent urination), polydipsia (excessive thirst), and polyphagia (excessive hunger), often triggered by stress or an illness. These symptoms are usually accompanied by fatigue, weight loss, and weakness. The diagnosis is confirmed by a fasting blood glucose (FBG) greater than or equal to 126 mg/dl, commonly accompanied by ketoacidosis. [Note: A FBG of 100–125 mg/dl is categorized as an impaired FBG.] Fasting is defined as no caloric intake for at least 8 hours. When the diagnosis of type 1 diabetes is uncertain by clinical presentation, testing for circulating islet-cell antibodies is recommended. [Note: The oral glucose tolerance test is not routinely used as a diagnostic tool for diabetes because it is difficult to perform in practice and the results are highly variable; however, it is used to screen pregnant women for gestational diabetes (see p. 342).]

B. Metabolic changes in type 1 diabetes

The metabolic abnormalities of type 1 diabetes mellitus result from a deficiency of insulin which profoundly affects metabolism in three tissues: liver, muscle, and adipose tissue (Figure 25.3).

1. **Hyperglycemia and ketoacidosis:** Elevated levels of blood glucose and ketones are the hallmarks of untreated type 1 diabetes melli-

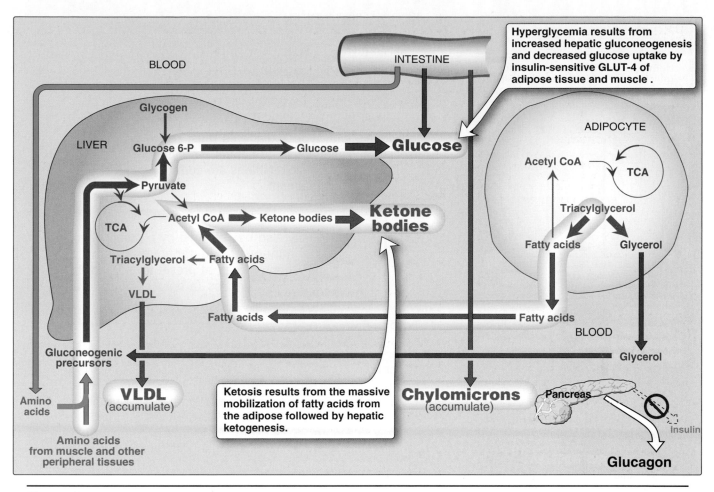

Figure 25.3
Intertissue relationships in type 1 diabetes.

tus (see Figure 25.3). Hyperglycemia is caused by increased hepatic production of glucose, combined with diminished peripheral utilization (muscle and adipose have the insulin-sensitive GLUT-4, see p. 97). Ketosis results from increased mobilization of fatty acids from adipose tissue, combined with accelerated hepatic fatty acid β-oxidation and synthesis of 3-hydroxybutyrate and acetoacetate. [Note: Acetyl coenzyme A from β-oxidation is the substrate for ketogenesis and the allosteric effector of *pyruvate carboxylase,* a gluconeogenic enzyme.] Diabetic ketoacidosis (DKA, a type of metabolic acidosis) occurs in 25–40% of those newly diagnosed with type 1 diabetes, and may recur if the patient becomes ill (most commonly with an infection) or does not comply with therapy. DKA is treated by replacing fluid and electrolytes, and administering short-acting insulin to gradually correct hyperglycemia without precipitating hypoglycemia.

2. **Hypertriacylglycerolemia:** Not all the fatty acids flooding the liver can be disposed of through oxidation or ketone body synthesis. These excess fatty acids are converted to triacylglycerol, which is packaged and secreted in very-low-density lipoproteins (VLDL, see p. 231). Chylomicrons are synthesized from dietary lipids by the intestinal mucosal cells following a meal (see p. 178). Because

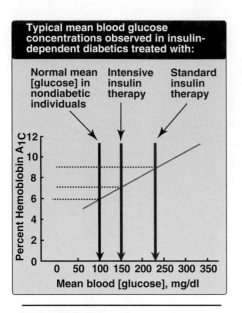

Figure 25.4
Correlation between mean blood glucose and HbA$_{1C}$ in patients with type 1 diabetes.

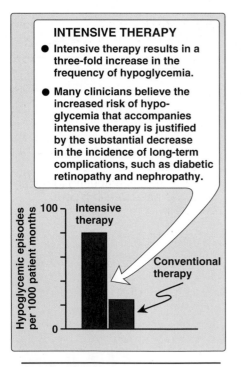

Figure 25.5
Effect of tight glucose control on hypoglycemic episodes in a population of patients on intensive therapy or conventional therapy.

lipoprotein degradation catalyzed by *lipoprotein lipase* in the capillary beds of muscle and adipose tissue (see. p. 228) is low in diabetics (synthesis of the enzyme is decreased when insulin levels are low), the plasma chylomicron and VLDL levels are elevated, resulting in hypertriacylglycerolemia (see Figure 25.3).

C. Treatment of type 1 diabetes

Individuals with type 1 diabetes must rely on exogenous insulin injected subcutaneously to control the hyperglycemia and ketoacidosis. Two therapeutic regimens are currently in use—standard and intensive insulin treatment.

> Insulin may also be delivered by a pump, which allows continuous subcutaneous infusion of insulin 24 hours a day at preset levels and the ability to program doses (a bolus) of insulin as needed at meal times.

1. **Standard treatment versus intensive treatment:** Standard treatment typically consists of one or two daily injections of recombinant human insulin. Mean blood glucose levels obtained are typically in the 225–275 mg/dl range, with a hemoglobin A$_{1C}$ (HbA$_{1C}$) level (see p. 34) of 8–9% of the total hemoglobin (blue arrow in Figure 25.4). [Note: The rate of formation of HbA$_{1C}$ is proportional to the average blood glucose concentration over the previous 3 months. Thus, HbA$_{1C}$ provides a measure of how well treatment has normalized blood glucose in the diabetic over that time.] In contrast to standard therapy, intensive treatment seeks to more closely normalize blood glucose through more frequent monitoring, and subsequent injections of insulin—typically three or more times a day. Mean blood glucose levels of 150 mg/dl can be achieved, with HbA$_{1C}$ approximately 7% of the total hemoglobin (red arrow: Figure 25.4). [Note: Normal mean blood glucose is approximately 100 mg/dl and HbA$_{1C}$ is 6% or less (black arrow, see Figure 25.4).] Thus, normalization of glucose values (euglycemia) is not achieved even in intensively treated patients. Nonetheless, patients on intensive therapy show a 50% or more reduction in the long-term microvascular complications of diabetes—retinopathy, nephropathy, and neuropathy—compared with patients receiving standard care. This confirms that the complications of diabetes are related to an elevation of plasma glucose.

2. **Hypoglycemia in type 1 diabetes:** One of the therapeutic goals in cases of diabetes is to decrease blood glucose levels in an effort to minimize the development of long-term complications of the disease (see p. 344 for a discussion of the chronic complications of diabetes). However, appropriate dosage of insulin is difficult to achieve. Hypoglycemia caused by excess insulin is the most common complication of insulin therapy, occurring in over 90% of patients. The frequency of hypoglycemic episodes, coma, and seizures is particularly high with intensive treatment regimens

designed to achieve tight control of blood glucose (Figure 25.5). Recall that in normal individuals hypoglycemia triggers a compensatory secretion of counter-regulatory hormones, most notably glucagon and epinephrine, which promote hepatic production of glucose. However, patients with type 1 diabetes also develop a deficiency of glucagon secretion. This defect occurs early in the disease and is almost universally present 4 years after diagnosis. These patients thus rely on epinephrine secretion to prevent severe hypoglycemia. However, as the disease progresses, type 1 diabetes patients show diabetic autonomic neuropathy and impaired ability to secrete epinephrine in response to hypoglycemia. The combined deficiency of glucagon and epinephrine secretion creates a condition sometimes called "hypoglycemia unawareness." Thus, patients with long-standing diabetes are particularly vulnerable to hypoglycemia. Hypoglycemia can also be caused by strenuous exercise. Exercise promotes glucose uptake into muscle and decreases the need for exogenous insulin. Patients are advised, therefore, to check blood glucose levels before or after intensive exercise to prevent or abort hypoglycemia.

3. **Contraindications for tight control:** Children are not put on a program of tight control of blood glucose because of the risk that episodes of hypoglycemia may adversely affect brain development. Elderly people typically do not go on tight control because hypoglycemia can cause strokes and heart attacks in this population. Also, the major goal of tight control is to prevent complications many years later. Tight control, then, is most worthwhile for otherwise healthy people who can expect to live at least ten more years.

III. TYPE 2 DIABETES

Type 2 diabetes is the most common form of the disease, afflicting approximately 90% of the diabetic population in the United States. [Note: Native Americans, Latinos, African Americans, and Asian Americans have the highest prevalence.] Typically, type 2 diabetes develops gradually without obvious symptoms. The disease is often detected by routine screening tests. However, many individuals with type 2 diabetes have symptoms of polyuria and polydipsia of several weeks duration. Polyphagia may be present, but is less common. Patients with type 2 diabetes have a combination of insulin resistance and dysfunctional β cells (Figure 25.6), but do not require insulin to sustain life, although insulin eventually will be required to control hyperglycemia and keep HbA$_{1c}$ below 7% in 90% of patients. The metabolic alterations observed in type 2 diabetes are milder than those described for type 1, in part, because insulin secretion in type 2 diabetes—although not adequate—does restrain ketogenesis and blunts the development of DKA. Diagnosis is based most commonly on the presence of hyperglycemia—that is, a fasting blood glucose concentration of equal to or greater than 126 mg/dl. Pathogenesis does not involve viruses or autoimmune antibodies. [Note: An acute complication of type 2 in the elderly is a hyperglycemic hyperosmolar state characterized by severe hyperglycemia and dehydration, and altered mental status.]

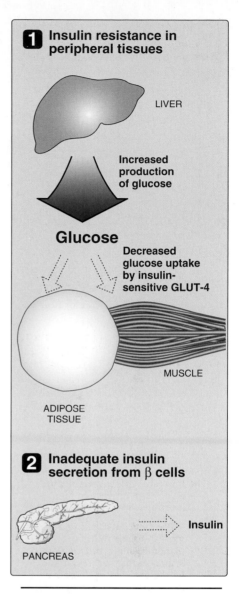

Figure 25.6
Major factors contributing to hyperglycemia observed in type 2 diabetes.

> Type 2 diabetes mellitus is characterized by hyperglycemia, insulin resistance, and relative impairment in insulin secretion.

A. Insulin resistance

Insulin resistance is the decreased ability of target tissues, such as liver, adipose, and muscle, to respond properly to normal (or elevated) circulating concentrations of insulin. For example, insulin resistance is characterized by uncontrolled hepatic glucose production, and decreased glucose uptake by muscle and adipose tissue.

1. **Insulin resistance and obesity:** Obesity is the most common cause of insulin resistance; however, most people with obesity and insulin resistance do not become diabetic. In the absence of a defect in β-cell function, nondiabetic, obese individuals can compensate for insulin resistance with elevated levels of insulin. For example, Figure 25.7A shows that insulin secretion is two to three times higher in obese subjects than it is in lean individuals. This higher insulin concentration compensates for the diminished effect of the hormone (as a result of insulin resistance), and produces blood glucose levels similar to those observed in lean individuals (Figure 25.7B).

2. **Insulin resistance and type 2 diabetes:** Insulin resistance alone will not lead to type 2 diabetes. Rather, type 2 diabetes develops in insulin-resistant individuals who also show impaired β-cell function. Insulin resistance and subsequent risk for the development of type 2 diabetes is commonly observed in the elderly, and in individuals who are obese, physically inactive, or in the 3–5% of pregnant women who develop gestational diabetes. These patients are unable to sufficiently compensate for insulin resistance with increased insulin release. Figure 25.8 shows the time course for the development of hyperglycemia and the loss of β-cell function.

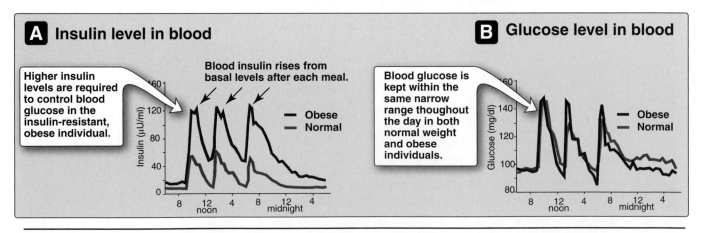

Figure 25.7
Blood insulin and glucose levels in normal weight and obese subjects.

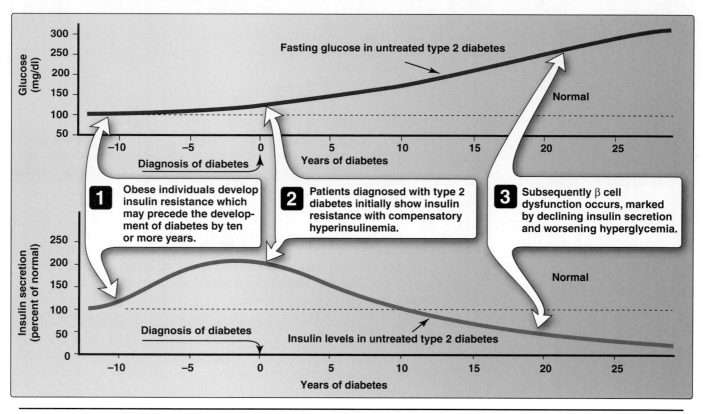

Figure 25.8
Progression of blood glucose and insulin levels in patients with type 2 diabetes.

3. **Causes of insulin resistance:** Insulin resistance increases with weight gain and, conversely, diminishes with weight loss. This suggests that fat accumulation is important in the development of insulin resistance. Adipose tissue is not simply an energy storage organ, but also a secretory organ. Regulatory substances produced by adipocytes include leptin (see p. 353), and adiponectin (see p. 353), all of which may contribute to the development of insulin resistance. In addition, the elevated levels of free fatty acids (FFA) that occur in obesity have also been implicated in the development of insulin resistance. [Note: FFA also arise from lipolysis in insulin-resistant adipose.]

B. Dysfunctional β cells

In type 2 diabetes, the pancreas initially retains β-cell capacity, resulting in insulin levels that vary from above normal to below normal. However, with time, the β cell becomes increasingly dysfunctional and fails to secrete enough insulin to correct the prevailing hyperglycemia. For example, insulin levels are high in typical, obese, type 2 diabetic patients, but not as high as in similarly obese individuals who are nondiabetic. Thus, the natural progression of the disease results in a declining ability to control hyperglycemia with endogenous secretion of insulin (Figure 25.9). Deterioration of β-cell function may be accelerated by the toxic effects of sustained hyperglycemia and elevated FFA.

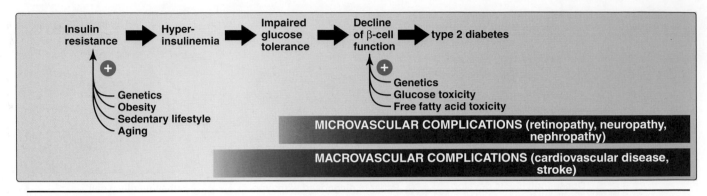

Figure 25.9
Typical progression of type 2 diabetes.

C. Metabolic changes in type 2 diabetes

The metabolic abnormalities of type 2 diabetes mellitus are the result of insulin resistance expressed primarily in liver, muscle, and adipose tissue (Figure 25.10).

1. **Hyperglycemia:** Hyperglycemia is caused by increased hepatic production of glucose, combined with diminished peripheral use. Ketosis is usually minimal or absent in type 2 patients because the presence of insulin—even in the presence of insulin resistance—diminishes hepatic ketogenesis. [Note: Metformin, an oral agent for the treatment of type 2 diabetes, inhibits hepatic gluconeogenesis[1].]

2. **Dyslipidemia:** In the liver, fatty acids are converted to triacylglycerols, which are packaged and secreted in VLDL. Chylomicrons are synthesized from dietary lipids by the intestinal mucosal cells following a meal (see p. 177). Because lipoprotein degradation catalyzed by *lipoprotein lipase* in adipose tissue (and muscle, see p. 228) is low in diabetics, the plasma chylomicron and VLDL levels are elevated, resulting in hypertriacylglycerolemia (see Figure 25.10). Low HDL levels are also associated with type 2 diabetes.

D. Treatment of type 2 diabetes

The goal in treating type 2 diabetes is to maintain blood glucose concentrations within normal limits, and to prevent the development of long-term complications. Weight reduction, exercise, and medical nutrition therapy (dietary modifications) often correct the hyperglycemia of newly diagnosed type 2 diabetes. Hypoglycemic agents or insulin therapy may be required to achieve satisfactory plasma glucose levels.

IV. CHRONIC EFFECTS AND PREVENTION OF DIABETES

As noted previously, available therapies moderate the hyperglycemia of diabetes, but fail to completely normalize metabolism. The long-standing elevation of blood glucose is associated with the chronic complica-

[1]See Chapter 24 in *Lippincott's Illustrated Reviews: Pharmacology* for a discussion of the use of hypoglycemic agents in the treatment of diabetes.

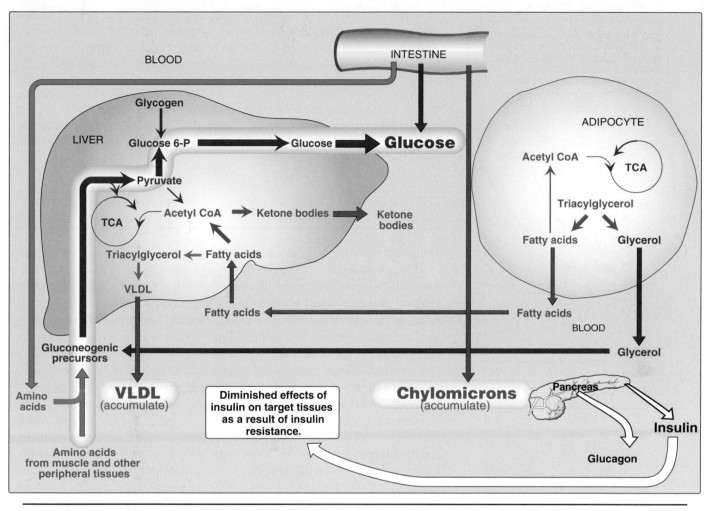

Figure 25.10
Intertissue relationships in type 2 diabetes.

tions of diabetes—premature atherosclerosis (including cardiovascular disease and stroke), retinopathy, nephropathy, and neuropathy. Intensive treatment with insulin (see p. 340) delays the onset and slows the progression of these long-term complications. For example, the incidence of retinopathy decreases as control of blood glucose improves and HbA_{1C} levels decrease (Figure 25.11). The benefits of tight control of blood glucose outweigh the increased risk of severe hypoglycemia in most patients. How hyperglycemia causes the chronic complications of diabetes is unclear. In cells where entry of glucose is not dependent on insulin, elevated blood glucose leads to increased intracellular glucose and its metabolites. For example, increased intracellular sorbitol contributes to the formation of cataracts (see p. 140) in diabetics. Furthermore, hyperglycemia promotes the non-enzymic condensation of glucose with cellular proteins in a reaction analogous to the formation of HbA_{1C} (see p. 34). These glycated proteins mediate some of the early microvascular changes of diabetes. There is currently no preventative treatment for type 1 diabetes. The risk for type 2 diabetes can be significantly decreased by a combined regimen of medical nutrition therapy, weight loss, exercise and aggressive control

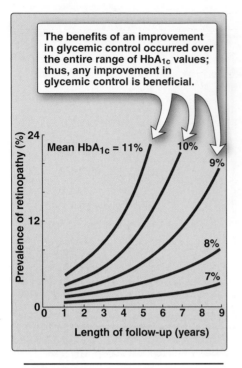

Figure 25.11
Relationship of glycemic control
and diabetic retinopathy.

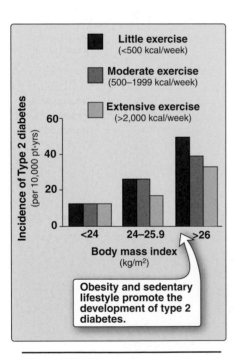

Figure 25.12
Effect of body weight and exercise
on the development of type 2
diabetes.

of hypertension and dyslipidemias. For example, Figure 25.12 shows the incidence of disease in normal and overweight individuals with varying degrees of exercise. The beneficial effect of intensive therapy on cardiovascular disease has not been shown in individuals with long-standing type 2 diabetes. In contrast, initial intensive control in individuals with newly diagnosed diabetes has long-term benefit in decreasing the risk of myocardial infarction, diabetes-related death, and overall death. The clinical evidence thus supports initiating intensive therapy with the goal of lowering HbA_{1C} levels to below 7.0% as early as possible in the course of diabetes.

V. CHAPTER SUMMARY

Diabetes mellitus is a heterogeneous group of syndromes characterized by an **elevation of fasting blood glucose** that is caused by a relative or absolute deficiency in insulin (Figure 25.13). Diabetes is the leading cause of **adult blindness** and **amputation**, and a major cause of **renal failure**, **nerve damage**, **heart attacks**, and **stroke**. The disease can be classified into two groups, type 1 and type 2. **Type 1** diabetics constitute approximately 10% of diabetics in the United States. The disease is characterized by an **absolute deficiency of insulin** caused by an **autoimmune attack** on the β **cells of the pancreas**. This destruction requires a **stimulus from the environment** (such as a viral infection) and a **genetic determinant** that allows the β cell to be recognized as "nonself." The **metabolic abnormalities** of type 1 diabetes mellitus include **hyperglycemia**, **ketoacidosis**, and **hypertriacylglycerolemia**. They result from a deficiency of insulin and a relative excess of glucagon. Type 1 diabetics must rely on **exogenous insulin** injected subcutaneously to control hyperglycemia and ketoacidosis. **Type 2** diabetes has a strong **genetic** component. It results from a combination of **insulin resistance** and **dysfunctional β cells**. Insulin resistance is the decreased ability of target tissues, such as liver, adipose tissue, and muscle, to respond properly to normal (or elevated) circulating concentrations of insulin. **Obesity** is the most common cause of insulin resistance. However, most people with obesity and insulin resistance do not become diabetic. In the absence of a defect in β-cell function, **nondiabetic, obese individuals** can compensate for insulin resistance with **elevated levels of insulin**. Insulin resistance alone will not lead to type 2 diabetes. Rather, type 2 diabetes develops in insulin-resistant individuals who also show impaired β-cell function. The **metabolic alterations** observed in type 2 diabetes are **milder** than those described for the insulin-dependent form of the disease, in part, because insulin secretion in type 2 diabetes—although not adequate—does restrain ketogenesis and blunts the development of diabetic ketoacidosis. Available treatments for diabetes moderate the hyperglycemia, but fail to completely normalize metabolism. The long-standing elevation of blood glucose is associated with the **chronic complications of diabetes**—**premature atherosclerosis**, **retinopathy**, **nephropathy**, and **neuropathy**.

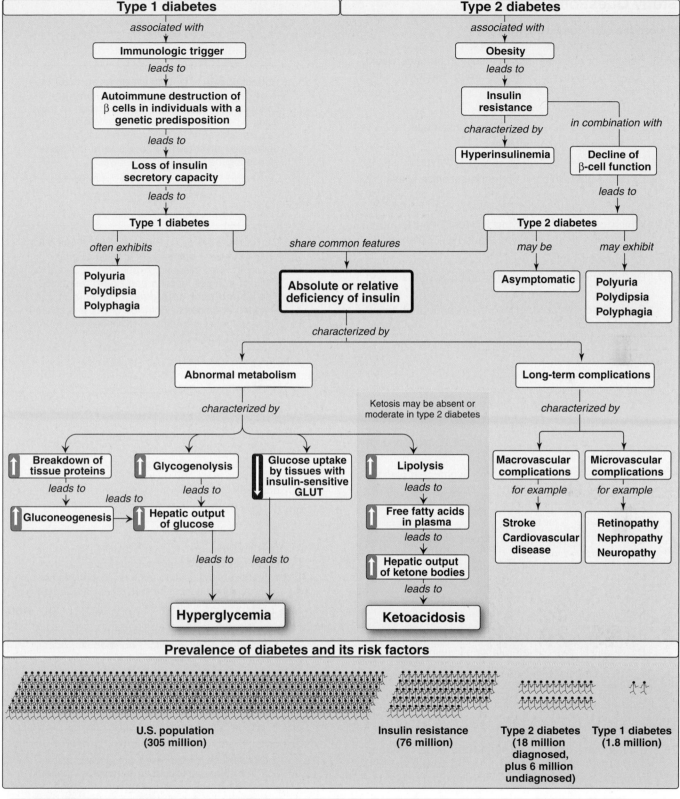

Figure 25.13
Key concept map for diabetes.

Study Questions

Choose the ONE correct answer.

25.1 Relative or absolute lack of insulin in humans would result in which one of the following reactions in the liver?

A. Increased glycogen synthesis.

B. Decreased gluconeogenesis from lactate.

C. Decreased glycogenolysis.

D. Increased formation of 3-hydroxybutyrate.

E. Decreased action of hormone-sensitive lipase.

> Correct answer = D. Low insulin levels favor the liver producing ketone bodies, using acetyl coenzyme A it generated by β-oxidation of fatty acids provided by the adipose. Low insulin also causes activation of hormone-sensitive lipase, decreased glycogen synthesis, and increased gluconeogenesis and glycogenolysis.

25.2 Which one of the following is most often found in untreated patients with type 1 and type 2 diabetes?

A. Hyperglycemia.

B. Extremely low levels of insulin synthesis and secretion.

C. Synthesis of an insulin with an abnormal amino acid sequence.

D. A simple pattern of genetic inheritance.

E. Ketoacidosis.

> Correct answer = A. Elevated blood glucose occurs in type 1 diabetes as a result of a lack of insulin. In type 2 diabetes, hyperglycemia is due to a defect in β-cell function and insulin resistance. The amino acid sequence of insulin is not changed in diabetes. Both forms of the disease show complex genetics. Ketoacidosis is more common in type 1 disease.

25.3 An obese individual with type 2 diabetes:

A. usually shows a sudden onset of symptoms.

B. usually has a lower plasma level of insulin than a normal individual.

C. usually shows significant improvement in glucose tolerance if body weight is reduced to normal.

D. usually benefits from receiving insulin about 6 hours after a meal.

E. usually has lower plasma levels of glucagon than a normal individual.

> Correct answer = C. Eighty percent of type 2 diabetics are obese, and almost all show some improvement in blood glucose with weight reduction. Symptoms usually develop gradually. These patients have elevated insulin levels, and usually do not require insulin (certainly not 6 hours after a meal). Glucagon levels are typically normal.

25.4 An individual with insulin resistance and normal β-cell function:

A. usually shows elevated fasting glucose levels.

B. usually shows elevated fasting insulin levels.

C. will eventually become diabetic.

D. is rarely obese.

E. is treated by injection of insulin.

> Correct answer = B. Insulin resistance is the decreased ability of target tissues, such as liver, adipose, and muscle, to respond properly to normal circulating concentrations of insulin. Obesity is the most common cause of insulin resistance. Most of the people with obesity and insulin resistance do not become diabetic. In the absence of a defect in β-cell function, nondiabetic, obese individuals can compensate for insulin resistance with elevated levels of insulin. The elevated insulin levels normalize fasting blood glucose levels. Insulin resistance without overt diabetes requires no pharmacologic treatment.

25.5 Explain why drugs that inhibit the α-glucosidase activity of the intestinal saccharidases aid in glycemic control in patients with diabetes.

> α-Glucosidase inhibitors prevent glucose production from those products of carbohydrate digestion in which glucose is attached through an α-glycosidic linkage, thus reducing the postprandial rise in blood glucose. Note that the digestion of lactose is unaffected because it has a β-linkage.

Obesity

26

I. OVERVIEW

Obesity is a disorder of body weight regulatory systems characterized by an accumulation of excess body fat. In primitive societies, in which daily life required a high level of physical activity and food was only available intermittently, a genetic tendency favoring storage of excess calories as fat may have had a survival value. Today, however, the sedentary lifestyle and abundance and wide variety of palatable, inexpensive foods in industrialized societies has undoubtedly contributed to an obesity epidemic. As adiposity has increased so has the risk of developing associated diseases, such as arthritis, diabetes, hypertension, cardiovascular disease, and cancer. Particularly alarming is the explosion of obesity in children and adolescents, which has shown a three-fold increase in prevalence over the last two decades. In the United States, the lifetime risk of becoming overweight or obese is approximately 50% and 25%, respectively. Obesity has increased globally. In fact, by some estimates, there are more obese than undernourished individuals worldwide.

II. ASSESSMENT OF OBESITY

The amount of body fat is difficult to measure directly, and is usually determined from an indirect measure—the body mass index (BMI)—which has been shown to correlate with the amount of body fat in most individuals. [Note: Exceptions are athletes who have large amounts of lean muscle mass.] Measuring the waist size with a tape measure is also used to screen for obesity, as this measurement reflects the amount of fat in the central abdominal area of the body. The presence of excess central fat is associated with an increased risk for morbidity and mortality.

A. Body mass index

The BMI (weight in kg)/(height in meters)^2 provides a measure of relative weight, adjusted for height. This allows comparisons both within and between populations. The healthy range for the BMI is between 18.5 and 24.9. Individuals with a BMI between 25 and 29.9 are considered overweight, those with a BMI equal to or greater than 30 are defined as obese, and a BMI over 40 is considered extremely obese. Anyone more than 100 pounds overweight is considered severely obese (Figure 26.1). These cutoffs are based on the studies examining the relationship of BMI to premature death, and are similar in men and women. Nearly two thirds of American adults are overweight, and more than one third are obese.

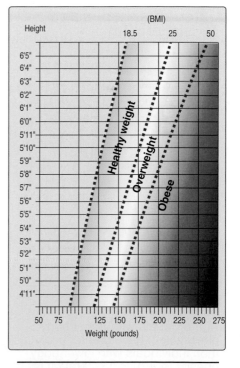

Figure 26.1
To use the BMI Chart, find height in the left-hand column. Move across the row to weight. Height and weight intersect at the individual's BMI.

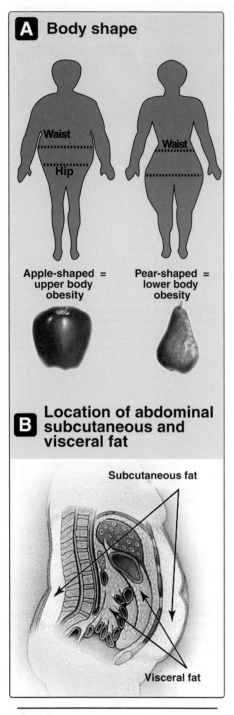

A Body shape

Waist

Waist

Hip

Apple-shaped = upper body obesity

Pear-shaped = lower body obesity

B Location of abdominal subcutaneous and visceral fat

Subcutaneous fat

Visceral fat

Figure 26.2
A. Individuals with upper body obesity (left) have greater health risks than individuals with lower body obesity (right). B. Visceral fat is located inside the abdominal cavity, packed in between the internal organs; subcutaneaous fat is found underneath the skin.

B. Anatomic differences in fat deposition

The anatomic distribution of body fat has a major influence on associated health risks. A waist to hip ratio of more than 0.8 for women and more than 1.0 for men is defined as android, "apple-shaped," or upper body obesity, and is associated with more fat deposition in the trunk (Figure 26.2A). In contrast, a lower waist to hip ratio reflects a preponderance of fat distributed in the hips and thighs and is called gynoid, "pear-shaped," or lower body obesity. It is defined as a waist to hip ratio of less than 0.8 for women and less than 1.0 for men. The pear shape, more commonly found in women, presents a much lower risk of metabolic disease, and some studies indicate it may actually be protective. Thus, the clinician can use simple indices of body shape to identify those who may be at higher risk for metabolic diseases associated with obesity.

1. **Subcutaneous and visceral depots:** About 80–90% of the fat stored in the human body is in subcutaneous depots, just under the skin, in the abdominal (upper body) and the gluteal-femoral (lower body) regions. In addition, 10–20% of body fat is stored in so-called visceral depots (omental and mesenteric), which are located within the abdominal cavity in close association with the digestive tract (Figure 26.2B). Excess fat in visceral stores (and also in abdominal subcutaneous fat) increases health risks associated with obesity.

C. Biochemical differences in regional fat depots

The regional types of fat described above are biochemically different. Subcutaneous adipocytes from the lower body (gluteal-femoral), particularly in women, are larger, very efficient at fat deposition, and tend to mobilize fatty acids more slowly than those from the abdominal subcutaneous depots. Visceral adipocytes are the most metabolically active. Both abdominal subcutaneous and visceral depots of obese subjects have high rates of lipolysis, and contribute to increased availability of free fatty acids. These metabolic differences may contribute to the higher risk found in individuals with upper body obesity.

1. **Endocrine function:** Adipose tissue, once thought to be a passive bystander in metabolism, is now known to play an active role in body weight regulatory systems. For example, the adipocyte is an endocrine cell that secretes a number of hormones, such as leptin, which regulates appetite as well as metabolism (see p. 353). Adiponectin, an adipocyte-derived cytokine, reduces levels of blood free fatty acids and has been associated with improved lipid profiles, better glycemic control, and reduced inflammation in diabetic patients.

2. **Importance of portal circulation:** One reason that visceral adipose depots may have such a large influence on metabolic dysfunction in obesity is that cytokines secreted by adipose tissue, as well as free fatty acids released from abdominal fat, enter the portal vein and, therefore, have direct access to the liver. Fatty acids

and inflammatory cytokines released from visceral adipose tissue are taken up by the liver. They may lead to insulin resistance (see p. 342) and increased synthesis of triacylglycerols, which are released as very-low-density lipoprotein (VLDL) particles and contribute to hypertriglyceridemia (see p. 353). By contrast, free fatty acids from subcutaneous body adipose depots enter the general circulation where they can be oxidized in muscle and, therefore, reach the liver in lower concentration.

D. Size and number of fat cells

As triacylglycerols are stored, adipocytes can expand to an average of two to three times their normal volume. (Figure 26.3). However, the ability of a fat cell to expand is limited. With prolonged overnutrition, preadipocytes within adipose tissue are stimulated to proliferate and differentiate into mature fat cells, increasing the number of adipocytes. Thus, most obesity is due to a combination of increased fat cell size (hypertrophy) and number (hyperplasia). Like other tissues, the adipose tissue undergoes continuous remodeling. Contrary to early dogma, we now know that adipocytes can die, but it is uncertain how fast this process occurs; some studies estimate that the average age of an adipocyte is 10 years.

Obese individuals can have up to five times the normal number of fat cells. If excess calories cannot be accommodated within adipose tissue, the excess fatty acids 'spillover' into other tissues, such as muscle and liver. The amount of this so-called 'ectopic fat' is strongly associated with insulin resistance. With weight loss in an obese individual, the size of the fat cells is reduced, but the number of fat cells is not usually affected. Thus, a normal body fat is achieved by decreasing the size of the fat cell below normal. Small fat cells are very efficient at reaccumulating fat, and this may drive appetite and weight regain.

III. BODY WEIGHT REGULATION

The body weight of most individuals tends to be relatively stable over time. This observation prompted the hypothesis that each individual has a biologically predetermined "set point" for body weight. The body attempts to add to adipose stores when the body weight falls below the set point, and to lose adipose stores when the body weight is higher than the set point. For example, with weight loss, appetite increases and energy expenditure falls, whereas with overfeeding, appetite falls and energy expenditure may slightly increase (Figure 26.4). However, a strict set point model does not explain why some individuals fail to revert to their starting weight after a period of overeating, or the current epidemic of obesity. It appears that factors in the environment (availability of food and exercise) influence a 'settling point' that is defended. Body weight, rather than being irrevocably set, seems to drift around a "settling point," reflecting a balance between environmental factors that influence food intake and energy expenditure, and biologic factors that control body weight.

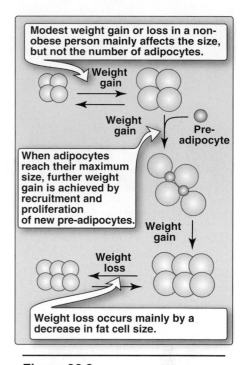

Figure 26.3
Hypertrophic and hyperplastic changes are thought to occur in severe obesity.

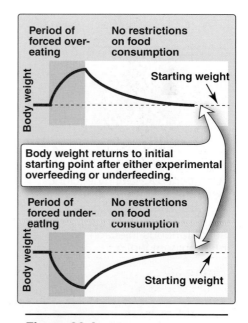

Figure 26.4
Weight changes following episodes of overfeeding or underfeeding followed by feeding with no restrictions.

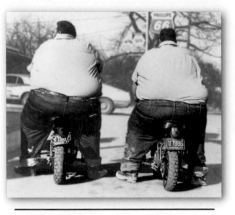

Figure 26.5
Identical twins with combined weight of 1,300 pounds. Note similarity in body shape.

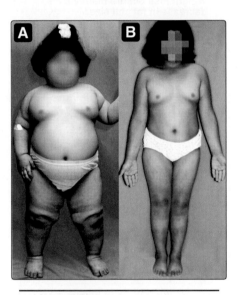

Figure 26.6
A. Patient with leptin deficiency before initiation of therapy at age 5 years. B. Patient at age 9 years after 48 months of therapy with subcutaneous injection of recombinant leptin.

A. Genetic contributions to obesity

It is now evident that genetic mechanisms play a major role in determining body weight. The importance of genetics as a determinant of obesity is indicated by the observation that children who are adopted usually show a body weight that correlates with their biologic rather than adoptive parents. Furthermore, identical twins have very similar BMI (Figure 26.5), whether reared together or apart, and their BMI are more similar than those of nonidentical, dizygotic twins.

1. **Mutations:** Rare, single gene mutations can cause human obesity. Mutations in the gene for the adipocyte hormone leptin or its receptor produce hyperphagia (increased appetite for and consumption of food) and massive obesity (Figure 26.6), underscoring the importance of the leptin system in regulation of human body weight (section IV). Most obese humans have elevated leptin levels but appear to be resistant to the appetite-regulating effects of this hormone.

B. Environmental and behavioral contributions

The epidemic of obesity occurring over the last decade cannot be simply explained by changes in genetic factors, which are stable on this short time scale. Clearly, environmental factors, such as the ready availability of palatable, energy-dense foods, play a role in the increased prevalence of obesity. Furthermore, sedentary lifestyles encouraged by TV watching, automobiles, computer usage, and energy-sparing devices in the workplace and at home, decrease physical activity and enhance the tendency to gain weight. Eating behaviors, such as snacking, portion size, variety of foods consumed, an individual's unique food preferences, and the number of people with whom one eats also influence food consumption. It is important to note, however, that in this same environment, many individuals do not become obese. The susceptibility to obesity appears to be explained, at least in part, by an interaction of an individual's genes and his or her environment, and can be influenced by additional factors such as maternal under- or overnutrition that may 'set' the body regulatory systems to defend a higher or lower level of body fat.

IV. MOLECULES THAT INFLUENCE OBESITY

The cause of obesity can be summarized in a deceptively simple statement of the first law of thermodynamics: Obesity results when energy intake exceeds energy expenditure. However, the mechanism underlying this imbalance involves a complex interaction of biochemical, neurologic, environmental, and psychologic factors. The basic neural and humoral pathways that regulate appetite, energy expenditure, and body weight involve systems that regulate short-term food intake (meal to meal), and signals for the long-term (day to day, week to week, year to year) regulation of body weight (Figure 26.7).

A. Long-term signals.

1. **Leptin:** Leptin is an adipocyte hormone that is secreted in proportion to the size of fat stores. When we consume fewer calories than we need, body fat declines and leptin production from the fat cell decreases. The body adapts by minimizing energy utilization (decreasing activity) and increasing appetite, closing the feedback loop that regulates body weight. Unfortunately, in many individuals, the leptin system may be better at preventing weight loss than preventing weight gain. Although a meal or overeating increases leptin and this should, in theory, also dampen appetite and prevent overconsumption of calories, other cues that stimulate appetite can apparently overcome the leptin system in many individuals.

2. **Insulin:** Obese individuals are also hyperinsulinemic. Like leptin, insulin acts on hypothalamic neurons to dampen appetite.

B. Short-term signals.

Short-term signals from the gastrointestinal tract control hunger and satiety, which affect the size and number of meals over a time course of minutes to hours. In the absence of food intake (between meals), the stomach produces ghrelin, an orexigenic (appetite-stimulating) hormone that drives hunger. During a meal, as food is consumed, gut hormones, including cholecystokinin (CCK) and peptide YY (PYY), among others, through actions on the gastric emptying and neural signals to the hypothalamus, cause satiety and meals are terminated. Within the hypothalamus, neuropeptides such as NPY and α-melanocyte stimulating hormone (α-MSH), and neurotransmitters such as serotonin and dopamine are important in regulating hunger and satiety. Long-term and short-term signals interact, as leptin can affect the sensitivity of hypothalamic neurons to short-term signals such as CCK. Thus, there are many and complex regulatory loops that control the size and number of meals in relationship to the status of body fat stores.

V. METABOLIC CHANGES OBSERVED IN OBESITY

The primary metabolic effects of obesity include dyslipidemias, glucose intolerance (hyperglycemia below that classified as diabetes, see p. 338), and insulin resistance, expressed primarily in the liver, muscle, and adipose tissue. These metabolic abnormalities reflect molecular signals originating from the increased mass of adipocytes.

A. Metabolic syndrome

Abdominal obesity is associated with a cluster of metabolic abnormalities that is referred to as the metabolic syndrome and includes glucose intolerance, insulin resistance, hyperinsulinemia, dyslipidemia (low high-density lipoprotein (HDL) and elevated triacylglycerols), and hypertension (Figure 26.8). The metabolic syndrome is also associated with a state of chronic systemic inflammation that contributes to the pathogenesis of insulin resistance and atherosclerosis. In obesity, low levels of the adipocyte hormone adiponectin

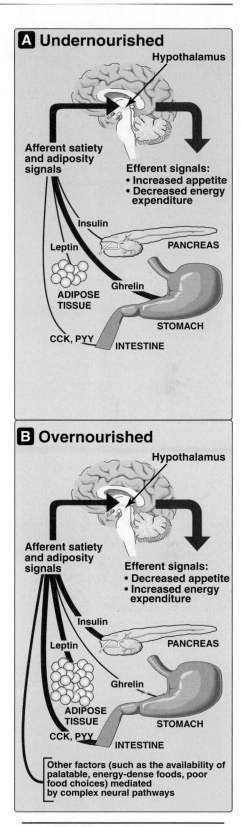

Figure 26.7
Some signals that influence appetite and satiety. CCK = cholecystokinin, PYY = peptide YY.

that normally dampens inflammation and sensitizes tissues, especially the liver, to insulin, may contribute to the metabolic syndrome and therefore the risk of type 2 diabetes and heart disease.

VI. OBESITY AND HEALTH

Obesity is correlated with an increased risk of death (Figure 26.9), and is a risk factor for a number of chronic conditions, including type 2 diabetes, dyslipidemias, hypertension, heart disease, some cancers, gallstones, arthritis, gout, and sleep apnea. The relationship between obesity and associated morbidities is stronger among individuals younger than 55 years. After age 74, there is no longer an association between increased BMI and mortality. Weight loss in obese individuals leads to decreased blood pressure, serum triacylglycerols, and blood glucose levels. HDL levels increase.

VII. WEIGHT REDUCTION

Weight reduction can help reduce the complications of obesity, including diabetes and hypertension. To achieve weight reduction, the obese patient must decrease energy intake or increase energy expenditure, though decreasing energy intake is thought to contribute more to inducing weight loss. Typically, a prescription for weight reduction combines dietary change, increased physical activity, and behavioral modification, which can include nutritional education and meal planning, recording and monitoring food intake through food diaries, modifying factors that lead to overeating, and relearning cues to satiety. Once weight loss is achieved, weight maintenance is a separate process that requires vigilance as the majority of patients regain weight after they stop their weight loss efforts.

A. Physical activity

An increase in physical activity can create an energy deficit. Although adding exercise to a hypocaloric regimen may not produce a greater weight loss initially, exercise is a key component of programs directed at maintaining a weight loss. In addition, physical activity increases cardiopulmonary fitness and reduces the risk of cardiovascular disease, independent of weight loss. Persons who combine caloric restriction and exercise with behavioral treatment may expect to lose about 5–10% of initial body weight over a period of 4–6 months. Studies show that individuals who maintain their exercise program regain less weight after their initial weight loss.

B. Caloric restriction

Dieting is the most commonly practiced approach to weight control. Because 1 pound of adipose tissue corresponds to approximately 3,500 kcal, one can estimate the effect of caloric restriction on the reduction in adipose tissue. Weight loss on calorie-restricted diets is determined primarily by energy intake and not nutrient composition. Caloric restriction is ineffective over the long term for many individuals. More than 90% of people who attempt to lose weight regain the lost weight when dietary intervention is suspended. Nonetheless, it is important to recognize that, although few individuals will reach their ideal weight with treatment, weight losses of

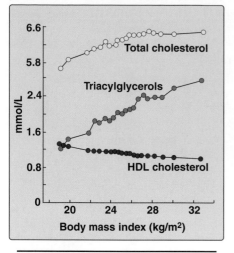

Figure 26.8
Body mass index and changes in blood lipids.

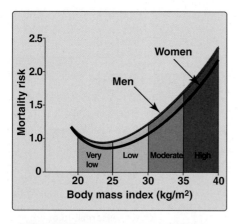

Figure 26.9
Body mass index and the relative risk of death.

10% of body weight over a 6-month period often reduce blood pressure and lipid levels, and enhance control of type 2 diabetes. The health benefits of relatively small weight losses should, therefore, be emphasized to the patient.

C. Pharmacologic treatment

Several weight-loss medications are currently approved by the U.S. Food and Drug Administration for use in adults with a BMI of 30 or higher[1]. Their effects on weight reduction tend to be modest, and weight regain upon termination of drug therapy is common.

D. Surgical treatment

Gastric bypass and restriction surgeries are effective in causing weight loss in severely obese individuals. Through mechanisms that remain poorly understood, these operations improve poor blood sugar control in diabetic individuals.

 [1]See Chapter 29 in **Lippincott's Illustrated Reviews: Pharmacology** for a more detailed discussion of drugs used to treat obesity.

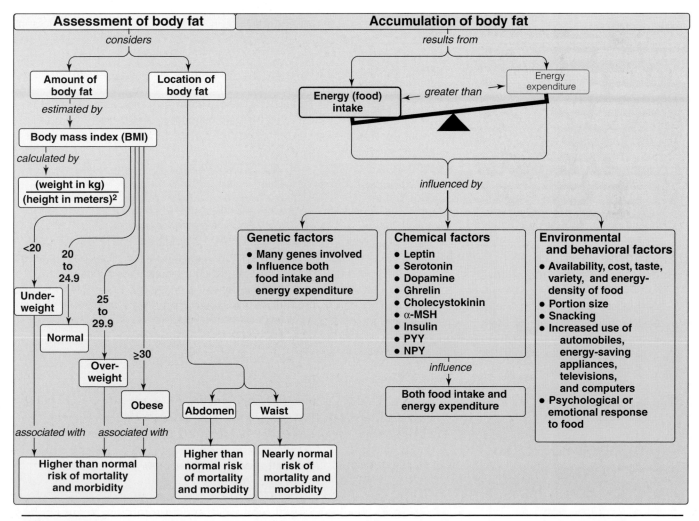

Figure 26.10
Key concept map for obesity.

VIII. CHAPTER SUMMARY

Obesity—the accumulation of excess body fat—results when energy intake exceeds energy expenditure. Obesity is increasing in industrialized countries because of a reduction in daily energy expenditure, and an increase in energy intake resulting from the increasing availability of palatable, inexpensive foods. The **body mass index (BMI)** is easy to determine and highly correlated to body fat. Nearly two thirds of American adults are **overweight** (BMI $\geq$ 25 kg/m^2) and more than 30% are **obese** (BMI > 30 kg/m^2). The anatomic distribution of body fat has a major influence on associated health risks. Excess fat located in the **central abdominal** area is associated with greater risk for hypertension, insulin resistance, diabetes, dyslipidemia, and coronary heart disease. A person's weight is determined by genetic and environmental factors. **Appetite** is influenced by **afferent**, or incoming, **signals**—neural signals, circulating hormones, and metabolites—that are integrated by the **hypothalamus**. These diverse signals prompt release of hypothalamic peptides and activate outgoing, efferent neural signals. **Obesity** is correlated with an **increased risk of death**, and is a risk factor for a number of chronic conditions. **Weight reduction** is achieved best with negative energy balance, that is, by **decreasing caloric intake**. Virtually all diets that limit particular groups of foods or macronutrients lead to short-term weight loss. Long-term maintenance of weight loss is difficult to achieve. Modest reduction in food intake occurs with **pharmacologic treatment. Surgical procedures** designed to limit food intake are an option for the severely obese patient who has not responded to other treatments.

Study Question

Choose the ONE correct answer.

26.1 A 40-year-old woman, 5 feet, 1 inch (155 cm) tall and weighing 188 pounds (85.5 kg), seeks your advice on how to lose weight. Her waist measured 41 inches and her hips 39 inches. A physical examination and blood laboratory data were all within the normal range. Her only child, who is 14 years old, her sister, and both of her parents are overweight. The patient recalls being obese throughout her childhood and adolescence. Over the past 15 years she had been on seven different diets for periods of 2 weeks to 3 months, losing from 5–25 pounds. On discontinuation of each diet, she regained weight, returning to 185–190 pounds. Which one of the following best describes this patient?

A. She is classified as overweight.

B. She shows an "apple" pattern of fat distribution.

C. She has approximately the same number of fat cells as a normal-weight individual, but each adipocyte is larger.

D. She would be expected to show lower than normal levels of circulating leptin.

E. She would be expected to show lower than normal levels of circulating triacylglycerols.

Correct answer = B. Her waist to hip ratio is 41/39 = 1.05. Apple shape is defined as a waist to hip ratio of more than 0.8 for women, and more than 1.0 for men. She has, therefore, an apple pattern of fat distribution, more commonly seen in males. Compared with other women of the same body weight who have a gynoid fat pattern, the presence of increased visceral or intra-abdominal adipose tissue places her at greater risk for diabetes, hypertension, dyslipidemia, and coronary heart disease. The calculated BMI indicates that the patient is classified as obese. Individuals with marked obesity and a history dating to early childhood have an adipose depot made up of too many adipocytes, each fully loaded with triacylglycerols. Plasma leptin in obese humans is usually normal for their fat mass, suggesting that resistance to leptin, rather than its deficiency, occurs in human obesity. The elevated circulating fatty acids characteristic of obesity are carried to the liver and converted to triacylglycerol and cholesterol. Excess triacylglycerol and cholesterol are released as VLDL, resulting in elevated serum triacylglycerols.

26.2 Calculate the BMI for the patient presented in question 26.1

BMI = weight (kg)/height (m^2) = 85.5/(1.55)^2 = 35.6 kg/m^2.

Nutrition

27

I. OVERVIEW

Nutrients are the constituents of food necessary to sustain the normal functions of the body. All energy is provided by three classes of nutrients: fats, carbohydrates, protein—and in some diets, ethanol (Figure 27.1). The intake of these energy-rich molecules is larger than that of the other dietary nutrients. Therefore, they are called macronutrients. This chapter focuses on the kinds and amounts of macronutrients that are needed to maintain optimal health and prevent chronic disease in adults. Those nutrients needed in lesser amounts, vitamins and minerals, are called micronutrients, and are considered in Chapter 28.

II. DIETARY REFERENCE INTAKES

Committees of U.S. and Canadian experts organized by the Food and Nutrition Board of the National Academy of Sciences have compiled Dietary Reference Intakes (DRI)—estimates of the amounts of nutrients required to prevent deficiencies and maintain optimal health and growth. The DRIs replace and expand on the Recommended Dietary Allowances (RDA), which have been published with periodic revisions since 1941. Unlike the RDA, the DRI establish upper limits on the consumption of some nutrients, and incorporate the role of nutrients in life-long health, going beyond deficiency diseases. Both the DRI and the RDA refer to long-term average daily nutrient intakes, because it is not necessary to consume the full RDA every day.

A. Definition of the DRI

The DRI consist of four dietary reference standards for the intake of nutrients designated for specific age groups, physiologic states, and gender (Figure 27.2).

1. **Estimated Average Requirement (EAR):** The EAR is the average daily nutrient intake level estimated to meet the requirement of one half of the healthy individuals in a particular life stage and gender group. It is useful in estimating the actual requirements in groups and individuals.

2. **Recommended Dietary Allowance (RDA):** The RDA is the average daily dietary intake level that is sufficient to meet the nutrient requirements of nearly all (97–98%) the individuals in a life stage and gender group. The RDA is not the minimal requirement for healthy individuals; rather, it is intentionally set to provide a margin of safety for most individuals. The EAR serves as the foundation for setting the RDA. If the standard deviation (SD) of the EAR

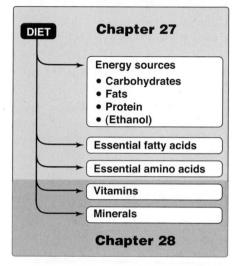

Figure 27.1
Essential nutrients obtained from the diet. [Note: Ethanol is not considered an essential component of the diet but may provide a significant contribution to the daily caloric intake of some individuals.]

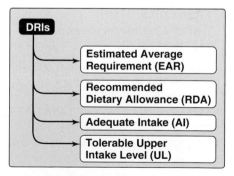

Figure 27.2
Components of the Dietary Reference Intakes (DRIs).

NUTRIENT	EAR, RDA or AI	UL
Thiamine	EAR, RDA	—
Riboflavin	EAR, RDA	—
Niacin	EAR, RDA	UL
Vitamin B$_6$	EAR, RDA	UL
Folate	EAR, RDA	UL
Vitamin B$_{12}$	EAR, RDA	—
Pantothenic acid	AI	—
Biotin	AI	—
Choline	AI	UL
Vitamin C	EAR, RDA	UL
Vitamin A	EAR, RDA	UL
Vitamin D	AI	UL
Vitamin E	EAR, RDA	UL
Vitamin K	AI	—
Boron	—	UL
Calcium	AI	UL
Chromium	AI	—
Copper	EAR, RDA	UL
Fluoride	AI	UL
Iodine	EAR, RDA	UL
Iron	EAR, RDA	UL
Magnesium	EAR, RDA	UL
Manganese	AI	UL
Molybdenum	EAR, RDA	UL
Nickel	—	UL
Phosphorus	EAR, RDA	UL
Selenium	EAR, RDA	UL
Vanadium	—	UL
Zinc	EAR, RDA	UL

Figure 27.3
Dietary Reference Intakes for vitamins and minerals in individuals one year and older. EAR = Estimated Average Requirement; RDA = Recommended Dietary Allowance; AI = Adequate Intake; UL = Tolerable Upper Intake Level; — = no value established.

is available and the requirement for the nutrient is normally distributed, the RDA is set at 2 SDs above the EAR, that is, RDA = EAR + 2SD$_{EAR}$.

3. **Adequate Intake (AI):** The AI is set instead of an RDA if sufficient scientific evidence is not available to calculate an EAR or RDA. The AI is based on estimates of nutrient intake by a group (or groups) of apparently healthy people that are assumed to be adequate. For example, the AI for young infants, for whom human milk is the recommended sole source of food for the first 4–6 months, is based on the estimated daily mean nutrient intake supplied by human milk for healthy, full-term infants who are exclusively breast-fed.

4. **Tolerable Upper Intake Level (UL):** The UL is the highest average daily nutrient intake level that is likely to pose no risk of adverse health effects to almost all individuals in the general population. As intake increases above the UL, the potential risk of adverse effects may increase. The UL is not intended to be a recommended level of intake. The UL are useful because of the increased availability of fortified foods and the increased use of dietary supplements. The UL applies to chronic daily use. For some nutrients, there may be insufficient data on which to develop a UL.

B. Using the DRI

Most nutrients have a set of DRI (Figure 27.3). Usually a nutrient has an EAR and a corresponding RDA. Most are set by age and gender, and may be influenced by special factors, such as pregnancy and lactation in women. When the data are not sufficient to estimate an EAR (or an RDA), then an AI is designated. The AI is judged by experts to meet the needs of all healthy individuals in a group, but is based on less data than an EAR and RDA. Intakes below the EAR need to be improved because the probability of adequacy is 50% or less (Figure 27.4). Intakes between the EAR and RDA likely need to be improved because the probability of adequacy is less than 98%, and intakes at or above the RDA can be considered adequate. Intake above the AI can be considered adequate. Intakes between the UL and the RDA can be considered to have no risk for adverse effects.

III. ENERGY REQUIREMENT IN HUMANS

The Estimated Energy Requirement is the average dietary energy intake predicted to maintain an energy balance (that is, when the calories consumed are equal to the energy expended) in a healthy adult of a defined age, gender, and height whose weight and level of physical activity are consistent with good health. Differences in the genetics, body composition, metabolism, and behavior of individuals make it difficult to accurately predict a person's caloric requirements. However, some simple approximations can provide useful estimates. For example, sedentary adults require about 30 kcal/kg/day to maintain body weight; moderately active adults require 35 kcal/kg/day; and very active adults require 40 kcal/kg/day. [Note: The daily average requirement for energy that is listed on food labels is either 2,000 or 2,500 kcal/day.]

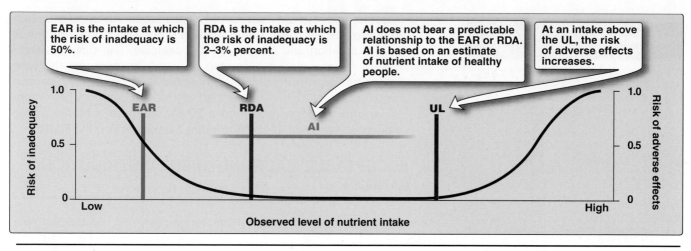

Figure 27.4
Comparison of the components of the Dietary Reference Intakes. EAR = Estimated Average Requirement; RDA = Recommended Dietary Allowance; AI = Adequate Intake; UL = Tolerable Upper Intake Level.

A. Energy content of food

The energy content of food is calculated from the heat released by the total combustion of food in a calorimeter. It is expressed in kilocalories (kcal, or Cal). The standard conversion factors for determining the metabolic caloric value of fat, protein, and carbohydrate are shown in Figure 27.5. Note that the energy content of fat is more than twice that of carbohydrate or protein, whereas the energy content of ethanol is intermediate between those of fat and carbohydrate. [Note: The joule is a unit of energy widely used in countries other than the United States. For uniformity, many scientists are promoting the use of joules (J), rather than calories. One cal = 4.2 J; 1 Cal (1 kcal, 1 food calorie) = 4.2 kJ. However, kcal still predominates and is used throughout this text.]

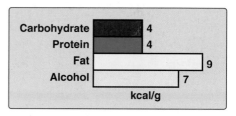

Figure 27.5
Average energy available from the major food components.

B. How energy is used in the body

The energy generated by metabolism of the macronutrients is used for three energy-requiring processes that occur in the body: resting metabolic rate, thermic effect of food (formerly termed specific dynamic action), and physical activity.

1. **Resting metabolic rate:** The energy expended by an individual in a resting, postabsorptive state is called the resting (formerly, basal) metabolic rate (RMR). It represents the energy required to carry out the normal body functions, such as respiration, blood flow, ion transport, and maintenance of cellular integrity. In an adult, the RMR is about 1,800 kcal for men (70 kg) and 1,300 kcal for women (50 kg). From 50–70% of the daily energy expenditure in sedentary individuals is attributable to the RMR (Figure 27.6).

2. **Thermic effect of food:** The production of heat by the body increases as much as 30% above the resting level during the digestion and absorption of food. This effect is called the thermic effect of food or diet-induced thermogenesis. Over a 24–hour period, the thermic response to food intake may amount to 5–10% of the total energy expenditure.

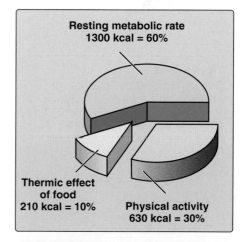

Figure 27.6
Estimated total energy expenditure in a typical 20-year-old woman, 165 cm (5 feet, 4 inches) tall, weighing 50 kg (110 lb), and engaged in light activity.

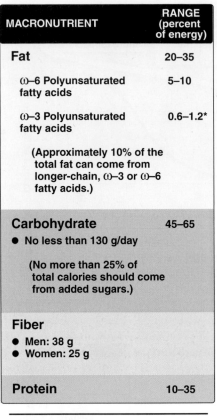

MACRONUTRIENT	RANGE (percent of energy)
Fat	**20–35**
ω–6 Polyunsaturated fatty acids	5–10
ω–3 Polyunsaturated fatty acids	0.6–1.2*
(Approximately 10% of the total fat can come from longer-chain, ω–3 or ω–6 fatty acids.)	
Carbohydrate	**45–65**
● No less than 130 g/day	
(No more than 25% of total calories should come from added sugars.)	
Fiber	
● Men: 38 g	
● Women: 25 g	
Protein	**10–35**

Figure 27.7
Acceptable macronutrient distribution ranges in adults. *A growing body of evidence suggests that higher levels of ω–3 polyunsaturated fatty acids provide protection against coronary heart disease.

3. **Physical activity:** Muscular activity provides the greatest variation in energy expenditure. The amount of energy consumed depends on the duration and intensity of the exercise. The daily expenditure of energy can be estimated by carefully recording the type and duration of all activities. In general, a sedentary person requires about 30–50% more than the resting caloric requirement for energy balance (see Figure 27.6), whereas a highly active individual may require 100% or more calories above the RMR.

IV. ACCEPTABLE MACRONUTRIENT DISTRIBUTION RANGES

Acceptable Macronutrient Distribution Ranges (AMDR) are defined as a range of intakes for a particular macronutrient that is associated with reduced risk of chronic disease while providing adequate amounts of essential nutrients. The AMDR for adults is 45–65% of their total calories from carbohydrates, 20–35% from fat, and 10–35% from protein (Figure 27.7). Note that there is a range of acceptable intakes for the macronutrients. The biologic properties of dietary fat, carbohydrate, and protein are described below.

V. DIETARY FATS

The incidence of a number of chronic diseases is significantly influenced by the kinds and amounts of nutrients consumed (Figure 27.8). Dietary fats most strongly influence the incidence of coronary heart disease (CHD); evidence linking dietary fat and the risk for cancer or obesity is much weaker.

> In the past, dietary recommendations emphasized decreasing the total amount of fat and cholesterol in the diet. Research now indicates that the type of fat is more important than the total amount of fat consumed.

A. Plasma lipids and CHD

Plasma cholesterol may arise from the diet or from endogenous biosynthesis. In either case, cholesterol is transported between the tissues in combination with protein and phospholipids as lipoproteins.

1. **Low-density lipoprotein (LDL) and high-density lipoprotein (HDL):** The level of plasma cholesterol is not precisely regulated, but rather varies in response to the diet. Elevated levels result in an increased risk for CHD (Figure 27.9). The risk increases progressively with higher values for serum total cholesterol. A much stronger correlation exists between the levels of blood LDL cholesterol and heart disease (see p. 232) In contrast, high levels of HDL cholesterol have been associated with a decreased risk for heart disease (see p. 235). Abnormal levels of plasma lipids (dyslipidemias) act in combination with smoking, obesity, seden-

tary lifestyle, insulin resistance, and other risk factors to increase the risk of CHD. Elevated plasma triacylglycerols are also a risk factor for CHD, but the association is weaker than that of LDL cholesterol with CHD.

2. **Beneficial effect of lowering plasma cholesterol:** Clinical trials have demonstrated that dietary or drug treatment of hyper-cholesterolemia is effective in decreasing LDL, increasing HDL, and reducing the risk for cardiovascular events. The diet-induced changes of plasma lipoprotein concentrations are modest, typically 10–20%, whereas treatment with "statin" drugs[1] decreases plasma cholesterol by 30–60% (see p. 224).

B. Dietary fats and plasma lipids

Triacylglycerols are quantitatively the most important class of dietary fats. The influence of triacylglycerols on blood lipids is determined by the chemical nature of their constituent fatty acids. The absence or presence and number of double bonds (saturated vs. mono- and polyunsaturated), the location of the double bonds (ω-6 vs ω-3), and the cis vs. trans configuration of the unsaturated fatty acids are the most important structural features that influence blood lipids.

1. **Saturated fat:** Triacylglycerols composed primarily of fatty acids whose hydrocarbon chains do not contain any double bonds are referred to as saturated fats. Consumption of saturated fats is positively associated with high levels of total plasma cholesterol and LDL cholesterol, and an increased risk of CHD. The main sources of saturated fatty acids are dairy and meat products and some vegetable oils, such as coconut and palm oils (a major source of fat in Latin America and Asia, although not in the United States, Figure 27.10). Most experts strongly advise limiting intake of saturated fats.

> Saturated fatty acids with carbon chain lengths of 14 (myristic) and 16 (palmitic) are most potent in increasing the serum cholesterol. Stearic acid (18 carbons—found in many foods including chocolate) has little effect on blood cholesterol.

2. **Monounsaturated fats:** Triacylglycerols containing primarily fatty acids with one double bond are referred to as monounsaturated fat. Unsaturated fatty acids are generally derived from vegetables and fish. When substituted for saturated fatty acids in the diet, monounsaturated fats lower both total plasma cholesterol and LDL cholesterol, but maintain or increase HDL cholesterol. This ability of monounsaturated fats to favorably modify lipoprotein levels may explain, in part, the observation that Mediterranean cultures, with diets rich in olive oil (high in monounsaturated oleic acid), show a low incidence of CHD.

[1]See Chapter 21 in ***Lippincott's Illustrated Reviews: Pharmacology*** for a more detailed discussion of antihyperlipidemic drugs.

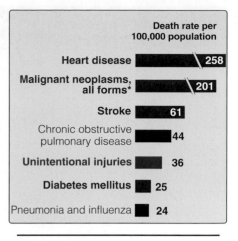

Figure 27.8
Influence of nutrition on some common causes of death in the United States in the year 2000. Red indicates causes of death in which the diet plays a significant role. Blue indicates causes of death in which excessive alcohol consumption plays a part. (*Diet plays a role in only some forms of cancer.)

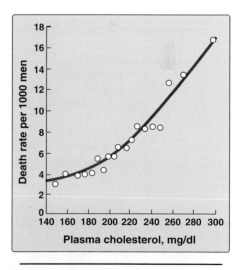

Figure 27.9
Correlation of the death rate from coronary heart disease with the concentration of plasma cholesterol. [Note: The data were obtained from a 6 year study of men with the death rate adjusted for age.]

Amount of saturated fat (grams per tablespoon)	Type of fat	Amount of unsaturated fat (grams per tablespoon)
■ Saturated fat		
0.8	Safflower oil	10.2 / 2
1.0	Canola oil	8.2 / 2.8 / 1.3
1.3	Flaxseed oil	2.5 / 2.2 / 8.0
1.4	Sunflower oil	2.7 / 8.9
1.7	Corn oil	3.3 / 7.9
1.8	Olive oil	10.0 / 1.1
1.9	Sesame oil	5.4 / 5.6
2.0	Soybean oil	3.2 / 6.9 / 0.9
2.3	Peanut oil	6.2 / 4.3
2.7	Salmon fat	3.9 / 4.8
3.2	Cream cheese	1.4
3.5	Cottonseed oil	2.4 / 7.0
3.8	Chicken fat	5.7 / 2.5
5.0	Lard (pork fat)	5.8 / 1.3
6.4	Beef tallow	5.4
7.2	Butter	3.3
8.1	Cocoa butter	4.5
11.1	Palm kernel oil	1.6
11.8	Coconut oil	0.8

■ Monounsaturated fat
□ Polyunsaturated fat (ω-6)
□ Polyunsaturated fat (ω-3)

Figure 27.10
Compositions of commonly encountered dietary lipids.

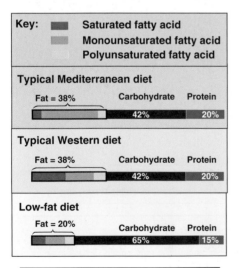

Figure 27.11
Composition of typical Mediterranean, Western, and low-fat diets.

Key:
■ Saturated fatty acid
■ Monounsaturated fatty acid
□ Polyunsaturated fatty acid

Typical Mediterranean diet
Fat = 38%   Carbohydrate 42%   Protein 20%

Typical Western diet
Fat = 38%   Carbohydrate 42%   Protein 20%

Low-fat diet
Fat = 20%   Carbohydrate 65%   Protein 15%

a. **The Mediterranean diet:** The Mediterranean diet is an example of a diet rich in monounsaturated fatty acids or MUFAs (from olive oil) and ω-3 fatty acids (from fish oils and some nuts), but low in saturated fat. For example, Figure 27.11 shows the composition of the Mediterranean diet in comparison with both a Western diet similar to that consumed in the United States and a typical low-fat diet. The Mediterranean diet contains seasonally fresh food, with an abundance of plant material, low amounts of red meat, and olive oil as the principal source of fat. The Mediterranean diet is associated with decreased serum total cholesterol and LDL cholesterol—but little change in HDL cholesterol—when compared with a typical Western diet higher in saturated fats. Plasma triacylglycerols are unchanged.

3. **Polyunsaturated fats:** Triacylglycerols containing primarily fatty acids with more than one double bond are referred to as polyunsaturated fats. The effects of polyunsaturated fatty acids (PUFAs) on cardiovascular disease is influenced by the location of the double bonds within the molecule.

a. ω-6 Fatty acids: These are long-chain, PUFAs, with the first double bond beginning at the sixth bond position when starting from the methyl end of the fatty acid molecule.

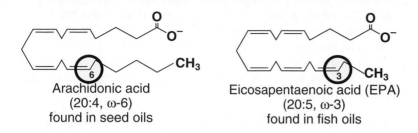

Arachidonic acid
(20:4, ω-6)
found in seed oils

Eicosapentaenoic acid (EPA)
(20:5, ω-3)
found in fish oils

[Note: They are also called n-6 fatty acids (see p. 183).] Consumption of fats containing ω-6 PUFAs, principally linoleic acid, 18:2(9,12), obtained from vegetable oils, lowers plasma cholesterol when substituted for saturated fats. Plasma LDL are lowered, but HDL, which protect against CHD, are also lowered. The powerful benefits of lowering LDL are only partially offset because of the decreased HDL. Nuts, avocados, olives, soybeans, and various oils, including sesame, cottonseed, and corn oil, are common sources of these fatty acids (see Figure 27.10). Linoleic acid, along with α-linolenic acid, 18:3(9,12,15), an ω-3 fatty acid (see below), are essential fatty acids required for fluidity of membrane structure and synthesis of eicosanoids (see p. 213). [Note: A deficiency of essential fatty acids is characterized by scaly dermatitis, hair loss, and poor wound healing.] A lower boundary level of 5% of calories meets the AI set for linoleic acid. An upper boundary for linoleic acid is set at 10% of total calories because of concern that oxidation of these polyunsaturated fatty acids may lead to deleterious products.

b. ω-3 Fatty acids: These are long-chain, PUFAs, with the first double bond beginning at the third bond position from the methyl end. Dietary ω-3 polyunsaturated fats suppress cardiac arrhythmias, reduce serum triacylglycerols, decrease the tendency for thrombosis, lower blood pressure, and substantially reduce risk of cardiovascular mortality (Figure 27.12), but they have little effect on LDL or HDL cholesterol levels. The ω-3 polyunsatyrated fats, principally α-linolenic acid, 18:3(9,12,15), are found in plants. The acceptable range for α-linolenic acid is 0.6-1.2% of total calories. Fish oil contains the long-chain, ω-3 docosahexaenoic acid (DHA) and eicosapentaenoic acid (EPA). Two fatty fish (for example, salmon) meals per week are recommended. [Note: The ω-3 long-chain PUFAs are included in infant formulas to promote brain development.]

4. Trans fatty acids: Trans fatty acids (Figure 27.13) are chemically classified as unsaturated fatty acids, but behave more like saturated fatty acids in the body, that is, they elevate serum LDL (but not HDL), and they increase the risk of CHD. Trans fatty acids do not occur naturally in plants, but occur in small amounts in ani-

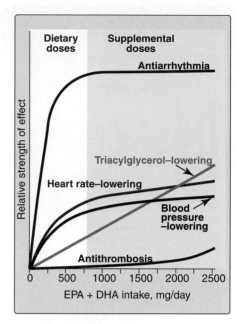

Figure 27.12
Dose responses of physiologic effects of fish oil intake.

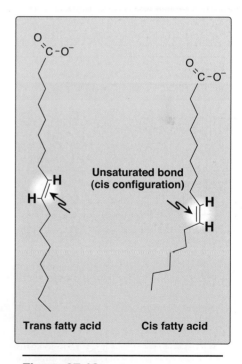

Figure 27.13
Structure of cis and trans fatty acids.

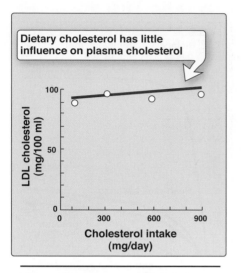

Figure 27.14
Response of plasma LDL concentrations to an increase in dietary cholesterol intake.

mals. However, trans fatty acids are formed during the hydrogenation of liquid vegetable oils, for example, in the manufacture of margarine and partially hydrogenated vegetable oil. Trans fatty acids are a major component of many commercial baked goods, such as cookies and cakes, and most deep-fried foods. Many manufacturers have reformulated their products to be free of trans fats. Starting in 2006, the U.S. Food and Drug Administration requires that Nutrition Facts labels portray trans fat content. Some municipalities, for example, New York City, have banned the use of trans fats in restaurants.

5. **Dietary cholesterol:** Cholesterol is found only in animal products. The effect of dietary cholesterol on plasma cholesterol (Figure 27.14) is less important than the amount and types of fatty acids consumed.

C. Other dietary factors affecting CHD

Moderate consumption of alcohol (for example, two drinks a day) decreases the risk of CHD, because there is a positive correlation between moderate alcohol consumption and the plasma concentration of HDL. However, because of the potential dangers of alcohol abuse, health professionals are reluctant to recommend increased alcohol consumption to their patients. Red wine may provide cardioprotective benefits in addition to those resulting from its alcohol content, for example, red wine contains phenolic compounds that inhibit lipoprotein oxidation (see p. 235). [Note: These antioxidants are also present in raisins and grape juice.] Figure 27.15 summarizes the effects of dietary fats.

TYPE OF FAT	METABOLIC EFFECTS		EFFECTS ON DISEASE PREVENTION
Trans fatty acid	⬆ LDL ⬇ HDL		⬆ Incidence of coronary heart disease
Saturated fatty acid	⬆ LDL Little effect on HDL		⬆ Incidence of coronary heart disease; may increase risk of prostate, colon cancer
Monounsaturated fatty acid	⬇ LDL ⬇ HDL		⬇ Incidence of coronary heart disease
Polyunsaturated fatty acids ω–6	⬇ LDL ⬇ HDL	Provide arachidonic acid which is an important precursor of prostaglandins and leukotrienes	⬇ Incidence of coronary heart disease
Polyunsaturated fatty acids ω–3	Little effect on LDL Little effect on HDL	Suppress cardiac arrhythmias, reduce serum triacylglycerols, decrease the tendency for thrombosis, lower blood pressure	⬇ Incidence of coronary heart disease ⬇ Risk of sudden cardiac death

Figure 27.15
Effects of dietary fats.

VI. DIETARY CARBOHYDRATES

The primary role of dietary carbohydrate is to provide energy. Although caloric intake in the United States has shown a modest increase since 1971, the incidence of obesity has dramatically increased (see p. 349). During this same period, carbohydrate consumption has significantly increased, leading some observers to link obesity with carbohydrate consumption. However, obesity has also been related to increasingly inactive lifestyles, and to calorie-dense foods served in expanded portion size. Carbohydrates are not inherently fattening.

A. Classification of carbohydrates

Carbohydrates in the diet are classified as either monosaccharides and disaccharides (simple sugars), polysaccharides (complex sugars), or fiber.

1. **Monosaccharides:** Glucose and fructose are the principal monosaccharides found in food. Glucose is abundant in fruits, sweet corn, corn syrup, and honey. Free fructose is found together with free glucose and sucrose in honey and fruits.

    a. **High fructose corn syrup:** High-fructose corn syrups (HFCS) are corn syrups that have undergone enzymatic processing to convert their glucose into fructose and have then been mixed with pure corn syrup (100% glucose) to produce a desired sweetness. In the United States, HFCS 55 (containing 55% fructose and 42% glucose) is commonly used as a substitute for sucrose in beverages, including soft drinks, with HFCS 42 used in processed foods. The composition and metabolism of HFCS and sucrose are similar, the major difference being that HFCS is ingested as a mixture of monosaccharides (Figure 27.16). Most studies have shown no significant difference between sucrose and HFCS syrup meals in either postprandial glucose or insulin responses.

2. **Disaccharides:** The most abundant disaccharides are sucrose (glucose + fructose), lactose (glucose + galactose), and maltose (glucose + glucose). Sucrose is ordinary "table sugar," and is abundant in molasses and maple syrup. Lactose is the principal sugar found in milk. Maltose is a product of enzymic digestion of polysaccharides. It is also found in significant quantities in beer and malt liquors. The term "sugar" refers to monosaccharides and disaccharides. "Added sugars" are those sugars and syrups added to foods during processing or preparation.

3. **Polysaccharides:** Complex carbohydrates are polysaccharides (most often polymers of glucose), which do not have a sweet taste. Starch is an example of a complex carbohydrate that is found in abundance in plants. Common sources include wheat and other grains, potatoes, dried peas and beans, and vegetables.

4. **Fiber:** Dietary fiber is defined as the nondigestible carbohydrates and lignin (a complex polymer of phenylpropanoid subunits) present intact in plants. Several different terms are used to

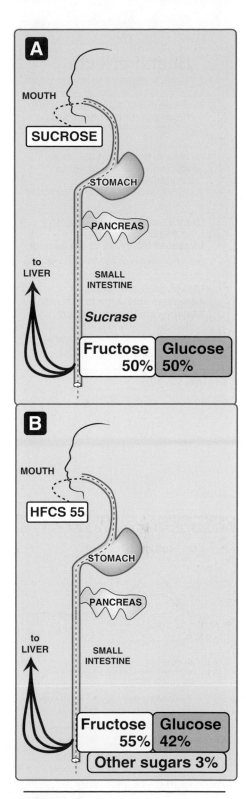

Figure 27.16
Digestion of HFCS 55 or sucrose leads to absorption of glucose plus fructose.

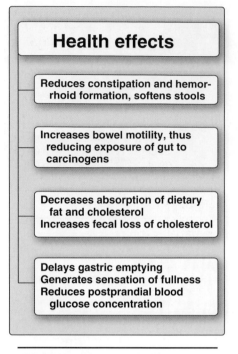

Health effects

Reduces constipation and hemor-
rhoid formation, softens stools

Increases bowel motility, thus
reducing exposure of gut to
carcinogens

Decreases absorption of dietary
fat and cholesterol
Increases fecal loss of cholesterol

Delays gastric emptying
Generates sensation of fullness
Reduces postprandial blood
glucose concentration

Figure 27.17
Actions of dietary fiber.

describe this complex group of compounds. For example, functional fiber is the isolated, extracted, or synthetic fiber that has proven health benefits. Total fiber is the sum of dietary fiber and functional fiber. Soluble fiber is the edible parts of plants that is resistant to digestion and absorption in the human small intestine, but is completely or partially fermented to short-chain fatty acids in the large intestine. Insoluble fiber passes through the digestive track largely intact. Dietary fiber provides little energy but has several beneficial effects. First, it adds bulk to the diet (Figure 27.17). Fiber can absorb 10–15 times its own weight in water, drawing fluid into the lumen of the intestine and increasing bowel motility. Soluble fiber delays gastric emptying and can result in a sensation of fullness. This delayed emptying also results in reduced peaks of blood glucose following a meal. Second, consumption of soluble fiber has now been shown to lower LDL cholesterol levels by increasing fecal bile acid excretion and interfering with bile acid absorption. For example, diets rich (25–50 g/day) in the soluble fiber oat bran are associated with a modest, but significant, reduction in risk for cardiovascular disease by lowering total and LDL cholesterol levels. Also, fiber-rich diets decrease the risk for constipation, hemorrhoids, and diverticulosis. The recommended daily fiber intake (AI) is 25 g/day for women and 38 g/day for men. However, most American diets are far lower in fiber—approximately 15 g/day.

B. Dietary carbohydrate and blood glucose

Some carbohydrate-containing foods produce a rapid rise followed by a steep fall in blood glucose concentration, whereas others result in a gradual rise followed by a slow decline—they differ in their glycemic response. The glycemic index (GI) quantitates these differences in the time course of postprandial glucose concentrations (Figure 27.18). Glycemic index is defined as the area under the blood glucose curves seen after ingestion of a meal with carbohydrate-rich food, compared with the area under the blood glucose curve observed after a meal consisting of the same amount (50g) of carbohydrate either as glucose or white bread. The clinical importance of glycemic index is controversial. Food with a low glycemic index tends to create a sense of satiety over a longer period of time, and may be helpful in limiting caloric intake. [Note: How much a typical serving size of a food raises blood glucose is referred to as the glycemic load (GL). A food, for example, carrots, can have a high GI and a low GL.]

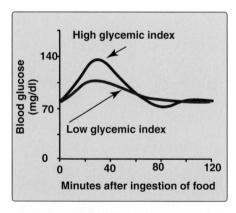

Figure 27.18
Blood glucose concentrations following ingestion of food with low or high glycemic index.

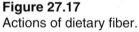

Many experts assert that high nutrient and fiber content, such as occurs in whole grains, fruits, and vegetables, is a better guide than glycemic index for selecting dietary carbohydrates.

C. Requirements for carbohydrate

Carbohydrates are not essential nutrients, because the carbon skeletons of most amino acids can be converted into glucose (see p. 261). However, the absence of dietary carbohydrate leads to ketone body production (see p. 262), and degradation of body protein whose constituent amino acids provide carbon skeletons for gluconeogenesis (see p. 118). The RDA for carbohydrate is set at 130 g/day for adults and children, based on the amount of glucose used by carbohydrate-dependent tissues, such as the brain and erythrocytes. However, this level of intake is usually exceeded to meet energy needs. Adults should consume 45–65% of their total calories from carbohydrates. It is recommended that added sugar represent no more than 25% of total energy because of concerns that sugar may displace nutrient-rich foods from the diet, potentially leading to deficiencies of certain micronutrients.

D. Simple sugars and disease

There is no direct evidence that the consumption of simple sugars is harmful. Contrary to folklore, diets high in sucrose do not lead to diabetes or hypoglycemia. Also contrary to popular belief, carbohydrates are not inherently fattening. They yield 4 kcal/g (the same as protein and less than one half that of fat, see Figure 27.5), and result in fat synthesis only when consumed in excess of the body's energy needs. However, there is an association between sucrose consumption and dental caries, particularly in the absence of fluoride treatment.

VII. DIETARY PROTEIN

Humans have no dietary requirement for protein, per se, but the protein in food does provide essential amino acids (see Figure 20.2, p. 262). Nine of the 20 amino acids needed for the synthesis of body proteins are essential—that is, they cannot be synthesized in humans.

A. Quality of proteins

The quality of a dietary protein is a measure of its ability to provide the essential amino acids required for tissue maintenance. Most government agencies have adopted the Protein Digestibility-Corrected Amino Acid Score (PDCAAS) as the standard by which to evaluate protein quality. PDCAAS is based on the profile of essential amino acids and the digestibility of the protein. The highest possible score under these guidelines is 1.00. This amino acid score provides a method to balance intakes of poorer-quality proteins with high-quality dietary proteins.

1. **Proteins from animal sources:** Proteins from animal sources (meat, poultry, milk, and fish) have a high quality because they contain all the essential amino acids in proportions similar to those required for synthesis of human tissue proteins (Figure 27.19). [Note: Gelatin prepared from animal collagen is an exception; it has a low biologic value as a result of deficiencies in several essential amino acids.]

Source	PDCAAS value
Animal proteins	
Egg	1.00
Milk protein	1.00
Beef/poultry/fish	0.82–0.92
Gelatin	0.08
Plant proteins	
Soybean protein	1.00
Kidney beans	0.68
Whole wheat bread	0.40

Figure 27.19
Relative quality of some common dietary proteins.

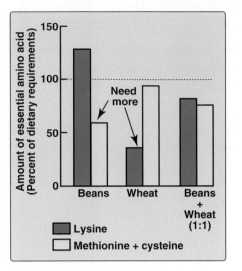

Figure 27.20
Combining two incomplete proteins that have complementary amino acid deficiencies results in a mixture with a higher biologic value.

2. Proteins from plant sources: Proteins from wheat, corn, rice, and beans have a lower quality than do animal proteins. However, proteins from different plant sources may be combined in such a way that the result is equivalent in nutritional value to animal protein. For example, wheat (lysine-deficient but methionine-rich) may be combined with kidney beans (methionine-poor but lysine-rich) to produce an improved biologic value. Thus, eating foods with different amino acids during the day can result in a dietary combination with a higher biologic value than either of the component proteins (Figure 27.20). [Note: Animal proteins can also complement the biologic value of plant proteins.]

B. Nitrogen balance

Nitrogen balance occurs when the amount of nitrogen consumed equals that of the nitrogen excreted in the urine, sweat, and feces. Most healthy adults are normally in nitrogen balance.

1. Positive nitrogen balance: This occurs when nitrogen intake exceeds nitrogen excretion. It is observed during situations in which tissue growth occurs, for example, in childhood, pregnancy, or during recovery from an emaciating illness.

2. Negative nitrogen balance: This occurs when nitrogen loss is greater than nitrogen intake. It is associated with inadequate dietary protein, lack of an essential amino acid, or during physiologic stresses, such as trauma, burns, illness, or surgery.

C. Requirement for protein in humans

The amount of dietary protein required in the diet varies with its biologic value. The greater the proportion of animal protein included in the diet, the less protein is required. The RDA for protein is computed for proteins of mixed biologic value at 0.8 g/kg of body weight for adults, or about 56 g of protein for a 70-kg individual. People who exercise strenuously on a regular basis may benefit from extra protein to maintain muscle mass; a daily intake of about 1 g/kg has been recommended for athletes. Women who are pregnant or lactating require up to 30 g/day in addition to their basal requirements. To support growth, infants should consume 2 g/kg/day.

CHARACTERISTIC	KWASHIORKOR	MARASMUS
Weight for age (% expected)	60–80	<60
Weight for height	Normal or decreased	Markedly decreased
Edema	Present	Absent
Mood	Irritable when picked up; apathetic when left alone	Alert, irritable
Appetite	Poor	Good

Figure 27.21
Features of protein-energy malnutrition in children.

1. **Consumption of excess protein:** There is no physiologic advantage to the consumption of more protein than the RDA. Protein consumed in excess of the body's needs is deaminated, and the resulting carbon skeletons are metabolized to provide energy or acetyl coenzyme A for fatty acid synthesis. When excess protein is eliminated from the body as urinary nitrogen, it is often accompanied by increased urinary calcium, increasing the risk of nephrolithiasis and osteoporosis.

2. **The protein-sparing effect of carbohydrate:** The dietary protein requirement is influenced by the carbohydrate content of the diet. When the intake of carbohydrates is low, amino acids are deaminated to provide carbon skeletons for the synthesis of glucose that is needed as a fuel by the central nervous system. If carbohydrate intake is less than 130 g/day, substantial amounts of protein are metabolized to provide precursors for gluconeogenesis. Therefore, carbohydrate is considered to be "protein-sparing," because it allows amino acids to be used for repair and maintenance of tissue protein rather than for gluconeogenesis.

D. Protein energy (calorie) malnutrition (PEM)

In developed countries, PEM is most frequently seen in patients with medical conditions that decrease appetite or alter how nutrients are digested or absorbed, or in hospitalized patients with major trauma or infections. [Note: Such highly catabolic patients frequently require intravenous (parenteral) or tube-based (enteral) administration of nutrients.] PEM may also be seen in children or the elderly who are malnourished. In developing countries, an inadequate intake of protein and/or energy is the primary cause of PEM. Affected individuals show a variety of symptoms, including a depressed immune system with a reduced ability to resist infection. Death from secondary infection is common. Two extreme forms of PEM are kwashiorkor and marasmus (Figure 27.21).

1. **Kwashiorkor:** Kwashiorkor occurs when protein deprivation is relatively greater than the reduction in total calories. Protein deprivation is associated with severely decreased synthesis of visceral protein. Kwashiorkor is frequently seen in children after weaning at about one year of age, when their diet consists predominantly of carbohydrates. Typical symptoms include stunted growth, edema, skin lesions, depigmented hair, anorexia, enlarged fatty liver, and decreased plasma albumin concentration. Edema results from the lack of adequate plasma proteins to maintain the distribution of water between blood and tissues. Edema may mask muscle loss.

2. **Marasmus:** Marasmus occurs when calorie deprivation is relatively greater than the reduction in protein. It usually occurs in children younger than 1 year of age when breast milk is supplemented with watery gruels of native cereals that are usually deficient in protein and calories. Typical symptoms include arrested growth, extreme muscle wasting (emaciation), weakness, and anemia (Figure 27.22). Victims of marasmus do not show the edema or changes in plasma proteins observed in kwashiorkor.

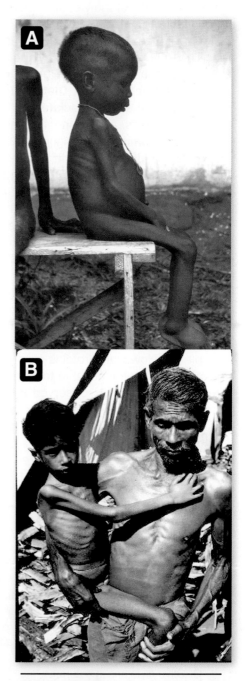

Figure 27.22
A.Listless child with kwashiorkor.
B.Child suffering with marasmus.

VIII. CHAPTER SUMMARY

Estimated Average Requirement (**EAR**) is the average daily nutrient intake level estimated to meet the require-ment of one half the healthy individuals in a particular life stage and gender group. The **Recommended Dietary Allowance** (**RDA**) is the average daily dietary intake level that is sufficient to meet the nutrient requirements of nearly all (97–98%) individuals. **Adequate Intake** (**AI**) is set instead of an RDA if sufficient scientific evidence is not available to calculate the RDA. The **Tolerable Upper Intake Level** (**UL**) is the highest average daily nutrient intake level that is likely to pose no risk of adverse health effects to almost all individuals in the general popula-tion. The energy generated by the metabolism of the **macronutrients** is used for three energy-requiring processes that occur in the body: **resting metabolic rate**, **thermic effect of food**, and **physical activity**. **Acceptable Macronutrient Distribution Ranges** (**AMDR**) are defined as the ranges of intake for a particular macronutrient that is associated with reduced risk of chronic disease while providing adequate amounts of essential nutrients. Adults should consume **45–65%** of their **total calories** from **carbohydrates**, **20–35%** from **fat**, and **10–35%** from **protein** (Figure 27.23). Elevated levels of cholesterol or LDL cholesterol result in increased risk for **cardiovascular disease**. In contrast, high levels of HDL cholesterol have been associated with a decreased risk for heart disease. Dietary or drug treatment of **hypercholesterolemia** is effective in decreasing LDL, increas-ing HDL, and reducing the risk for cardiovascular events. Consumption of **saturated fats** is strongly associated with high levels of total plasma and LDL cholesterol. When substituted for saturated fatty acids in the diet, **monounsaturated fats** lower both total plasma and LDL cholesterol, but increase HDL. Consumption of fats con-taining **ω-6 polyunsaturated fatty acids** lowers plasma LDL, but HDL, which protect against coronary heart dis-ease, are also lowered. Dietary **ω-3 polyunsaturated fats** suppress cardiac arrhythmias and reduce serum triacylglycerols, decrease the tendency for thrombosis, and substantially reduce the risk of cardiovascular mortal-ity. **Carbohydrates** provide **energy** and **fiber** to the diet. When they are consumed as part of a diet in which caloric intake is equal to energy expenditure, they do not promote obesity. Dietary **protein** provides **essential amino acids**. The **quality of a protein** is a measure of its ability to provide the essential amino acids required for tissue maintenance. Proteins from animal sources, in general, have a higher-quality protein than that derived from plants. However, proteins from different plant sources may be combined in such a way that the result is equivalent in nutritional value to animal protein. **Positive nitrogen balance** occurs when nitrogen intake exceeds nitrogen excretion. It is observed in situations in which tissue growth occurs, for example, in childhood, preg-nancy, or during recovery from an emaciating illness. **Negative nitrogen balance** occurs when nitrogen losses are greater than nitrogen intake. It is associated with inadequate dietary protein, lack of an essential amino acid, or during physiologic stresses such as trauma, burns, illness, or surgery. **Kwashiorkor** is caused by inadequate intake of protein and is characterized by edema. **Marasmus** results from chronic deficiency of calories.

Study Questions

Choose the ONE correct answer.

27.1 Which one of the following statements concerning dietary lipid is correct?

A. Corn oil and soybean oil are examples of fats rich in saturated fatty acids.

B. Triacylglycerols obtained from plants generally contain less unsaturated fatty acids than those from animals.

C. Olive oil is rich in saturated fats.

D. Fatty acids containing double bonds in the trans configuration, unlike the naturally occurring cis isomers, raise plasma cholesterol levels.

E. Coconut and palm oils are rich in polyunsaturated fats.

Correct answer = D. Trans fatty acids raise plasma cholesterol levels. Corn oil and soybean oil are examples of fats rich in polyunsaturated fatty acids. Triacylglycerols obtained from plants generally contain more unsaturated fatty acids than those from animals. Olive oil, the staple of the Mediterranean diet, is rich in monounsatu-rated fats. Coconut and palm oils are unusual plant oils in that they are rich in saturated fats.

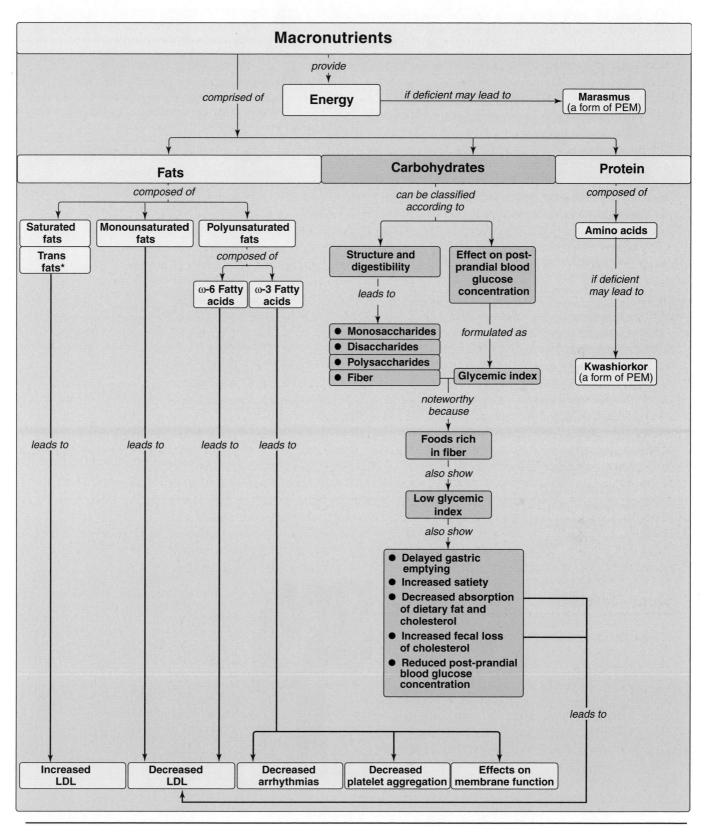

Figure 27.23
Key concept map for the macronutrients. *Note: Trans fatty acids are chemically classified as monounsaturated. PEM = protein energy malnutrition.

27.2 Given the information that a 70-kg man is consuming a daily average of 275 g of carbohydrate, 75 g of protein, and 65 g of lipid, one can draw which of the following conclusions?

A. Total energy intake per day is approximately 3,000 kcal.

B. About 20% of the calories are derived from lipids.

C. The diet does not contain a sufficient amount of dietary fiber.

D. The proportions of carbohydrate, protein, and lipid in the diet conform to the recommendations of academic groups and government agencies.

E. The individual is in nitrogen balance.

Correct answer = D. The total energy intake is (275 g carbohydrate × 4 kcal/g) + (75 g protein × 4 kcal/g) + (65 g lipid × 9 kcal/g) = 1100 + 300 + 585 = 1,985 total kcal/day. The percentage calories from carbohydrate is 1,100/1,985 = 55; percentage calories from protein is 300/1,985 = 15; and percentage calories derived from lipid is 585/1,985 = 30. These are very close to current recommendations. The amount of fiber or nitrogen balance cannot be deduced from the data presented. If the protein is of low biologic value, a negative nitrogen balance is possible.

27.3 A sedentary 50-year-old man, weighing 80 kg (176 pounds), requests a physical examination. He denies any health problems. Routine blood analysis is unremarkable except for plasma cholesterol of 280 mg/dl. The man refuses drug therapy for his hypercholesterolemia. Analysis of a 1-day dietary recall showed the following:

Kilocalories	3,475 kcal	Cholesterol	822 mg
Protein	102 g	Saturated fat	69 g
Carbohydrate	383 g	Total Fat	165 g
Fiber crude	6 g		

Changes in which one of the following dietary components would have the greatest effect in lowering plasma cholesterol?

A. Cholesterol.

B. Saturated fat.

C. Polyunsaturated fat.

D. Monounsaturated fat.

E. Carbohydrate.

Correct answer = B. The intake of saturated fat most strongly influences plasma cholesterol in this diet. The patient is consuming a high-calorie, high-fat diet with 40% of the fat as saturated fat. The most important dietary recommendations are: lower total caloric intake, substitute monounsaturated and polyunsaturated fats for saturated fats, and increase dietary fiber. A decrease in dietary cholesterol would be helpful, but is not a primary objective.

27.4 Which of the findings in the child shown at right would support a diagnosis of kwashiorkor?

A. Shows increased serum albumin.

B. Shows a good appetite.

C. Appears plump due to increased adipose tissue.

D. Displays abdominal and peripheral edema.

E. Has markedly decreased weight for height.

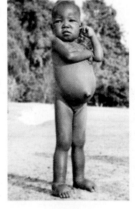

The correct answer = D. Kwashiorkor is caused by inadequate protein intake in the presence of fair to good energy (calorie) intake. Typical findings in a patient with Kwashiorkor include abdominal and peripheral edema (note the swollen belly and legs of the child) caused largely by a decreased serum albumin concentration. Anorexia is almost always present. Weight for height can be normal. Treatment includes a diet adequate in calories and protein.

Vitamins

28

I. OVERVIEW

Vitamins are chemically unrelated organic compounds that cannot be synthesized in adequate quantities by humans and, therefore, must be supplied by the diet. Nine vitamins (folic acid, cobalamin, ascorbic acid, pyridoxine, thiamine, niacin, riboflavin, biotin, and pantothenic acid) are classified as water-soluble, whereas four vitamins (vitamins A, D, K, and E) are termed fat-soluble (Figure 28.1). Vitamins are required to perform specific cellular functions, for example, many of the water-soluble vitamins are precursors of coenzymes for the enzymes of intermediary metabolism. In contrast to the water-soluble vitamins, only one fat soluble vitamin (vitamin K) has a coenzyme function. These vitamins are released, absorbed, and transported with the fat of the diet. They are not readily excreted in the urine, and significant quantities are stored in the liver and adipose tissue. In fact, consumption of vitamins A and D in excess of the Dietary Reference Intakes (DRIs) can lead to accumulation of toxic quantities of these compounds.

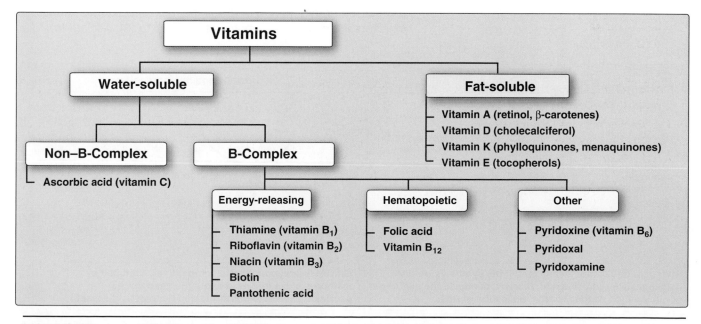

Figure 28.1
Classification of the vitamins.

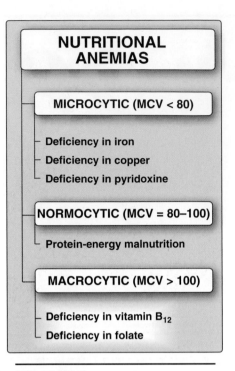

Figure 28.2
Classification of nutritional anemias by cell size. The normal mean corpuscular volume (MCV) for people older than age 18 is between 80 and 100 μm³. [Note: Microcytic anemia is also seen with lead poisoning.]

II. FOLIC ACID

Folic acid (or folate), which plays a key role in one-carbon metabolism, is essential for the biosynthesis of several compounds. Folic acid deficiency is probably the most common vitamin deficiency in the United States, particularly among pregnant women and alcoholics.

A. Function of folic acid

Tetrahydrofolate (reduced folate) receives one-carbon fragments from donors such as serine, glycine, and histidine and transfers them to intermediates in the synthesis of amino acids, purines, and thymidine monophosphate (TMP)—a pyrimidine found in DNA.

B. Nutritional anemias

Anemia is a condition in which the blood has a lower than normal concentration of hemoglobin, which results in a reduced ability to transport oxygen. Nutritional anemias—those caused by inadequate intake of one or more essential nutrients—can be classified according to the size of the red blood cells or mean corpuscular volume observed in the individual (Figure 28.2). Microcytic anemia, caused by lack of iron, is the most common form of nutritional anemia. The second major category of nutritional anemia, macrocytic, results from a deficiency in folic acid or vitamin B_{12}. [Note: These macrocytic anemias are commonly called megaloblastic because a deficiency of folic acid or vitamin B_{12} causes accumulation of large, immature red cell precursors, known as megaloblasts, in the bone marrow and the blood.]

1. **Folate and anemia:** Inadequate serum levels of folate can be caused by increased demand (for example, pregnancy and lactation), poor absorption caused by pathology of the small intestine, alcoholism, or treatment with drugs that are *dihydrofolate reductase* inhibitors, for example, methotrexate (Figure 28.3). A folate-free diet

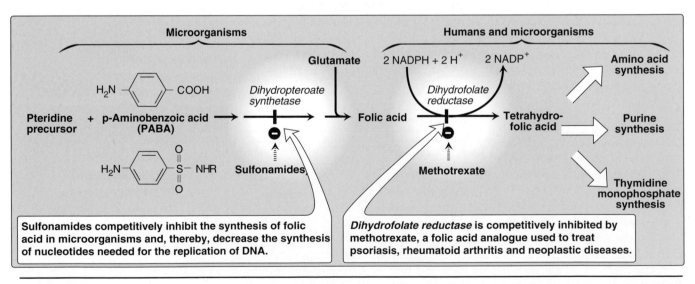

Figure 28.3
Inhibition of tetrahydrofolate synthesis by sulfonamides and methotrexate.

can cause a deficiency within a few weeks. A primary result of folic acid deficiency is megaloblastic anemia (Figure 28.4), caused by diminished synthesis of purines and TMP, which leads to an inability of cells (including red cell precursors) to make DNA and, therefore, they cannot divide. [Note: It is important to evaluate the cause of the megaloblastic anemia prior to instituting therapy, because vitamin B$_{12}$ deficiency indirectly causes symptoms of this disorder (see p. 377).]

2. **Folate and neural tube defects in the fetus:** Spina bifida and anencephaly, the most common neural tube defects, affect approximately 4,000 pregnancies in the United State annually. Folic acid supplementation before conception and during the first trimester has been shown to significantly reduce the defects. Therefore, all women of childbearing age are advised to consume 0.4 mg/day of folic acid to reduce the risk of having a pregnancy affected by neural tube defects. Adequate folate nutrition must occur at the time of conception because critical folate-dependent development occurs in the first weeks of fetal life—at a time when many women are not yet aware of their pregnancy. The U.S. Food and Drug Administration has authorized the addition of folic acid to enriched grain products, resulting in a dietary supplementation of about 0.1 mg/day. It is estimated that this supplementation will allow approximately 50% of all reproductive-aged women to receive 0.4 mg of folate from all sources. However, there is an association of high-dose supplementation with folic acid (>0.8 mg/day) and an increased risk of cancer. Thus, supplementation is not recommended for most middle-aged or older adults.

III. COBALAMIN (VITAMIN B$_{12}$)

Vitamin B$_{12}$ is required in humans for two essential enzymatic reactions: the remethylation of homocysteine to methionine and the isomerization of methylmalonyl coenzyme A (CoA) that is produced during the degradation of some amino acids (isoleucine, valine, threonine, and methionine), and fatty acids with odd numbers of carbon atoms (Figure 28.5). When the vitamin is deficient, unusual fatty acids accumulate and become incorporated into cell membranes, including those of the nervous system. This may account for some of the neurologic manifestations of vitamin B$_{12}$ deficiency.

A. Structure of cobalamin and its coenzyme forms

Cobalamin contains a corrin ring system that differs from the porphyrins in that two of the pyrrole rings are linked directly rather than through a methene bridge. Cobalt is held in the center of the corrin ring by four coordination bonds from the nitrogens of the pyrrole groups. The remaining coordination bonds of the cobalt are with the nitrogen of 5,6-dimethylbenzimidazole and with cyanide in commercial preparations of the vitamin in the form of cyanocobalamin (Figure 28.6). The coenzyme forms of cobalamin are 5'-deoxyadenosylcobalamin, in which cyanide is replaced with 5'-deoxyadenosine (forming an unusual carbon–cobalt bond), and methylcobalamin, in which cyanide is replaced by a methyl group (see Figure 28.6).

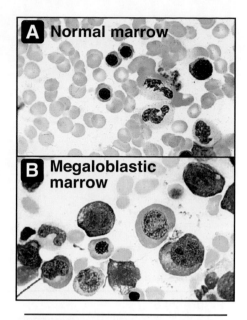

Figure 28.4
Bone marrow histology in normal and folate-deficient individuals.

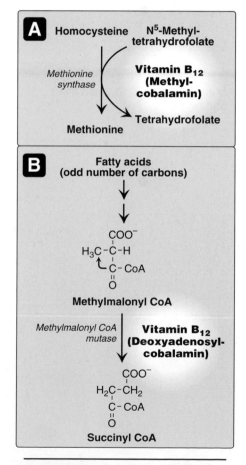

Figure 28.5
Reactions requiring coenzyme forms of vitamin B$_{12}$.

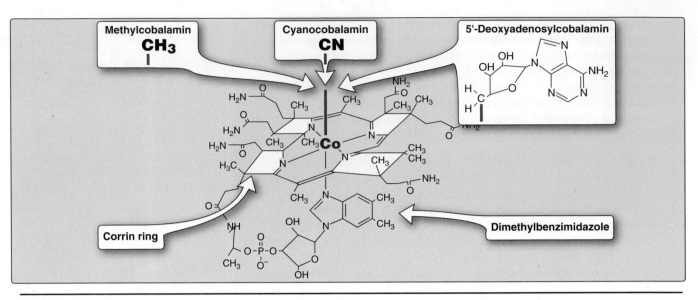

Figure 28.6
Structure of vitamin B_{12} (cyanocobalamin) and its coenzyme forms (methylcobalamin and 5'-deoxyadenosyl-cobalamin).

B. Distribution of cobalamin

Vitamin B_{12} is synthesized only by microorganisms; it is not present in plants. Animals obtain the vitamin preformed from their natural bacterial flora or by eating foods derived from other animals. Cobalamin is present in appreciable amounts in liver, whole milk, eggs, oysters, fresh shrimp, pork, and chicken.

C. Folate trap hypothesis

The effects of cobalamin deficiency are most pronounced in rapidly dividing cells, such as the erythropoietic tissue of bone marrow and the mucosal cells of the intestine. Such tissues need both the N^5,N^{10}-methylene and N^{10}-formyl forms of tetrahydrofolate for the synthesis of nucleotides required for DNA replication (see pp. 293 and 303). However, in vitamin B_{12} deficiency, the utilization of the N^5-methyl form of tetrahydrofolate in the B_{12}-dependent methylation of homocysteine to methionine is impaired. Because the methylated form cannot be converted directly to other forms of tetrahydrofolate, folate is trapped in the N^5-methyl form, which accumulates. The levels of the other forms decrease. Thus, cobalamin deficiency is hypothesized to lead to a deficiency of the tetrahydrofolate forms needed in purine and TMP synthesis, resulting in the symptoms of megaloblastic anemia.

D. Clinical indications for vitamin B_{12}

In contrast to other water-soluble vitamins, significant amounts (4–5 mg) of vitamin B_{12} are stored in the body. As a result, it may take several years for the clinical symptoms of B_{12} deficiency to develop in individuals who have had a partial or total gastrectomy (who, therefore, become intrinsic factor-deficient, see p. 377) and can no longer absorb the vitamin.

1. **Pernicious anemia:** Vitamin B_{12} deficiency is rarely a result of an absence of the vitamin in the diet. It is much more common to find

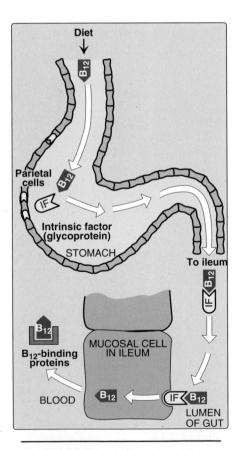

Figure 28.7
Absorption of vitamin B_{12}. IF = intrinsic factor.

deficiencies in patients who fail to absorb the vitamin from the intestine. Malabsorption of cobalamin in the elderly is most often due to reduced secretion of gastric acid and less efficient absorption of vitamin B_{12} from foods. A severe malabsorption of vitamin B_{12} leads to pernicious anemia. This disease is most commonly a result of an autoimmune destruction of the gastric parietal cells that are responsible for the synthesis of a glycoprotein called intrinsic factor. Normally, vitamin B_{12} obtained from the diet binds to intrinsic factor in the intestine (Figure 28.7). The cobalamin–intrinsic factor complex travels through the gut and eventually binds to specific receptors on the surface of mucosal cells of the ileum. The bound cobalamin is transported into the mucosal cell and, subsequently, into the general circulation, where it is carried by B_{12}-binding proteins. Lack of intrinsic factor prevents the absorption of vitamin B_{12}, resulting in pernicious anemia. Patients with cobalamin deficiency are usually anemic, but later in the development of the disease they show neuropsychiatric symptoms. However, central nervous system (CNS) symptoms may occur in the absence of anemia. The CNS effects are irreversible and occur by mechanisms that appear to be different from those described for megaloblastic anemia. The disease is treated by giving high-dose B_{12} orally, or intramuscular (IM) injection of cyanocobalamin. Therapy must be continued throughout the lives of patients with pernicious anemia. Deficiency of vitamin B_{12} can be measured by the level of methylmalonic acid in blood, which is elevated in individuals with low intake or decreased absorption of the vitamin.

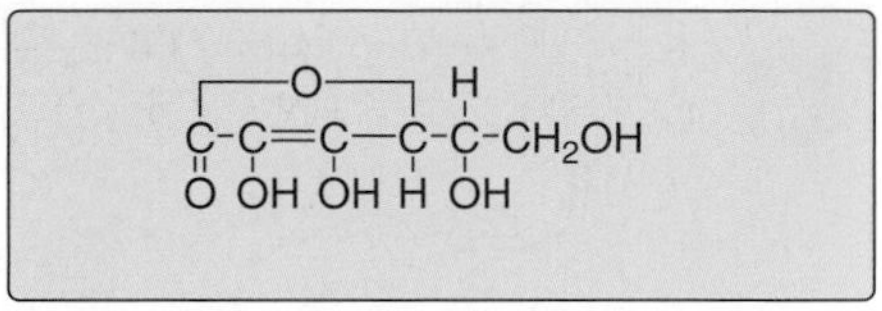

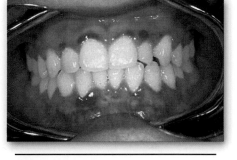

Figure 28.8
Structure of ascorbic acid.

> Folic acid can partially reverse the hematologic abnormalities of B_{12} deficiency and, therefore, can mask a cobalamin deficiency. Thus, therapy of megaloblastic anemia is often initiated with folic acid and vitamin B_{12} until the cause of the anemia can be determined.

Figure 28.9
Hemorrhage and swollen gums of a patient with scurvy.

IV. ASCORBIC ACID (VITAMIN C)

The active form of vitamin C is ascorbic acid (Figure 28.8). The main function of ascorbate is as a reducing agent in several different reactions. Vitamin C has a well-documented role as a coenzyme in hydroxylation reactions, for example, hydroxylation of prolyl and lysyl residues of collagen (see p. 47). Vitamin C is, therefore, required for the maintenance of normal connective tissue, as well as for wound healing. Vitamin C also facilitates the absorption of dietary iron from the intestine.

A. Deficiency of ascorbic acid

A deficiency of ascorbic acid results in scurvy, a disease characterized by sore and spongy gums, loose teeth, fragile blood vessels, swollen joints, and anemia (Figure 28.9). Many of the deficiency symptoms can be explained by a deficiency in the hydroxylation of collagen, resulting in defective connective tissue.

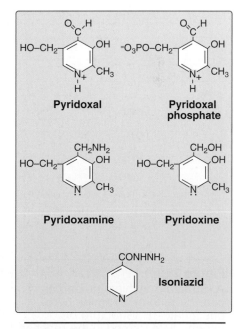

Figure 28.10
Structures of vitamin B_6 and and the antituberculosis drug isoniazid.

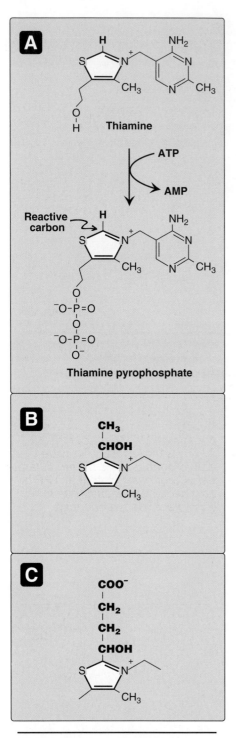

Figure 28.11
A. Structure of thiamine and its coenzyme form, thiamine pyrophosphate. B. Structure of intermediate formed in the reaction catalyzed by *pyruvate dehydrogenase*. C. Structure of intermediate formed in the reaction catalyzed by α-*ketoglutarate dehydrogenase*.

B. Prevention of chronic disease

Vitamin C is one of a group of nutrients that includes vitamin E (see p. 391) and β-carotene (see p. 382), which are known as antioxidants. Consumption of diets rich in these compounds is associated with a decreased incidence of some chronic diseases, such as coronary heart disease and certain cancers. However, clinical trials involving supplementation with the isolated antioxidants have failed to determine any convincing beneficial effects.

V. PYRIDOXINE (VITAMIN B₆)

Vitamin B_6 is a collective term for pyridoxine, pyridoxal, and pyridoxamine, all derivatives of pyridine. They differ only in the nature of the functional group attached to the ring (Figure 28.10). Pyridoxine occurs primarily in plants, whereas pyridoxal and pyridoxamine are found in foods obtained from animals. All three compounds can serve as precursors of the biologically active coenzyme, pyridoxal phosphate. Pyridoxal phosphate functions as a coenzyme for a large number of enzymes, particularly those that catalyze reactions involving amino acids.

Reaction type	Example
Transamination	Oxaloacetate + glutamate $\rightleftarrows$ aspartate + α-ketoglutarate
Deamination	Serine → pyruvate + NH_3
Decarboxylation	Histidine → histamine + CO_2
Condensation	Glycine + succinyl CoA → δ-aminolevulinic acid

A. Clinical indications for pyridoxine:

Isoniazid (isonicotinic acid hydrazide), a drug frequently used to treat tuberculosis, can induce a vitamin B_6 deficiency by forming an inactive derivative with pyridoxal phosphate. Dietary supplementation with B_6 is, thus, an adjunct to isoniazid treatment. Otherwise, dietary deficiencies in pyridoxine are rare but have been observed in newborn infants fed formulas low in B_6, in women taking oral contraceptives, and in alcoholics.

B. Toxicity of pyridoxine

Pyridoxine is the only water-soluble vitamin with significant toxicity. Neurologic symptoms (sensory neuropathy) occur at intakes above 200 mg/day, an amount more than 100 times the RDA. Substantial improvement, but not complete recovery, occurs when the vitamin is discontinued.

VI. THIAMINE (VITAMIN B₁)

Thiamine pyrophosphate is the biologically active form of the vitamin, formed by the transfer of a pyrophosphate group from adenosine triphosphate (ATP) to thiamine (Figure 28.11). Thiamine pyrophosphate serves as a coenzyme in the formation or degradation of α-ketols by *transketo-*

lase (Figure 28.12A), and in the oxidative decarboxylation of α-keto acids (Figure 28.12B).

A. Clinical indications for thiamine

The oxidative decarboxylation of pyruvate and α-ketoglutarate, which plays a key role in energy metabolism of most cells, is particularly important in tissues of the nervous system. In thiamine deficiency, the activity of these two *dehydrogenase*-catalyzed reactions is decreased, resulting in a decreased production of ATP and, thus, impaired cellular function. [Note: Thiamine deficiency is diagnosed by an increase in erythrocyte *transketolase* activity observed on addition of thiamine pyrophosphate.]

1. **Beriberi:** This is a severe thiamine-deficiency syndrome found in areas where polished rice is the major component of the diet. Signs of infantile beriberi include tachycardia, vomiting, convulsions, and, if not treated, death. The deficiency syndrome can have a rapid onset in nursing infants whose mothers are deficient in thiamine. Adult beriberi is characterized by dry skin, irritability, disordered thinking, and progressive paralysis.

2. **Wernicke-Korsakoff syndrome:** In the United States, thiamine deficiency, which is seen primarily in association with chronic alcoholism, is due to dietary insufficiency or impaired intestinal absorption of the vitamin. Some alcoholics develop Wernicke-Korsakoff syndrome—a thiamine deficiency state characterized by apathy, loss of memory, ataxia, and a rhythmic to-and-fro motion of the eyeballs (nystagmus). The neurologic consequences of Wernicke's syndrome are treatable with thiamine supplementation.

VII. NIACIN

Niacin, or nicotinic acid, is a substituted pyridine derivative. The biologically active coenzyme forms are nicotinamide adenine dinucleotide (NAD$^+$) and its phosphorylated derivative, nicotinamide adenine

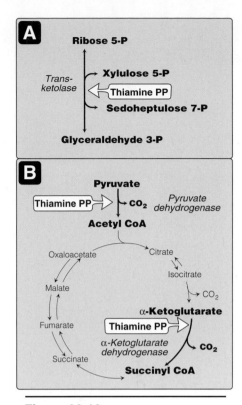

Figure 28.12
Reactions that use thiamine pyrophosphate (TPP) as coenzyme. A. *Transketolase*. B. *Pyruvate dehydrogenase* and α-*ketoglutarate dehydrogenase*. Note that TPP is also used by *branched-chain α-keto acid dehydrogenase*.

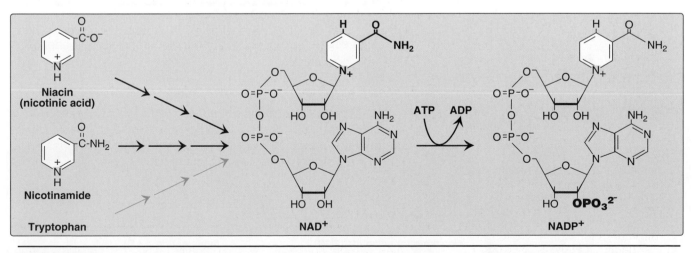

Figure 28.13
Structure and biosynthesis of NAD$^+$ and NADP$^+$. Note that a metabolite of tryptophan (quinolinate) can also be used in the synthesis of NAD$^+$.

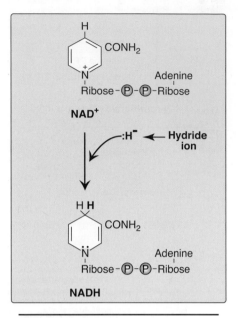

Figure 28.14
Reduction of NAD⁺ to NADH.

dinucleotide phosphate (NADP⁺, Figure 28.13). Nicotinamide, a derivative of nicotinic acid that contains an amide instead of a carboxyl group, also occurs in the diet. Nicotinamide is readily deaminated in the body and, therefore, is nutritionally equivalent to nicotinic acid. NAD⁺ and NADP⁺ serve as coenzymes in oxidation-reduction reactions in which the coenzyme undergoes reduction of the pyridine ring by accepting a hydride ion (hydrogen atom plus one electron, Figure 28.14). The reduced forms of NAD⁺ and NADP⁺ are NADH and NADPH, respectively.

A. Distribution of niacin

Niacin is found in unrefined and enriched grains and cereal, milk, and lean meats, especially liver. [Note: Corn is low in both niacin and tryptophan. Corn-based diets can cause pellagra (see below).]

B. Clinical indications for niacin

1. **Deficiency of niacin:** A deficiency of niacin causes pellagra, a disease involving the skin, gastrointestinal tract, and CNS. The symptoms of pellagra progress through the three Ds: dermatitis, diarrhea, dementia—and, if untreated, death.

2. **Treatment of hyperlipidemia:** Niacin (at doses of 1.5 g/day or 100 times the Recommended Dietary Allowance or RDA) strongly inhibits lipolysis in adipose tissue—the primary producer of circulating free fatty acids. The liver normally uses these circulating fatty acids as a major precursor for triacylglycerol synthesis. Thus, niacin causes a decrease in liver triacylglycerol synthesis, which is required for very-low-density lipoprotein (VLDL, see p. 231) production. Low-density lipoprotein (LDL, the cholesterol-rich lipoprotein) is derived from VLDL in the plasma. Thus, both plasma triacylglycerol (in VLDL) and cholesterol (in VLDL and LDL) are lowered. Therefore, niacin is particularly useful in the treatment of Type IIb hyperlipoproteinemia, in which both VLDL and LDL are elevated. [Note: Niacin raises HDL levels.]

VIII. RIBOFLAVIN (VITAMIN B₂)

The two biologically active forms are flavin mononucleotide (FMN) and flavin adenine dinucleotide (FAD), formed by the transfer of an adenosine

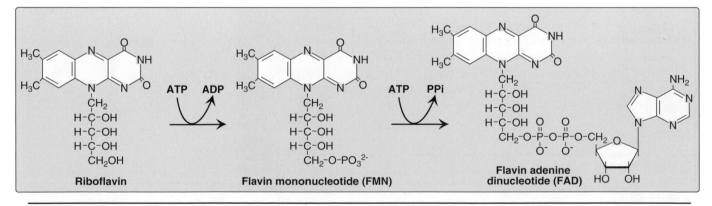

Figure 28.15
Structure and biosynthesis of flavin mononucleotide and flavin adenine dinucleotide.

monophosphate moiety from ATP to FMN (Figure 28.15). FMN and FAD are each capable of reversibly accepting two hydrogen atoms, forming FMNH$_2$ or FADH$_2$. FMN and FAD are bound tightly—sometimes covalently—to flavoenzymes that catalyze the oxidation or reduction of a substrate. Riboflavin deficiency is not associated with a major human disease, although it frequently accompanies other vitamin deficiencies. Deficiency symptoms include dermatitis, cheilosis (fissuring at the corners of the mouth), and glossitis (the tongue appearing smooth and purplish).

IX. BIOTIN

Biotin is a coenzyme in carboxylation reactions, in which it serves as a carrier of activated carbon dioxide (see Figure 10.3, p. 119, for the mechanism of biotin-dependent carboxylations). Biotin is covalently bound to the ε-amino groups of lysine residues in biotin-dependent enzymes (Figure 28.16). Biotin deficiency does not occur naturally because the vitamin is widely distributed in food. Also, a large percentage of the biotin requirement in humans is supplied by intestinal bacteria. However, the addition of raw egg white to the diet as a source of protein induces symptoms of biotin deficiency, namely, dermatitis, glossitis, loss of appetite, and nausea. Raw egg white contains a glycoprotein, avidin, which tightly binds biotin and prevents its absorption from the intestine. With a normal diet, however, it has been estimated that 20 eggs/day would be required to induce a deficiency syndrome. Thus, inclusion of an occasional raw egg in the diet does not lead to biotin deficiency, although eating raw eggs is generally not recommended due to the possibility of salmonella infection.

> Multiple *carboxylase* deficiency results from a defect in the ability to link biotin to *carboxylases* or to remove it from *carboxylases* during their degradation. Treatment is biotin supplementation.

X. PANTOTHENIC ACID

Pantothenic acid is a component of coenzyme A (CoA), which functions in the transfer of acyl groups (Figure 28.17). CoA contains a thiol group that carries acyl compounds as activated thiol esters. Examples of such structures are succinyl CoA, fatty acyl CoA, and acetyl CoA. Pantothenic acid is also a component of the acyl carrier protein (ACP) domain of *fatty acid synthase* (see p. 184). Eggs, liver, and yeast are the most important sources of pantothenic acid, although the vitamin is widely distributed. Pantothenic acid deficiency is not well characterized in humans, and no RDA has been established.

XI. VITAMIN A

The retinoids, a family of molecules that are related to retinol (vitamin A), are essential for vision, reproduction, growth, and maintenance of epithelial tissues. Retinoic acid, derived from oxidation of dietary retinol, mediates most of the actions of the retinoids, except for vision, which depends on retinal, the aldehyde derivative of retinol.

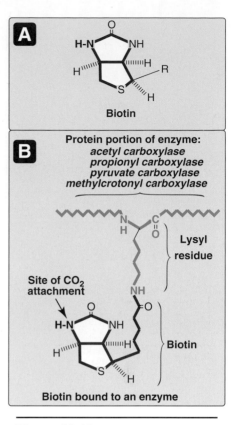

Figure 28.16
A. Structure of biotin. B. Biotin covalently bound to a lysyl residue of a biotin-dependent enzyme.

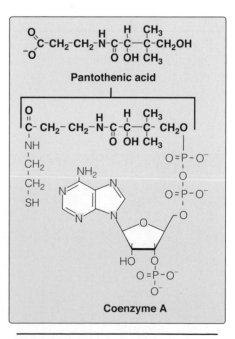

Figure 28.17
Structure of coenzyme A.

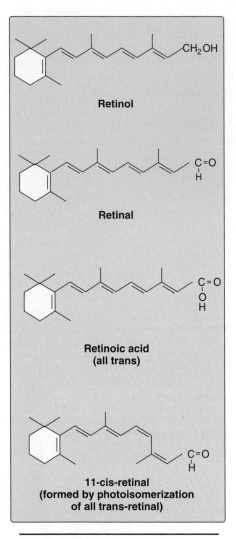

Figure 28.18
Structure of the retinoids.

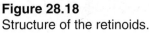

A. Structure of vitamin A

Vitamin A is often used as a collective term for several related biologically active molecules (Figure 28.18). The term retinoids includes both natural and synthetic forms of vitamin A that may or may not show vitamin A activity.

1. **Retinol:** A primary alcohol containing a β-ionone ring with an unsaturated side chain, retinol is found in animal tissues as a retinyl ester with long-chain fatty acids.

2. **Retinal:** This is the aldehyde derived from the oxidation of retinol. Retinal and retinol can readily be interconverted.

3. **Retinoic acid:** This is the acid derived from the oxidation of retinal. Retinoic acid cannot be reduced in the body, and, therefore, cannot give rise to either retinal or retinol.

4. **β-Carotene:** Plant foods contain β-carotene, which can be oxidatively cleaved in the intestine to yield two molecules of retinal. In humans, the conversion is inefficient, and the vitamin A activity of β-carotene is only about one twelfth that of retinol.

B. Absorption and transport of vitamin A

1. **Transport to the liver:** Retinyl esters present in the diet are hydrolyzed in the intestinal mucosa, releasing retinol and free fatty acids (Figure 28.19). Retinol derived from esters and from the cleavage and reduction of carotenes is re-esterified to long-chain fatty acids in the intestinal mucosa and secreted as a component of chylomicrons into the lymphatic system (see Figure 28.19). Retinyl esters contained in chylomicron remnants are taken up by, and stored in, the liver.

2. **Release from the liver:** When needed, retinol is released from the liver and transported to extrahepatic tissues by the plasma retinol-binding protein (RBP). The retinol–RBP complex attaches to specific receptors on the surface of the cells of peripheral tissues, permitting retinol to enter. Many tissues contain a cellular retinol-binding protein that carries retinol to sites in the nucleus where the vitamin acts in a manner analogous to that of steroid hormones.

C. Mechanism of action of vitamin A

Retinol is oxidized to retinoic acid. Retinoic acid binds with high affinity to specific receptor proteins present in the nucleus of target tissues, such as epithelial cells (Figure 28.20). The activated retinoic acid–receptor complex interacts with nuclear chromatin to regulate retinoid-specific RNA synthesis, resulting in control of the production of specific proteins that mediate several physiologic functions. For example, retinoids control the expression of the gene for keratin in most epithelial tissues of the body. The specific retinoic acid–receptor proteins are part of the superfamily of transcriptional regulators that includes the steroid and thyroid hormones and 1,25-dihydroxycholecalciferol, all of which function in a similar way (see p. 240).

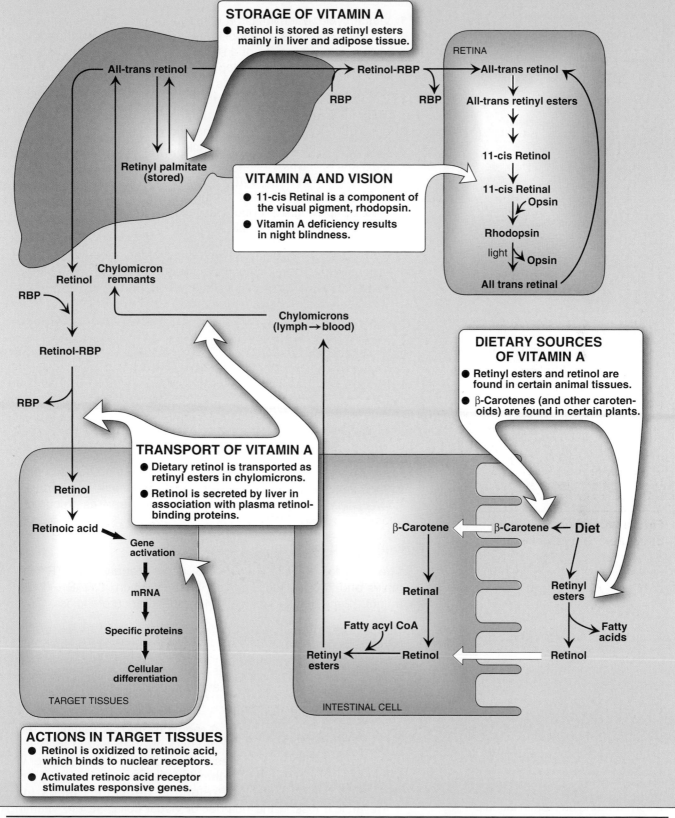

Figure 28.19
Absorption, transport, and storage of vitamin A and its derivatives. RBP = retinol-binding protein.

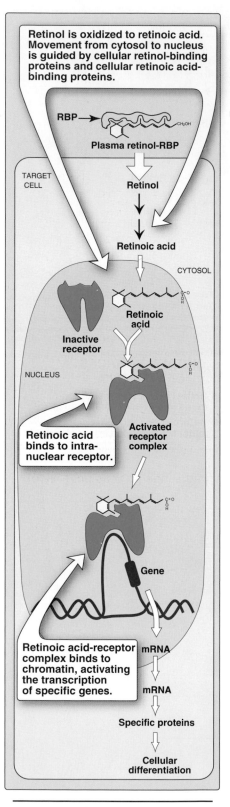

Figure 28.20
Action of retinoids Note: Retinoic acid-receptor complex is a dimer, but is shown as monomer for simplicity. [RBP = retinol-binding protein.]

D. Functions of vitamin A

1. **Visual cycle:** Vitamin A is a component of the visual pigments of rod and cone cells. Rhodopsin, the visual pigment of the rod cells in the retina, consists of 11-cis retinal specifically bound to the protein opsin. When rhodopsin is exposed to light, a series of photochemical isomerizations occurs, which results in the bleaching of the visual pigment and release of all-trans retinal and opsin. This process triggers a nerve impulse that is transmitted by the optic nerve to the brain. Regeneration of rhodopsin requires isomerization of all-trans retinal back to 11-cis retinal. All-trans retinal, after being released from rhodopsin, is reduced to all-trans retinol, esterfied, and isomerized to 11-cis retinol that is oxidized to 11-cis retinal. The latter combines with opsin to form rhodopsin, thus completing the cycle. Similar reactions are responsible for color vision in the cone cells.

2. **Growth:** Vitamin A deficiency results in a decreased growth rate in children. Bone development is also slowed.

3. **Reproduction:** Retinol and retinal are essential for normal reproduction, supporting spermatogenesis in the male and preventing fetal resorption in the female. Retinoic acid is inactive in maintaining reproduction and in the visual cycle, but promotes growth and differentiation of epithelial cells; thus, animals given vitamin A only as retinoic acid from birth are blind and sterile.

4. **Maintenance of epithelial cells:** Vitamin A is essential for normal differentiation of epithelial tissues and mucus secretion.

E. Distribution of vitamin A

Liver, kidney, cream, butter, and egg yolk are good sources of preformed vitamin A. Yellow and dark green vegetables and fruits are good dietary sources of the carotenes, which serve as precursors of vitamin A.

F. Requirement for vitamin A

The RDA for adults is 900 retinol activity equivalents (RAE) for males and 700 RAE for females. In comparison, 1 RAE = 1 mg of retinol, 12 mg of β-carotene, or 24 mg of other carotenoids.

G. Clinical indications

Although chemically related, retinoic acid and retinol have distinctly different therapeutic applications. Retinol and its precursor are used as dietary supplements, whereas various forms of retinoic acid are useful in dermatology.

1. **Dietary deficiency:** Vitamin A, administered as retinol or retinyl esters, is used to treat patients who are deficient in the vitamin (Figure 28.21). Night blindness is one of the earliest signs of vitamin A deficiency. The visual threshold is increased, making it difficult to see in dim light. Prolonged deficiency leads to an irreversible loss in the number of visual cells. Severe vitamin A deficiency leads to xerophthalmia, a pathologic dryness of the conjunctiva and cornea. If untreated, xerophthalmia results in

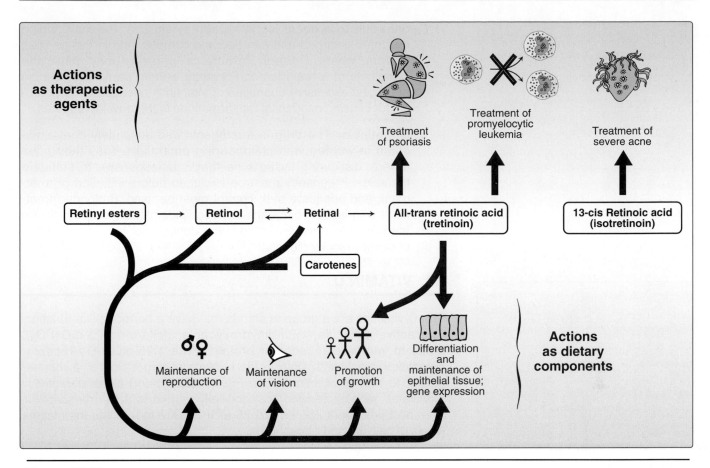

Figure 28.21
Summary of actions of retinoids. Compounds in boxes are available as dietary components or as pharmacologic agents.

corneal ulceration and, ultimately, in blindness because of the formation of opaque scar tissue. The condition is most frequently seen in children in developing tropical countries. Over 500,000 children worldwide are blinded each year by xerophthalmia caused by insufficient vitamin A in the diet.

2. **Acne and psoriasis:** Dermatologic problems such as acne and psoriasis are effectively treated with retinoic acid or its derivatives (see Figure 28.21). Mild cases of acne, Darier disease (keratosis follicularis), and skin aging are treated with topical application of tretinoin (all-trans retinoic acid), as well as benzoyl peroxide and antibiotics. [Note: Tretinoin is too toxic for systemic administration and is confined to topical application.] In patients with severe, recalcitrant, cystic acne unresponsive to conventional therapies, the drug of choice is isotretinoin (13-cis retinoic acid) administered orally. Retinoic acid is also used in the treatment of promyelocytic leukemia.

H. Toxicity of retinoids

1. **Vitamin A:** Excessive intake of vitamin A produces a toxic syndrome called hypervitaminosis A. Amounts exceeding 7.5 mg/day of retinol should be avoided. Early signs of chronic hypervitaminosis A are reflected in the skin, which becomes dry and pru-

ritic (due to a decrease in keratin synthesis), the liver, which becomes enlarged and can become cirrhotic, and in the nervous system, where a rise in intracranial pressure may mimic the symptoms of a brain tumor. Pregnant women particularly should not ingest excessive quantities of vitamin A because of its potential for causing congenital malformations in the developing fetus.

2. **Isotretinoin:** The drug is teratogenic and absolutely contraindicated in women with childbearing potential unless they have severe, disfiguring cystic acne that is unresponsive to standard therapies. Pregnancy must be excluded before initiation of treatment, and adequate birth control must be used. Prolonged treatment with isotretinoin leads to hyperlipidemia and an increase in the LDL/HDL ratio, providing some concern for an increased risk of cardiovascular disease.

XII. VITAMIN D

The D vitamins are a group of sterols that have a hormone-like function. The active molecule, 1,25-dihydroxycholecalciferol (1,25-diOH-D$_3$), binds to intracellular receptor proteins. The 1,25-diOH-D$_3$–receptor complex interacts with DNA in the nucleus of target cells in a manner similar to that of vitamin A (see Figure 28.20), and either selectively stimulates gene expression or specifically represses gene transcription. The most prominent actions of 1,25-diOH-D$_3$ are to regulate the plasma levels of calcium and phosphorus.

A. Distribution of vitamin D

1. **Diet:** Ergocalciferol (vitamin D$_2$), found in plants, and cholecalciferol (vitamin D$_3$), found in animal tissues, are sources of preformed vitamin D activity (Figure 28.22). Ergocalciferol and cholecalciferol differ chemically only in the presence of an additional double bond and methyl group in the plant sterol.

2. **Endogenous vitamin precursor:** 7-Dehydrocholesterol, an intermediate in cholesterol synthesis, is converted to cholecalciferol in the dermis and epidermis of humans exposed to sunlight. Preformed vitamin D is a dietary requirement only in individuals with limited exposure to sunlight.

B. Metabolism of vitamin D

1. **Formation of 1,25-diOH-D$_3$:** Vitamins D$_2$ and D$_3$ are not biologically active, but are converted in vivo to the active form of the D vitamin by two sequential hydroxylation reactions (Figure 28.23). The first hydroxylation occurs at the 25-position, and is catalyzed by a specific *hydroxylase* in the liver. The product of the reaction, 25-hydroxycholecalciferol (25-OH-D$_3$, calcidol), is the predominant form of vitamin D in the plasma and the major storage form of the vitamin. 25-OH-D$_3$ is further hydroxylated at the 1 position by *25-hydroxycholecalciferol 1-hydroxylase* found primarily in the kidney, resulting in the formation of 1,25-diOH-D$_3$ (calcitriol). [Note: This *hydroxylase*, as well as the liver *25-hydroxylase*, are cytochrome P450 (CYP) proteins (see p. 149).]

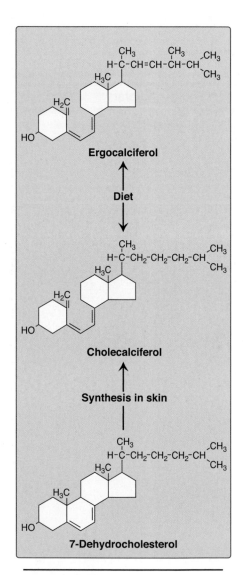

Figure 28.22
Sources of vitamin D.

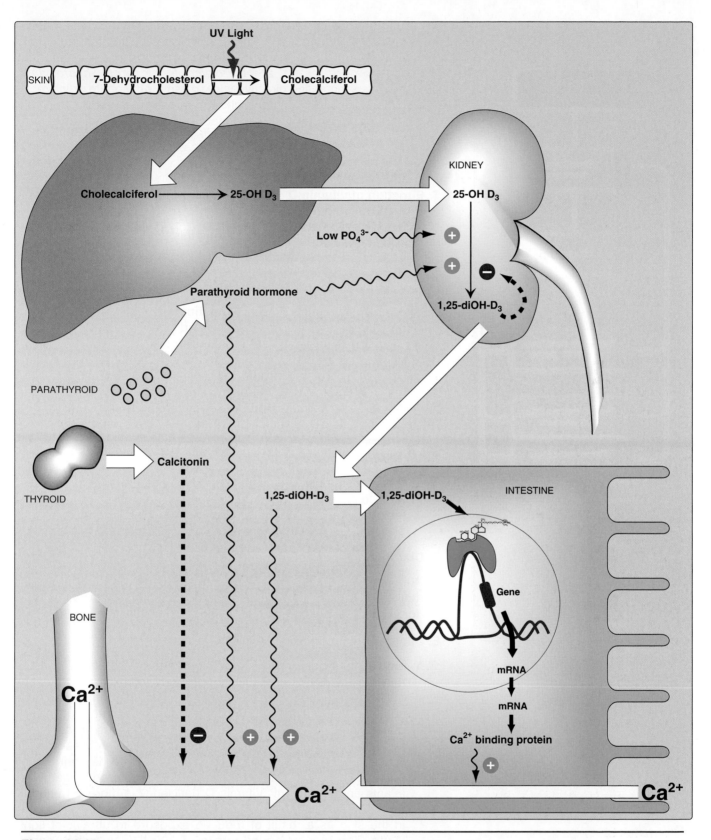

Figure 28.23
Metabolism and actions of vitamin D. [Note: Calcitonin, a thyroid hormone, decreases blood calcium by inhibiting mobilization from bone and reabsorption by the kidney.]

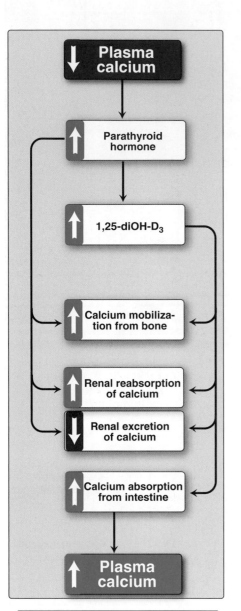

Figure 28.24
Response to low plasma calcium.

2. **Regulation of 25-hydroxycholecalciferol 1-hydroxylase:** 1,25-diOH-D$_3$ is the most potent vitamin D metabolite. Its formation is tightly regulated by the level of plasma phosphate and calcium ions (Figure 28.24). *25-Hydroxycholecalciferol 1-hydroxylase* activity is increased directly by low plasma phosphate or indirectly by low plasma calcium, which triggers the release of parathyroid hormone (PTH). Hypocalcemia caused by insufficient dietary calcium thus results in elevated levels of plasma 1,25-diOH-D$_3$. *1-Hydroxylase* activity is also decreased by excess 1,25-diOH-D$_3$, the product of the reaction.

C. Function of vitamin D

The overall function of 1,25-diOH-D$_3$ is to maintain adequate plasma levels of calcium. It performs this function by: 1) increasing uptake of calcium by the intestine, 2) minimizing loss of calcium by the kidney, and 3) stimulating resorption of bone when necessary (see Figure 28.23).

1. **Effect of vitamin D on the intestine:** 1,25-diOH-D$_3$ stimulates intestinal absorption of calcium and phosphate. 1,25-diOH-D$_3$ enters the intestinal cell and binds to a cytosolic receptor. The 1,25-diOH-D$_3$–receptor complex then moves to the nucleus where it selectively interacts with the cellular DNA. As a result, calcium uptake is enhanced by an increased synthesis of a specific calcium-binding protein. Thus, the mechanism of action of 1,25-diOH-D$_3$ is typical of steroid hormones (see p. 240).

2. **Effect of vitamin D on bone:** 1,25-diOH-D$_3$ stimulates the mobilization of calcium and phosphate from bone by a process that requires protein synthesis and the presence of PTH. The result is an increase in plasma calcium and phosphate. Thus, bone is an important reservoir of calcium that can be mobilized to maintain plasma levels.

D. Distribution and requirement of vitamin D

Vitamin D occurs naturally in fatty fish, liver, and egg yolk. Milk, unless it is artificially fortified, is not a good source of the vitamin. AI for vitamin D is 200 IU to age 50, and 400-600 IU after age 50.

E. Clinical indications

1. **Nutritional rickets:** Vitamin D deficiency causes a net demineralization of bone, resulting in rickets in children and osteomalacia in adults (Figure 28.25). Rickets is characterized by the continued formation of the collagen matrix of bone, but incomplete mineralization, resulting in soft, pliable bones. In osteomalacia, demineralization of pre-existing bones increases their susceptibility to fracture. Insufficient exposure to daylight and/or deficiencies in vitamin D consumption occur predominantly in infants and the elderly. Vitamin D deficiency is more common in the northern latitudes, because less vitamin D synthesis occurs in the skin as a result of reduced exposure to ultraviolet light. [Note: The recommended intake of 200 IU/day (which corresponds to 5 μg of cholecalciferol) may be insufficient, because higher doses of 800 IU/day have been shown to reduce the inci-

dence of osteoporotic fractures.] Sufficient levels of serum 25-hydroxycholecalciferol (>75 nmol/L) have been linked to fall prevention in older people as well as to increased muscle strength and bone mass.

2. **Renal osteodystrophy:** Chronic renal failure results in decreased ability to form the active form of vitamin D. Supplementation with calcitriol is an effective therapy. [Note: Vitamin D supplementation is accompanied by phosphate reduction therapy to prevent hyperphosphatemia (due to renal failure) and precipitation of calcium phosphate crystals.]

3. **Hypoparathyroidism:** Lack of parathyroid hormone causes hypocalcemia and hyperphosphatemia. These patients may be treated with calcitriol and calcium supplementation.

F. Toxicity of vitamin D

Like all fat-soluble vitamins, vitamin D can be stored in the body and is only slowly metabolized. High doses (100,000 IU for weeks or months) can cause loss of appetite, nausea, thirst, and stupor. Enhanced calcium absorption and bone resorption results in hypercalcemia, which can lead to deposition of calcium in many organs, particularly the arteries and kidneys. The UL is 2000 IU/day.

XIII. VITAMIN K

The principal role of vitamin K is in the posttranslational modification of various blood clotting factors, in which it serves as a coenzyme in the carboxylation of certain glutamic acid residues present in these proteins. Vitamin K exists in several forms, for example, in plants as phylloquinone (or vitamin K_1), and in intestinal bacterial flora as menaquinone (or vitamin K_2). A synthetic form of vitamin K, menadione, is available.

A. Function of vitamin K

1. **Formation of γ-carboxyglutamate (Gla):** Vitamin K is required in the hepatic synthesis of prothrombin and blood clotting factors II, VII, IX, and X. These proteins are synthesized as inactive precursor molecules. Formation of the clotting factors requires the vitamin K–dependent carboxylation of glutamic acid residues to Gla residues (Figure 28.26). This forms a mature clotting factor that contains Gla and is capable of subsequent activation. The reaction requires O_2, CO_2, and the hydroquinone form of vitamin K. The formation of Gla is sensitive to inhibition by dicumarol, an anticoagulant occurring naturally in spoiled sweet clover, and by warfarin, a synthetic analog of vitamin K.

2. **Interaction of prothrombin with platelets:** The Gla residues of prothrombin are good chelators of positively charged calcium ions, because of the two adjacent, negatively charged carboxylate groups. The prothrombin–calcium complex is then able to bind to phospholipids essential for blood clotting on the surface of platelets. Attachment to the platelet increases the rate at which the proteolytic conversion of prothrombin to thrombin can occur (Figure 28.27).

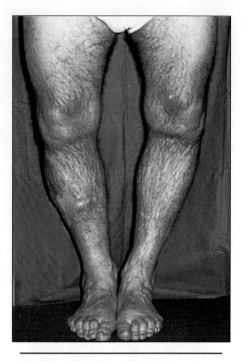

Figure 28.25
Bowed legs of middle-aged man with osteomalacia, a nutritional vitamin D deficiency that results in malformation of the skeleton.

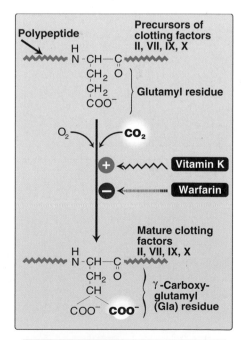

Figure 28.26
Carboxylation of glutamate to form γ-carboxyglutamate (Gla).

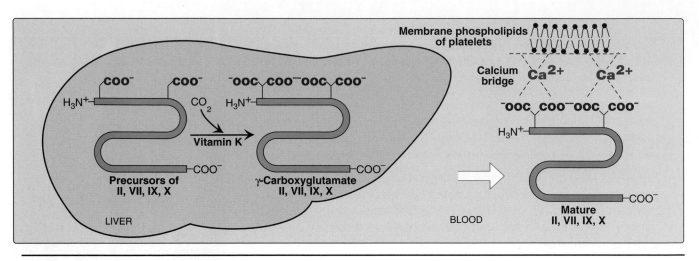

Figure 28.27
Role of vitamin K in blood coagulation.

3. **Role of Gla residues in other proteins:** Gla is also present in other proteins (for example, osteocalcin of bone, and in proteins such as protein C involved in limiting the formation of blood clots).

B. Distribution and requirement of vitamin K

Vitamin K is found in cabbage, kale, spinach, egg yolk, and liver. There is also extensive synthesis of the vitamin by the bacteria in the gut. AI for vitamin K is 120 μg/day for adult males and 90 μg for adult females.

C. Clinical indications

1. **Deficiency of vitamin K:** A true vitamin K deficiency is unusual because adequate amounts are generally produced by intestinal bacteria or obtained from the diet. If the bacterial population in the gut is decreased, for example, by antibiotics, the amount of endogenously formed vitamin is depressed, and this can lead to hypoprothrombinemia in the marginally malnourished individual, for example, a debilitated geriatric patient. This condition may require supplementation with vitamin K to correct the bleeding tendency. In addition, certain second-generation cephalosporins, for example, cefoperazone, cefamandole, and moxalactam cause hypoprothrombinemia, apparently by a warfarin-like mechanism. Consequently, their use in treatment is usually supplemented with vitamin K.

2. **Deficiency of vitamin K in the newborn:** Newborns have sterile intestines and so initially lack the bacteria that synthesize vitamin K. Because human milk provides only about one fifth of the daily requirement for vitamin K, it is recommended that all newborns receive a single intramuscular dose of vitamin K as prophylaxis against hemorrhagic disease.

D. Toxicity of vitamin K

Prolonged administration of large doses of synthetic vitamin K (menadione) can produce hemolytic anemia and jaundice in the infant, due to toxic effects on the membrane of red blood cells; therefore, it is no longer used to treat vitamin K deficiency. No UL has been set for vitamin K.

XIV. VITAMIN E

The E vitamins consist of eight naturally occurring tocopherols, of which α-tocopherol is the most active (Figure 28.28). The primary function of vitamin E is as an antioxidant in prevention of the nonenzymic oxidation of cell components, for example, polyunsaturated fatty acids, by molecular oxygen and free radicals.

A. Distribution and requirements of vitamin E

Vegetable oils are rich sources of vitamin E, whereas liver and eggs contain moderate amounts. The RDA for α-tocopherol is 15 mg for adults. The vitamin E requirement increases as the intake of polyunsaturated fatty acid increases.

B. Deficiency of vitamin E

Vitamin E deficiency is almost entirely restricted to premature infants. When observed in adults, it is usually associated with defective lipid absorption or transport. The signs of human vitamin E deficiency include sensitivity of erythrocytes to peroxide, and the appearance of abnormal cellular membranes.

C. Clinical indications

Vitamin E is not recommended for the prevention of chronic disease, such as coronary heart disease or cancer. Clinical trials using vitamin E supplementation have been uniformly disappointing. For example, subjects in the Alpha-Tocopherol, Beta-Carotene Cancer Prevention Study trial who received high doses of vitamin E not only lacked cardiovascular benefit but also had an increased incidence of stroke.

D. Toxicity of vitamin E

Vitamin E is the least toxic of the fat-soluble vitamins, and no toxicity has been observed at doses of 300 mg/day.

> Populations consuming diets high in fruits and vegetables show decreased incidence of some chronic diseases. However, clinical trials have failed to show a definitive benefit from supplements of vitamins A, C, or E; multivitamins with folic acid; or antioxidant combinations for the prevention of cancer or cardiovascular disease.

The vitamins are summarized in Figure 28.29.

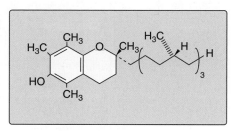

Figure 28.28
Structure of vitamin E.

VITAMIN	OTHER NAMES	ACTIVE FORM	FUNCTION
Folic acid	—	Tetrahydro-folic acid	Transfer one-carbon units; Synthesis of methionine, purines, and thymidine monophosphate
Vitamin B$_{12}$	Cobalamin	Methylcobalamin Deoxyadenosyl cobalamin	Coenzyme for reactions: Homocysteine $\rightarrow$ methionine Methylmalonyl CoA $\rightarrow$ succinyl CoA
Vitamin C	Ascorbic acid	Ascorbic acid	Antioxidant Coenzyme for hydroxylation reactions, for example: In procollagen: Proline $\rightarrow$ hydroxyproline Lysine $\rightarrow$ hydroxylysine
Vitamin B$_6$	Pridoxine Pyridoxamine Pyridoxal	Pyridoxal phosphate	Coenzyme for enzymes, particularly in amino acid metabolism
Vitamin B$_1$	Thiamine	Thiamine pyrophosphate	Coenzyme of enzymes catalyzing: Pyruvate $\rightarrow$ acetyl CoA α-Ketoglutarate $\rightarrow$ Succinyl CoA Ribose 5-P + xylulose 5-P $\rightarrow$ Sedoheptulose 7-P + Glyceraldehyde 3-P Branched-chain amino acid oxidation
Niacin	Nicotinic acid Nicotinamide	NAD$^+$, NADP$^+$	Electron transfer
Vitamin B$_2$	Riboflavin	FMN, FAD	Electron transfer
Biotin	—	Enzyme-bound biotin	Carboxylation reactions
Pantothenic acid	—	Coenzyme A	Acyl carrier

WATER-SOLUBLE

FAT-SOLUBLE

VITAMIN	OTHER NAMES	ACTIVE FORM	FUNCTION
Vitamin A	Retinol Retinal Retinoic acid β-Carotene	Retinol Retinal Retinoic acid	Maintenance of reproduction Vision Promotion of growth Differentiation and maintenance of epithelial tissues Gene expression
Vitamin D	Cholecalciferol Ergocalciferol	1,25-Dihydroxy-cholecalciferol	Calcium uptake
Vitamin K	Menadione Menaquinone Phylloquinone	Menadione Menaquinone Phylloquinon	γ-Carboxylation of glutamate residue in clotting and other proteins
Vitamin E	α-Tocopherol	Any of several tocopherol derivatives	Antioxidant

Figure 28.29 (continued on next page)
Summary of vitamins.

DEFICIENCY	SIGNS AND SYMPTOMS	TOXICITY	NOTES
Megaloblastic anemia Neural tube defects	Anemia Birth defects	None	Administration of high levels of folate can mask vitamin B_{12} deficiency
Pernicious anemia Dementia Spinal degeneration	Megaloblastic anemia Neuropsychiatric symptoms	None	Pernicious anemia is treated with IM or high-dose oral vitamin B_{12}
Scurvy	Sore, spongy gums Loose teeth Poor wound healing	None	Benefits of supplementation not established in controlled trials
Rare	Glossitis Neuropathy	Yes	Deficiency can be induced by isoniazid Sensory neuropathy occurs at high doses
Beriberi Wernicke-Korsakoff syndrome (most common in alcoholics)	Tachycardia, vomiting, convulsions Apathy, loss of memory, eye movements	None	—
Pellagra	Dermatitis Diarrhea Dementia	None	High doses of niacin used to treat hyperlipidemia
Rare	Dermatitis Angular stomatitis	None	—
Rare	—	None	Consumption of large amounts of raw egg whites (which contains a protein, avidin, that binds biotin) can induce a biotin deficiency
Rare	—	None	—
			WATER-SOLUBLE
			FAT-SOLUBLE
infertility Night blindness Retardation of growth Xerophthalmia	Increased visual threshold Dryness of cornea	Yes	β-Carotene not acutely toxic, but supplementation is not recommended Excess vitamin A can increase incidence of fractures
Rickets (in children) Osteomalacia (in adults)	Soft, pliable bones	Yes	Vitamin D is not a true vitamin because it can be synthesized in skin. Application of sunscreen lotions or presence of dark skin color decreases this synthesis.
Newborn Rare in adults	Bleeding	Rare	Vitamin K produced by intestinal bacteria. Vitamin K deficiency common in newborns Intramuscular treatment with vitamin K is recommended at birth
Rare	Red blood cell fragility leads to hemolytic anemia	None	Benefits of supplementation not established in controlled trials

Figure 28.29 (continued from previous page)
Summary of vitamins.

Study Questions

Choose the ONE correct answer.

28.1 Which one of the following statements concerning vitamin B$_{12}$ is correct?

A. The cofactor form is vitamin B$_{12}$ itself.

B. It is involved in the transfer of amino groups.

C. It requires a specific glycoprotein for its absorption.

D. It is present in plant products.

E. Its deficiency is most often caused by a lack of the vitamin in the diet.

> Correct answer = C. Vitamin B$_{12}$ requires intrinsic factor for its absorption. A deficiency of vitamin B$_{12}$ is most often caused by a lack of intrinsic factor. However, high does of the vitamin, given orally, are sufficiently absorbed to serve as treatment for pernicious anemia. The cofactor forms are methylcobalamin and deoxyadenosylcobalamin. Vitamin B$_6$, not vitamin B$_{12}$, is involved in the transfer of amino groups. B$_{12}$ is found in food derived from animal sources.

28.2 Retinol:

A. can be enzymically formed from retinoic acid.

B. in its ester form is transported from the intestine to the liver in chylomicrons.

C. is the light-absorbing portion of rhodopsin.

D. is phosphorylated and dephosphorylated during the visual cycle.

E. mediates most of the actions of the retinoids.

> Correct answer = B. Retinyl esters are incorporated into chylomicrons. Retinoic acid cannot be reduced to retinol. Retinal, the aldehyde form of retinol, is the chromophore for rhodopsin. Retinal is photoisomerized during the visual cycle. Retinoic acid, not retinol, is the most important retinoid.

28.3 Which one of the following statements concerning vitamin D is correct?

A. Chronic renal failure requires the oral administration of 1,25-dihydroxycholecalciferol.

B. It is required in the diet of individuals exposed to sunlight.

C. 25-Hydroxycholecalciferol is the active form of the vitamin.

D. Vitamin D opposes the effect of parathyroid hormone.

E. A deficiency in vitamin D results in an increased secretion of calcitonin.

> Correct answer = A. Renal failure results in the decreased ability to form the active form of the vitamin, which must be supplied. The vitamin is not required in individuals exposed to sunlight. 1,25-Dihydroxycholecalciferol is the active form of the vitamin. Vitamin D and parathyroid hormone both increase serum calcium. A deficiency of vitamin D decreases the secretion of calcitonin.

28.4 Vitamin K:

A. plays an essential role in preventing thrombosis.

B. increases the coagulation time in newborn infants with hemorrhagic disease.

C. is present in high concentration in cow or breast milk.

D. is synthesized by intestinal bacteria.

E. is a water-soluble vitamin.

> Correct answer = D. Vitamin K is essential for clot formation, decreases coagulation time, and is present in low concentrations in milk. It is one of four fat-soluble vitamins.

28.5 Deficiency of which vitamin results in: beri-beri; scurvy; pellagra; night blindness; rickets or osteomalacia; pernicious anemia; megaloblastic anemia; bleeding?

> Thiamin; vitamin C; niacin; vitamin A, vitamin D; vitamin B12 (due primarily to a deficiency of intrinsic factor), both B12 and folate; vitamin K.

Storage and Expression of Genetic Information

DNA Structure, Replication, and Repair

29

I. OVERVIEW

Nucleic acids are required for the storage and expression of genetic information. There are two chemically distinct types of nucleic acids: deoxyribonucleic acid (DNA) and ribonucleic acid (RNA, see Chapter 30). DNA, the repository of genetic information, is present not only in chromosomes in the nucleus of eukaryotic organisms, but also in mitochondria and the chloroplasts of plants. Prokaryotic cells, which lack nuclei, have a single chromosome, but may also contain nonchromosomal DNA in the form of plasmids. The genetic information found in DNA is copied and transmitted to daughter cells through DNA replication. The DNA contained in a fertilized egg encodes the information that directs the development of an organism. This development may involve the production of billions of cells. Each cell is specialized, expressing only those functions that are required for it to perform its role in maintaining the organism. Therefore, DNA must be able to not only replicate precisely each time a cell divides, but also to have the information that it contains be selectively expressed. Transcription (RNA synthesis) is the first stage in the expression of genetic information (see Chapter 30). Next, the code contained in the nucleotide sequence of messenger RNA molecules is translated (protein synthesis, see Chapter 31), thus completing gene expression. The regulation of gene expression is discussed in Chapter 32.

> The flow of information from DNA to RNA to protein is termed the "central dogma" of molecular biology (Figure 29.1), and is descriptive of all organisms, with the exception of some viruses that have RNA as the repository of their genetic information.

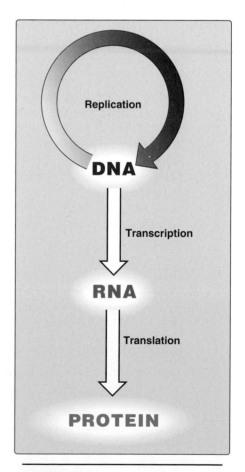

Figure 29.1
The "central dogma" of molecular biology.

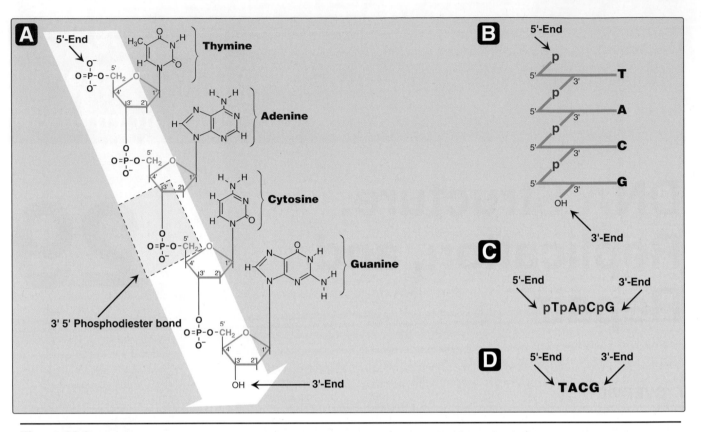

Figure 29.2
A. DNA chain with the nucleotide sequence shown written in the 5'→ 3' direction. A 3' →5'-phosphodiester bond is shown highlighted in the blue box, and the deoxyribose-phosphate backbone is shaded in yellow.
B. The DNA chain written in a more stylized form, emphasizing the ribose–phosphate backbone.
C. A simpler representation of the nucleotide sequence. D. The simplest (and most common) representation, with the abbreviations for the bases written in the conventional 5'→3' direction.

II. STRUCTURE OF DNA

DNA is a polymer of deoxyribonucleoside monophosphates covalently linked by 3'→5'–phosphodiester bonds. With the exception of a few viruses that contain single-stranded (ss) DNA, DNA exists as a double-stranded (ds) molecule, in which the two strands wind around each other, forming a double helix. In eukaryotic cells, DNA is found associated with various types of proteins (known collectively as nucleoprotein) present in the nucleus, whereas in prokaryotes, the protein–DNA complex is present in a nonmembrane-bound region known as the nucleoid.

A. 3'→5'-Phosphodiester bonds

Phosphodiester bonds join the 3'-hydroxyl group of the deoxypentose of one nucleotide to the 5'-hydroxyl group of the deoxypentose of an adjacent nucleotide through a phosphate group (Figure 29.2). The resulting long, unbranched chain has polarity, with both a 5'-end (the end with the free phosphate) and a 3'-end (the end with the free hydroxyl) that are not attached to other nucleotides. The bases located along the resulting deoxyribose–phosphate backbone are, by convention, always written in sequence from the 5'-end of the chain to the 3'-end. For example, the sequence of bases in the DNA shown in Figure 29.2 is read "thymine, adenine, cytosine, guanine" (5'-TACG-3'). Phosphodiester linkages between nucleotides (in DNA or RNA) can be cleaved hydrolytically by chemicals, or hydrolyzed enzymatically by a family of *nucleases*: *deoxyribonucleases* for DNA and *ribonucleases* for RNA. [Note: Only RNA is cleaved by alkali.]

B. Double helix

In the double helix, the two chains are coiled around a common axis called the axis of symmetry. The chains are paired in an antiparallel manner, that is, the 5'-end of one strand is paired with the 3'-end of the other strand (Figure 29.3). In the DNA helix, the hydrophilic deoxyribose–phosphate backbone of each chain is on the outside of the molecule, whereas the hydrophobic bases are stacked inside. The overall structure resembles a twisted ladder. The spatial relationship between the two strands in the helix creates a major (wide) groove and a minor (narrow) groove. These grooves provide access for the binding of regulatory proteins to their specific recognition sequences along the DNA chain. Certain anticancer drugs, such as dactinomycin (actinomycin D), exert their cytotoxic effect by intercalating into the narrow groove of the DNA double helix, thus interfering with DNA and RNA synthesis.[1]

1. **Base pairing:** The bases of one strand of DNA are paired with the bases of the second strand, so that an adenine is always paired with a thymine and a cytosine is always paired with a guanine. [Note: The base pairs are perpendicular to the axis of the helix (see Figure 29.3).] Therefore, one polynucleotide chain of the DNA double helix is always the complement of the other. Given the sequence of bases on one chain, the sequence of bases on the complementary chain can be determined (Figure 29.4). [Note: The specific base pairing in DNA leads to the Chargaff Rule: In any sample of dsDNA, the amount of adenine equals the amount of thymine, the amount of guanine equals the amount of cytosine, and the total amount of purines equals the total amount of pyrimidines.] The base pairs are held together by hydrogen bonds: two between A and T and three between G and C (Figure 29.5). These hydrogen bonds, plus the hydrophobic interactions between the stacked bases, stabilize the structure of the double helix.

2. **Separation of the two DNA strands in the double helix:** The two strands of the double helix separate when hydrogen bonds between the paired bases are disrupted. Disruption can occur in the laboratory if the pH of the DNA solution is altered so that the nucleotide bases ionize, or if the solution is heated. [Note: Phosphodiester bonds are not broken by such treatment.] When DNA is heated, the temperature at which one half of the helical structure is lost is defined as the melting temperature (T_m). The loss of helical structure in DNA, called denaturation, can be monitored by measuring its absorbance at 260 nm. [Note: ssDNA has a higher relative absorbance at this wavelength than does dsDNA.] Because there are three hydrogen bonds between G and C but

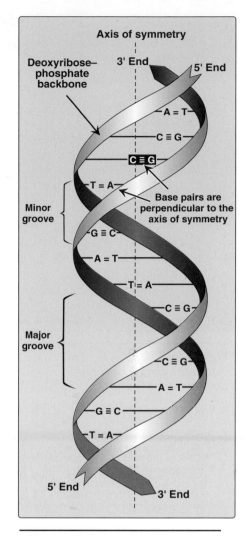

Figure 29.3
DNA double helix, illustrating some of its major structural features.

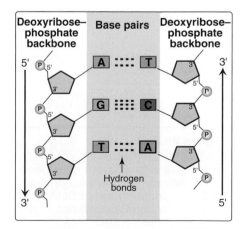

Figure 29.4
Two complementary DNA sequences.

[1]See Chapter 39 in *Lippincott's Illustrated Reviews: Pharmacology* for a discussion of the anticancer drug, actinomycin D.

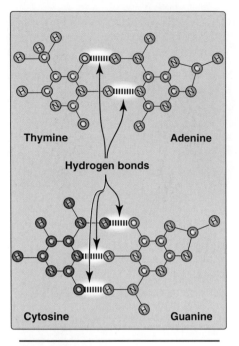

Figure 29.5
Hydrogen bonds between
complementary bases.

only two between A and T, DNA that contains high concentrations of A and T denatures at a lower temperature than G- and C-rich DNA (Figure 29.6). Under appropriate conditions, complementary DNA strands can reform the double helix by the process called renaturation (or reannealing).

3. **Structural forms of the double helix:** There are three major structural forms of DNA: the B form, described by Watson and Crick in 1953, the A form, and the Z form. The B form is a right-handed helix with ten residues per 360° turn of the helix, and with the planes of the bases perpendicular to the helical axis. Chromosomal DNA is thought to consist primarily of B-DNA (Figure 29.7 illustrates a space-filling model of B-DNA). The A form is produced by moderately dehydrating the B form. It is also a right-handed helix, but there are 11 base pairs per turn, and the planes of the base pairs are tilted 20° away from the perpendicular to the helical axis. The conformation found in DNA–RNA hybrids or RNA–RNA double-stranded regions is probably very close to the A form. Z-DNA is a left-handed helix that contains about 12 base pairs per turn (see Figure 29.7). [Note: The deoxyribose–phosphate backbone "zigzags," hence, the name "Z"-DNA.] Stretches of Z-DNA can occur naturally in regions of DNA that have a sequence of alternating purines and pyrimidines, for example, poly GC. Transitions between the B and Z helical forms of DNA may play a role in regulating gene expression.

C. Linear and circular DNA molecules

Each chromosome in the nucleus of a eukaryote contains one long, linear molecule of dsDNA, which is bound to a complex mixture of proteins (histone and non-histone, see p. 409) to form chromatin. Eukaryotes have closed, circular DNA molecules in their mitochondria, as do plant chloroplasts. A prokaryotic organism typically contains a single, double-stranded, supercoiled, circular chromosome. Each prokaryotic chromosome is associated with non-histone proteins that can condense the DNA to form a nucleoid. In addition, most species of bacteria also contain small, circular, extrachromosomal DNA molecules called plasmids. Plasmid DNA carries genetic information, and undergoes replication that may or may not be synchronized to chromosomal division.[2]

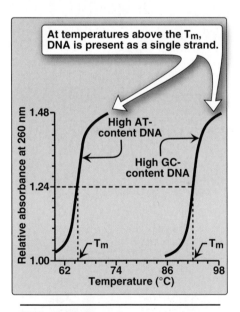

Figure 29.6
Melting temperatures (T_m) of DNA molecules with different nucleotide compositions. (At a wavelength of 260 nm, single-stranded DNA has a higher relative absorbance than does double-stranded DNA.)

> Plasmids may carry genes that convey antibiotic resistance to the host bacterium, and may facilitate the transfer of genetic information from one bacterium to another.

[Note: The use of plasmids as vectors in recombinant DNA technology is described in Chapter 33.]

 [2]See Chapter 7 in *Lippincott's Illustrated Reviews: Microbiology* for a discussion of plasmids.

III. STEPS IN PROKARYOTIC DNA SYNTHESIS

When the two strands of the DNA double helix are separated, each can serve as a template for the replication of a new complementary strand. This produces two daughter molecules, each of which contains two DNA strands with an antiparallel orientation (see Figure 29.3). This process is called semiconservative replication because, although the parental duplex is separated into two halves (and, therefore, is not "conserved" as an entity), each of the individual parental strands remains intact in one of the two new duplexes (Figure 29.8). The enzymes involved in the DNA replication process are template-directed *polymerases* that can synthesize the complementary sequence of each strand with extraordinary fidelity. The reactions described in this section were first known from studies of the bacterium <u>Escherichia</u> <u>coli</u> (<u>E. coli</u>), and the description given below refers to the process in prokaryotes. DNA synthesis in higher organisms is less well understood, but involves the same types of mechanisms. In either case, initiation of DNA replication commits the cell to continue the process until the entire genome has been replicated.

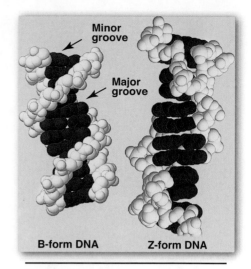

Figure 29.7
Structures of B-DNA and Z-DNA.

A. Separation of the two complementary DNA strands

In order for the two strands of the parental double helical DNA to be replicated, they must first separate (or "melt") over a small region, because the *polymerases* use only ssDNA as a template. In prokaryotic organisms, DNA replication begins at a single, unique nucleotide sequence—a site called the origin of replication (Figure 29.9A). [Note: This is referred to as a consensus sequence, because the order of nucleotides is essentially the same at each site.] This site includes a short sequence composed almost exclusively of AT base pairs that facilitate melting. In eukaryotes, replication begins at multiple sites along the DNA helix (Figure 29.9B). Having multiple origins of replication provides a mechanism for rapidly replicating the great length of the eukaryotic DNA molecules.

B. Formation of the replication fork

As the two strands unwind and separate, they form a "V" where active synthesis occurs. This region is called the replication fork. It moves along the DNA molecule as synthesis occurs. Replication of dsDNA is bidirectional—that is, the replication forks move in opposite directions from the origin, generating a replication bubble (see Figure 29.9).

1. **Proteins required for DNA strand separation:** Initiation of DNA replication requires the recognition of the origin of replication by a group of proteins that form the prepriming complex. These proteins are responsible for maintaining the separation of the parental strands, and for unwinding the double helix ahead of the advancing replication fork. These proteins include the following:

   a. **DnaA protein:** *DnaA* protein binds to specific nucleotide sequences at the origin of replication, causing short, tandemly arranged (one after the other) AT-rich regions in the origin to melt. Melting is ATP-dependent, and results in strand separation with the formation of localized regions of ssDNA.

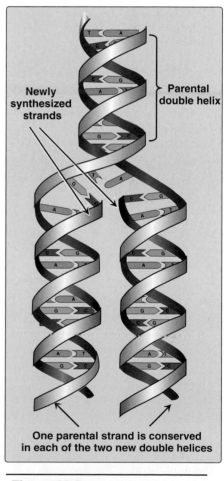

Figure 29.8
Semiconservative replication of DNA.

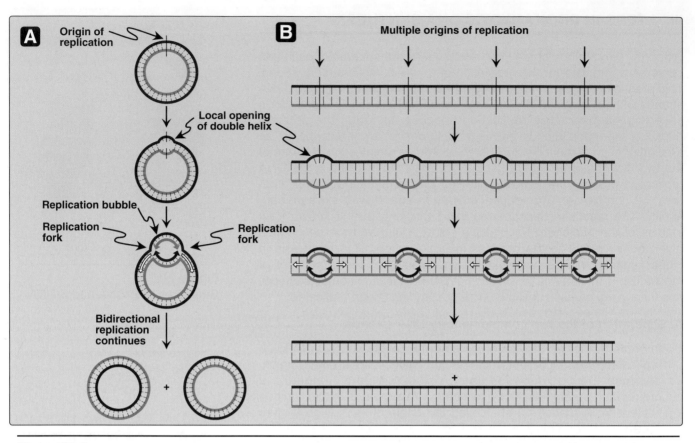

Figure 29.9
Replication of DNA: origins and replication forks. A. Small prokaryotic circular DNA. B. Very long eukaryotic DNA.

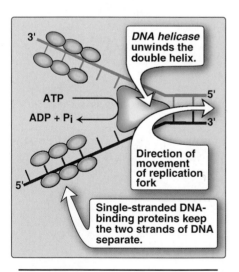

Figure 29.10
Proteins responsible for maintaining the separation of the parental strands and unwinding the double helix ahead of the advancing replication fork.

b. **DNA helicases:** These enzymes bind to ssDNA near the replication fork, and then move into the neighboring double-stranded region, forcing the strands apart—in effect, unwinding the double helix. *Helicases* require energy provided by ATP (Figure 29.10). [Note: *DnaB* is the principal *helicase* of replication in E. coli. Its binding to DNA requires *DnaC*.]

c. **Single-stranded DNA-binding (SSB) proteins:** These proteins bind to the ssDNA generated by *helicases* (see Figure 29.10). They bind cooperatively—that is, the binding of one molecule of SSB protein makes it easier for additional molecules of SSB protein to bind tightly to the DNA strand. The SSB proteins are not enzymes, but rather serve to shift the equilibrium between dsDNA and ssDNA in the direction of the single-stranded forms. These proteins not only keep the two strands of DNA separated in the area of the replication origin, thus providing the single-stranded template required by *polymerases*, but also protect the DNA from *nucleases* that degrade ssDNA.

2. **Solving the problem of supercoils:** As the two strands of the double helix are separated, a problem is encountered, namely, the appearance of positive supercoils (also called supertwists) in the region of DNA ahead of the replication fork (Figure 29.11). The

accumulating positive supercoils interfere with further unwinding of the double helix. [Note: Supercoiling can be demonstrated by tightly grasping one end of a helical telephone cord while twisting the other end. If the cord is twisted in the direction of tightening the coils, the cord will wrap around itself in space to form positive supercoils. If the cord is twisted in the direction of loosening the coils, the cord will wrap around itself in the opposite direction to form negative supercoils.] To solve this problem, there is a group of enzymes called *DNA topoisomerases*, which are responsible for removing supercoils in the helix.

a. **Type I DNA topoisomerases:** These enzymes reversibly cut one strand of the double helix. They have both *nuclease* (strand-cutting) and *ligase* (strand-resealing) activities. They do not require ATP, but rather appear to store the energy from the phosphodiester bond they cleave, reusing the energy to reseal the strand (Figure 29.12). Each time a transient "nick" is created in one DNA strand, the intact DNA strand is passed through the break before it is resealed, thus relieving ("relaxing") accumulated supercoils. *Type I topoisomerases* relax negative supercoils (that is, those that contain fewer turns of the helix than relaxed DNA) in E. coli, and both negative and positive supercoils (that is, those that contain fewer or more turns of the helix than relaxed DNA) in eukaryotic cells.

b. **Type II DNA topoisomerases:** These enzymes bind tightly to the DNA double helix and make transient breaks in both strands. The enzyme then causes a second stretch of the DNA double helix to pass through the break and, finally, reseals the break (Figure 29.13). As a result, both negative and positive supercoils can be relieved by this ATP-requiring process. *Type II DNA topoisomerases* are also required in both prokaryotes and eukaryotes for the separation of interlocked molecules of DNA following chromosomal replication. *DNA gyrase*, a *Type II topoisomerase* found in bacteria and plants, has the unusual property of being able to introduce negative supercoils into relaxed circular DNA using energy from the hydrolysis of ATP. This facilitates the future replication of DNA because the negative supercoils neutralize the positive supercoils introduced during opening of the double helix. It also aids in the transient strand separation required during transcription (see p. 417).

> Anticancer agents, such as etoposide,[3] target human *topoisomerase II*. Bacterial *DNA gyrase* is a unique target of a group of antimicrobial agents called quinolones, for example, ciprofloxacin.[4]

[3]See Chapter 39 in *Lippincott's Illustrated Reviews: Pharmacology* for a discussion of etoposide as an anticancer agent.
[4]See Chapter 33 in *Lippincott's Illustrated Reviews: Pharmacology* for a discussion of the quinolones.

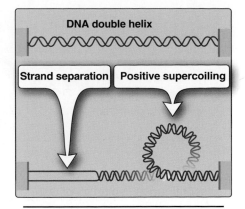

Figure 29.11
Positive supercoiling resulting from DNA strand separation.

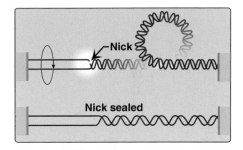

Figure 29.12
Action of *Type I DNA topoisomerases*.

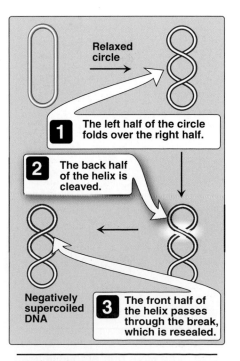

Figure 29.13
Action of *Type II DNA topoisomerase*.

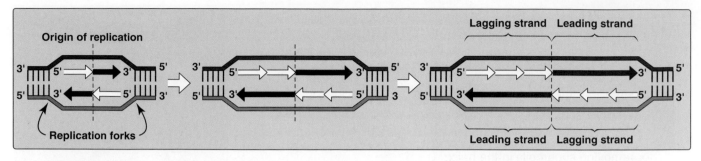

Figure 29.14
Discontinuous synthesis of DNA.

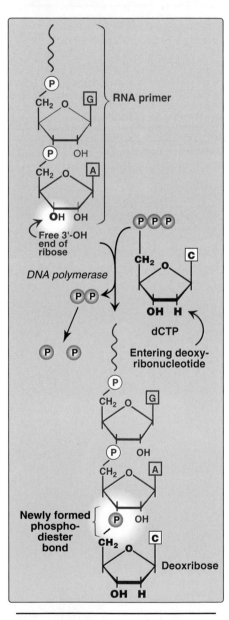

Figure 29.15
Use of an RNA primer to initiate DNA synthesis.

C. Direction of DNA replication

The *DNA polymerases* responsible for copying the DNA templates are only able to "read" the parental nucleotide sequences in the 3'→5' direction, and they synthesize the new DNA strands only in the 5'→3' (antiparallel) direction. Therefore, beginning with one parental double helix, the two newly synthesized stretches of nucleotide chains must grow in opposite directions—one in the 5'→3' direction toward the replication fork and one in the 5'→3' direction away from the replication fork (Figure 29.14). This feat is accomplished by a slightly different mechanism on each strand.

1. **Leading strand:** The strand that is being copied in the direction of the advancing replication fork is called the leading strand and is synthesized continuously.

2. **Lagging strand:** The strand that is being copied in the direction away from the replication fork is synthesized discontinuously, with small fragments of DNA being copied near the replication fork. These short stretches of discontinuous DNA, termed Okazaki fragments, are eventually joined (ligated) to become a single, continuous strand. The new strand of DNA produced by this mechanism is termed the lagging strand.

D. RNA primer

DNA polymerases cannot initiate synthesis of a complementary strand of DNA on a totally single-stranded template. Rather, they require an RNA primer—that is, a short, double-stranded region consisting of RNA base-paired to the DNA template, with a free hydroxyl group on the 3'-end of the RNA strand (Figure 29.15). This hydroxyl group serves as the first acceptor of a deoxynucleotide by action of *DNA polymerase*. [Note: Recall that *glycogen synthase* also requires a primer (see p. 126).]

1. **Primase:** A specific *RNA polymerase*, called *primase (DnaG)*, synthesizes the short stretches of RNA (approximately ten nucleotides long) that are complementary and antiparallel to the DNA template. In the resulting hybrid duplex, the U in RNA pairs with A in DNA. As shown in Figure 29.16, these short RNA sequences are constantly being synthesized at the replication fork on the lagging strand, but only one RNA sequence at the origin of replication is required on the leading strand. The substrates for

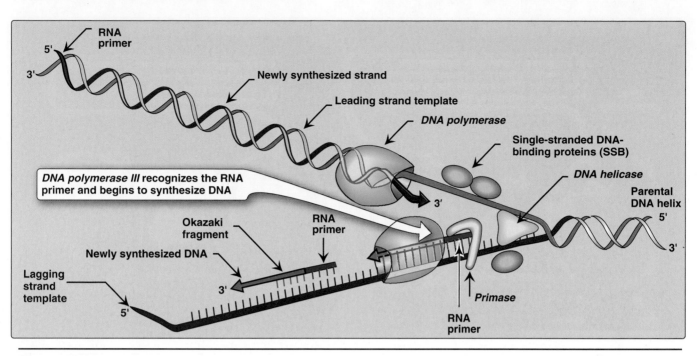

Figure 29.16
Elongation of the leading and lagging strands.

this process are 5'-ribonucleoside triphosphates, and pyrophosphate is released as each ribonucleoside monophosphate is added through formation of a 3'→5' phosphodiester bond. [Note: The RNA primer is later removed as described on p. 405.]

2. **Primosome:** The addition of *primase* converts the prepriming complex of proteins required for DNA strand separation (see p. 399) to a primosome. The primosome makes the RNA primer required for leading strand synthesis, and initiates Okazaki fragment formation in lagging strand synthesis. As with DNA synthesis, the direction of synthesis of the primer is 5'→3'.

E. Chain elongation

Prokaryotic (and eukaryotic) *DNA polymerases* elongate a new DNA strand by adding deoxyribonucleotides, one at a time, to the 3'-end of the growing chain (see Figure 29.16). The sequence of nucleotides that are added is dictated by the base sequence of the template strand with which the incoming nucleotides are paired.

1. **DNA polymerase III:** DNA chain elongation is catalyzed by *DNA polymerase III*. Using the 3'-hydroxyl group of the RNA primer as the acceptor of the first deoxyribonucleotide, *DNA polymerase III* begins to add nucleotides along the single-stranded template that specifies the sequence of bases in the newly synthesized chain. *DNA polymerase III* is a highly "processive" enzyme—that is, it remains bound to the template strand as it moves along, and does not diffuse away and then rebind before adding each new nucleotide. The processivity of *DNA polymerase III* is the result of

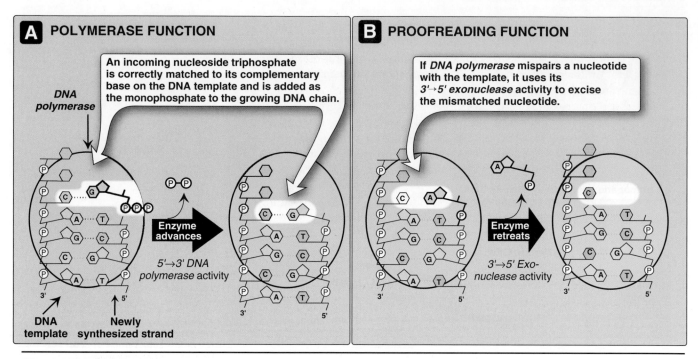

Figure 29.17
3'→5'-Exonuclease activity enables *DNA polymerase III* to "proofread" the newly synthesized DNA strand.

its β subunit forming a ring that encircles and moves along the template strand of the DNA, thus serving as a sliding DNA clamp. The new strand grows in the 5'→3' direction, antiparallel to the parental strand (see Figure 29.16). The nucleotide substrates are 5'-deoxyribonucleoside triphosphates. Pyrophosphate (PP$_i$) is released when each new deoxynucleoside monophosphate is added to the growing chain (see Figure 29.15). Hydrolysis of PP$_i$ to 2P$_i$ means that a total of two high-energy bonds are used to drive the addition of each deoxynucleotide.

> The production of PP$_i$ with subsequent hydrolysis to 2P$_i$, as seen in the synthesis of DNA and RNA, is a common theme in biochemistry. Removal of the PP$_i$ product drives a reaction in the forward direction, making it essentially irreversible.

All four deoxyribonucleoside triphosphates (dATP, dTTP, dCTP, and dGTP) must be present for DNA elongation to occur. If one of the four is in short supply, DNA synthesis stops when that nucleotide is depleted.

2. **Proofreading of newly synthesized DNA:** It is highly important for the survival of an organism that the nucleotide sequence of DNA be replicated with as few errors as possible. Misreading of the template sequence could result in deleterious, perhaps lethal, mutations. To ensure replication fidelity, *DNA polymerase III* has, in addition to its *5'→3' polymerase* activity, a "proofreading" activity

(*3'→5' exonuclease*, Figure 29.17). As each nucleotide is added to the chain, *DNA polymerase III* checks to make certain the added nucleotide is, in fact, correctly matched to its complementary base on the template. If it is not, the *3'→5' exonuclease* activity corrects the mistake. [Note: The enzyme requires an improperly base-paired 3'-hydroxy terminus and, therefore, does not degrade correctly paired nucleotide sequences.] For example, if the template base is cytosine and the enzyme mistakenly inserts an adenine instead of a guanine into the new chain, the *3'→5' exonuclease* activity hydrolytically removes the misplaced nucleotide. The *5'→3' polymerase* activity then replaces it with the correct nucleotide containing guanine (see Figure 29.17). [Note: The proofreading *exonuclease* activity requires movement in the 3'→5' direction, not 5'→3' like the *polymerase* activity. This is because the excision must be done in the reverse direction from that of synthesis.]

F. Excision of RNA primers and their replacement by DNA

DNA polymerase III continues to synthesize DNA on the lagging strand until it is blocked by proximity to an RNA primer. When this occurs, the RNA is excised and the gap filled by *DNA polymerase I*.

1. **5'→3' Exonuclease activity:** In addition to having the *5'→3' polymerase* activity that synthesizes DNA, and the *3'→5' exonuclease* activity that proofreads the newly synthesized DNA chain like *DNA polymerase III*, *DNA polymerase I* also has a *5'→3' exonuclease* activity that is able to hydrolytically remove the RNA primer. [Note: These activities are *exonucleases* because they remove one nucleotide at a time from the end of the DNA chain, rather than cleaving the chain internally as do the *endonucleases* (Figure 29.18).] First, *DNA polymerase I* locates the space ("nick") between the 3'-end of the DNA newly synthesized by *DNA polymerase III* and the 5'-end of the adjacent RNA primer. Next, *DNA polymerase I* hydrolytically removes the RNA nucleotides "ahead" of itself, moving in the 5'→3' direction (*5'→3' exonuclease* activity). As it removes the RNA, *DNA polymerase I* replaces it with deoxyribonucleotides, synthesizing DNA in the 5'→3' direction (*5'→3' polymerase* activity). As it synthesizes the DNA, it also "proofreads" the new chain using *3'→5' exonuclease* activity. This removal/synthesis/proofreading continues, one nucleotide at a time, until the RNA primer is totally degraded and the gap is filled with DNA (Figure 29.19).

2. **Differences between 5'→3' and 3'→5' exonucleases:** The *5'→3' exonuclease* activity of *DNA polymerase I* differs from the *3'→5' exonuclease* used by both *DNA polymerase I* and *III* in two important ways. First, *5'→3' exonuclease* can remove one nucleotide at a time from a region of DNA that is properly base-paired. The nucleotides it removes can be either ribonucleotides or deoxyribonucleotides. Second, *5'→3' exonuclease* can also remove groups of altered nucleotides in the 5'→3' direction, removing from one to ten nucleotides at a time. This ability is important in the repair of some types of damaged DNA.

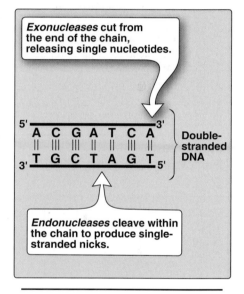

Figure 29.18
Endonuclease versus *exonuclease* activity.

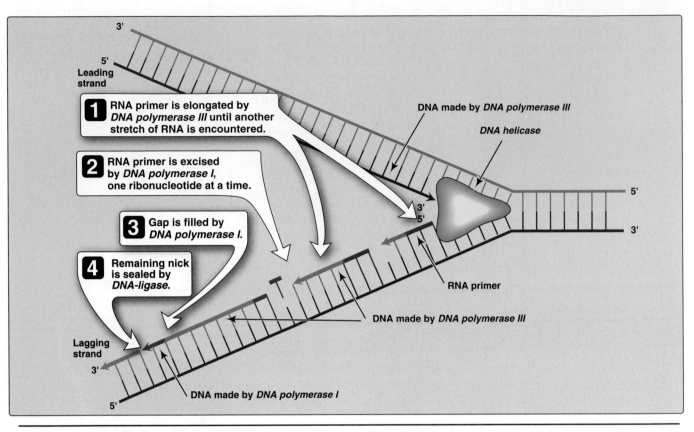

Figure 29.19
Removal of RNA primer and filling of the resulting "gaps" by *DNA polymerase I*.

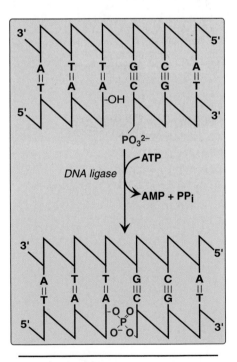

Figure 29.20
Formation of a phosphodiester bond by *DNA ligase*. [Note: AMP is linked to *ligase* then the 5'phosphate and released.]

G. DNA ligase

The final phosphodiester linkage between the 5'-phosphate group on the DNA chain synthesized by *DNA polymerase III* and the 3'-hydroxyl group on the chain made by *DNA polymerase I* is catalyzed by *DNA ligase* (Figure 29.20). The joining of these two stretches of DNA requires energy, which in most organisms is provided by the cleavage of ATP to AMP + PP_i.

IV. EUKARYOTIC DNA REPLICATION

The process of eukaryotic DNA replication closely follows that of prokaryotic DNA synthesis. Some differences, such as the multiple origins of replication in eukaryotic cells versus single origins of replication in prokaryotes, have already been noted. Eukaryotic single-stranded DNA-binding proteins and ATP-dependent *DNA helicases* have been identified, whose functions are analogous to those of the prokaryotic enzymes previously discussed. In contrast, RNA primers are removed by *RNase H* and *FEN1* rather than by a *DNA polymerase*.

A. The eukaryotic cell cycle

The events surrounding eukaryotic DNA replication and cell division (mitosis) are coordinated to produce the cell cycle (Figure 29.21). The period preceding replication is called the G_1 phase (Gap1). DNA replication occurs during the S (synthesis) phase. Following

DNA synthesis, there is another period (G₂ phase, or Gap2) before mitosis (M). Cells that have stopped dividing, such as mature neurons, are said to have gone out of the cell cycle into the G₀ phase. Cells can leave the G₀ phase and reenter the early G₁ phase to resume division. [Note: The cell cycle is controlled at a series of "checkpoints" that prevent entry into the next phase of the cycle until the preceding phase has been completed. Two key classes of proteins that control the progress of a cell through the cell cycle are the cyclins and *cyclin-dependent kinases* (*Cdk*).]

B. Eukaryotic DNA polymerases

At least five key eukaryotic *DNA polymerases* have been identified and categorized on the basis of molecular weight, cellular location, sensitivity to inhibitors, and the templates or substrates on which they act. They are designated by Greek letters rather than by Roman numerals (Figure 29.22).

1. **Pol α:** *Pol α* is a multisubunit enzyme. One subunit has *primase* activity, which initiates strand synthesis on the leading strand and at the beginning of each Okazaki fragment on the lagging strand. The *primase* subunit synthesizes a short RNA primer that is extended by the *pol α 5'→3' polymerase* activity, generating a short piece of DNA.

2. **Pol ε and pol δ:** *Pol ε* is thought to be recruited to complete DNA synthesis on the leading strand whereas *pol δ* elongates the Okazaki fragments of the lagging strand, each using *3'→5' exonuclease* activity to proofread the newly synthesized DNA. [Note: *DNA polymerase ε* associates with the protein, proliferating cell nuclear antigen (PCNA), which serves as a sliding DNA clamp in much the same way the β subunit of *DNA polymerase III* does in <u>E. coli</u>, thus ensuring high processivity.].

3. **Pol β and pol γ:** *Pol β* is involved in "gap filling" in DNA repair (see below). *Pol γ* replicates mitochondrial DNA.

C. Telomeres

Telomeres are complexes of noncoding DNA plus proteins located at the ends of linear chromosomes. They maintain the structural integrity of the chromosome, preventing attack by *nucleases*, and allow repair systems to distinguish a true end from a break in dsDNA. In humans, telomeric DNA consists of several thousand tandem repeats of a noncoding hexameric sequence, AG3T2, base-paired to a complementary region of Cs and As. The GT-rich strand is longer than its CA complement, leaving ssDNA a few hundred nucleotides in length at the 3'-end. The single-stranded region is thought to fold back on itself, forming a loop structure that is stabilized by protein.

1. **Telomere shortening:** Eukaryotic cells face a special problem in replicating the ends of their linear DNA molecules. Following removal of the RNA primer from the extreme 5'-end of the lagging strand, there is no way to fill in the remaining gap with DNA. Consequently, in most normal human somatic cells, telomeres shorten with each successive cell division. Once telomeres are

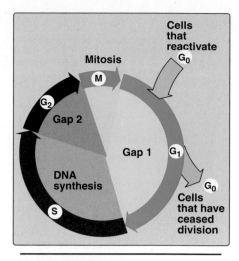

Figure 29.21
The eukaryotic cell cycle.

POLYM-ERASE	FUNCTION	PROOF-READING*
Pol α (alpha)	● **Contains primase** ● **Initiates DNA synthesis**	–
Pol β (beta)	● **Repair**	–
Pol γ (gamma)	● **Replicates mitochondrial DNA**	+
Pol δ (delta)	● **Thought to elongate Okazaki fragments of the lagging strand**	+
Pol ε (epsilon)	● **Thought to elongate the leading strand**	+

Figure 29.22
Activities of eukaryotic *DNA polymerases* (*pols*). *3'→5' exonuclease activity.

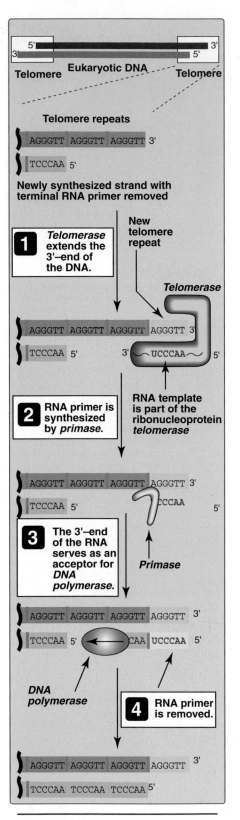

Figure 29.23
Mechanism of action of *telomerase*.

shortened beyond some critical length, the cell is no longer able to divide and is said to be senescent. In germ cells and other stem cells, as well as in cancer cells, telomeres do not shorten and the cells do not senesce. This is a result of the presence of a ribonucleoprotein, *telomerase*, which maintains telomeric length in these cells.

2. **Telomerase:** This complex contains a protein that acts as a *reverse transcriptase*, and a short piece of RNA that acts as a template. The CA-rich RNA template base-pairs with the GT-rich, single-stranded 3'-end of telomeric DNA (Figure 29.23). The *reverse transcriptase* uses the RNA template to synthesize DNA in the usual 5'→3' direction, extending the already longer 3'-end. *Telomerase* then translocates to the newly synthesized end, and the process is repeated. Once the GT-rich strand has been lengthened, *primase* can use it as a template to synthesize an RNA primer. The RNA primer is extended by *DNA polymerase*, and the primer is removed.

> Telomeres may be viewed as mitotic clocks in that their length in most cells is inversely related to the number of times the cells have divided. The study of telomeres is providing insight into the biology of aging and cancer.

D. Reverse transcriptases

Reverse transcriptases, as seen with *telomerase,* are RNA-directed *DNA polymerases*. A *reverse transcriptase* is involved in the replication of retroviruses, such as human immunodeficiency virus (HIV).[5] These viruses carry their genome in the form of ssRNA molecules. Following infection of a host cell, the viral enzyme, *reverse transcriptase*, uses the viral RNA as a template for the 5'→3' synthesis of viral DNA, which then becomes integrated into host chromosomes. *Reverse transcriptase* activity is also seen with transposons, DNA elements that can move about the genome (see p. 461). In eukaryotes, such elements are transcribed to RNA, the RNA is used as a template for DNA synthesis by a *reverse transcriptase* encoded by the transposon, and the DNA is randomly inserted into the genome. [Note: Transposons that involve an RNA intermediate are called retrotransposons or retroposons.]

E. Inhibition of DNA synthesis by nucleoside analogs

DNA chain growth can be blocked by the incorporation of certain nucleoside analogs that have been modified in the sugar portion of the nucleoside (Figure 29.24).[6] For example, removal of the hydroxyl

[5]See Chapter 38 in *Lippincott's Illustrated Reviews: Microbiology* for a discussion of retroviruses.

[6]See Chapter 38 in *Lippincott's Illustrated Reviews: Pharmacology* for a discussion of nucloside analogs.

group from the 3'-carbon of the deoxyribose ring as in 2',3'-dideoxyinosine (ddI, also known as didanosine), or conversion of the deoxyribose to another sugar such as arabinose, prevents further chain elongation. By blocking DNA replication, these compounds slow the division of rapidly growing cells and viruses. Cytosine arabinoside (cytarabine, or araC) has been used in anticancer chemotherapy, whereas adenine arabinoside (vidarabine, or araA) is an antiviral agent. Chemically modifying the sugar moiety, as seen in zidovudine (AZT, ZDV), also terminates DNA chain elongation. [Note: These drugs are generally supplied as nucleosides, which are then converted to the active nucleotides by cellular "salvage" enzymes (see p. 296).]

V. ORGANIZATION OF EUKARYOTIC DNA

A typical human cell contains 46 chromosomes, whose total DNA is approximately 1m long! It is difficult to imagine how such a large amount of genetic material can be effectively packaged into a volume the size of a cell nucleus so that it can be efficiently replicated and its genetic information expressed. To do so requires the interaction of DNA with a large number of proteins, each of which performs a specific function in the ordered packaging of these long molecules of DNA. Eukaryotic DNA is associated with tightly bound basic proteins, called histones. These serve to order the DNA into fundamental structural units, called nucleosomes, that resemble beads on a string. Nucleosomes are further arranged into increasingly more complex structures that organize and condense the long DNA molecules into chromosomes that can be segregated during cell division. [Note: The complex of DNA and protein found inside the nuclei of eukaryotic cells is called chromatin.]

A. Histones and the formation of nucleosomes

There are five classes of histones, designated H1, H2A, H2B, H3, and H4. These small proteins are positively charged at physiologic pH as a result of their high content of lysine and arginine. Because of their positive charge, they form ionic bonds with negatively charged DNA. Histones, along with positively charged ions such as Mg^{2+}, help neutralize the negatively charged DNA phosphate groups.

1. **Nucleosomes:** Two molecules each of H2A, H2B, H3, and H4 form the structural core of the individual nucleosome "beads." Around this core, a segment of the DNA double helix is wound nearly twice, forming a negatively supertwisted helix (Figure 29.25). [Note: The N-terminal ends of these histones can be acetylated, methylated, or phosphorylated. These reversible covalent modifications influence how tightly the histones bind to the DNA, thereby affecting the expression of specific genes (see p. 422).] Neighboring nucleosomes are joined by "linker" DNA approximately 50 base pairs long. Histone H1, of which there are several related species, is not found in the nucleosome core, but instead binds to the linker DNA chain between the nucleosome beads. H1 is the most tissue-specific and species-specific of the histones. It facilitates the packing of nucleosomes into the more compact structures.

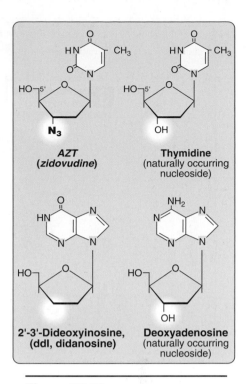

Figure 29.24
Examples of nucleoside analogs that lack a 3'-hydroxyl group. [Note: ddI is converted to its active form (ddATP).]

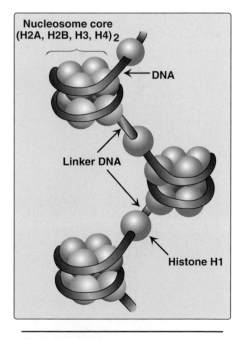

Figure 29.25
Organization of human DNA, illustrating the structure of nucleosomes.

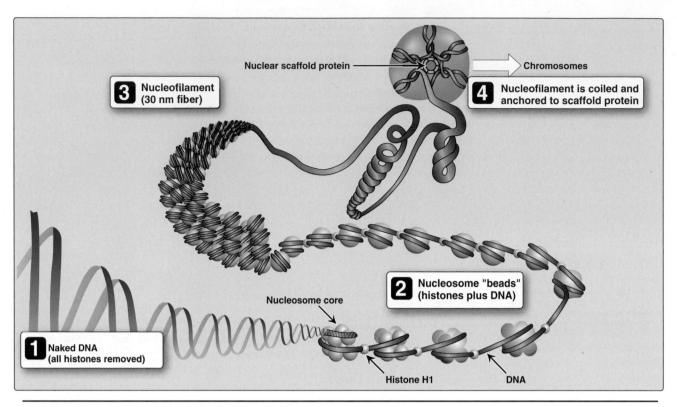

Figure 29.26
Structural organization of eukaryotic DNA.

2. **Higher levels of organization:** Nucleosomes can be packed more tightly to form a polynucleosome (also called a nucleofilament). This structure assumes the shape of a coil, often referred to as a 30-nm fiber. The fiber is organized into loops that are anchored by a nuclear scaffold containing several proteins. Additional levels of organization lead to the final chromosomal structure (Figure 29.26).

B. Fate of nucleosomes during DNA replication

In order to be replicated, the highly structured and constrained chromatin must be relaxed. Although the nucleosomes are displaced, dissociation of the nucleosome core from the DNA is incomplete, with all the parental histones remaining loosely associated with only one of the parental DNA strands. Synthesis of new histones occurs simultaneously with DNA replication, and nucleosomes containing the newly synthesized histones associate with only one of the new daughter helices. Therefore, the parental histone octamers are conserved.

VI. DNA REPAIR

Despite the elaborate proofreading system employed during DNA synthesis, errors—including incorrect base-pairing or insertion of one to a few extra nucleotides—can occur. In addition, DNA is constantly being subjected to environmental insults that cause the alteration or removal of nucleotide bases. The damaging agents can be either chemicals, for example, nitrous acid, or radiation, for example, ultraviolet light, which can fuse two pyrimidines adjacent to each other in the DNA, and high-energy ionizing radiation, which can cause double-strand breaks. Bases are also altered or lost spontaneously from mammalian DNA at a rate of many thousands per cell per day. If the damage is not repaired, a permanent change (mutation) is introduced that can result in any of a number of deleterious effects, including loss of control over the proliferation of the mutated cell, leading to cancer. Luckily, cells are remarkably efficient at repairing damage done to their DNA. Most of the repair systems involve recognition of the damage (lesion) on the DNA, removal or excision of the damage, replacement or filling the gap left by excision using the sister strand as a template for DNA synthesis, and ligation. These repair systems thus perform excision repair, with the removal of one to tens of nucleotides. [Note: Repair reduces the error rate from one in ten million bases to one in a billion.]

A. Methyl-directed mismatch repair

Sometimes replication errors escape the proofreading function during DNA synthesis, causing a mismatch of one to several bases. In E. coli, mismatch repair is mediated by a group of proteins known as the Mut proteins (Figure 29.27). Homologous proteins are present in humans.

1. **Identification of the mismatched strand:** When a mismatch occurs, the Mut proteins that identify the mispaired nucleotide(s) must be able to discriminate between the correct strand and the strand with the mismatch. Discrimination is based on the degree of methylation. GATC sequences, which are found approximately once every thousand nucleotides, are methylated on the adenine residue. This methylation is not done immediately after synthesis, so the newly synthesized DNA is hemimethylated (that is, the parental strand is methylated but the daughter strand is not). The methylated parental strand is assumed to be correct, and it is the daughter strand that gets repaired. [Note: The exact mechanism by which the daughter strand is identified in eukaryotes is not yet known.]

2. **Repair of damaged DNA:** When the strand containing the mismatch is identified, an *endonuclease* nicks the strand and the mismatched nucleotide(s) is/are removed by an *exonuclease*. Additional nucleotides at the 5'- and 3'-ends of the mismatch are also removed. The gap left by removal of the nucleotides is filled, using the sister strand as a template, by a *DNA polymerase*. The 3'-hydroxyl of the newly synthesized DNA is joined to the 5'-phosphate of the remaining stretch of the original DNA strand by *DNA ligase* (see p. 406).

> Mutation to the proteins involved in mismatch repair in humans is associated with hereditary nonpolyposis colorectal cancer (HNPCC), also known as Lynch syndrome. With HNPCC, there is an increased risk for developing colon cancer (as well as other cancers), but only about 5% of all colon cancer is the result of mutations in mismatch repair.

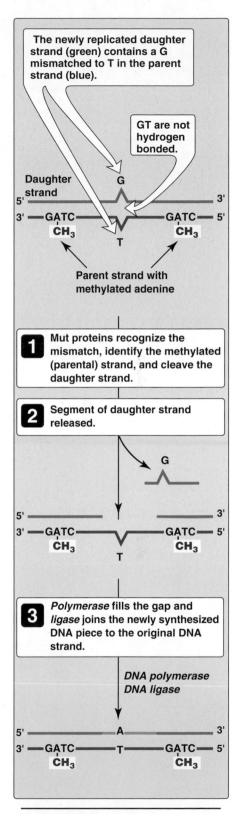

Figure 29.27
Methyl-directed mismatch repair.

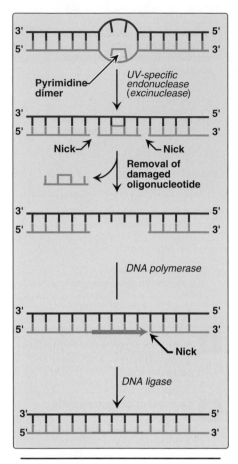

Figure 29.28
Nucleotide excision repair of
pyrimidine dimers in E. coli DNA.

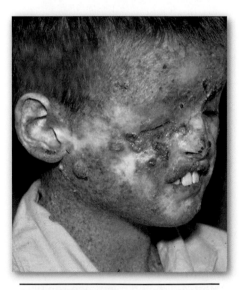

Figure 29.29
Patient with xeroderma pigmentosum.

B. Repair of damage caused by ultraviolet (UV) light

Exposure of a cell to UV light can result in the covalent joining of two adjacent pyrimidines (usually thymines), producing a dimer. These thymine dimers prevent *DNA polymerase* from replicating the DNA strand beyond the site of dimer formation. Thymine dimers are excised in bacteria by UvrABC proteins in a process known as nucleotide excision repair as illustrated in Figure 29.28. A related pathway involving XP proteins is present in humans.

1. **Recognition and excision of dimers by UV-specific endonuclease:** First, a *UV-specific endonuclease* (called *uvrABC excinuclease*) recognizes the dimer, and cleaves the damaged strand on both the 5'-side and 3'-side of the dimer. A short oligonucleotide containing the dimer is released, leaving a gap in the DNA strand that formerly contained the dimer. This gap is filled in using the same process described previously.

2. **UV radiation and cancer:** Pyrimidine dimers can be formed in the skin cells of humans exposed to unfiltered sunlight. In the rare genetic disease xeroderma pigmentosum (XP), the cells cannot repair the damaged DNA, resulting in extensive accumulation of mutations and, consequently, early and numerous skin cancers (Figure 29.29). XP can be caused by defects in any of the several genes that code for the XP proteins required for nucleotide excision repair of UV damage in humans.

C. Correction of base alterations (base excision repair)

The bases of DNA can be altered, either spontaneously, as is the case with cytosine, which slowly undergoes deamination (the loss of its amino group) to form uracil, or by the action of deaminating or alkylating compounds. For example, nitrous acid, which is formed by the cell from precursors, such as the nitrosamines, nitrites, and nitrates, is a potent compound that deaminates cytosine, adenine (to hypoxanthine), and guanine (to xanthine). Bases can also be lost spontaneously. For example, approximately 10,000 purine bases are lost this way per cell per day. Lesions involving base alterations or loss can be corrected by base excision repair (Figure 29.30).

1. **Removal of abnormal bases:** Abnormal bases, such as uracil, which can occur in DNA either by deamination of cytosine or improper use of dUTP instead of dTTP during DNA synthesis, are recognized by specific *glycosylases* that hydrolytically cleave them from the deoxyribose–phosphate backbone of the strand. This leaves an apyrimidinic site (or apurinic, if a purine was removed), both referred to as AP sites.

2. **Recognition and repair of an AP site:** Specific *AP-endonucleases* recognize that a base is missing and initiate the process of excision and gap-filling by making an endonucleolytic cut just to the 5'-side of the AP site. A *deoxyribose phosphate lyase* removes the single, base-free, sugar phosphate residue. A *DNA polymerase* and *DNA ligase* complete the repair process.

D. Repair of double-strand breaks

High-energy radiation or oxidative free radicals (see p. 148) can cause double-strand breaks in DNA, which are potentially lethal to the cell. Such breaks also occur naturally during gene rearrangements. dsDNA breaks cannot be corrected by the previously described strategy of excising the damage on one strand and using the remaining strand as a template for replacing the missing nucleotide(s). Instead, they are repaired by one of two systems. The first is nonhomologous end-joining repair, in which the ends of two DNA fragments are brought together by a group of proteins that effect their religation. However, some DNA is lost in the process. Consequently, this mechanism of repair is error prone and mutagenic. Defects in this repair system are associated with a predisposition to cancer and immunodeficiency syndromes. The second repair system, homologous recombination repair, uses the enzymes that normally perform genetic recombination between homologous chromosomes during meiosis. This system is much less error prone than nonhomologous end-joining joining because any DNA that was lost is replaced using homologous DNA as a template.

VII. CHAPTER SUMMARY

DNA contains many deoxyribonucleoside monophosphates covalently linked by **3'→5'-phosphodiester bonds** (Figure 29.31). The resulting long, unbranched chain has **polarity**, with both a 5'-end and a 3'-end. The sequence of nucleotides is read 5'→3'. DNA exists as a **double-stranded** molecule, in which the two chains are paired in an **antiparallel** manner, and wind around each other, forming a **double helix**. **Adenine** pairs with **thymine** and **cytosine** pairs with **guanine**. Each strand of the double helix serves as a **template** for constructing a **complementary** daughter strand (**semiconservative replication**). DNA replication occurs in the **S phase** of the cell cycle and begins at the **origin of replication**. The strands are separated locally, forming two **replication forks**. Replication of dsDNA is **bidirectional**. **Helicase** unwinds the double helix. As the two strands of the double helix are separated, **positive supercoils** are produced in the region of DNA ahead of the replication fork. **DNA topoisomerases Types I and II** remove supercoils. **DNA polymerases synthesize** new DNA strands only in the **5'→3'** direction. Therefore, one of the newly synthesized stretches of nucleotide chains must grow in the 5'→3' direction toward the replication fork (**leading strand**), and one in the 5'→3' direction away from the replication fork (**lagging strand**). DNA polymerases require a **primer**. The primer for de novo DNA synthesis is a short stretch of RNA synthesized by **primase**. The leading strand only needs one RNA primer, whereas the lagging strand needs many. In E. coli DNA chain elongation is catalyzed by **DNA polymerase III**, using **5'-deoxyribonucleoside triphosphates** as substrates. The enzyme "**proofreads**" the newly synthesized DNA, removing terminal mismatched nucleotides with its **3'→5' exonuclease** activity. RNA primers are removed by **DNA polymerase I**, using its **5'→3' exonuclease** activity. This enzyme fills the gaps with DNA, proofreading as it synthesizes. The final phosphodi-

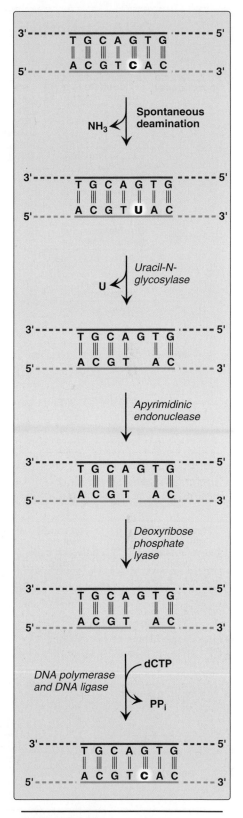

Figure 29.30
Correction of base alterations by base excision repair.

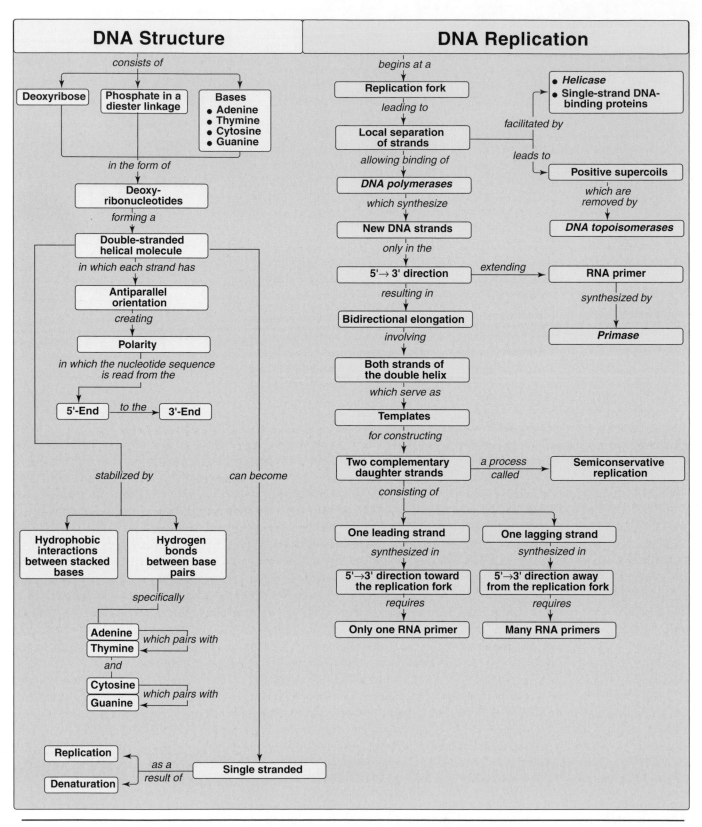

Figure 29.31 (continued on next page)
Key concept map for DNA structure, replication, and repair. (continued on next page)

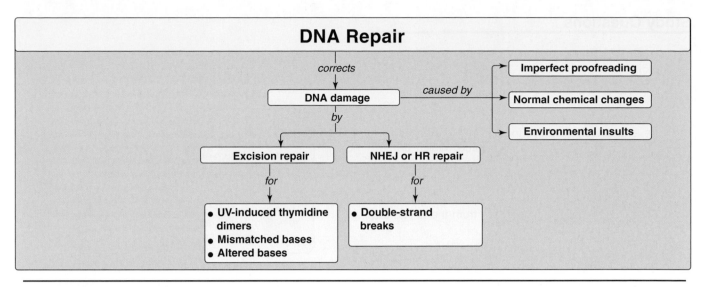

Figure 29.31 (continued from previous page)
Key concept map for DNA structure, replication, and repair. NHEJ = nonhomologous end-joining;
HR = homologous recombination.

ester linkage is catalyzed by **DNA ligase**. There are at least five **eukaryotic DNA polymerases**. **Pol** α is a multi-subunit enzyme, one subunit of which is a **primase**. Pol α $5'{\rightarrow}3'$ polymerase activity adds a short piece of DNA to the RNA primer. **Pol** ε is thought to complete DNA synthesis on the leading strand whereas **pol** δ elongates each lagging strand fragment. Both ε and δ use $3'{\rightarrow}5'$ **exonuclease** activity to **proofread**. **Pol** β is involved with DNA repair, and pol γ replicates mitochondrial DNA. **Nucleoside analogs** containing modified sugars can be used to block DNA chain growth. They are useful in anticancer and antiviral chemotherapy. **Telomeres** are stretches of **highly repetitive DNA** complexed with protein that protect the **ends** of linear chromosomes. As most cells divide and age, these sequences are shortened, contributing to senescence. In cells that do not senesce (for example, germline and cancer cells), **telomerase** employs its enzyme component **reverse transcriptase** to extend the telomeres, using its **RNA as a template**. There are five classes of **positively charged histone proteins**. Two each of histones H2A, H2B, H3, and H4 form a structural core around which DNA is wrapped creating a **nucleosome**. The DNA connecting the nucleosomes, called **linker DNA**, is bound to histone H1. Nucleosomes can be packed more tightly to form a nucleofilament. Additional levels of organization create a chromosome. Most DNA damage can be corrected by **excision repair** involving recognition and removal of the damage by repair proteins, followed by replacement by DNA polymerase and joining by ligase. **Ultraviolet light** can cause thymine dimers that are recognized and removed by **uvrABC** proteins of nucleotide excision repair. Defects in the **XP proteins** needed for thymine dimer repair in humans result in **xeroderma pigmentosum**. **Mismatched** bases are repaired by a similar process of recognition and removal by **Mut proteins** in E. coli. The extent of **methylation** is used for strand identification in prokaryotes. Defective mismatch repair by homologous proteins in humans is associated with **hereditary nonpolyposis colorectal cancer**. Abnormal bases (such as uracil) are removed by **glycosylases in base excision repair**, and the sugar phosphate at the AP site is cut out. Double-strand breaks in DNA are repaired by **nonhomologous end-joining** (error prone) and **homologous recombination**.

Study Questions

Choose the ONE correct answer.

29.1 A 10-year-old girl is brought to the dermatologist by her parents. She has many freckles on her face, neck, arms, and hands, and the parents report that she is unusually sensitive to sunlight. Two basal cell carcinomas are identified on her face. Which of the following processes is most likely to be defective in this patient?

A. Repair of double-strand breaks.

B. Removal of mismatched bases from the 3'-end of Okazaki fragments.

C. Removal of pyrimidine dimers from DNA.

D. Removal of uracil from DNA.

Correct answer = C. The sensitivity to sunlight, extensive freckling on parts of the body exposed to the sun, and presence of skin cancer at a young age indicates that the patient most likely suffers from xeroderma pigmentosum. These patients are deficient in any one of several XP proteins required for nucleotide excision repair of ultraviolet-damaged DNA. Double-strand breaks are repaired by nonhomologous end-joining or homologous recombination. Uracil is removed from damaged DNA molecules by a specific glycosylase.

29.2 Telomeres are complexes of DNA and protein that protect the ends of linear chromosomes. In most normal human somatic cells, telomeres shorten with each division. In stem cells and in cancer cells, however, telomeric length is maintained. In the synthesis of telomeres:

A. telomerase, a ribonucleoprotein, provides both the RNA and the polymerase needed for synthesis.

B. the RNA of telomerase serves as a primer.

C. the polymerase of telomerase is a DNA-directed DNA polymerase.

D. the shorter, 3'→5' strand gets extended.

E. the direction of synthesis is 3'→5'.

Correct answer = A. Telomerase is a ribonucleoprotein particle required for telomere maintenance. Telomerase contains an RNA that serves as the template, not the primer, for the synthesis of telomeric DNA by the reverse transcriptase of telomerase. As a reverse transcriptase, it synthesizes DNA using its RNA template and so is an RNA-directed DNA polymerase. The direction of synthesis, as with all DNA synthesis, is 5'→3', and it is the already longer 5'→3' strand that gets extended.

29.3 While studying the structure of a small gene that was recently sequenced during the Human Genome Project, an investigator notices that one strand of the DNA molecule contains 20 As, 25 Gs, 30 Cs, and 22 Ts. How many of each base is found in the complete double-stranded molecule?

A. A = 40, G = 50, C = 60, T = 44.

B. A = 44, G = 60, C = 50, T = 40.

C. A = 45, G = 45, C = 52, T = 52.

D. A = 50, G = 47, C = 50, T = 47.

E. A = 42, G = 55, C = 55, T = 42.

Correct answer = E. The two DNA strands are complementary to each other, with A base-paired with T, and G base-paired with C. So, for example, the 20 As on the first strand would be paired with 20 Ts on the second strand, the 25 Gs on the first strand would be paired with 25 Cs on the second strand, and so forth. When these are all added together, the correct numbers of each base are indicated in choice E. Notice that, in the correct answer, A = T and G = C.

29.4 The extent of DNA synthesis in a cell could most specifically be determined by measuring the incorporation of radiolabeled:

A. leucine.

B. phosphate.

C. ribose

D. thymidine

E. uracil

Correct answer = D. Thymidine is incorporated only into DNA, and thus would reflect the extent of DNA synthesis. Leucine is an amino acid, not a nucleotide base. Phosphate is not exclusive to DNA. Ribose is found in RNA, whereas deoxyribose is found in DNA. Uracil is normally found only in RNA. If present in DNA, likely as a result of deamination of cytosine, it is removed by uracil glycosylase during base excision repair.

RNA Structure, Synthesis, and Processing

30

I. OVERVIEW

The genetic master plan of an organism is contained in the sequence of deoxyribonucleotides in its deoxyribonucleic acid (DNA). However, it is through the ribonucleic acid (RNA)—the "working copies" of the DNA—that the master plan is expressed (Figure 30.1). The copying process, during which a DNA strand serves as a template for the synthesis of RNA, is called transcription. Transcription produces messenger RNAs that are translated into sequences of amino acids (polypeptide chains or proteins), and ribosomal RNAs, transfer RNAs, and additional small RNA molecules that perform specialized structural, catalytic, and regulatory functions and are not translated, that is, they are noncoding RNAs (ncRNAs). The final product of gene expression, therefore, can be RNA or protein, depending upon the gene. A central feature of transcription is that it is highly selective. For example, many transcripts are made of some regions of the DNA. In other regions, few or no transcripts are made. This selectivity is due, at least in part, to signals embedded in the nucleotide sequence of the DNA. These signals instruct the *RNA polymerase* where to start, how often to start, and where to stop transcription. A variety of regulatory proteins is also involved in this selection process. The biochemical differentiation of an organism's tissues is ultimately a result of the selectivity of the transcription process. [Note: This selectivity of transcription is in contrast to the "all or none" nature of genomic replication.] Another important feature of transcription is that many RNA transcripts that initially are faithful copies of one of the two DNA strands may undergo various modifications, such as terminal additions, base modifications, trimming, and internal segment removal, which convert the inactive primary transcript into a functional molecule.

II. STRUCTURE OF RNA

There are three major types of RNA that participate in the process of protein synthesis: ribosomal RNA (rRNA), transfer RNA (tRNA), and messenger RNA (mRNA). Like DNA, these three types of RNA are unbranched polymeric molecules composed of nucleoside monophosphates joined together by phosphodiester bonds (see p. 396). However, they differ from DNA in several ways, for example, they are considerably

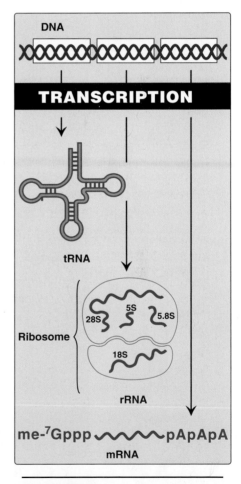

Figure 30.1
Expression of genetic information by transcription. [Note: RNAs shown are eukaryotic.] me-^{7}Gppp = 7-methylguanosine triphosphate "cap," AAA = poly-A tail, each described on p. 418.

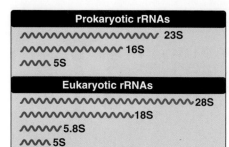

Figure 30.2
Prokaryotic and eukaryotic rRNAs.

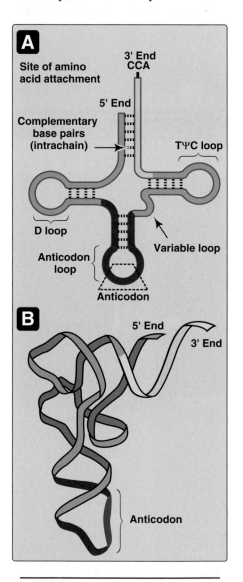

Figure 30.3
A. Characteristic tRNA secondary structure. B. Folded (tertiary) tRNA structure found in cells. D = dihydrouracil. Ψ = pseudouracil.

smaller than DNA, contain ribose instead of deoxyribose and uracil instead of thymine, and exist as single strands that are capable of folding into complex structures. The three major types of RNA also differ from each other in size, function, and special structural modifications. [Note: In eukaryotes, additional small ncRNA molecules found in the nucleolus (snoRNAs) and nucleus (snRNAs) perform specialized functions as described on pp. 425 and 426.]

A. Ribosomal RNA

rRNAs are found in association with several proteins as components of the ribosomes—the complex structures that serve as the sites for protein synthesis (see p. 436). There are three distinct size species of rRNA (23S, 16S, and 5S) in prokaryotic cells (Figure 30.2). In the eukaryotic cytosol, there are four rRNA species (28S, 18S, 5.8S, and 5S). [Note: "S" is the Svedberg unit, which is related to the molecular weight and shape of the compound.] Together, rRNAs make up about 80% of the total RNA in the cell. [Note: Some RNAs function as catalysts, for example, rRNA in protein synthesis (see p. 439). RNA with catalytic activity is termed a "ribozyme".]

B. Transfer RNA

tRNAs are the smallest (4S) of the three major types of RNA molecules. There is at least one specific type of tRNA molecule for each of the 20 amino acids commonly found in proteins. Together, tRNAs make up about 15% of the total RNA in the cell. The tRNA molecules contain a high percentage of unusual bases (for example, dihydrouracil, see Figure 22.2, p. 292) and have extensive intrachain base-pairing (Figure 30.3) that leads to characteristic secondary and tertiary structure. Each tRNA serves as an "adaptor" molecule that carries its specific amino acid—covalently attached to its 3'-end—to the site of protein synthesis. There it recognizes the genetic code sequence on an mRNA, which specifies the addition of its amino acid to the growing peptide chain (see p. 432).

C. Messenger RNA

mRNA comprises only about 5% of the RNA in the cell, yet is by far the most heterogeneous type of RNA in size and base sequence. The mRNA carries genetic information from the nuclear DNA to the cytosol, where it is used as the template for protein synthesis. If the mRNA carries information from more than one gene, it is said to be polycistronic. Polycistronic mRNA is characteristic of prokaryotes. If the mRNA carries information from just one gene, it is said to be monocistronic and is characteristic of eukaryotes. In addition to the protein coding regions that can be translated, mRNA contains untranslated regions at its 5'- and 3'-ends (Figure 30.4). Special structural characteristics of eukaryotic (but not prokaryotic) mRNA include a long sequence of adenine nucleotides (a "poly-A tail") on the 3'-end of the RNA chain, plus a "cap" on the 5'-end consisting of a molecule of 7-methylguanosine attached "backward" (5'→5') through a triphosphate linkage as shown in Figure 30.4. The mechanisms for modifying mRNA to create these special structural characteristics are discussed on p. 425.

III. TRANSCRIPTION OF PROKARYOTIC GENES

The structure of *RNA polymerase*, the signals that control transcription, and the varieties of modification that RNA transcripts can undergo differ among organisms, and particularly from prokaryotes to eukaryotes. Therefore, the discussions of prokaryotic and eukaryotic transcription are presented separately.

A. Properties of prokaryotic RNA polymerase

In bacteria, one species of *RNA polymerase* synthesizes all of the RNA except for the short RNA primers needed for DNA replication (RNA primers are synthesized by a specialized enzyme, *primase*, see p. 402). *RNA polymerase* is a multisubunit enzyme that recognizes a nucleotide sequence (the promoter region) at the beginning of a length of DNA that is to be transcribed. It next makes a complementary RNA copy of the DNA template strand, and then recognizes the end of the DNA sequence to be transcribed (the termination region). RNA is synthesized from its 5'-end to its 3'-end, antiparallel to its DNA template strand (see p. 397). The template is copied as it is in DNA synthesis, in which a G on the DNA specifies a C in the RNA, a C specifies a G, a T specifies an A, but an A specifies a U instead of a T (Figure 30.5). The RNA, then, is complementary to the DNA template (antisense) strand and identical to the coding (sense) strand, with U replacing T. Within the DNA molecule, regions of both strands can serve as templates for transcription. For a given gene, however, only one of the two DNA strands can be the template. Which strand is used is determined by the location of the promoter for that gene. Transcription by *RNA polymerase* involves a core enzyme and several auxiliary proteins:

1. **Core enzyme:** Four of the enzyme's peptide subunits, 2α, 1β, and 1β', are required for enzyme assembly (2α), template binding (β'), and the *5'→3' RNA polymerase* activity (β), and are referred to as the core enzyme (Figure 30.6). However, this enzyme lacks specificity, that is, it cannot recognize the promoter region on the DNA template. [Note: The *in vivo* function of a fifth subunit, Ω, is unclear.]

2. **Holoenzyme:** The σ subunit ("sigma factor") enables *RNA polymerase* to recognize promoter regions on the DNA. The σ subunit plus the core enzyme make up the holoenzyme. [Note: Different σ factors recognize different groups of genes.]

B. Steps in RNA synthesis

The process of transcription of a typical gene of E. coli can be divided into three phases: initiation, elongation, and termination. A transcription unit extends from the promoter to the termination region, and the initial product of transcription by *RNA polymerase* is termed the primary transcript.

1. **Initiation:** Transcription begins with the binding of the *RNA polymerase* holoenzyme to a region of the DNA known as the promoter, which is not transcribed. The prokaryotic promoter contains

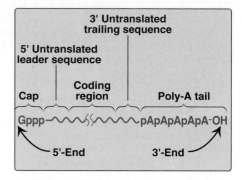

Figure 30.4
Structure of eukaryotic messenger RNA.

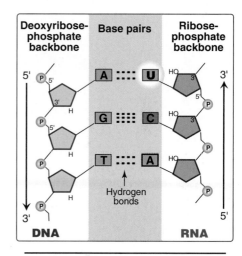

Figure 30.5
Antiparallel, complementary base pairs between DNA and RNA.

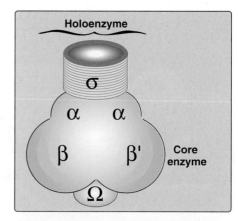

Figure 30.6
Components of prokaryotic *RNA polymerase*.

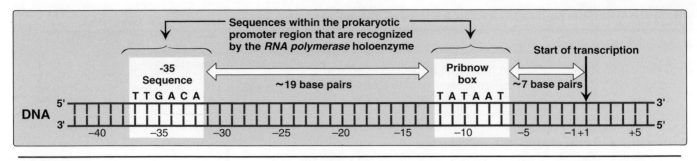

Figure 30.7
Structure of the prokaryotic promoter region.

characteristic consensus sequences (Figure 30.7). [Note: Consensus sequences are idealized sequences in which the base shown at each position is the base most frequently (but not necessarily always) encountered at that position.] Those that are recognized by prokaryotic *RNA polymerase* σ factors include:

a. **–35 sequence:** A consensus sequence (5'-TTGACA-3'), centered about 35 bases to the left of the transcription start site (see Figure 30.7), is the initial point of contact for the holoenzyme, and a closed complex is formed. [Note: The regulatory sequences that control transcription are, by convention, designated by the 5'→3' nucleotide sequence on the nontemplate strand. A base in the promoter region is assigned a negative number if it occurs prior to (to the left of, toward the 5'-end of, or "upstream" of) the transcription start site. Therefore, the TTGACA sequence is centered at approximately base –35. The first base at the transcription start site is assigned a position of +1. There is no base designated "0."]

b. **Pribnow box:** The holoenzyme moves and covers a second consensus sequence (5'-TATAAT-3'), centered at about –10 (see Figure 30.7), which is the site of initial DNA melting (unwinding). Melting of a short stretch (about 14 bases) converts the closed complex to an open one known as a transcription bubble. [Note: A mutation in either the –10 or the –35 sequence can affect the transcription of the gene controlled by the mutant promoter.]

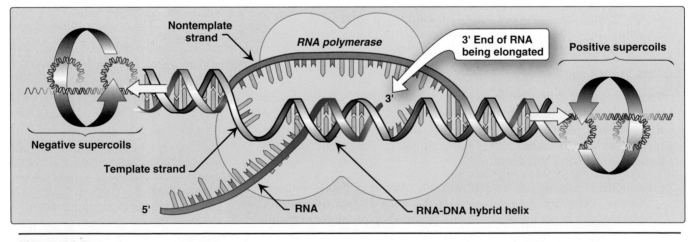

Figure 30.8
Local unwinding of DNA caused by *RNA polymerase* and formation of an open initiation complex.

2. **Elongation:** Once the promoter region has been recognized and bound by the holoenzyme, local unwinding of the DNA helix continues (Figure 30.8), mediated by the *polymerase*. [Note: Unwinding generates supercoils in the DNA that can be relieved by *DNA topoisomerases* (see p. 401.] *RNA polymerase* begins to synthesize a transcript of the DNA sequence, and several short pieces of RNA are made and discarded. The elongation phase is said to begin when the transcript (typically starting with a purine) exceeds ten nucleotides in length. Sigma is then released, and the core enzyme is able to leave ("clear") the promoter and move along the template strand in a processive manner. During transcription, a short DNA-RNA hybrid helix is formed (see Figure 30.8). Like *DNA polymerase*, *RNA polymerase* uses nucleoside triphosphates as substrates and releases pyrophosphate each time a nucleoside monophosphate is added to the growing chain. As with replication, transcription is always in the 5'→3' direction. In contrast to *DNA polymerase*, *RNA polymerase* does not require a primer and does not appear to have proofreading activity.

3. **Termination:** The elongation of the single-stranded RNA chain continues until a termination signal is reached. Termination can be intrinsic (spontaneous) or dependent upon the participation of a protein known as the ρ (rho) factor.

   a. **ρ-Independent termination**: Seen with most prokaryotic genes, this requires that a sequence in the DNA template generate a sequence in the nascent (newly made) RNA that is self-complementary (Figure 30.9). This allows the RNA to fold back on itself, forming a GC-rich stem (stabilized by H-bonds) plus a loop. This structure is known as a "hairpin". Additionally, just beyond the hairpin, the RNA transcript contains a string of Us at the 3'-end. The bonding of these Us to the complementary As of the DNA template is weak. This facilitates the separation of the newly synthesized RNA from its DNA template, as the double helix "zips up" behind the *RNA polymerase*.

   b. **ρ-Dependent termination**: This requires the participation of an additional protein, rho (ρ), which is a hexameric *adenosine triphosphatase* (*ATPase*) with *helicase* activity. ρ binds a C-rich "rho recognition site" near the 3'-end of the nascent RNA and, using its *ATPase* activity, moves along the RNA until it reaches the *RNA polymerase* paused at the termination site. The *ATP-dependent helicase* activity of ρ separates the RNA-DNA hybrid helix, causing the release of the RNA.

4. **Action of antibiotics:** Some antibiotics prevent bacterial cell growth by inhibiting RNA synthesis. For example, rifampin inhibits the initiation of transcription by binding to the β subunit of prokaryotic *RNA polymerase*, thus interfering with the formation of the first phosphodiester bond (Figure 30.10). Rifampin is useful in the treatment of tuberculosis.[1] Dactinomycin (known to biochemists as actinomycin D) was the first antibiotic to find therapeutic application in tumor chemotherapy.[2] It binds to the DNA template and interferes with the movement of *RNA polymerase* along the DNA.

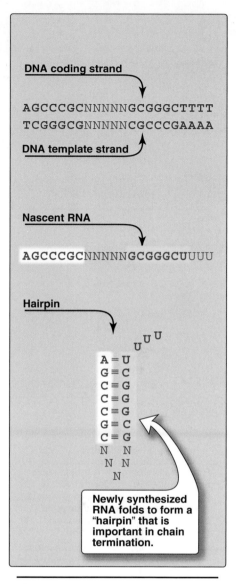

Figure 30.9
Rho-independent termination of transcription. A. DNA template sequence generates a self-complementary sequence in the nascent RNA. B. Hairpin structure formed by the RNA. "N" represents a noncomplementary base.

[1]See Chapter 34 in *Lippincott's Illustrated Reviews: Pharmacology* for a discussion of rifampin in the treatment of tuberculosis.
[2]See Chapter 39 in *Lippincott's Illustrated Reviews: Pharmacology* for a discussion of dactinomycin in treating cancer.

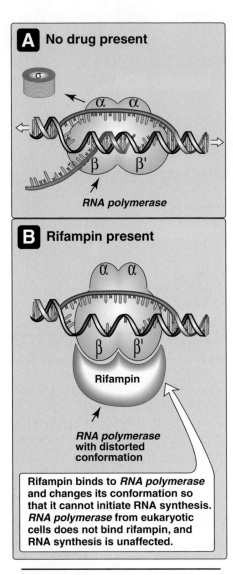

Figure 30.10
Inactivation of prokaryotic *RNA polymerase* by rifampin.

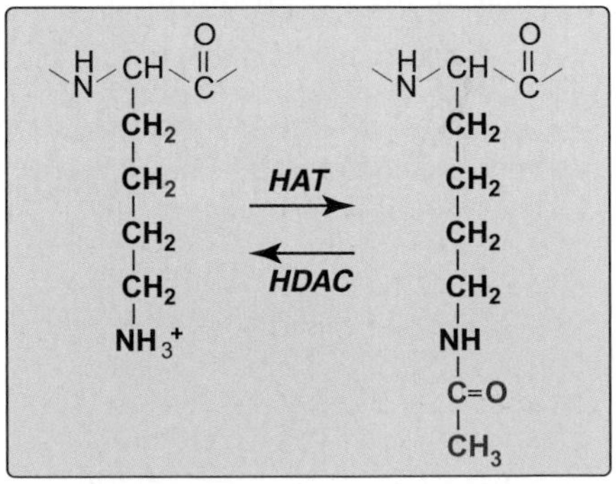

Figure 30.11
Acetylation/deacetylation of a lysine residue in a histone protein. *HAT = histone acetyltransferase; HDAC = histone deacetylase.*

IV. TRANSCRIPTION OF EUKARYOTIC GENES

The transcription of eukaryotic genes is a far more complicated process than transcription in prokaryotes. Eukaryotic transcription involves separate *polymerases* for the synthesis of rRNA, tRNA, and mRNA. In addition, a large number of proteins called transcription factors (TFs) are involved. TFs bind to distinct sites on the DNA—either within the core promoter region, close (proximal) to it, or some distance away (distal). They are required both for the assembly of a transcription complex at the promoter and the determination of which genes are to be transcribed. [Note: Each eukaryotic *RNA polymerase* has its own promoters and TFs.] For TFs to recognize and bind to their specific DNA sequences, the chromatin structure in that region must be altered (remodeled) to allow access to the DNA. The role of transcription in the regulation of gene expression is discussed in Chapter 32.

A. Chromatin structure and gene expression

The association of DNA with histones to form nucleosomes (see p. 409) affects the ability of the transcription machinery to access the DNA to be transcribed. Most actively transcribed genes are found in a relatively relaxed form of chromatin called euchromatin, whereas most inactive segments of DNA are found in highly condensed heterochromatin. [Note: The interconversion of these forms is called chromatin remodeling.] A major mechanism by which chromatin is remodeled is through acetylation of lysine residues at the amino terminus of histone proteins (Figure 30.11). Acetylation, mediated by *histone acetyltransferases (HATs)*, eliminates the positive charge on the lysine and thereby decreases the interaction of the histone with the negatively charged DNA. Removal of the acetyl group by *histone deacetylases (HDACs)* restores the positive charge, and fosters stronger interactions between histones and DNA.

B. Nuclear RNA polymerases of eukaryotic cells

There are three distinct classes of *RNA polymerase* in the nucleus of eukaryotic cells. All are large enzymes with multiple subunits. Each class of *RNA polymerase* recognizes particular types of genes.

1. **RNA polymerase I:** This enzyme synthesizes the precursor of the 28S, 18S, and 5.8S rRNA in the nucleolus.

2. **RNA polymerase II:** This enzyme synthesizes the nuclear precursors of mRNA that are subsequently translated to produce proteins. *Polymerase II* also synthesizes certain small ncRNAs, such as snRNA (see p. 426), snoRNA (see p. 425) and miRNA (see p. 459).

   a. **Promoters and transcription factors for RNA polymerase II:** In some genes transcribed by *RNA polymerase II*, a sequence of nucleotides that is nearly identical to that of the Pribnow box (see p. 420) is found centered about 25 nucleotides upstream of the transcription start site. This promoter consensus sequence is called the TATA or Hogness box. Between 70 and

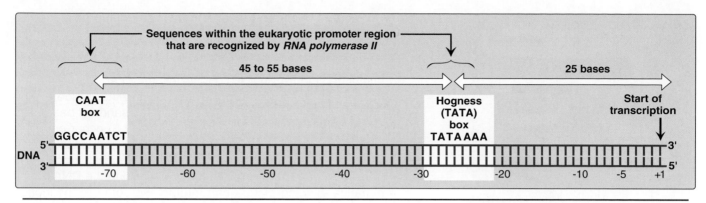

Figure 30.12
Eukaryotic gene promoter consensus sequences.

80 nucleotides upstream of the transcription start site often is found a second consensus sequence known as the CAAT box (Figure 30.12). In other genes, for example, those that are always ("constitutively") expressed, no TATA box is typically present. Instead, a GC-rich region (GC box) may be found. [Note: No one consensus sequence is found in all core promoters.] Because these sequences are on the same molecule of DNA as the gene being transcribed, they are called cis-acting elements. Such sequences serve as binding sites for TFs, which in turn interact with each other and with *RNA polymerase II*.

> Transcription factors bind DNA through a variety of motifs, such as the helix-loop-helix, zinc fingers, and leucine zippers (see p. 18).]

Because TFs are encoded by different genes, synthesized in the cytosol, and must transit to their sites of action, they are called trans-acting factors. General TFs are the minimal requirements for recognition of the promoter, recruitment of *RNA polymerase II* to the promoter, and initiation of transcription (Figure 30.13A). [Note: In contrast to the holoenzyme of prokaryotes, eukaryotic *RNA polymerase II* does not itself recognize and bind the promoter. Instead, TFIID recognizes and binds the TATA box, and TFIIF brings the *polymerase* to the promoter. The *helicase* activity of TFIIH melts the DNA and its *kinase* activity phosphorylates *polymerase*, allowing it to clear the promoter.] Specific TFs (transcriptional activators) bind to sequences within and outside of the core promoter. They are required to modulate the frequency of initiation, to mediate the response to signals such as hormones (see p. 456), and to regulate which genes are expressed at a given point in time. A typical protein-coding eukaryotic gene has binding sites for many such factors. In addition to binding DNA, specific TFs also bind other proteins ("coactivators"), recruiting them to the transcription complex. [Note: Coactivators include the *HAT* enzymes involved in chromatin remodeling (see p. 422).]

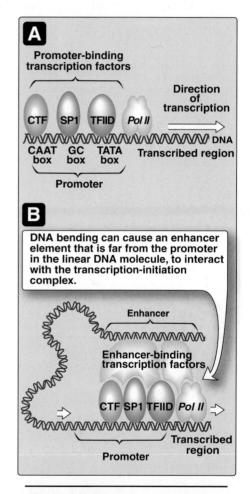

Figure 30.13
A. Eukaryotic general transcription factors (CTF, SP1, TFIID) bind to consensus sequences found in promoters for *RNA polymerase II* . Additional general transcription factors (TFIIs) are required for assembly of the initiation complex and recruitment of polymerase. B. Enhancer stimulation of *RNA polymerase II*.

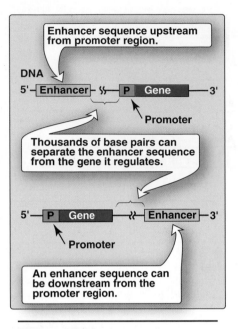

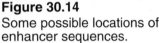

Figure 30.14
Some possible locations of enhancer sequences.

b. Role of enhancers in eukaryotic gene regulation: Enhancers are special cis-acting DNA sequences that increase the rate of initiation of transcription by *RNA polymerase II*. Enhancers are on the same chromosome as the gene whose transcription they stimulate (Figure 30.13B). However, they can 1) be located upstream (to the 5'-side) or downstream (to the 3'-side) of the transcription start site; 2) be close to or thousands of base pairs away from the promoter (Figure 30.14); and 3) occur on either strand of the DNA. Enhancers contain DNA sequences called "response elements" that bind specific TFs that function as transcriptional activators. By bending or looping the DNA, these enhancer-binding factors can interact with other transcription factors bound to a promoter and with *RNA polymerase II*, thereby stimulating transcription (see Figure 30.13B). [Note: Silencers are similar to enhancers in that they act over long distances; however, they reduce gene expression.]

c. Inhibitors of RNA polymerase II: This enzyme is inhibited by α-amanitin—a potent toxin produced by the poisonous mushroom <u>Amanita</u> <u>phalloides</u> (sometimes called "death cap"). α-Amanitin forms a tight complex with the *polymerase*, thereby inhibiting mRNA synthesis and, ultimately, protein synthesis.

3. RNA polymerase III: This enzyme synthesizes tRNA, 5S rRNA, and some snRNA and snoRNA.

B. Mitochondrial RNA polymerase

Mitochondria contain a single *RNA polymerase* that more closely resembles bacterial *RNA polymerase* than the eukaryotic enzyme.

V. POSTTRANSCRIPTIONAL MODIFICATION OF RNA

A primary transcript is the initial, linear, RNA copy of a transcription unit—the segment of DNA between specific initiation and termination sequences. The primary transcripts of both prokaryotic and eukaryotic tRNA and rRNA are posttranscriptionally modified by cleavage of the original transcripts by *ribonucleases*. tRNAs are then further modified to help give each species its unique identity. In contrast, prokaryotic mRNA is generally identical to its primary transcript, whereas eukaryotic mRNA is extensively modified both co- and posttranscriptionally.

A. Ribosomal RNA

rRNAs of both prokaryotic and eukaryotic cells are generated from long precursor molecules called pre-rRNAs. The 23S, 16S, and 5S rRNA of prokaryotes are produced from a single pre-rRNA molecule, as are the 28S, 18S, and 5.8S rRNA of eukaryotes (Figure 30.15). [Note: Eukaryotic 5S rRNA is synthesized by *RNA polymerase III* and modified separately.] The pre-rRNAs are cleaved by *ribonucleases* to yield intermediate-sized pieces of rRNA, which are further processed (trimmed by *exonucleases* and modified at some bases and riboses) to produce the required RNA species. [Note: In eukaryotes, rRNA genes are found in long, tandem arrays. rRNA synthesis and processing occur in the nucleolus, with base and sugar modifi-

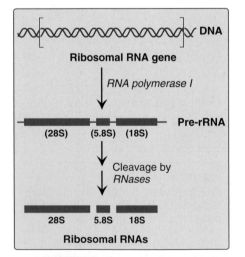

Figure 30.15
Posttranscriptional processing of eukaryotic ribosomal RNA by *ribonucleases* (*RNases*).

cations facilitated by small nucleolar RNAs (snoRNA). Some of the proteins destined to become components of the ribosome associate with pre-rRNA prior to and during its modification.]

B. Transfer RNA

Both eukaryotic and prokaryotic tRNA are also made from longer precursor molecules that must be modified (Figure 30.16). Sequences at both ends of the molecule are removed and, if present, an intron (see below) is removed from the anticodon loop by *nucleases*. Other posttranscriptional modifications include addition of a –CCA sequence by *nucleotidyltransferase* to the 3'-terminal end of tRNA, and modification of bases at specific positions to produce the "unusual bases" characteristic of tRNA (see p. 292).

C. Eukaryotic mRNA

The collection of all the primary transcripts synthesized in the nucleus by *RNA polymerase II* is known as heterogeneous nuclear RNA (hnRNA). The pre-mRNA components of hnRNA undergo extensive co- and posttranscriptional modification in the nucleus. These modifications usually include:

1. **5' "Capping":** This is the first of the processing reactions for pre-mRNA (Figure 30.17). The cap is a 7-methylguanosine attached "backward" to the 5'-terminal end of the mRNA, forming an unusual 5'→5' triphosphate linkage. Creation of the cap requires removal of the γ phosphate from the 5'-triphosphate of the pre-mRNA, followed by addition of GMP (from GTP) by the nuclear enzyme *guanylyltransferase*. Methylation of this terminal guanine occurs in the cytosol, and is catalyzed by *guanine-7-methyltransferase*. S-adenosylmethionine is the source of the methyl group

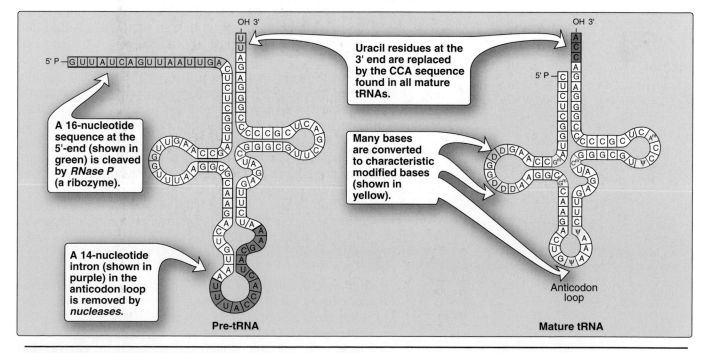

Figure 30.16
A. Primary tRNA transcript. B. Functional tRNA after posttranscriptional modification. Modified bases include D (dihydrouracil), ψ (pseudouracil), and ᵐ, which means that the base has been methylated.

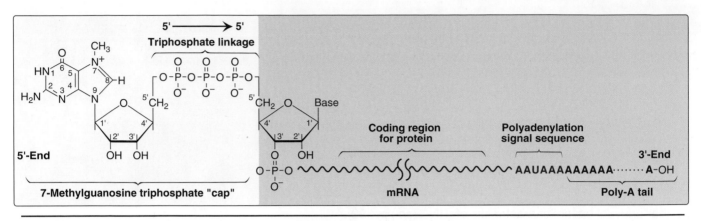

Figure 30.17
Posttranscriptional modification of mRNA showing the 7-methylguanosine cap and poly-A tail.

(see p. 264). Additional methylation steps may occur. The addition of this 7-methylguanosine "cap" helps stabilize the mRNA, and permits initiation of translation (see p. 439). Eukaryotic mRNAs lacking the cap are not efficiently translated.

2. **Addition of a poly-A tail:** Most eukaryotic mRNA (with several notable exceptions, including those coding for the histones) have a chain of 40–200 adenine nucleotides attached to the 3'-end (see Figure 30.17). This poly-A tail is not transcribed from the DNA, but rather is added after transcription by the nuclear enzyme, *polyadenylate polymerase*, using ATP as the substrate. The mRNA is cleaved downstream of a consensus sequence, called the polyadenylation signal sequence (AAUAAA), found near the 3'-end of the RNA, and the poly-A tail is added to the new 3'-end. These tails help stabilize the mRNA, facilitate its exit from the nucleus, and aid in translation. After the mRNA enters the cytosol, the poly-A tail is gradually shortened.

3. **Removal of introns:** Maturation of eukaryotic mRNA usually involves the removal of RNA sequences (introns, or intervening sequences), which do not code for protein from the primary transcript. The remaining coding sequences, the exons, are joined together to form the mature mRNA. The process of removing introns and joining exons is called splicing. The molecular complex that accomplishes these tasks is known as the spliceosome. A few eukaryotic primary transcripts contain no introns, for example, those from histone genes. Others contain a few introns, whereas some, such as the primary transcripts for the α chains of collagen, contain more than 50 intervening sequences that must be removed before mature mRNA is ready for translation.

   a. **Role of snRNAs:** In association with proteins, uracil-rich small nuclear RNAs (snRNA) form small nuclear ribonucleoprotein particles (snRNPs, or "snurps" designated as U1, U2, etc.) that mediate splicing. They facilitate the removal of introns by forming base pairs with the consensus sequences at each end of the intron (Figure 30.18).

Systemic lupus erythematosus, an often fatal inflammatory disease, results from an autoimmune response in which individuals produce antibodies against their own nuclear proteins such as snRNPs.

b. Mechanism of splicing: The binding of snRNPs brings the sequences of the neighboring exons into the correct alignment for splicing. The 2'-OH group of an adenosine (A) residue (known as the branch site) in the intron attacks the phosphate at the 5'-end of the intron (splice donor site), forming an unusual 2'→5' phosphodiester bond and creating a "lariat" structure (see Figure 30.18). The newly freed 3'-OH of exon 1 attacks the 5'-phosphate at the splice acceptor site, forming a phosphodiester bond that joins exons 1 and 2. The excised intron is released as a lariat, which is typically degraded. [Note: The GU and AG sequences at the beginning and end, respectively, of introns are invariant.] After introns have been removed and exons joined, the mature mRNA molecules leave the nucleus and pass into the cytosol through pores in the nuclear membrane. [Note: The introns in tRNA (see Figure 30.16) are removed by a different mechanism.]

c. Effect of splice site mutations: Mutations at splice sites can lead to improper splicing and the production of aberrant proteins. It is estimated that 15% of all genetic diseases are a result of mutations that affect RNA splicing. For example, mutations that cause the incorrect splicing of β-globin mRNA are responsible for some cases of β–thalassemia—a disease in which the production of the β-globin protein is defective (see p. 38).

4. Alternative splicing of mRNA molecules: The pre-mRNA molecules from some genes can be spliced in alternative ways in different tissues. This produces multiple variations of the mRNA and, therefore, of its protein product (Figure 30.19). This appears to be a mechanism for producing a diverse set of proteins from a limited set of genes. For example, in eukaryotic cells the mRNA for tropomyosin, an actin filament-binding protein of the cytoskeleton (and of the contractile apparatus in muscle cells), undergoes extensive tissue-specific alternative splicing with production of multiple isoforms of the tropomyosin protein.

VI. CHAPTER SUMMARY

There are three major types of RNA that participate in the process of protein synthesis: **ribosomal RNA (rRNA)**, **transfer RNA (tRNA)**, and **messenger RNA (mRNA)** (Figure 30.20). They are unbranched polymers of nucleotides, but differ from DNA by containing **ribose** instead of deoxyribose and **uracil** instead of thymine. **rRNA** is a component of the **ribosomes**. **tRNA** serves as an "adaptor" molecule that carries a spe-

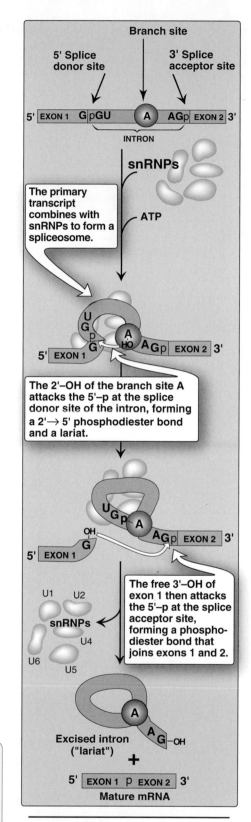

Figure 30.18
Splicing. snRNP = small nuclear ribonucleoprotein particle.

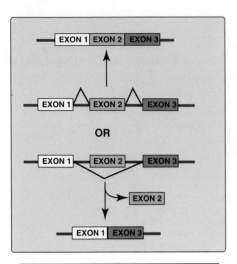

Figure 30.19
Alternative splicing patterns in eukaryotic mRNA.

cific amino acid to the site of protein synthesis. **mRNA** carries genetic information from the nuclear DNA to the cytosol, where it is used as the template for protein synthesis. The process of RNA synthesis is called **transcription**, and its substrates are **ribonucleoside triphosphates**. The enzyme that synthesizes RNA is **RNA polymerase,** which is a multisubunit enzyme. In **prokaryotic** cells, the **core enzyme** has five subunits—2α, 1β, $1\beta'$, and 1Ω—and possesses **5'→3' polymerase activity** that **elongates** the growing RNA strand. This enzyme requires an additional subunit—sigma (σ) **factor**—that recognizes the nucleotide sequence (**promoter** region) at the beginning of a length of DNA that is to be transcribed. This region contains characteristic **consensus nucleotide sequences** that are highly conserved and include the **Pribnow box** and the **−35 sequence**. Another protein—rho (ρ) **factor**—is required for **termination** of transcription of some genes. There are three distinct classes of RNA polymerase in the nucleus of eukaryotic cells. **RNA polymerase I** synthesizes the precursor of large rRNA in the nucleolus. **RNA polymerase II** synthesizes the precursors for mRNA and some ncRNAs in the nucleoplasm, and **RNA polymerase III** produces the precursors of **tRNA** in the nucleoplasm. In both prokaryotes and eukaryotes, RNA polymerase does not require a primer, and has no proofreading activity. **Promoters** for genes transcribed by **RNA polymerase II** contain consensus sequences, such as the **TATA** or **Hogness box**, the **CAAT box**, and the **GC box.** They serve as binding sites for proteins called **general transcription factors**, which, in turn, interact with each other and with RNA polymerase II. **Enhancers** are DNA sequences that increase the rate of initiation of transcription by binding **specific transcription factors** that serve as transcription activators. Eukaryotic transcription requires that the **chromatin** be accessible. **A primary transcript** is a linear copy of a **transcription unit**—the segment of DNA between specific initiation and termination sequences. The primary transcripts of both prokaryotic and eukaryotic tRNA and rRNA are **posttranscriptionally modified** by cleavage of the original transcripts by ribonucleases. **rRNA** of both prokaryotic and eukaryotic cells are synthesized from long precursor molecules called **preribosomal RNA**. These precursors are cleaved and trimmed by ribonucleases, producing the three largest rRNA, and bases and sugars are modified. Eukaryotic 5S rRNA is synthesized by *RNA polymerase III* , and is modified separately. Prokaryotic mRNA is generally identical to its primary transcript, whereas eukaryotic mRNA is extensively modified co- and posttranscriptionally. For example, a **7-methylguanosine "cap"** is attached to the 5'-terminal end of the mRNA through a 5'→5' linkage. A **long poly-A tail**—not transcribed from the DNA—is attached to the 3'-end of most mRNA. Most eukaryotic mRNAs also contain **intervening sequences (introns)** that must be removed to make the mRNA functional. Their removal, as well as the **joining of expressed sequences (exons)**, requires a **spliceosome** composed of **small, nuclear ribonucleoprotein particles** that mediate the process of **splicing**. Eukaryotic mRNA is monocistronic, containing information from just one gene. Prokaryotic and eukaryotic tRNA are also made from longer precursor molecules. If present, an intron is removed by nucleases, and both ends of the molecule are trimmed by ribonucleases. A **3'-CCA** sequence is added, and bases at specific positions are modified, producing "unusual" bases.

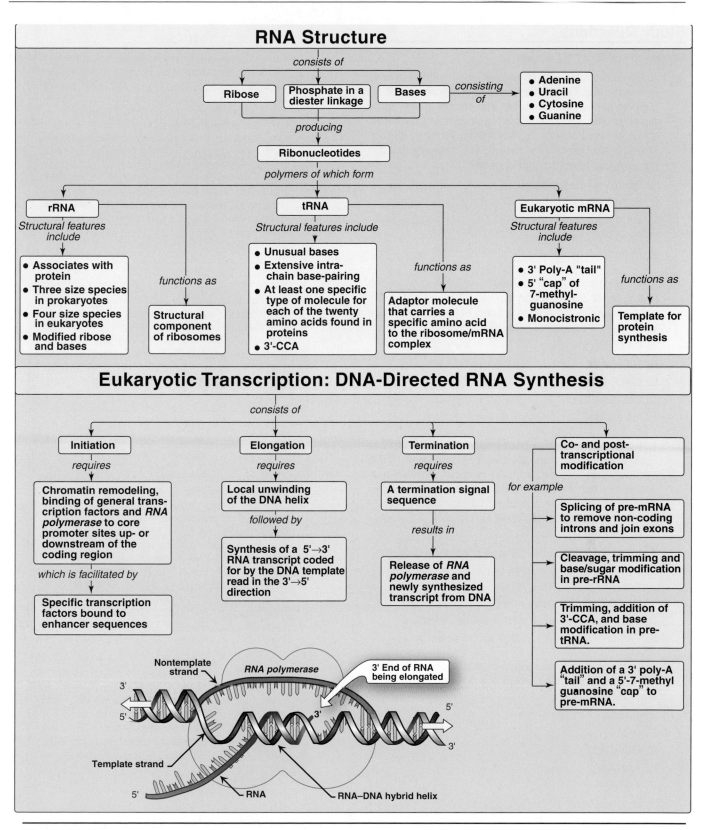

Figure 30.20
Key concept map for RNA structure and synthesis.

Study Questions

Choose the ONE correct answer.

30.1 A 1-year-old male with chronic anemia is found to have β-thalassemia. Genetic analysis shows that one of his β-globin genes has a mutation that creates a new splice acceptor site 19 nucleotides upstream of the normal splice acceptor site of the first intron. Which of the following best describes the new mRNA molecule that can be produced from this mutant gene?

A. Exon 1 will be too short.

B. Exon 1 will be too long.

C. Exon 2 will be too short.

D. Exon 2 will be too long.

E. Exon 2 will be missing.

Correct answer = D. Because the mutation creates an additional splice acceptor site (the 3'-end) upstream of the normal acceptor site of intron 1, the 19 nucleotides that are usually found at the 3'-end of the excised intron 1 lariat can remain behind as part of exon 2. Exon 2 can, therefore, have these extra 19 nucleotides at its 5'-end. The presence of these extra nucleotides in the coding region of the mutant mRNA molecule will prevent the ribosome from translating the message into a normal β-globin protein molecule. Those mRNA for which the normal splice site is used to remove the first intron will be normal, and their translation will produce normal β-globin protein.

30.2 The base sequence of the strand of DNA used as the template for transcription is GATCTAC. What is the base sequence of the RNA product? (All sequences are written 5'→ 3' according to standard convention.)

A. CTAGATG.

B. GTAGATC.

C. GAUCUAC.

D. CUAGAUG.

E. GUAGAUC.

Correct answer = E. The RNA product has a sequence that is complementary to the template strand and identical to the coding strand of DNA. Uracil (U) is found in RNA in place of the thymine (T) in DNA. Thus, the DNA template 5'-GATCTAC-3' would produce the RNA product 3'-CUAGAUG-5' or, written correctly in the standard direction, 5'-GUAGAUC-3'.

30.3 A 4-year-old child who becomes easily tired and has trouble walking is diagnosed with Duchenne muscular dystrophy, an X-linked recessive disorder. Genetic analysis shows that the patient's gene for the muscle protein dystrophin contains a mutation in its promoter region. Of the choices listed, which would be the most likely effect of this mutation?

A. Initiation of dystrophin transcription will be defective.

B. Termination of dystrophin transcription will be defective.

C. Capping of dystrophin mRNA will be defective.

D. Splicing of dystrophin mRNA will be defective.

E. Tailing of dystrophin mRNA will be defective.

Correct answer = A. Mutations in the promoter typically prevent formation of the RNA polymerase II transcription complex, resulting in a decrease in the initiation of mRNA synthesis. A deficiency of dystrophin mRNA will result in a deficiency in the production of the dystrophin protein. Capping, splicing and tailing defects are not a consequence of promoter mutations. They can, however, result in mRNA with decreased stability (capping and tailing defects), or a mRNA in which too many or too few introns have been removed (splicing defects)

30.4 A mutation to this sequence in eukaryotic mRNA will affect the process by which the 3'-end poly-A tail is added to the mRNA.

A. CAAT

B. CCA

C. GGGGCG

D. AAUAAA

E. TATAAA

Correct answer = D. An endonuclease cleaves mRNA just downstream of this polyadenylation signal, creating a new 3'-end to which the *pol A polymerase* adds the poly-A tail using ATP as the substrate in a template-independent process. CAAT, GGGGCGT, and TATAAA are sequences found in promoters for *RNA polymerase II*. CCA is added to the 3'-end of tRNA by *nucleotidyl transferase*.

Protein Synthesis

31

I. OVERVIEW

Genetic information, stored in the chromosomes and transmitted to daughter cells through DNA replication, is expressed through transcription to RNA and, in the case of messenger RNA (mRNA), subsequent translation into proteins (polypeptide chains, Figure 31.1). The pathway of protein synthesis is called translation because the "language" of the nucleotide sequence on the mRNA is translated into the "language" of an amino acid sequence. The process of translation requires a genetic code, through which the information contained in the nucleic acid sequence is expressed to produce a specific sequence of amino acids. Any alteration in the nucleic acid sequence may result in an incorrect amino acid being inserted into the polypeptide chain, potentially causing disease or even death of the organism. Newly made proteins undergo a number of processes to achieve their functional form. They must fold properly, and misfolding can result in degradation of the protein. Many proteins are covalently modified to activate them or alter their activities. Finally, proteins are targeted to their final intra- or extracellular destinations by signals present in the proteins themselves.

II. THE GENETIC CODE

The genetic code is a dictionary that identifies the correspondence between a sequence of nucleotide bases and a sequence of amino acids. Each individual "word" in the code is composed of three nucleotide bases. These genetic words are called codons.

A. Codons

Codons are presented in the mRNA language of adenine (A), guanine (G), cytosine (C), and uracil (U). Their nucleotide sequences are always written from the 5'-end to the 3'-end. The four nucleotide bases are used to produce the three-base codons. There are, therefore, 64 different combinations of bases, taken three at a time (a triplet code) as shown in Figure 31.2.

1. **How to translate a codon:** This table (or "dictionary") can be used to translate any codon and, thus, to determine which amino acids are coded for by an mRNA sequence. For example, the codon 5'-AUG-3' codes for methionine (see Figure 31.2). [Note: AUG is

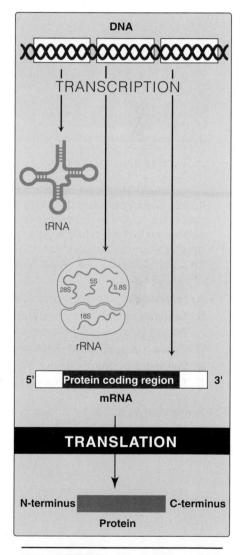

Figure 31.1
Protein synthesis or translation.

431

5' - BASE	MIDDLE BASE				3' - BASE
	U	**C**	**A**	**G**	
U	Phe	Ser	Tyr	Cys	U
	Phe	Ser	Tyr	Cys	C
	Leu	Ser	Stop	Stop	A
	Leu	Ser	Stop	Trp	G
C	Leu	Pro	His	Arg	U
	Leu	Pro	His	Arg	C
	Leu	Pro	Gln	Arg	A
	Leu	Pro	Gln	Arg	G
A	Ile	Thr	Asn	Ser	U
	Ile	Thr	Asn	Ser	C
	Ile	Thr	Lys	Arg	A
	Met	Thr	Lys	Arg	G
G	Val	Ala	Asp	Gly	U
	Val	Ala	Asp	Gly	C
	Val	Ala	Glu	Gly	A
	Val	Ala	Glu	Gly	G

1 These four rows show 16 amino acids whose codons begin (5') with A.

2 This column shows 16 amino acids whose codons have the middle base U.

3 These four, separated rows show 16 amino acids whose codons end (3') with G.

4 The codon 5'-AUG-3' designates methionine (Met).

Figure 31.2
Use of the genetic code table to translate the codon AUG.

the initiation (start) codon for translation.] Sixty-one of the 64 codons code for the 20 common amino acids.

2. **Termination ("stop" or "nonsense") codons:** Three of the codons, UAG, UGA, and UAA, do not code for amino acids, but rather are termination codons. When one of these codons appears in an mRNA sequence, synthesis of the polypeptide coded for by that mRNA stops.

B. Characteristics of the genetic code

Usage of the genetic code is remarkably consistent throughout all living organisms. It is assumed that once the standard genetic code evolved in primitive organisms, any mutation that altered its meaning would have caused the alteration of most, if not all, protein sequences, resulting in lethality. Characteristics of the genetic code include the following:

1. **Specificity:** The genetic code is specific (unambiguous), that is, a particular codon always codes for the same amino acid.

2. **Universality:** The genetic code is virtually universal, that is, its specificity has been conserved from very early stages of evolution, with only slight differences in the manner in which the code is translated. [Note: An exception occurs in mitochondria, in which a few codons have meanings different than those shown in Figure 31.2, for example, UGA codes for Trp.]

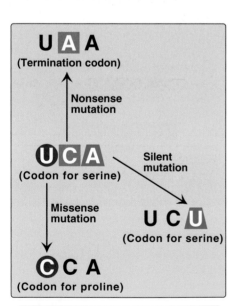

Figure 31.3
Possible effects of changing a single nucleotide base in the coding region of an mRNA chain.

3. **Degeneracy:** The genetic code is degenerate (sometimes called redundant). Although each codon corresponds to a single amino acid, a given amino acid may have more than one triplet coding for it. For example, arginine is specified by six different codons (see Figure 31.2). Only Met and Trp have just one coding triplet.

4. **Nonoverlapping and commaless:** The genetic code is nonoverlapping and commaless, that is, the code is read from a fixed starting point as a continuous sequence of bases, taken three at a time. For example, AGCUGGAUACAU is read as AGC/UGG/AUA/CAU without any "punctuation" between the codons.

C. Consequences of altering the nucleotide sequence:

Changing a single nucleotide base on the mRNA chain (a "point mutation") can lead to any one of three results (Figure 31.3):

1. **Silent mutation:** The codon containing the changed base may code for the same amino acid. For example, if the serine codon UCA is given a different third base—U—to become UCU, it still codes for serine. This is termed a "silent" mutation.

2. **Missense mutation:** The codon containing the changed base may code for a different amino acid. For example, if the serine codon UCA is given a different first base—C—to become CCA, it will code for a different amino acid, in this case, proline. The substitution of an incorrect amino acid is called a "missense" mutation.

3. **Nonsense mutation:** The codon containing the changed base may become a termination codon. For example, if the serine codon UCA is given a different second base—A—to become UAA, the new codon causes termination of translation at that point, and the production of a shortened (truncated) protein. The creation of a termination codon at an inappropriate place is called a "nonsense" mutation.

4. **Other mutations:** These can alter the amount or structure of the protein produced by translation.

   a. **Trinucleotide repeat expansion:** Occasionally, a sequence of three bases that is repeated in tandem will become amplified in number, so that too many copies of the triplet occur. If this happens within the coding region of a gene, the protein will contain many extra copies of one amino acid. For example, amplification of the CAG codon leads to the insertion of many extra glutamine residues in the huntingtin protein, causing the neurodegenerative disorder, Huntington disease (Figure 31.4). The additional glutamines result in unstable proteins that cause the accumulation of protein aggregates. If the trinucleotide repeat expansion occurs in the untranslated regions of a gene, the result can be a decrease in the amount of protein produced as seen, for example, in fragile X syndrome and myotonic dystrophy. [Note: In fragile X syndrome, the most common cause of intellectual disability, the expansion results in gene silencing through DNA hypermethylation (see p. 460).]

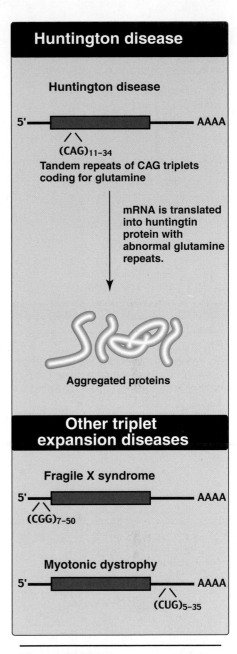

Figure 31.4
Role of tandem triplet repeats in mRNA causing Huntington disease and other triplet expansion diseases.

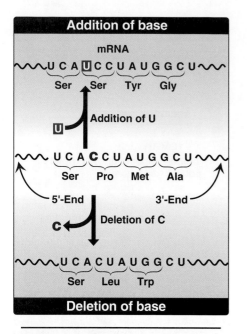

Figure 31.5
Frame-shift mutations as a result of addition or deletion of a base can cause an alteration in the reading frame of mRNA.

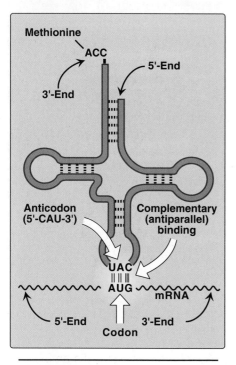

Figure 31.6
Complementary, antiparallel binding of the anticodon for methionyl-tRNA (CAU) to the mRNA codon for methionine (AUG), the initiation codon for translation.

b. Splice site mutations: Mutations at splice sites (see p. 427) can alter the way in which introns are removed from pre-mRNA molecules, producing aberrant proteins. [Note: In myotonic dystrophy gene silencing is the result of splicing alterations.]

c. Frame-shift mutations: If one or two nucleotides are either deleted from or added to the coding region of a message sequence, a frame-shift mutation occurs and the reading frame is altered. This can result in a product with a radically different amino acid sequence, or a truncated product due to the creation of a termination codon (Figure 31.5). If three nucleotides are added, a new amino acid is added to the peptide or, if three nucleotides are deleted, an amino acid is lost. Loss of three nucleotides maintains the reading frame, but can result in serious pathology. For example, cystic fibrosis (CF), a hereditary disease that primarily affects the pulmonary and digestive systems, is most commonly caused by deletion of three nucleotides from the coding region of a gene, resulting in the loss of phenylalanine at the 508th position (ΔF508) in the protein encoded by that gene. This ΔF508 mutation prevents normal folding of the CF transmembrane conductance regulator (CFTR) protein, leading to its destruction by the proteasome (see p. 247). CFTR normally functions as a chloride channel in epithelial cells, and its loss results in the production of thick, sticky secretions in the lungs and pancreas, leading to lung damage and digestive deficiencies (see p. 248). In over 70% of Caucasians with CF, the ΔF508 mutation is the cause of the disease.

III. COMPONENTS REQUIRED FOR TRANSLATION

A large number of components are required for the synthesis of a protein. These include all the amino acids that are found in the finished product, the mRNA to be translated, transfer RNA (tRNA) for each of the amino acids, functional ribosomes, energy sources, and enzymes, as well as protein factors needed for initiation, elongation, and termination steps of polypeptide chain synthesis.

A. Amino acids

All the amino acids that eventually appear in the finished protein must be present at the time of protein synthesis. [Note: If one amino acid is missing (for example, if the diet does not contain an essential amino acid, see p. 261), translation stops at the codon specifying that amino acid. This demonstrates the importance of having all the essential amino acids in sufficient quantities in the diet to ensure continued protein synthesis.]

B. Transfer RNA

At least one specific type of tRNA is required for each amino acid. In humans, there are at least 50 species of tRNA, whereas bacteria contain 30–40 species. Because there are only 20 different amino acids commonly carried by tRNA, some amino acids have more than one specific tRNA molecule. This is particularly true of those amino acids that are coded for by several codons.

1. **Amino acid attachment site:** Each tRNA molecule has an attachment site for a specific (cognate) amino acid at its 3'-end (Figure 31.6). The carboxyl group of the amino acid is in an ester linkage with the 3'-hydroxyl of the ribose portion of the adenosine (A) nucleotide in the —CCA sequence at the 3'-end of the tRNA. [Note: When a tRNA has a covalently attached amino acid, it is said to be charged; when it does not, it is said to be uncharged. The amino acid attached to the tRNA molecule is said to be activated.]

2. **Anticodon:** Each tRNA molecule also contains a three-base nucleotide sequence—the anticodon—that pairs with a specific codon on the mRNA (see Figure 31.6). This codon specifies the insertion into the growing peptide chain of the amino acid carried by that tRNA.

C. Aminoacyl-tRNA synthetases

This family of enzymes is required for attachment of amino acids to their corresponding tRNAs. Each member of this family recognizes a specific amino acid and all the tRNAs that correspond to that amino acid (isoaccepting tRNAs). *Aminoacyl-tRNA synthetases* catalyze a two-step reaction that results in the covalent attachment of the carboxyl group of an amino acid to the 3'-end of its corresponding (cognate) tRNA. The overall reaction requires adenosine triphosphate (ATP), which is cleaved to adenosine monophosphate (AMP) and inorganic pyrophosphate (PP$_i$) (Figure 31.7). The extreme specificity of the *synthetase* in recognizing both the amino acid and its cognate tRNA contributes to the high fidelity of translation of the genetic message. In addition, the *synthetases* have a "proofreading" or "editing" activity that can remove amino acids from the enzyme or the tRNA molecule.

D. Messenger RNA

The specific mRNA required as a template for the synthesis of the desired polypeptide chain must be present. [Note: Interactions between proteins that bind the 5'-cap (eIF-4 proteins) and the 3'-tail (poly-A binding proteins) of eukaryotic mRNA mediate circularization of the mRNA and likely prevent the use of incompletely processed mRNA in translation.]

E. Functionally competent ribosomes

Ribosomes are large complexes of protein and ribosomal RNA (rRNA, Figure 31.8). They consist of two subunits—one large and one small—whose relative sizes are given in terms of their sedimentation coefficients, or S (Svedberg) values. [Note: Because the S values are determined both by shape as well as molecular mass, their numeric values are not strictly additive. For example, the prokaryotic 50S and 30S ribosomal subunits together form a 70S ribosome. The eukaryotic 60S and 40S subunits form an 80S ribosome.]

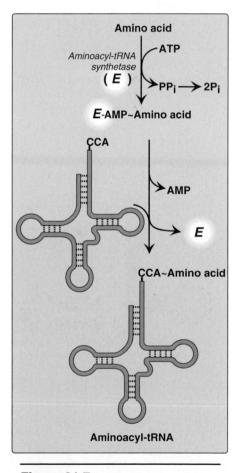

Figure 31.7
Attachment of a specific amino acid to its corresponding tRNA by *aminoacyl-tRNA synthetase* (*E*).

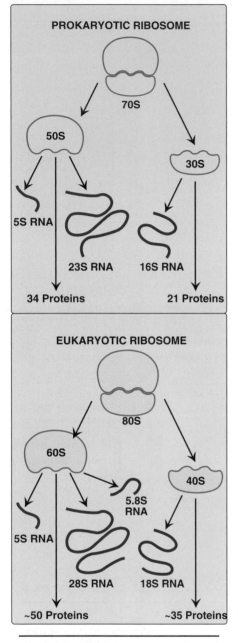

Figure 31.8
Ribosomal composition. (The number of proteins in the eukaryotic ribosomal subunits varies somewhat from species to species.)

Prokaryotic and eukaryotic ribosomes are similar in structure, and serve the same function, namely, as the macromolecular complexes in which the synthesis of proteins occurs.

> The small ribosomal subunit binds mRNA and is responsible for the accuracy of translation by ensuring correct base-pairing between the codon in the mRNA and the anticodon of the tRNA. The large ribosomal subunit catalyzes formation of the peptide bonds that link amino acid residues in a protein.

1. **Ribosomal RNA:** As discussed on p. 418, prokaryotic ribosomes contain three size species of rRNA, whereas eukaryotic ribosomes contain four (see Figure 31.8). The rRNAs are generated from a single pre-rRNA by the action of *ribonucleases*, and some bases and riboses are modified.

2. **Ribosomal proteins:** Ribosomal proteins are present in considerably greater numbers in eukaryotic ribosomes than in prokaryotic ribosomes. These proteins play a number of roles in the structure and function of the ribosome and its interactions with other components of the translation system.

3. **A, P, and E sites on the ribosome:** The ribosome has three binding sites for tRNA molecules—the A, P, and E sites—each of which extends over both subunits. Together, they cover three neighboring codons. During translation, the A site binds an incoming aminoacyl-tRNA as directed by the codon currently occupying this site. This codon specifies the next amino acid to be added to the growing peptide chain. The P-site codon is occupied by peptidyl-tRNA. This tRNA carries the chain of amino acids that has already been synthesized. The E site is occupied by the empty tRNA as it is about to exit the ribosome. (See Figure 31.13 for an illustration of the role of the A, P, and E sites in translation.)

4. **Cellular location of ribosomes:** In eukaryotic cells, the ribosomes are either "free" in the cytosol or are in close association with the endoplasmic reticulum (which is then known as the "rough" endoplasmic reticulum, or RER). The RER-associated ribosomes are responsible for synthesizing proteins that are to be exported from the cell, as well as those that are destined to become incorporated into plasma, endoplasmic reticulum, or Golgi membranes, or imported into lysosomes (see p. 169 for an overview of the latter process). Cytosolic ribosomes synthesize proteins required in the cytosol itself, or destined for the nucleus, mitochondria, and peroxisomes. [Note: Mitochondria contain their own set of ribosomes and their own unique, circular DNA. Most mitochondrial proteins, however, are encoded by nuclear DNA, synthesized in the cytosol, and posttranslationally targeted to mitochondria.]

F. Protein factors

Initiation, elongation, and termination (or release) factors are required for peptide synthesis. Some of these protein factors perform a catalytic function, whereas others appear to stabilize the synthetic machinery. [Note: A number of the factors are G proteins, and thus are active when bound to GTP and inactive when bound to GDP.]

G. ATP and GTP are required as sources of energy

Cleavage of four high-energy bonds is required for the addition of one amino acid to the growing polypeptide chain: two from ATP in the *aminoacyl-tRNA synthetase* reaction—one in the removal of PP$_i$, and one in the subsequent hydrolysis of the PP$_i$ to inorganic phosphate by *pyrophosphatase*—and two from GTP—one for binding the aminoacyl-tRNA to the A site and one for the translocation step (see Figure 31.13, p. 440). [Note: Additional ATP and GTP molecules are required for initiation in eukaryotes, whereas an additional GTP molecule is required for termination in both eukaryotes and prokaryotes.]

IV. CODON RECOGNITION BY tRNA

Correct pairing of the codon in the mRNA with the anticodon of the tRNA is essential for accurate translation (see Figure 31.6). Some tRNAs recognize more than one codon for a given amino acid.

A. Antiparallel binding between codon and anticodon

Binding of the tRNA anticodon to the mRNA codon follows the rules of complementary and antiparallel binding, that is, the mRNA codon is "read" 5'→3' by an anticodon pairing in the "flipped" (3'→5') orientation (Figure 31.9). [Note: Nucleotide sequences are ALWAYS assumed to be written in the 5' to 3' direction unless otherwise noted.]

B. Wobble hypothesis

The mechanism by which tRNAs can recognize more than one codon for a specific amino acid is described by the "wobble" hypothesis in which the base at the 5'-end of the anticodon (the "first" base of the anticodon) is not as spatially defined as the other two bases. Movement of that first base allows nontraditional (less stringent) base-pairing with the 3'-base of the codon (the "last" base of the codon). This movement is called "wobble" and allows a single tRNA to recognize more than one codon. Examples of these flexible pairings are shown in Figure 31.9. The result of wobble is that there need not be 61 tRNA species to read the 61 codons that code for amino acids.

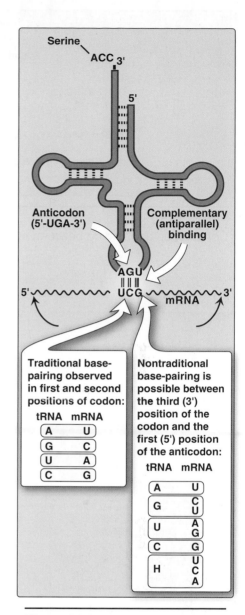

Figure 31.9
Wobble: Nontraditional base-pairing between the 5'-nucleotide (first nucleotide) of the anticodon with the 3'-nucleotide (last nucleotide) of the codon. H = hypoxanthine (the product of adenine deamination).

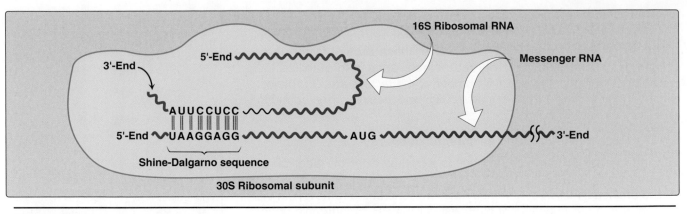

Figure 31.10
Complementary binding between prokaryotic mRNA Shine-Dalgarno sequence and 16S rRNA.

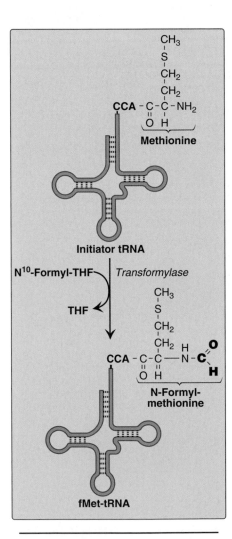

Figure 31.11
Generation of the initiator N-formyl-methionyl-tRNA (fMet-tRNA).

V. STEPS IN PROTEIN SYNTHESIS

The process of protein synthesis translates the three-letter alphabet of nucleotide sequences on mRNA into the 20-letter alphabet of amino acids that constitute proteins. The mRNA is translated from its 5'-end to its 3'-end, producing a protein synthesized from its amino-terminal end to its carboxyl-terminal end. Prokaryotic mRNAs often have several coding regions, that is, they are polycistronic (see p. 418). Each coding region has its own initiation and termination codon and produces a separate species of polypeptide. In contrast, each eukaryotic mRNA has only one coding region, that is, it is monocistronic. The process of translation is divided into three separate steps: initiation, elongation, and termination. Eukaryotic protein synthesis resembles that of prokaryotes in most aspects. Individual differences are noted in the text.

> One important difference is that translation and transcription are coupled in prokaryotes, with translation starting before transcription is completed. Coupling is a consequence of the lack of a nuclear membrane in prokaryotes.

A. Initiation

Initiation of protein synthesis involves the assembly of the components of the translation system before peptide bond formation occurs. These components include the two ribosomal subunits, the mRNA to be translated, the aminoacyl-tRNA specified by the first codon in the message, GTP (which provides energy for the process), and initiation factors that facilitate the assembly of this initiation complex (see Figure 31.13). [Note: In prokaryotes, three initiation factors are known (IF-1, IF-2, and IF-3), whereas in eukaryotes, there are over ten (designated eIF to indicate eukaryotic origin). Eukaryotes also require ATP for initiation.] There are two mechanisms by which the ribosome recognizes the nucleotide sequence (AUG) that initiates translation:

1. **Shine-Dalgarno sequence:** In E. coli, a purine-rich sequence of nucleotide bases, known as the Shine-Dalgarno (SD) sequence, is located six to ten bases upstream of the initiating AUG codon on the mRNA molecule—that is, near its 5'-end. The 16S rRNA component of the 30S ribosomal subunit has a nucleotide sequence near its 3'-end that is complementary to all or part of the SD sequence. Therefore, the 5' end of the mRNA and the 3'-end of the 16S rRNA can form complementary base pairs, thus facilitating the positioning of the small (30S) ribosomal subunit on the mRNA in close proximity to the initiating AUG codon (Figure 31.10). Eukaryotic messages do not have SD sequences. In eukaryotes, the 40S ribosomal subunit (aided by members of the eIF-4 family of proteins) binds close to the cap structure at the 5-end of the mRNA and moves down the mRNA until it encounters the initiator AUG. This "scanning" process requires ATP.

2. **Initiation codon:** The initiating AUG is recognized by a special initiator tRNA. Recognition is facilitated by IF-2-GTP in prokaryotes and eIF-2-GTP (plus additional eIFs) in eukaryotes. The charged initiator tRNA enters the P site on the small subunit. [Note: The initiator tRNA is the only tRNA recognized by eIF-2, and the only tRNA to go directly to the P site.] In bacteria and in mitochondria, the initiator tRNA carries an N-formylated methionine (Figure 31.11). After methionine is attached to the initiator tRNA, the formyl group is added by the enzyme *transformylase*, which uses N^{10}-formyl tetrahydrofolate (see p. 267) as the carbon donor. In eukaryotes, the initiator tRNA carries a methionine that is not formylated. [Note: In both prokaryotic and eukaryotic cells, this N-terminal methionine is usually removed before translation is completed.] The large ribosomal subunit then joins the complex, and a functional ribosome is formed with the charged initiating tRNA in the P site, and the A site empty. The GTP on (e)IF-2 gets hydrolyzed to GDP. A guanine nucleotide exchange factor facilitates the reactivation of (e)IF-2-GDP.

B. Elongation

Elongation of the polypeptide chain involves the addition of amino acids to the carboxyl end of the growing chain. During elongation, the ribosome moves from the 5'-end to the 3'-end of the mRNA that is being translated. Delivery of the aminoacyl-tRNA whose codon appears next on the mRNA template in the ribosomal A site is facilitated in E. coli by elongation factors EF-Tu-GTP and EF-Ts, and requires GTP hydrolysis. [Note: In eukaryotes, comparable elongation factors are EF-1α–GTP and EF-1βγ. Both EF-Ts and EF-1βγ function as nucleotide exchange factors.] The formation of the peptide bond is catalyzed by *peptidyltransferase*, an activity intrinsic to the 23S rRNA found in the large (50S) ribosomal subunit (Figure 31.12). [Note: Because this rRNA catalyzes the reaction, it is referred to as a ribozyme.] After the peptide bond has been formed, what was attached to the tRNA at the P site is now linked to the amino acid on the tRNA at the A site. The ribosome then advances three nucleotides toward the 3'-end of the mRNA. This process is known as translocation and, in prokaryotes, requires the

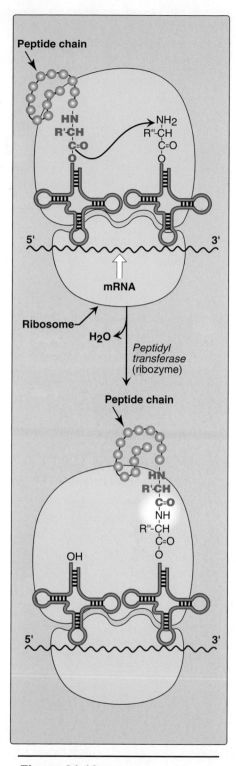

Figure 31.12
Formation of a peptide bond. [Note: The tRNA carrying the peptide chain is in the P site of the ribosome, and the tRNA carrying the next amino acid to be incorporated is in the A site.]

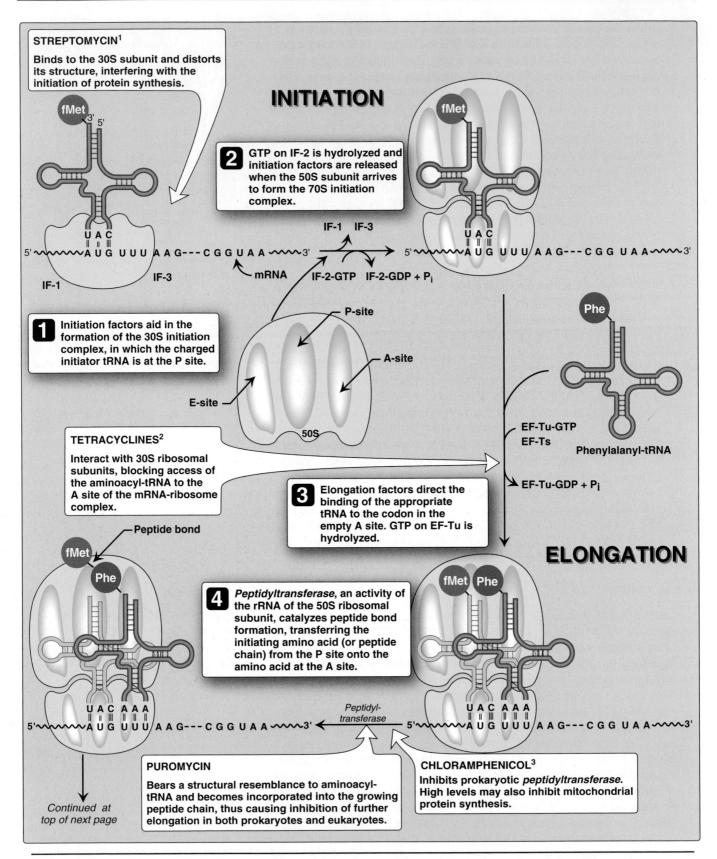

STREPTOMYCIN[1]

Binds to the 30S subunit and distorts its structure, interfering with the initiation of protein synthesis.

INITIATION

fMet

2 GTP on IF-2 is hydrolyzed and initiation factors are released when the 50S subunit arrives to form the 70S initiation complex.

IF-1   IF-3

5'—AUG UUU AAG---CGG UAA——3'

mRNA   IF-2-GTP   IF-2-GDP + P_i

IF-1   IF-3

1 Initiation factors aid in the formation of the 30S initiation complex, in which the charged initiator tRNA is at the P site.

P-site

A-site

E-site

50S

Phe

EF-Tu-GTP
EF-Ts

Phenylalanyl-tRNA

EF-Tu-GDP + P_i

TETRACYCLINES[2]

Interact with 30S ribosomal subunits, blocking access of the aminoacyl-tRNA to the A site of the mRNA-ribosome complex.

3 Elongation factors direct the binding of the appropriate tRNA to the codon in the empty A site. GTP on EF-Tu is hydrolyzed.

ELONGATION

Peptide bond

fMet
Phe

fMet   Phe

4 *Peptidyltransferase*, an activity of the rRNA of the 50S ribosomal subunit, catalyzes peptide bond formation, transferring the initiating amino acid (or peptide chain) from the P site onto the amino acid at the A site.

UAC AAA   UAC AAA

5'—AUG UUU AAG---CGG UAA——3'   *Peptidyl-transferase*   5'—AUG UUU AAG---CGG UAA——3'

Continued at top of next page

PUROMYCIN

Bears a structural resemblance to aminoacyl-tRNA and becomes incorporated into the growing peptide chain, thus causing inhibition of further elongation in both prokaryotes and eukaryotes.

CHLORAMPHENICOL[3]

Inhibits prokaryotic *peptidyltransferase*. High levels may also inhibit mitochondrial protein synthesis.

Figure 31.13 (*Continued on the next page*)
Steps in prokaryotic protein synthesis (translation).

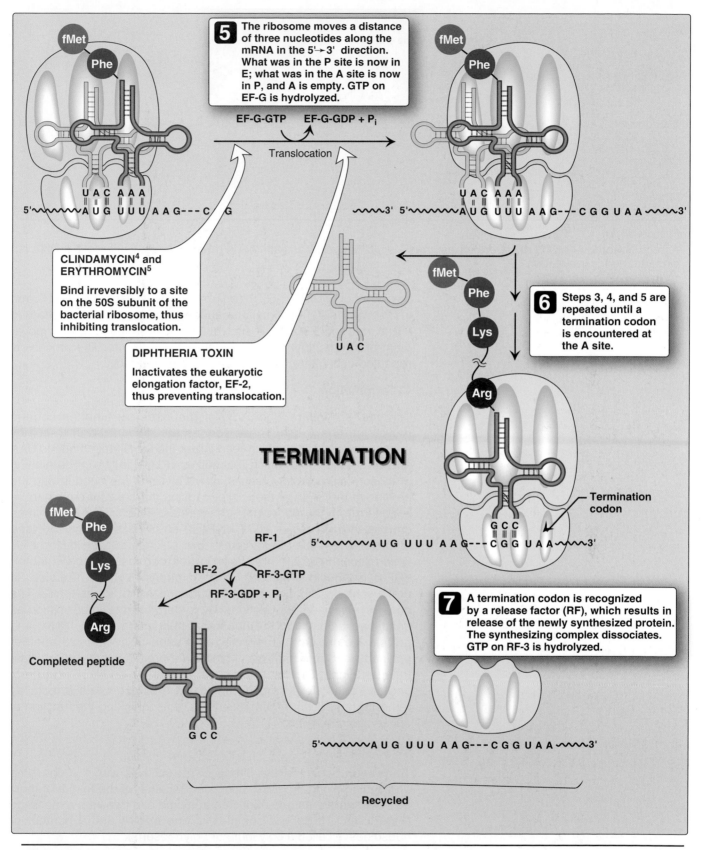

Figure 31.13 (*Continued from the previous page*)

[1-5]See Chapter 32 in *Lippincott's Illustrated Reviews: Pharmacology* for a more detailed discussion of antibiotics that inhibit bacterial protein synthesis.

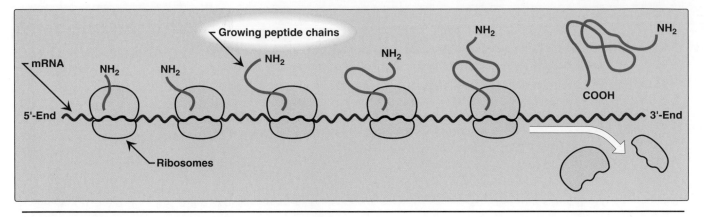

Figure 31.14
A polyribosome consists of several ribosomes simultaneously translating one mRNA. [Note: Eukaryotic mRNA is circularized for translation.]

participation of EF-G-GTP (eukaryotic cells use EF-2-GTP) and GTP hydrolysis. Translocation causes movement of the uncharged tRNA from the P to the E site (before being released), and movement of the peptidyl-tRNA from the A to the P site. The process is repeated until a termination codon is encountered.

C. Termination

Termination occurs when one of the three termination codons moves into the A site. These codons are recognized in E. coli by release factors: RF-1, which recognizes the termination codons UAA and UAG, and RF-2, which recognizes UGA and UAA. The binding of these release factors results in hydrolysis of the bond linking the peptide to the tRNA at the P site, causing the nascent protein to be released from the ribosome. A third release factor, RF-3-GTP then causes the release of RF-1 or RF-2 as GTP is hydrolyzed (see Figure 31.13). [Note: Eukaryotes have a single release factor, eRF, which recognizes all three termination codons. A second factor, eRF-3, is thought to function like the prokaryotic RF-3.] The steps in prokaryotic protein synthesis are summarized in Figure 31.13. The newly synthesized polypeptide may undergo further modification as described below, and the ribosomal subunits, mRNA, tRNA, and protein factors can be recycled and used to synthesize another polypeptide. Some antibiotic inhibitors of protein synthesis are illustrated in Figure 31.13, as is diphtheria toxin. In addition, ricin (from castor beans) is a very potent toxin that exerts its effects by removing an adenine from 28S rRNA, thus inhibiting the function of eukaryotic ribosomes.

D. Polysomes

Translation begins at the 5'-end of the mRNA, with the ribosome proceeding along the RNA molecule. Because of the length of most mRNAs, more than one ribosome at a time can translate a message (Figure 31.14). Such a complex of one mRNA and a number of ribosomes is called a polysome or polyribosome.

E. Protein targeting

Although most protein synthesis is initiated in the cytoplasm of eukaryotic cells, many proteins are destined to perform their functions extracellularly or within specific cellular organelles. Such proteins usually contain amino acid sequences that direct these proteins to their final locations. For example, proteins destined for secretion from the cell are targeted during their synthesis (cotranslationally) targeted to the RER (see p. 436) by the presence of an N-terminal hydrophobic signal sequence. Proteins targeted after synthesis (posttranslationally) include nuclear proteins, which contain a short, basic "nuclear localization signal," and mitochondrial proteins, which contain an amphipathic, α-helical "mitochondrial entry sequence."

F. Regulation of translation

Gene expression is most commonly regulated at the transcriptional level; however, translation may also be regulated. An important mechanism by which this is accomplished in eukaryotes is by covalent modification of eIF-2: phosphorylated eIF-2 is inactive. In both eukaryotes and prokaryotes, regulation can also be achieved through proteins that bind mRNA and either inhibit its use by blocking translation or extend its use by protecting it from degradation. For a more detailed discussion of the regulation of translation, see p. 454.

VI. CO- AND POSTTRANSLATIONAL MODIFICATION OF POLYPEPTIDE CHAINS

Many polypeptide chains are covalently modified, either while they are still attached to the ribosome (cotranslational) or after their synthesis has been completed (posttranslational). These modifications may include removal of part of the translated sequence, or the covalent addition of one or more chemical groups required for protein activity. Some types of posttranslational modifications are listed below.

A. Trimming

Many proteins destined for secretion from the cell are initially made as large, precursor molecules that are not functionally active. Portions of the protein chain must be removed by specialized endoproteases, resulting in the release of an active molecule. The cellular site of the cleavage reaction depends on the protein to be modified. Some precursor proteins are cleaved in the endoplasmic reticulum or the Golgi apparatus, others are cleaved in developing secretory vesicles (for example, insulin, see Figure 23.4, p. 309), and still others, such as collagen (see p. 47), are cleaved after secretion. Zymogens are inactive precursors of secreted enzymes (including the proteases required for digestion). They become activated through cleavage when they reach their proper sites of action. For example, the pancreatic zymogen, trypsinogen, becomes activated to *trypsin* in the small intestine (see Figure 19.5, p. 249). The synthesis of proteases as zymogens protects the cell from being digested by its own products.

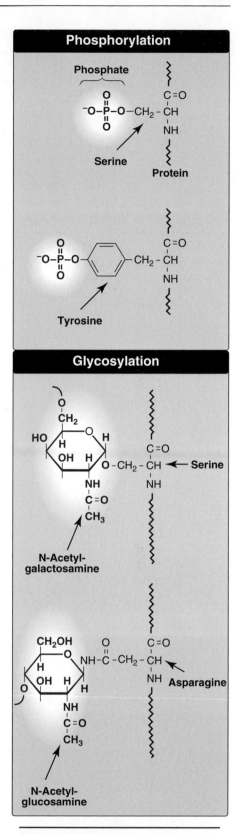

Figure 31.15 *(continued on next page)* Covalent modifications of some amino acid residues.

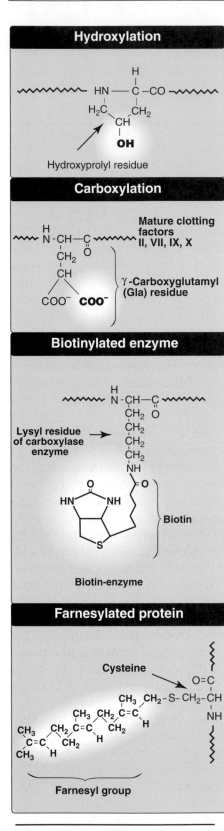

Figure 31.15 *(continued from previous page)* Covalent modifications of some amino acid residues.

B. Covalent attachments

Proteins may be activated or inactivated by the covalent attachment of a variety of chemical groups. Examples include (Figure 31.15):

1. **Phosphorylation:** Phosphorylation occurs on the hydroxyl groups of serine, threonine, or, less frequently, tyrosine residues in a protein. This phosphorylation is catalyzed by one of a family of protein *kinases* and may be reversed by the action of cellular protein *phosphatases*. The phosphorylation may increase or decrease the functional activity of the protein. Several examples of these phosphorylation reactions have been previously discussed (for example, see Chapter 11, p. 125, for the regulation of synthesis and degradation of glycogen).

2. **Glycosylation:** Many of the proteins that are destined to become part of a plasma membrane or to be secreted from the cell, have carbohydrate chains attached to the amide nitrogen of asparagine (N-linked) or the hydroxyl groups of serine, threonine, or hydroxylysine (O-linked). N-glycosylation occurs in the endoplasmic reticulum and O-glycosyation in the Golgi. (The process of producing such glycoproteins was discussed on p. 165.) Glycosylation is also used to target proteins to the matrix of lysosomes. Lysosomal acid hydrolases are modified by the phosphorylation of mannose residues at carbon 6 (see p. 169).

3. **Hydroxylation:** Proline and lysine residues of the α chains of collagen are extensively hydroxylated by vitamin C–dependent *hydroxylases* in the endoplasmic reticulum (see p. 47).

4. **Other covalent modifications:** These may be required for the functional activity of a protein. For example, additional carboxyl groups can be added to glutamate residues by vitamin K–dependent carboxylation (see p. 389). The resulting γ-carboxyglutamate (Gla) residues are essential for the activity of several of the blood-clotting proteins. Biotin is covalently bound to the ε-amino groups of lysine residues of biotin-dependent enzymes that catalyze carboxylation reactions, such as *pyruvate carboxylase* (see p. 119). Attachment of lipids, such as farnesyl groups, can help anchor proteins to membranes. Histone proteins can be reversibly acetylated (see p. 409).

C. Protein folding

Proteins must fold to assume their functional state. Folding can be spontaneous (as a result of the primary structure), or facilitated by proteins known as "chaperones" (see p. 20).

D. Protein degradation

Proteins that are defective, for example, misfolded, or destined for rapid turnover are often marked for destruction by ubiquitination—the attachment of chains of a small, highly conserved protein, called ubiquitin (see p. 246). Proteins marked in this way are rapidly degraded by a cellular component known as the proteasome, which is a macromolecular, ATP-dependent, proteolytic system located in the cytosol. [Note: The ΔF508 mutation seen in CF causes misfolding of the CFTR protein, resulting in its proteasomal degradation.]

VII. CHAPTER SUMMARY

Codons are composed of three nucleotide bases presented in the mRNA language of **A**, **G**, **C**, and **U**. They are always written **5'→3'**. Of the 64 possible three-base combinations, 61 code for the 20 common amino acids and three signal termination of protein synthesis (**translation**). Altering the nucleotide sequence in a codon can cause **silent mutations** (the altered codon codes for the original amino acid), **missense mutations** (the altered codon codes for a different amino acid), or **nonsense mutations** (the altered codon is a termination codon). Characteristics of the genetic code include **specificity**, **universality**, and **degeneracy**, and it is **nonoverlapping** and **commaless**. Requirements for protein synthesis include all the amino acids that eventually appear in the finished protein, at least one specific type of tRNA for each amino acid, one **aminoacyl-tRNA synthetase for** each amino acid, the mRNA coding for the protein to be synthesized, fully competent **ribosomes**, **protein factors** needed for initiation, elongation, and termination of protein synthesis, and **ATP** and **GTP** as energy sources. tRNA has an attachment site for a specific amino acid at its 3'-end, and an anticodon region that can recognize the codon specifying the amino acid the tRNA is carrying. **Ribosomes** are large complexes of protein and rRNA. They consist of **two subunits**. Each ribosome has three binding sites for tRNA molecules—the A, P, and E sites that cover three neighboring codons. The **A-site** codon binds an **incoming aminoacyl-tRNA**, the **P-site** codon is occupied by **peptidyl-tRNA**, and the **E site** is occupied by the **empty tRNA** as it is about to exit the ribosome. Recognition of an mRNA codon is accomplished by the tRNA **anticodon**. The anticodon binds to the codon following the rules of **complementarity** and **antiparallel** binding. (Nucleotide sequences are ALWAYS assumed to be written in the 5' to 3' direction unless otherwise noted.) The **"wobble" hypothesis** states that the first (5') base of the anticodon is not as spatially defined as the other two bases. Movement of that first base allows nontraditional base-pairing with the last (3') base of the codon, thus allowing a single tRNA to recognize more than one codon for a specific amino acid. For **initiation of protein synthesis**, the components of the translation system are assembled, and mRNA associates with the small ribosomal subunit. The process requires **initiation factors**. In **prokaryotes**, a purine-rich region of the mRNA (the **Shine-Dalgarno sequence**) base-pairs with a complementary sequence on 16S rRNA, resulting in the positioning of the small subunit on the mRNA so that translation can begin. The **5'-cap on eukaryotic mRNA** is used to position the small subunit on the mRNA. The **initiation codon** is **AUG**; **N-formylmethionine** is the initiating amino acid in prokaryotes, whereas methionine is in eukaryotes. The polypeptide chain is elongated by the addition of amino acids to the carboxyl end of its growing chain. The process requires elongation factors. The formation of the peptide bond is catalyzed by **peptidyltransferase**, which is an activity intrinsic to the rRNA of the large subunit. Following peptide bond formation, the ribosome advances along the mRNA in the **5'→3' direction** to the next codon (translocation). Because of the length of most mRNAs, more than one ribosome at a time can translate a message, forming a **polysome**. Termination begins when one of the three termination codons moves into the A site. These codons are recognized by **release factors**. The newly synthesized protein is released from the ribosomal complex, and the ribosome is dissociated from the mRNA. Initiation, elongation, and termination are driven by the hydrolysis of GTP; initiation in eukaryotes also requires ATP for scanning. Numerous **antibiotics** interfere with the process of protein synthesis. Many polypeptide chains are covalently modified during or after translation. Such modifications include **removal of amino acids**, **phosphorylation,** which may activate or inactivate the protein, **glycosylation**, which plays a role in protein targeting, or **hydroxylation** such as that seen in collagen. Proteins must fold to achieve their functional form. Folding can be spontaneous or facilitated by **chaperones**. Proteins that are defective, for example misfolded, or destined for rapid turnover are marked for destruction by the attachment of chains of a small, highly conserved protein called **ubiquitin**. Ubiquitinated proteins are rapidly degraded by a cytosolic complex known as the **proteasome**.

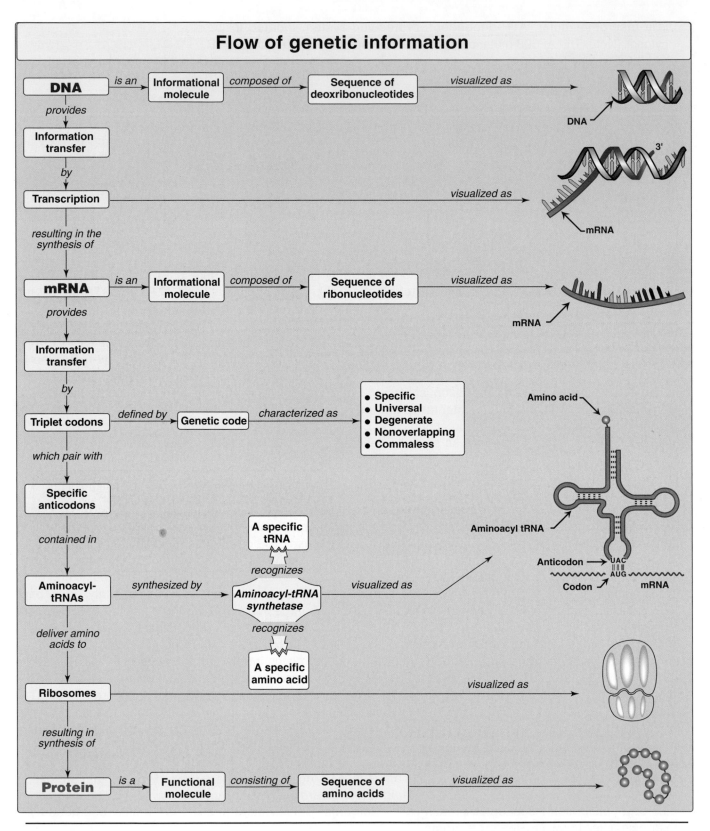

Figure 31.16
Key concept map for protein synthesis.

Study Questions

Choose the ONE correct answer.

31.1 A 20-year-old anemic man is found to have an abnormal form of β-globin (Hemoglobin Constant Spring) that is 172 amino acids long, rather than the 141 found in the normal protein. Which of the following point mutations is consistent with this abnormality?

A. UAA → CAA.

B. UAA → UAG.

C. CGA → UGA.

D. GAU → GAC.

E. GCA → GAA.

Correct answer = A. Mutating the normal stop codon for β-globin from UAA to CAA causes the ribosome to insert a glutamine at that point. It will continue extending the protein chain until it comes upon the next stop codon further down the message, resulting in an abnormally long protein. A change from UAA to UAG would simply change one termination codon for another and would have no effect on the protein. The replacement of CGA (arginine) with UGA (stop) would cause the protein to be too short. GAU and GAC both encode aspartate and would cause no change in the protein. Changing GCA (alanine) to GAA (glutamate) would not change the size of the protein product.

31.2 A pharmaceutical company is studying a new antibiotic that inhibits bacterial protein synthesis. When this antibiotic is added to an in vitro protein synthesis system that is translating the mRNA sequence AUGUUUUUUUAG, the only product formed is the dipeptide fMet-Phe. What step in protein synthesis is most likely inhibited by the antibiotic?

A. Initiation.

B. Binding of charged tRNA to the ribosomal A site.

C. Peptidyltransferase activity.

D. Ribosomal translocation.

E. Termination.

Correct answer = D. Because fMet-Phe is made, the ribosomes must be able to complete initiation, bind Phe-tRNA to the A site, and use peptidyltransferase activity to form the first peptide bond. Because the ribosome is not able to proceed any further, ribosomal movement (translocation) is most likely the inhibited step. The ribosome is, therefore, frozen before it reaches the termination codon of this message.

31.3 A tRNA molecule that is supposed to carry cysteine (tRNA^{cys}) is mischarged, so that it actually carries alanine (ala-tRNA^{cys}). Assuming no correction occurs, what will be the fate of this alanine residue during protein synthesis?

A. It will be incorporated into a protein in response to an alanine codon.

B. It will be incorporated into a protein in response to a cysteine codon.

C. It will remain attached to the tRNA, as it cannot be used for protein synthesis.

D. It will be incorporated randomly at any codon.

E. It will be chemically converted to cysteine by cellular enzymes.

Correct answer = B. Once an amino acid is attached to a tRNA molecule, only the anticodon of that tRNA determines the specificity of incorporation. The mischarged alanine will, therefore, be incorporated in the protein at a position determined by a cysteine codon.

31.4 In a patient with cystic fibrosis caused by the ΔF508 mutation, the mutant cystic fibrosis transmembrane conductance regulator (CFTR) protein folds incorrectly. The patient's cells modify this abnormal protein by attaching ubiquitin molecules to it. What is the fate of this modified CFTR protein?

A. It performs its normal function, as the ubiquitin largely corrects for the effect of the mutation.

B. It is secreted from the cell.

C. It is placed into storage vesicles.

D. It is degraded by the proteasome.

E. It is repaired by cellular enzymes.

Correct answer = D. Ubiquitination usually marks old, damaged, or misfolded proteins for destruction by the proteasome. There is no known cellular mechanism for repair of damaged proteins.

31.5 Many antimicrobials inhibit protein translation. Which of the following antimicrobials is correctly paired with its mechanism of action?

    A. Tetracyclines inhibit peptidyltransferase.

    B. Diphtheria toxin binds to the 30S ribosomal subunit.

    C. Puromycin inactivates EF-2.

    D. Clindamycin binds to the 30S ribosomal subunit.

    E. Erythromycin binds to the 50S ribosomal subunit.

> Correct answer = E. Erythromycin and clindamycin both bind the 50S ribosomal subunit. Tetracyclines inhibit the 30S ribosomal subunit (chloramphenicol inhibits peptidyl transferase). Diphtheria toxin binds EF-2, inactivating it through ADP ribosylation. Puromycin has structure similar to that of aminoacyl-tRNA. It is incorporated into the growing chain, and inhibits further elongation of the peptide chain.

31.6 Translation of a synthetic polyribonucleotide containing the repeating sequence CAA in a cell-free protein-synthesizing system produces three homopolypeptides: polyglutamine, polyasparagine, and polythreonine. If the codon for glutamine and asparagine are CAA and AAC, respectively, which of the following triplets is the codon for threonine?

    A. AAC.

    B. CAA.

    C. CAC.

    D. CCA.

    E. ACA.

> Correct answer = E. The synthetic polynucleotide sequence of CAACAACAACAA . . could be read by the in vitro protein synthesizing system starting at the first C, the first A, or the second A. In the first case, the first triplet codon would be CAA, which codes glutamine; in the second case, the first triplet codon would be AAC, which codes for asparagine; in the last case, the first triplet codon would be ACA, which codes for threonine.

31.7 Which of the following is required for both prokaryotic and eukaryotic protein synthesis?

    A. Binding of the small ribosomal subunit to the Shine-Dalgarno sequence.

    B. fMet~tRNA.

    C. Movement of the mRNA out of the nucleus and into the cytoplasm.

    D. Recognition of the 5'-cap by initiation factors.

    E. Translocation of the peptidyl-tRNA from the A site to the P site.

> Correct answer = E. In both prokaryotes and eukaryotes, continued translation (elongation) requires movement of the peptidyl-tRNA from the A site to the P site to allow the next aminoacyl-tRNA to enter the A site. Only prokaryotes have a Shine-Dalgarno sequence and use fMet, whereas only eukaryotes have a nucleus and co- and posttranscriptionally process their mRNA.

31.8 Why is the genetic code described as both degenerate and unambiguous?

> A given amino acid can be coded for by more than one codon (degenerate code), but a given codon codes for just one particular amino acid (unambiguous code).

31.9 α1-Antitrypsin (A1AT) deficiency can result in emphysema, a lung pathology, because the action of elastase, a serine protease, is unopposed. Deficiency of A1AT in the lungs is the consequence of its retention in (rather than secretion from) the liver, the site of its synthesis. Proteins such as A1AT that are designed to be secreted are best characterized by which of the following statements?

    A. Their synthesis is initiated on the smooth endoplasmic reticulum.

    B. They contain a mannose 6-phosphate targeting signal.

    C. They always contain methionine as the N-terminal amino acid.

    D. They are produced from translation products that have an N-terminal hydrophobic signal sequence.

    E. They contain no sugars with O-glycosidic linkages because their synthesis does not involve the Golgi apparatus.

> Answer = D. Synthesis of secreted proteins is begun on free (cytosolic) ribosomes. As the N-terminal hydrophobic signal sequence of the peptide emerges from the ribosome, it is bound by the signal recognition particle, taken to the rough endoplasmic reticulum (RER), threaded into the lumen, and removed as translation continues. The proteins move through the RER and the Golgi, and undergo processing such as N-glycosylation (RER) and O-glycosylation (Golgi). In the Golgi, they are packaged in secretory vesicles and released from the cell. The smooth endoplasmic reticulum is associated with synthesis of lipids, not proteins, and has no ribosomes attached. Phosphorylation at carbon 6 of terminal mannose residues in glycoproteins targets these proteins (acid hydrolases) to lysosomes. The N-terminal methionine is removed from most proteins during processing.

Regulation of Gene Expression

32

I. OVERVIEW

Gene expression refers to the multistep process that ultimately results in the production of a functional gene product, either ribonucleic acid (RNA) or protein. The first step in gene expression—the use of deoxyribonucleic acid (DNA) for the synthesis of RNA (transcription)—is the primary site of regulation in both prokaryotes and eukaryotes. In eukaryotes, however, gene expression also involves extensive posttranscriptional and posttranslational processes, as well as actions that influence access to particular regions of the DNA. Each of these steps can be regulated to provide additional control over the kinds and amounts of functional products that are produced.

Not all genes are regulated. For example, genes described as constitutive encode products required for basic cellular functions, and so are continually expressed; they are also known as "housekeeping" genes. Regulated genes, however, are expressed only under certain conditions. They may be expressed in all cells or in only a subset of cells, for example, hepatocytes. The ability to regulate gene expression, that is, to determine if, how much, and when particular gene products will be made, gives the cell control over structure and function. It is the basis for cellular differentiation, morphogenesis, and adaptability of any organism. Control of gene expression is best understood in prokaryotes, but many themes are repeated in eukaryotes. Figure 32.1 lists some common strategies employed in gene regulation.

II. REGULATORY SEQUENCES AND MOLECULES

Regulation of transcription—the initial step in all gene expression—is controlled by regulatory sequences of DNA, usually embedded in the noncoding regions of the genome. The interaction between these DNA segments and regulatory molecules, such as transcription factors, can engage or repress the transcriptional machinery, influencing the kinds and amounts of products that are produced. These DNA sequences flanking a gene are called cis-acting because they influence expression of genes only on the same chromosome (see p. 423). A trans-acting

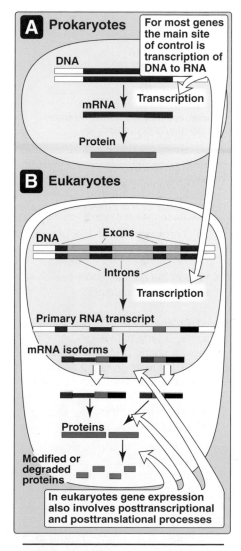

Figure 32.1
Control of gene expression.

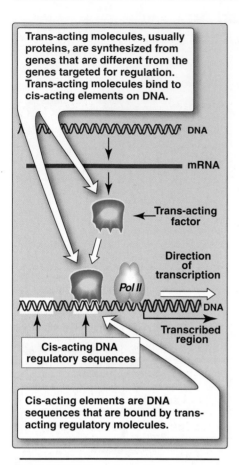

Trans-acting molecules, usually proteins, are synthesized from genes that are different from the genes targeted for regulation. Trans-acting molecules bind to cis-acting elements on DNA.

DNA

mRNA

Trans-acting factor

Direction of transcription

Pol II

DNA

Transcribed region

Cis-acting DNA regulatory sequences

Cis-acting elements are DNA sequences that are bound by trans-acting regulatory molecules.

Figure 32.2
Cis-acting elements and trans-acting molecules. *Pol II = RNA polymerase II.*

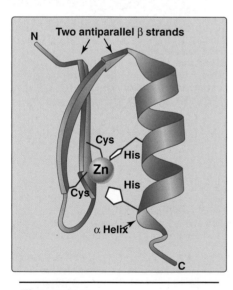

N   Two antiparallel β strands

Cys
His
Zn
His
Cys
α Helix
C

Figure 32.3
Zinc finger is a common motif in proteins that bind DNA.

factor is the regulatory molecule itself, which can diffuse through the cell from its site of synthesis to its DNA-binding site (Figure 32.2). For example, a protein transcription factor (a trans-acting molecule) which regulates a gene on chromosome 6 might itself have been transcribed from a gene on chromosome 11. The binding of proteins to DNA is through structural motifs such as the zinc finger (Figure 32.3), leucine zipper, or helix-turn-helix in the protein. [Note: Some trans-acting factors can negatively affect gene expression.]

III. REGULATION OF PROKARYOTIC GENE EXPRESSION

In prokaryotes such as <u>Escherichia</u> <u>coli</u> (<u>E. coli</u>), regulation of gene expression occurs primarily at the level of transcription and, in general, is mediated by the binding of trans-acting proteins to cis-acting regulatory elements on their single DNA molecule (chromosome). [Note: Regulating the first step in the expression of a gene is an efficient approach, as energy is not wasted making unneeded gene products.] Transcriptional control in prokaryotes can involve the initiation or premature termination of transcription.

A. Transcription of mRNA from bacterial operons

In bacteria, the structural genes that code for proteins involved in a particular metabolic pathway are often found sequentially grouped on the chromosome along with the cis-acting regulatory elements that determine the transcription of these genes. The transcription product is a single polycistronic messenger RNA (mRNA) (see p. 418). The genes are thus coordinately controlled, that is, turned on or off as a unit. This entire package is referred to as an operon.

B. Role of operators in prokaryotic transcription

Prokaryotic operons contain an operator—a segment of DNA that regulates the activity of the structural genes of the operon. If the operator is not bound by a repressor molecule, *RNA polymerase* passes over the operator and reaches the protein-coding genes which it transcribes to mRNA. If a repressor molecule is bound to the operator, the *polymerase* is blocked and does not produce mRNA. As long as the repressor is bound to the operator, no proteins are made. However, when an inducer molecule is present, it binds to the repressor, causing the repressor to change shape so that it no longer binds the operator. When this happens, the *RNA polymerase* can proceed with transcription. One of the best-understood examples is the lactose operon of <u>E. coli</u>, which illustrates both positive and negative regulation (Figure 32.4).

C. The lactose operon

The lactose (lac) operon contains the genes that code for three proteins involved in the catabolism of the disaccharide, lactose: The <u>lacZ</u> gene codes for *β-galactosidase*, which hydrolyzes lactose to galactose and glucose; the <u>lacY</u> gene, which codes for a *permease* that facilitates the movement of lactose into the cell; and the <u>lacA</u> gene that codes for *thiogalactoside transacetylase* whose exact physiologic function is unknown. All of these proteins are produced

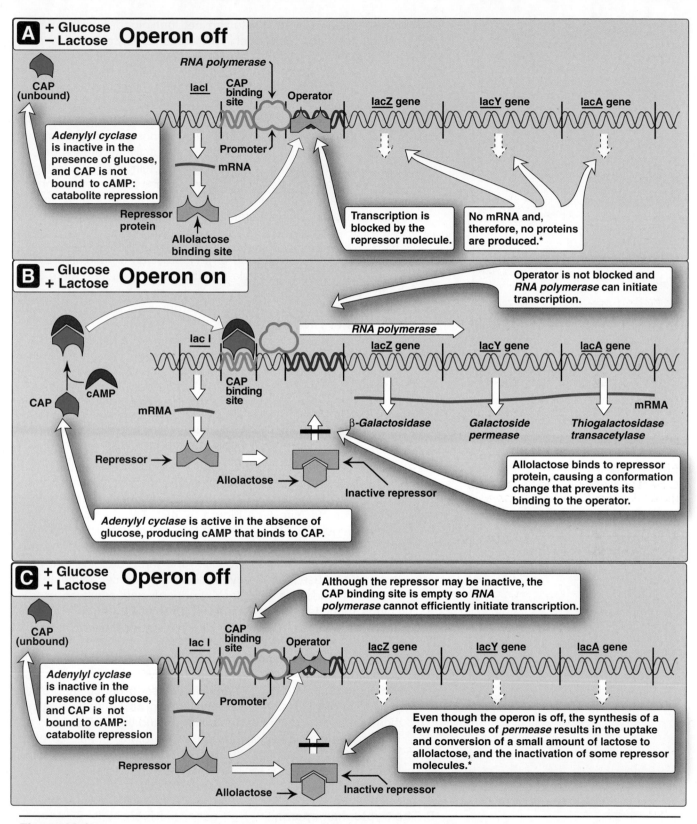

Figure 32.4
The lactose operon of E. coli. *[Note: Even when the operon has been turned off by catabolite repression, the repressor transiently dissociates from the operator at a slow rate, allowing a very low level of expression. The synthesis of a few molecules of *permease* (and β-*galactosidase*) allows the organism to respond rapidly should glucose become unavailable.]

when lactose is available to the cell but glucose is not. [Note: Bacteria use glucose as a fuel in preference to any other sugar.] The regulatory portion of the operon is upstream of the three structural genes, and consists of the promoter (P) region where *RNA polymerase* binds, and two additional sites, the operator (O) site and the CAP site, where regulatory proteins bind. The lacZ, lacY, and lacA genes are expressed only when the O site is empty, and the CAP site is bound by a complex of cyclic adenosine monophosphate (cAMP, see p. 94) and the catabolite gene activator protein or CAP (sometimes called the cAMP regulatory protein or CRP, see Figure 32.4). A regulatory gene, the lacI gene, codes for the repressor protein (a trans-acting factor) that binds to the operator site. [Note: The lacI gene has its own promoter.]

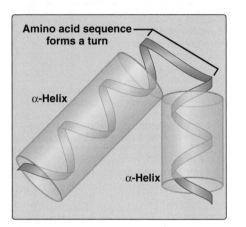

Figure 32.5
Helix-turn-helix motif.

1. **When glucose is the only sugar available:** In this case, the lac operon is repressed (turned off). Repression is mediated by the repressor protein binding via a helix-turn-helix motif (Figure 32.5) to the operator site, which is downstream of the promoter region (see Figure 32.4A). Binding of the repressor interferes with the progress of *RNA polymerase*, and blocks transcription of the structural genes. This is an example of negative regulation.

2. **When only lactose is available:** In this case, the lac operon is induced (maximally expressed or turned on). A small amount of lactose is converted to an isomer, allolactose. This compound is an inducer that binds to the repressor protein, changing its conformation so that it can no longer bind to the operator. In the absence of glucose, *adenylyl cyclase* is active, and sufficient quantities of cAMP are made and bind to the CAP protein. The cAMP–CAP trans-acting complex binds to the CAP-binding site, causing *RNA polymerase* to more efficiently initiate transcription at the promoter site (see Figure 32.4B). This is an example of positive regulation. The transcript is a single polycistronic mRNA molecule that contains three sets of start and stop codons. Translation of the mRNA produces the three proteins that allow lactose to be used for energy production by the cell. [Note: In contrast to the inducible lacZ, lacY, and lacA genes, whose expression is regulated, the lacI gene is constitutive. Its gene product, the repressor protein, is active unless the inducer is present.]

3. **When both glucose and lactose are available:** In this case, transcription of the lac operon is negligible, even if lactose is present at a high concentration. *Adenylyl cyclase* is deactivated in the presence of glucose—a process known as catabolite repression—so no cAMP–CAP complex forms and the CAP-binding site remains empty. *RNA polymerase* is, therefore, unable to effectively initiate transcription, even though the repressor may not be bound to the operator region. Consequently, the three structural genes are not expressed (see Figure 32.4C).

D. The tryptophan operon

The tryptophan (trp) operon codes for five proteins that are required for the synthesis of the amino acid, tryptophan. As with the lac operon, the trp operon is subject to both positive and negative con-

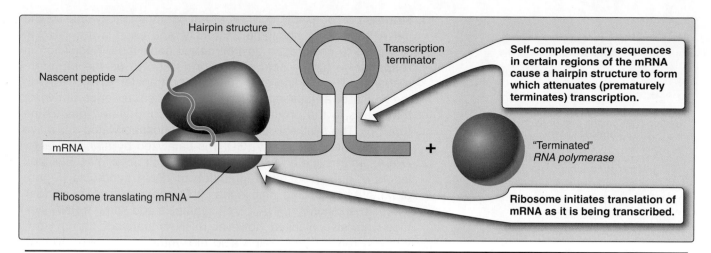

Figure 32.6
Attenuation of transcription of the trp operon when tryptophan is plentiful.

trol. Negative control includes trp itself binding to the repressor protein and facilitating the binding of the repressor to the operator. Repression by trp is not always complete, however, and so unlike the lac operon, the trp operon is also regulated by a process known as attenuation. With attenuation, transcription is initiated but is terminated well before completion (Figure 32.6). If trp is plentiful, transcription initiation that escaped repression by trp is attenuated (stopped) by the formation at the 5'-end of the mRNA of a hairpin (stem-loop) structure like that seen in ρ-independent termination (see p. 421). Transcription and translation are coupled processes in prokaryotes (see p. 438), and, therefore, attenuation also results in the formation of a truncated, nonfunctional peptide product that is rapidly degraded. [Note: If trp is scarce, the operon is expressed. The 5'-end of the mRNA contains two adjacent codons for trp. The lack of trp causes ribosomes to stall at these codons, covering regions of the mRNA required for formation of the attenuation hairpin. This prevents attenuation and thus allows transcription to continue.]

> Transcriptional attenuation can occur in prokaryotes because translation of an mRNA begins before its synthesis is complete. In eukaryotes this does not occur because, as a result of having a membrane-bound nucleus, transcription and translation are spatially and temporally separate processes.

E. Coordination of transcription and translation in prokaryotes

Whereas transcriptional regulation of mRNA production is primary in bacteria, regulation at the level of ribosomal RNA (rRNA) and protein synthesis also occurs, and plays important roles in the microbe's ability to adapt to environmental stress.

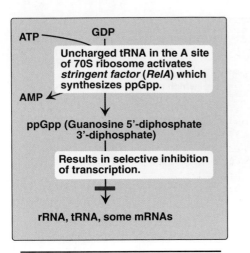

Figure 32.7
Regulation of transcription by the stringent response to amino acid starvation.

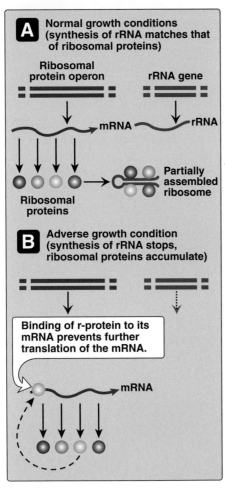

Figure 32.8
Regulation of translation by an excess of ribosomal proteins.

1. **Stringent response:** E. coli has seven operons that synthesize the rRNA needed for ribosome assembly, and each is regulated in response to changes in environmental conditions. Regulation in response to amino acid starvation is known as the stringent response. The binding of an uncharged transfer RNA (tRNA) to the A site of a ribosome (see p. 436) triggers a series of events that leads to the production of polyphosphorylated guanosine (ppGpp). The synthesis of this unusual phosphorylated derivative of guanosine diphosphate (GDP) is catalyzed by *stringent factor (RelA)*, an enzyme physically associated with ribosomes. Elevated levels of ppGpp result in inhibition of rRNA synthesis (Figure 32.7), but how ppGpp inhibits the rRNA operons is as yet unclear. [Note: In addition to rRNA, tRNA synthesis and some mRNA synthesis are also inhibited; however, mRNAs that code for enzymes that are required for amino acid biosynthesis are not inhibited. Thus, transcriptional control by the stringent response ultimately results in down-regulation of protein synthesis until amino acids are again available.]

2. **Regulatory ribosomal proteins:** Operons for ribosomal proteins (r-proteins) can be inhibited by an excess of their own protein products. For each operon, one specific r-protein functions in the repression of translation of the polycistronic mRNA from that operon (Figure 32.8). The r-protein does so by binding to the Shine-Dalgarno (SD) sequence located on the mRNA just upstream of the initiating AUG codon (see p. 439), and acting as a physical impediment to the binding of the small ribosomal subunit to the SD sequence. One r-protein thus inhibits synthesis of all the r-proteins of the operon. This same r-protein also binds to rRNA, and with a higher affinity than for mRNA. If the concentration of rRNA falls, the r-protein then is available to bind its own mRNA and inhibit its translation. This coordinated regulation keeps the synthesis of r-proteins in balance with the transcription of rRNA, so that each is present in appropriate amounts for the formation of ribosomes.

IV. REGULATION OF EUKARYOTIC GENE EXPRESSION

The higher degree of complexity of eukaryotic genomes, as well as the presence of a nuclear membrane, necessitates a wider range of regulatory processes. As with the prokaryotes, the primary site of regulation is at the level of transcription. Again, the theme of trans-acting molecules binding to cis-acting elements is seen. Operons, however, are not found in eukaryotes, which must use alternative strategies to solve the problem of how to coordinately regulate all the genes required for a specific response. In eukaryotes, gene expression is also regulated at multiple levels other than transcription. For example, the major modes of post-transcriptional regulation at the mRNA level are alternative mRNA splicing, control of mRNA stability, and control of translational efficiency. Additional regulation at the protein level occurs by mechanisms that modulate stability, processing, or targeting of the protein.

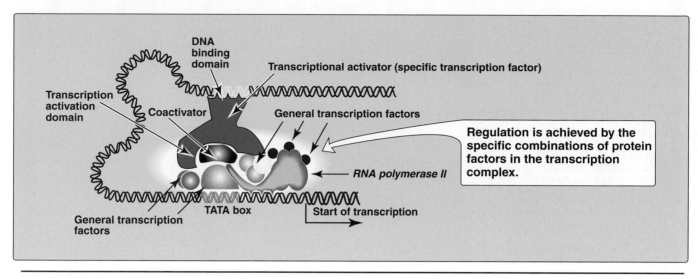

Figure 32.9
Combinatorial control of transcription.

A. Trans-acting molecules

Specific transcription factors are trans-acting DNA-binding proteins that function as transcriptional activators. They have at least two binding domains: the DNA-binding domain described above (see p. 450), and the transcription activation domain. The transcription activation domain allows the binding of other proteins, such as coactivators (for example, *histone acetyltransferases, or HATs,* see Figure 30.11 on p. 422). These facilitate formation of the transcription initiation complex (*RNA polymerase II* plus the general transcription factors, see p. 423) at the promoter, and thus activate transcription (Figure 32.9). Regulation is achieved by the formation of a multiprotein complex bound to DNA, with protein–protein and protein–DNA interactions controlling assembly of the complex. Although activation domains recruit a variety of proteins, the specific effect of any one of them is dependent upon the protein composition of the complex. This is known as combinatorial control. [Note: DNA-binding proteins can also inhibit transcription.]

B. Cis-acting regulatory elements

The need to coordinately regulate a group of genes to effect a particular response is of key importance in multicellular organisms including humans. An underlying theme occurs repeatedly: A protein binds to a regulatory element for each of the genes in the group and coordinately affects the expression of those genes, even if they are on different chromosomes. For example, hormone-response elements (HREs) are cis-acting DNA sequences that bind trans-acting protein factors and regulate gene expression in response to hormonal signals. In general, hormones bind either to intracellular receptors (steroid hormones are an example, see p. 240), or to cell-surface receptors (the peptide hormone, glucagon, is an example, see p. 314).

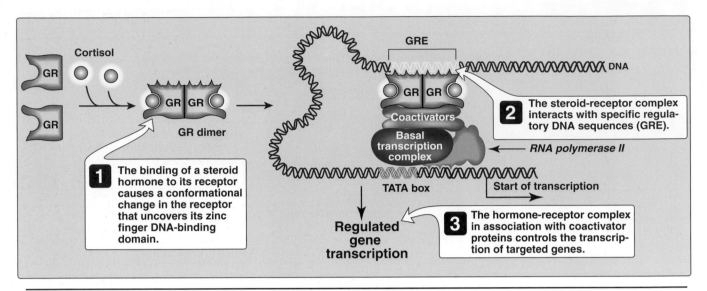

Figure 32.10
Transcriptional regulation by intracellular steroid hormone receptors. GRE = glucocorticoid-response element (an example of a hormone response element); GR = glucocorticoid receptor.

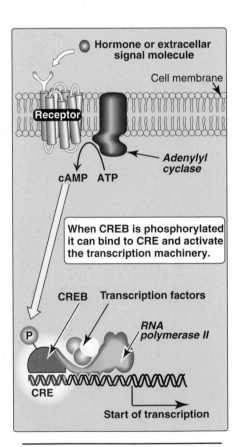

Figure 32.11
Transcriptional regulation by receptors located in the cell membrane.

1. **Regulatory signals mediated by intracellular receptors:** Members of the nuclear receptor superfamily, which includes the glucocorticoid, mineralocorticoid, sex hormone, vitamin D, retinoic acid, and thyroid hormone receptors, all directly influence activity of transcription factors by alteration of the DNA-binding affinity of the factors. This signal transduction pathway is direct, because the receptor and the transcription factor are the same molecule. For example, hydrophobic steroid hormones such as cortisol (a glucocorticoid) bind to soluble receptors (Figure 32.10). Binding of the steroid hormone ligand causes a conformational change in the receptor that activates it. The receptor–ligand complex enters the nucleus, dimerizes, and, in association with coactivators, binds via a zinc finger motif to nuclear DNA at a cis-acting regulatory element, the glucocorticoid-response element (GRE)—an example of an HRE. Each of the cortisol-responsive genes is under the control of its own GRE. Binding of the receptor–hormone complex to the GRE allows coordinate expression of a group of target genes, even when these genes are located on different chromosomes. The GRE can be located upstream or downstream of the genes it regulates, and is able to function at great distances from those genes. The GRE, then, can function as a true enhancer (see p. 424). [Note: If associated with corepressors, hormone-receptor complexes inhibit transcription.]

2. **Regulatory signals mediated by cell-surface receptors:** Cell-surface receptors include those for insulin, epinephrine, and glucagon. Glucagon, for example, is a peptide hormone that binds its G protein-coupled plasma membrane receptor. This extracellular signal is then transduced to intracellular cAMP (Figure 32.11; also see Figure 8.7 on p. 95), which can affect protein expression (and activity) through *protein kinase A*–mediated covalent modification. In response to a rise in cAMP, a trans-acting factor (cAMP-response element-binding protein, or CREB) is phosphorylated

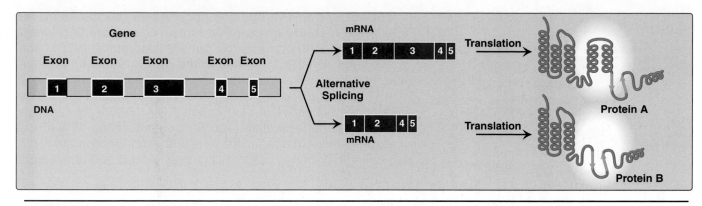

Figure 32.12
Alternative splicing produces multiple related proteins, or isoforms, from a single gene.

and activated. Active CREB binds via a leucine zipper to a cis-acting element, the cAMP-response element (CRE), resulting in the transcription of target genes with CREs in their promoters. [Note: The genes for *phosphoenolpyruvate carboxykinase* and *glucose 6-phosphatase*, key enzymes of gluconeogenesis (see p. 117), are examples of genes up-regulated by the cAMP/CRE/CREB system.]

C. Regulation by co- and posttranscriptional processing of mRNA

Eukaryotic mRNA undergoes several modifications before it is exported from the nucleus to the cytoplasm for use in protein synthesis (see p. 418). Capping at the 5'-end, polyadenylation at the 3'-end, and splicing are essential processing events for the production of a functional eukaryotic messenger from most pre-mRNA (see p. 425), and variations in these events can affect gene expression. In addition, messenger stability also affects gene expression.

1. **Splice-site choice:** Tissue-specific protein products (protein isoforms) can be made from the same pre-mRNA through differential cotranscriptional processing, particularly the use of alternative splice sites (Figure 32.12). For example, tropomyosin (TM) is an actin filament-binding protein that regulates the functions of actin in both muscle and nonmuscle cells. Its pre-mRNA undergoes differential splicing to yield a number of tissue-specific TM isoforms (see p. 427).

> Over 60% percent of the approximately 30,000 genes in the human genome undergo differential splicing. The use of alternative polyadenylation and transcription start sites is also seen in many genes. This explains, at least in part, how 30,000 genes can give rise to over 100,000 proteins.

2. **mRNA editing:** Even after mRNA has been fully processed, it may undergo additional posttranscriptional modification in which a base in the mRNA is altered. This is known as RNA editing. An

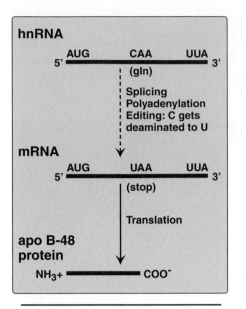

Figure 32.13
RNA editing of apo B in the intestine and generation of the apo B-48 protein needed for chylomicron synthesis.

important example in humans occurs with the transcript for apoprotein (apo) B—an essential protein component of chylomicrons (see p. 228) and very low density lipoproteins (VLDL, see p. 231). Apo B mRNA is made in the liver and the small intestine; however, in the intestine only, the C residue in the codon (CAA) for glutamine is deaminated to U, changing the sense codon to a nonsense or stop codon (UAA, Figure 32.13). This results in a shorter protein (apo B-48, representing 48% of the message) being made in the intestine (and incorporated into chylomicrons) than is made in the liver (apo B-100, full-length, incorporated into VLDL).

3. **mRNA stability:** How long an mRNA remains in the cytosol before it is degraded influences how much protein product can be produced from it. Regulation of iron metabolism and the gene-silencing process of RNA interference provide good examples of the importance of mRNA stability in the regulation of gene expression.

   a. **Iron metabolism:** Transferrin is a plasma protein that transports iron. Transferrin binds to cell-surface receptors (transferrin receptors, or TfRs) that are internalized and provide target cells with iron. The mRNA for the TfR has cis-acting iron-responsive elements (IREs) at its 3'-end. The IREs have a stem–loop structure that can be bound by trans-acting iron regulatory proteins (IRPs, Figure 32.14). When the iron concentration in the cell is low, the IRPs bind to the IREs and stabilize the mRNA for TfR, allowing TfR synthesis. When intracellular iron levels are high, the IRPs preferentially bind iron instead of IREs. The lack of IRPs bound to the mRNA hastens its degradation, resulting in decreased TfR synthesis. [Note: The mRNA for apoferritin, a protein of iron storage, also has IREs; however, they are at the 5'-end of the mRNA.

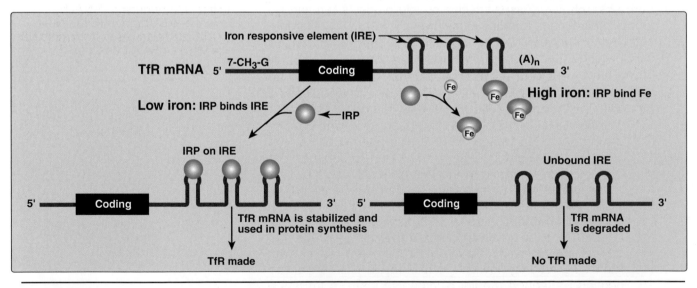

Figure 32.14
Regulation of transferrin receptor (TfR) synthesis. IRE = iron-responsive element; IRP = iron-responsive element binding protein.

When iron levels in the cell are low, IRPs bind the IREs and prevent the use of the mRNA; thus, less iron is able to be stored, allowing more iron to be transported to cells. As iron accumulates in the cell, however, the IRP protein becomes iron–bound, and loses its affinity for the IRE on mRNA, resulting in production of apoferritin molecules available to store the excess iron.]

b. RNA interference (RNAi): RNAi is a mechanism of gene silencing through decreased expression of mRNA, either by repression of translation or by increased degradation. It is thought to play a key role in such fundamental process as cell proliferation, differentiation, and apoptosis. RNAi is mediated by short (~22 bp), noncoding RNAs called microRNAs (miRNAs), which arise from far longer, genomically encoded nuclear transcripts that are partially processed in the nucleus then transported to the cytoplasm. There, an *endonuclease* (*Dicer*) completes the processing and generates short, double stranded (ds) miRNA. A single strand (the guide or antisense strand) of the ds miRNA associates with a cytosolic protein complex known as the RNA-induced silencing complex, or RISC. The guide strand hybridizes with a complementary sequence on a full length target mRNA, bringing RISC to the mRNA. This can result in repression of translation of the mRNA or its degradation by an *endonuclease* (*Argonaute/Ago/Slicer*) of the RISC. The extent of complementarity appears to be the determining factor. RNAi can also be triggered by ds short interfering RNAs (siRNAs) introduced into a cell from exogenous sources. [Note: In vertebrates, the function of siRNAs that may arise from endogenous sources is as yet unclear.] The medical and research applications of RNAi are growing rapidly.

1) RNAi therapy: Modulation of gene expression by providing siRNA to trigger RNAi has enormous therapeutic potential. The first clinical trial of RNAi-based therapy involved patients with age-related macular degeneration (AMD), the leading form of adult blindness in the world. AMD is triggered by overproduction of vascular endothelial growth factor (VEGF). In patients with AMD, too much VEGF leads to the sprouting of excess blood vessels behind the retina. The blood vessels leak, clouding and often entirely destroying vision; hence, AMD is also referred to as "wet" macular degeneration. The siRNA drug—a short dsRNA that specifically targets the mRNA of VEGF and promotes its degradation—is injected into the eye. One siRNA molecule can destroy hundreds of mRNA, resulting in the suppression of thousands of VEGF proteins, thus preventing damaging angiogenesis in the retina. [Note: The first clinical trial, involving about two dozen patients, showed promising results; however, subsequent trials were suspended.] Although the list of potential disease targets is extensive, the development of RNAi-based drugs is hindered by the problem of targeted RNAi delivery.

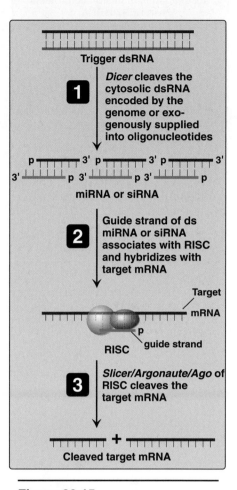

Figure 32.15
RNA interference or RNAi by cleavage of target mRNA. [Note: RNAi can also result from inhibition of target mRNA translation.]

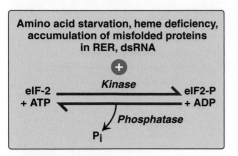

Figure 32.16
Regulation of translation initiation
in eukaryotes by phosphorylation
of eIF-2. RER = rough endoplasmic
reticulum.

4. Translation of mRNA: Regulation of gene expression can also
occur at the level of translation. One mechanism by which translation is regulated is through phosphorylation of the eukaryotic
translation initiation factor, eIF-2 (Figure 32.16). Phosphorylation
of eIF-2 inhibits its function and so inhibits translation at the initiation step (see p. 443). Phosphorylation is catalyzed by *kinases*
that are activated in response to environmental conditions such
as amino acid starvation, heme deficiency, the presence of
dsRNA, and the accumulation of misfolded proteins in the rough
endoplasmic reticulum. [Note: Phosphorylation of eIF-2 prevents
its reactivation by inhibiting GDP–GTP exchange.]

D. Regulation through modifications to DNA

Gene expression in eukaryotes is also influenced by the availability
of DNA to the transcriptional apparatus, the amount of DNA, and the
arrangement of DNA. [Note: Localized transitions between the B and
Z forms of DNA (see p. 398) can also affect gene expression.]

1. Access to DNA: In eukaryotes, DNA is found complexed with histone and nonhistone proteins to form chromatin (see p. 409).
Transcriptionally active, decondensed chromatin (euchromatin)
differs from the more condensed, inactive form (heterochromatin)
in a number of ways. Active chromatin contains histone proteins
that have been covalently modified at their amino terminal ends
by acetylation or phosphorylation (see p. 422 for a discussion of
histone acetylation/deacetylation by the *histone acetyltransferase*
and *histone deacetylase* enzymes). Such modifications decrease
the positive charge of these basic proteins, thus decreasing the
strength of their association with negatively charged DNA. This
chromatin remodeling relaxes the nucleosome (see p. 409), allowing transcription factors access to specific regions on the DNA. A
second difference between transcriptionally active and inactive
chromatin is the extent of methylation of cytosine bases in CG-
rich regions (CpG islands) in the promoter region of many genes.
Methylation is by *methyltransferases* that use S-adenosylmethionine as the methyl donor (Figure 32.17). Evidence supports the idea that transcriptionally active genes are less
methylated (hypomethylated) than their inactive counterparts,
suggesting that DNA hypermethylation silences gene expression.

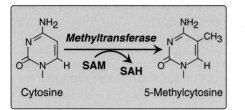

Figure 32.17
The methylation of cytosine in
eukaryotic DNA. SAM = S-adenosylmethionine; SAH = S-adenosyl
homocysteine.

2. Amount of DNA: A change in the number of copies of a gene can
affect the amount of gene product produced. An increase in copy
number—gene amplification—has contributed to increased
genomic complexity and is still a normal developmental process in
certain nonmammalian species. In mammalian cells, however,
gene amplification is seen in response to particular chemothera-
peutic drugs such as methotrexate, an inhibitor of the enzyme
dihydrofolate reductase (*DHFR*), required for the synthesis of
thymidine triphosphate (TTP) in the pyrimidine biosynthetic pathway (see p. 304). TTP is essential for DNA synthesis. Gene amplification results in an increase in the number of *DHFR* genes and
resistance to the drug, allowing TTP to be made.

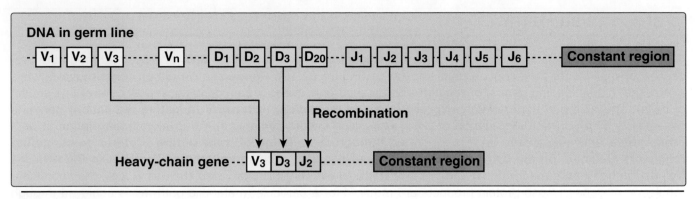

Figure 32.18
DNA rearrangements in the generation of immunoglobulins.

3. **Arrangement of DNA:** The process by which immunoglobulins (antibodies) are produced by B lymphocytes involves permanent rearrangements of the DNA in these cells. The immunoglobulins (for example, IgG) consist of two light and two heavy chains, with each chain containing regions of variable and constant amino acid sequence. The variable region is the result of somatic recombination of segments within both the light- and the heavy-chain genes. During B-lymphocyte development, single variable (V), diversity (D), and joining (J) gene segments are brought together through gene rearrangement to form a unique variable region (Figure 32.18). This process allows the generation of 10^9–10^{11} different immunoglobulins from a single gene, providing the diversity needed for the recognition of an enormous number of antigens. [Note: The shift from the membrane-bound form to the secreted form of immunoglobulins involves polyA-site choice (see p. 426).]

4. **Mobile DNA elements:** Transposons (Tn) are mobile segments of DNA that move in an essentially random manner from one site to another on the same or a different chromosome. Movement is mediated by *transposase*, an enzyme encoded by the Tn itself. Movement can be direct, in which *transposase* cuts out and then inserts the Tn at a new site, or replicative, in which the transposon is copied and the copy inserted elsewhere while the original remains in place. In eukaryotes, including humans, replicative transposition frequently involves an RNA intermediate, in which case the Tn is called a retrotransposon (see p. 408). Transposition has expanded the genome, but also has the potential to alter gene expression and even to cause disease. Although the vast majority of retrotransposons in the human genome have lost the ability to move, a small percentage is still active. Their transposition is thought to be the basis for some rare cases of hemophilia A and Duchenne muscular dystrophy. [Note: The growing problem of antibiotic-resistant bacteria is a consequence, at least in part, of the exchange of plasmids among bacterial cells. If the plasmids contain transposons carrying antibiotic resistance genes, the recipient bacteria gain resistance to one or more antimicrobial drugs.]

V. CHAPTER SUMMARY

Gene expression results in the production of a functional gene product (either RNA or protein) through the processes of replication, transcription, and translation (Figure 32.19). **Genes** can be either **constitutive** (always expressed, housekeeping genes) or **regulated** (expressed only under certain conditions in all cells or in a subset of cells). The ability to appropriately **express (positive regulation)** or **repress (negative regulation)** genes is essential in all organisms. **Regulation** of gene expression occurs primarily at the level of **transcription** in both **prokaryotes** and **eukaryotes**, and is mediated through the **binding** of **trans-acting proteins to cis-acting regulatory elements on the DNA**. In **eukaryotes**, regulation also occurs through **modifications to the DNA**, as well as through **posttranscriptional** and **posttranslational** events. In **prokaryotes** such as E. coli, the coordinate regulation of genes whose protein products are required for a particular metabolic pathway is achieved through **operons** (groups of genes sequentially arranged on the chromosome along with the regulatory elements that determine their transcription). The **lac operon** contains the Z, Y, and A structural genes, the protein products of which are needed for the catabolism of lactose. When **glucose is available**, the **operon is repressed** by the binding of the repressor protein (the product of the lacI gene) to the operator, thus preventing transcription. When **only lactose is present**, the **operon is induced** by an isomer of lactose (**allolactose**) that binds the repressor protein, preventing it from binding to the operator. In addition, **cAMP binds the CAP protein**, and the complex **binds the DNA** at the CAP site. This **increases promoter efficiency** and results in the expression of the structural genes through the production of a **polycistronic mRNA**. When both **glucose and lactose are present**, glucose prevents formation of cAMP and **transcription** of these genes is **negligible**. The **trp operon** contains genes needed for the synthesis of tryptophan, and like the lac operon, it is regulated by **positive** and **negative control**. Unlike the lac operon, it is **also regulated by attenuation**, in which mRNA synthesis that escaped repression by trp is terminated before completion. **Transcription** of **rRNA** and **tRNA** is selectively **inhibited** in prokaryotes by the **stringent response to amino acid starvation**. **Translation** is also a site of **prokaryotic gene regulation**: when ribosomal proteins are in excess, they bind the Shine-Dalgarno sequence on their own polycistronic mRNA, preventing ribosomes from binding. **Gene regulation** is **more complex in eukaryotes**. **Operons** are **not present**, but **coordinate regulation** of the transcription of genes located on different chromosomes can be achieved through the **binding of trans-acting proteins to cis-acting elements**. In **multicellular organisms**, **hormones** can **cause coordinated regulation**, either through the **binding** of the **hormone receptor–hormone complex** itself **to the DNA** (as with steroid hormones) or through the **binding of a protein** that is activated in **response to a second messenger** (as with glucagon). In each case, binding to DNA is mediated through structural motifs such as the **zinc-finger**. **Co- and posttranscriptional regulation** is also seen in **eukaryotes**, and includes **splice-site choice**, **polyA-site choice**, **mRNA editing**, and variations in **mRNA stability** as seen with transferrin receptor synthesis and with RNA interference. **Regulation at the translational level** can be caused by the **phosphorylation (inhibition) of eIF-2**. Gene expression in eukaryotes is also influenced by availability of DNA to the transcriptional apparatus, the amount of DNA, and the arrangement of the DNA.

Study Questions

Choose the one correct answer.

32.1 Which of the following mutations is most likely to result in reduced expression of the lac operon?

A. i⁻ (no repressor protein made)

B. Oᶜ (operator cannot bind repressor protein)

C. Cya⁻ (no adenylyl cyclase made)

D. Functionally impaired glucose transporter

Correct answer = C. In the absence of glucose, adenylyl cyclase makes cAMP, which forms a complex with the CAP protein. The cAMP–CAP complex binds the CAP site on the DNA, causing RNA polymerase to bind more efficiently to the lac operon promoter, thus increasing expression of the operon. With cya⁻ mutations, adenylyl cyclase is not made, and so the operon is unable to be turned on even when glucose is absent and lactose is present. The absence of a repressor protein or decreased ability of the repressor to bind the operator results in constitutive (constant) expression of the lac operon.

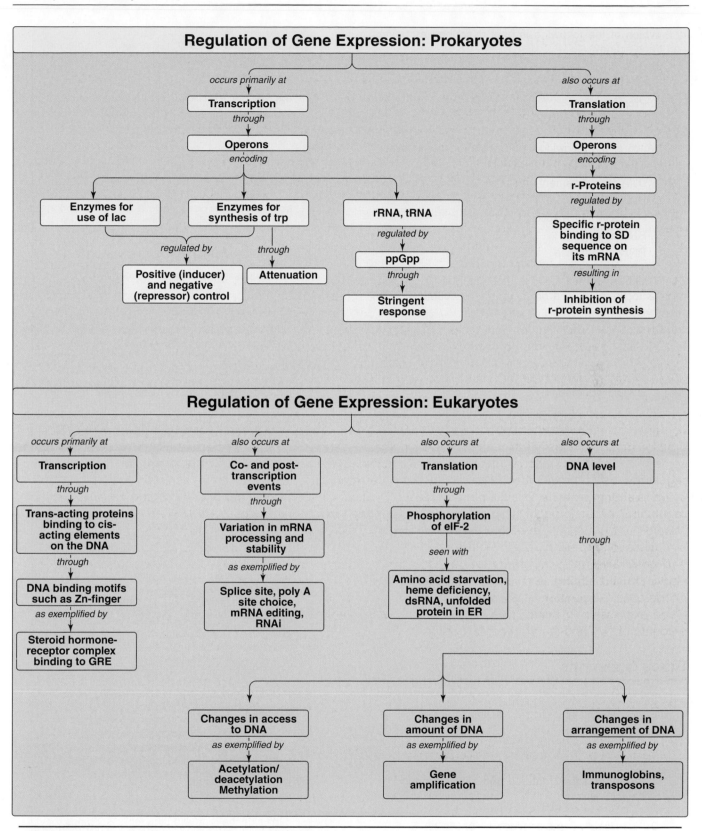

Figure 32.19
Summary of key concepts for the regulation of gene expression.

32.2 Which of the following is best described as being trans-acting?

A. CAP site

B. Operator

C. Promoter

D. Repressor

Correct answer = D. A repressor is a molecule that transits to the DNA, binds, and reduces the expression of that DNA; it is said to be trans-acting. The CAP site, operator, and promoter are part of the DNA itself, and so are said to be cis-acting.

32.3 Which of the following is the basis for the intestine-specific expression of apoprotein B-48?

A. DNA rearrangement and loss

B. DNA transposition

C. RNA alternative splicing

D. RNA editing

E. RNA interference

Correct answer = D. The production of apoB-48 in the intestine and apoB-100 in liver is the result of RNA editing in the intestine, where a sense codon is changed to a nonsense codon by posttranscriptional deamination of C to U. DNA rearrangement and transposition, as well as RNA interference and alternate splicing, do alter gene expression, but are not the basis of apoB-48 tissue-specific production.

32.4 Which of the following is most likely to be true in hemochromatosis, a disease of iron accumulation in the body?

A. The mRNA for the transferrin receptor (TfR) is stabilized by the binding of IRPs to 3' stem-loop structures known as IREs.

B. The mRNA for the TfR is not bound by IRPs, and is rapidly degraded.

C. The mRNA for apoferritin is not bound by IRPs at its 5' stem-loop IRE, and is translated.

D. The mRNA for apoferritin is bound by IRPs, and is not translated.

E. Both B and C

Correct answer = E. When iron levels in the body are high, as is seen with hemochromatosis, there is increased synthesis of the iron-storage molecule, apoferritin, and decreased synthesis of the transferrin receptor (TfR) that mediates iron uptake by cells. These effects are the result of trans-acting iron regulatory proteins (IRPs) binding iron rather than binding cis-acting iron-responsive elements (IREs), resulting in degradation of the mRNA for TfR, and increased translation of the mRNA for apoferritin.

32.5 After several weeks of chemotherapy with methotrexate, a cancer patient's tumor begins to show signs of resistance to treatment. Which of the following mechanisms is most likely to explain this resistance to methotrexate?

A. Overproduction of dihydrofolate reductase.

B. Overproduction of xanthine oxidase.

C. Deficiency of PRPP synthase.

D. Deficiency of thymidine kinase.

E. Deficiency of thymidylate synthase.

Correct answer = A. Methotrexate interferes with folate metabolism by acting as a competitive inhibitor of the enzyme dihydrofolate reductase. This starves cells for tetrahydrofolate, and makes them unable to synthesize purines and dTMP. This is especially toxic to rapidly growing cancer cells. Overproduction of dihydrofolate reductase, usually caused by amplification of its gene, can overcome the inhibition of the enzyme at the methotrexate concentrations used for chemotherapy, and can result in resistance of the tumor to treatment by this drug.

32.6 The ZYA region of the lac operon will be efficiently transcribed if:

A. glucose and lactose are available.

B. cAMP levels are low.

C. the operator is mutated and can't be bound by the repressor.

D. the repressor is mutated and can't be bound by the inducer.

Correct answer = C. The lac operon is negatively regulated by the repressor protein binding to the operator region and preventing RNA polymerase from transcribing the Z, Y, and A genes of the operon. If glucose is present, the operon is off as a result of catabolite repression. It is only when glucose is gone, cAMP levels are increased, and lactose is available that the operon is maximally induced. If the inducer can't bind the repressor, the repressor binds the operator and represses transcription.

Biotechnology and Human Disease

33

I. OVERVIEW

In the past, efforts to understand genes and their expression have been confounded by the immense size and complexity of human deoxyribonucleic acid (DNA). The human genome contains approximately three billion (10^9) base pairs (bp) that encode 20,000 to 30,000 protein-coding genes located on 23 pairs of chromosomes. It is now possible to determine the nucleotide sequence of long stretches of DNA, and the entire sequence of the human genome has been determined. This effort (called the Human Genome Project) was made possible by several techniques that have already contributed to our understanding of many genetic diseases (Figure 33.1). These include, first, the discovery of *restriction endonucleases* that permit the dissection of huge DNA molecules into defined fragments. Second, the development of cloning techniques, providing a mechanism for amplification of specific nucleotide sequences. Finally, the ability to synthesize specific probes, which has allowed the identification and manipulation of nucleotide sequences of interest. These and other experimental approaches have permitted the identification of both normal and mutant nucleotide sequences in DNA. This knowledge has led to the development of methods for the diagnosis of genetic diseases, and initial successes in the treatment of patients by gene therapy.

II. RESTRICTION ENDONUCLEASES

One of the major obstacles to molecular analysis of genomic DNA is the immense size of the molecules involved. The discovery of a special group of bacterial enzymes, called *restriction endonucleases* (restriction enzymes), which cleave double-stranded (ds) DNA into smaller, more manageable fragments, has opened the way for DNA analysis. Because each enzyme cleaves DNA at a specific nucleotide sequence, restriction enzymes are used experimentally to obtain precisely defined DNA segments called restriction fragments.

A. Specificity of restriction endonucleases

Restriction endonucleases recognize short stretches of DNA (four to eight bp) that contain specific nucleotide sequences. These sequences, which differ for each restriction enzyme, are palin-

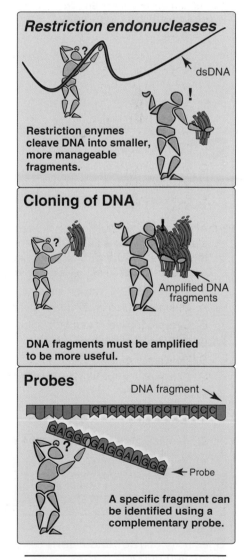

Restriction endonucleases

dsDNA

Restriction enymes cleave DNA into smaller, more manageable fragments.

Cloning of DNA

Amplified DNA fragments

DNA fragments must be amplified to be more useful.

Probes

DNA fragment

Probe

A specific fragment can be identified using a complementary probe.

Figure 33.1
Three techniques that facilitate analysis of human DNA.

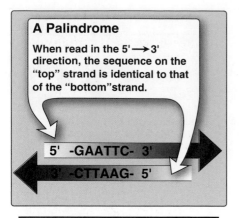

A Palindrome

When read in the 5'→3' direction, the sequence on the "top" strand is identical to that of the "bottom"strand.

5' -GAATTC- 3'
3' -CTTAAG- 5'

Figure 33.2
Recognition sequence of *restriction endonuclease EcoRI* shows two-fold rotational symmetry.

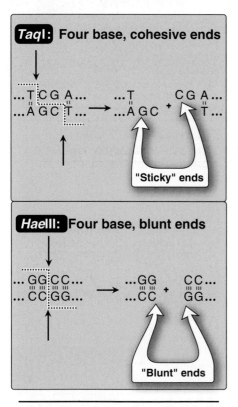

*Taq*I: Four base, cohesive ends

...TCGA...   ...T   CGA...
...AGCT... →   ...AGC +   T...

"Sticky" ends

*Hae*III: Four base, blunt ends

...GGCC...   ...GG   CC...
...CCGG... →   ...CC +   GG...

"Blunt" ends

Figure 33.3
Specificity of *Taq*I and *Hae*III *restriction endonucleases.*

dromes, that is, they exhibit twofold rotational symmetry (Figure 33.2). This means that, within a short region of the double helix, the nucleotide sequence on the two strands is identical if each is read in the 5'→3' direction. Therefore, if you turn the page upside down—that is, rotate it 180 degrees around its axis of symmetry—the sequence remains the same.

> In bacteria, *restriction endonucleases* "restrict" the expression of non-bacterial DNA through cleavage. Bacterial DNA is protected by methylation of bases at the restriction site

B. Nomenclature

A restriction enzyme is named according to the organism from which it was isolated. The first letter of the name is from the genus of the bacterium. The next two letters are from the name of the species. An additional letter indicates the type or strain, and a final number is appended to indicate the order in which the enzyme was discovered in that particular organism. For example, *Hae*III is the third *restriction endonuclease* isolated from the bacterium Haemophilus aegyptius.

C. "Sticky" and "blunt" ends

Restriction enzymes cleave dsDNA so as to produce a 3'-hydroxyl group on one end and a 5'-phosphate group on the other. Some *restriction endonucleases*, such as *Taq*I, form staggered cuts that produce "sticky" or cohesive ends—that is, the resulting DNA fragments have single-stranded (ss) sequences that are complementary to each other (Figure 33.3). Other *restriction endonucleases*, such as *Hae*III, produce fragments that have "blunt" ends that are double-stranded and therefore do not form hydrogen bonds with each other. Using the enzyme *DNA ligase* (see p. 406), sticky ends of a DNA fragment of interest can be covalently joined with other DNA fragments that have sticky ends produced by cleavage with the same *restriction endonuclease* (Figure 33.4). Another *ligase*, encoded by bacteriophage T4, can covalently join blunt-ended fragments.

D. Restriction sites

A DNA sequence that is recognized and cut by a restriction enzyme is called a restriction site. *Restriction endonucleases* cleave dsDNA into fragments of different sizes. For example, an enzyme that recognizes a specific four-base-pair sequence produces many cuts in the DNA molecule, one every 4^4 bp. In contrast, an enzyme requiring a unique sequence of six base pairs produces fewer cuts (one every 4^6 bp) and, hence, longer pieces. Hundreds of these enzymes, having different cleavage specificities (varying in both nucleotide sequences and length of recognition sites), are commercially available as analytic reagents.

III. DNA CLONING

Introduction of a foreign DNA molecule into a replicating cell permits the cloning or amplification (that is, the production of many identical copies) of that DNA. In some cases, a single DNA fragment can be isolated and purified prior to cloning. More commonly, to clone a nucleotide sequence of interest, the total cellular DNA is first cleaved with a specific restriction enzyme, creating hundreds of thousands of fragments. Each of the resulting DNA fragments is joined to a DNA vector molecule (referred to as a cloning vector) to form a hybrid or recombinant molecule. Each recombinant DNA molecule conveys its inserted DNA fragment into a single host cell, for example, a bacterium, where it is replicated. [Note: The process of introducing foreign DNA into a cell is called transformation for bacteria and yeast and transfection for higher eukaryotes.] As the host cell multiplies, it forms a clone in which every bacterium carries copies of the same inserted DNA fragment, hence the name "cloning." The cloned DNA is eventually released from its vector by cleavage (using the appropriate *restriction endonuclease*) and is isolated. By this mechanism, many identical copies of the DNA of interest can be produced. [Note: An alternative to biologic cloning—the polymerase chain reaction—is described on p. 479.]

A. Vectors

A vector is a molecule of DNA to which the fragment of DNA to be cloned is joined. Essential properties of a vector include: 1) it must be capable of autonomous replication within a host cell; 2) it must contain at least one specific nucleotide sequence recognized by a *restriction endonuclease*; and 3) it must carry at least one gene that confers the ability to select for the vector, such as an antibiotic resistance gene. Commonly used vectors include plasmids and viruses.

1. **Prokaryotic plasmids:** Prokaryotic organisms typically contain single, large, circular chromosomes. In addition, most species of bacteria also normally contain small, circular, extrachromosomal DNA molecules called plasmids[1] (Figure 33.5). Plasmid DNA undergoes replication that may or may not be synchronized to chromosomal division. Plasmids may carry genes that convey antibiotic resistance to the host bacterium, and may facilitate the transfer of genetic information from one bacterium to another. Plasmids can be readily isolated from bacterial cells, their circular DNA cleaved at specific sites by *restriction endonucleases*, and up to 10 kb of foreign DNA (cut with the same restriction enzyme) inserted. The recombinant plasmid can be introduced into a bacterium, and large numbers of copies of the plasmid produced. The bacteria are grown in the presence of antibiotics, thus selecting for cells containing the hybrid plasmids, which provide antibiotic resistance (Figure 33.6). [Note: The experiment is conducted to favor only one DNA fragment being inserted into each plasmid and only one plasmid being taken up by each bacterium.]

[1]See Chapter 7 in *Lippincott's Illustrated Reviews: Microbiology* for a discussion of plasmids.

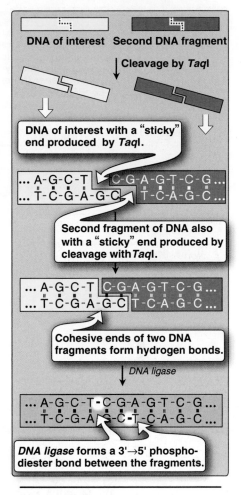

Figure 33.4
Formation of recombinant DNA from restriction fragments with "sticky" ends.

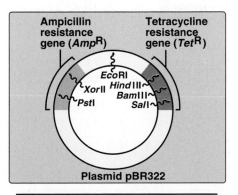

Figure 33.5
A restriction map of plasmid pBR322 indicating the positions of its antibiotic resistance genes and the sites of nucleotide sequences recognized by specific *restriction endonucleases*.

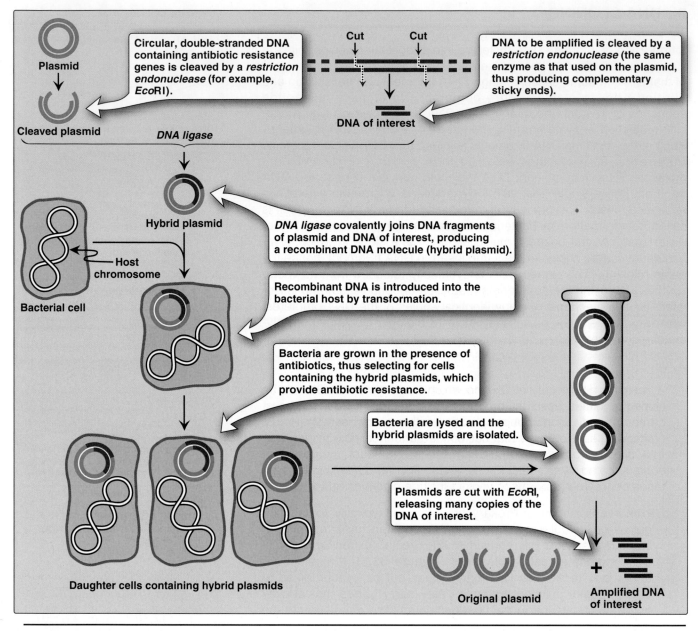

Figure 33.6
Summary of gene cloning.

2. **Other vectors:** The development of improved vectors that can more efficiently accommodate larger DNA segments, or express the passenger genes in different cell types, has aided molecular genetics research. In addition to the prokaryotic plasmids described above, naturally occurring viruses that infect bacteria (bacteriophage λ, for example) or mammalian cells (retroviruses, for example), as well as artificial constructs such as cosmids and bacterial or yeast artificial chromosomes (BACs or YACs, respectively), are currently in wide use as cloning vectors. [Note: BACs and YACs can accept DNA inserts of 100-200 kilobases (kb) and 200-500 kb, respectively.]

B. DNA libraries

A DNA library is a collection of cloned restriction fragments of the DNA of an organism. Two kinds of libraries are commonly used: genomic libraries and complementary DNA (cDNA) libraries. Genomic libraries ideally contain a copy of every DNA nucleotide sequence in the genome. In contrast, cDNA libraries contain those DNA sequences that only appear as processed mRNA molecules, and these differ from one cell type to another. [Note: cDNA lacks introns and the control regions of the genes, whereas these are present in genomic DNA.]

1. **Genomic DNA libraries:** A genomic library is created by digestion of the total DNA of the organism with a *restriction endonuclease* and subsequent ligation to an appropriate vector. The recombinant DNA molecules replicate within host bacteria. The amplified DNA fragments thus represent the entire genome of the organism and are called a genomic library. Regardless of the restriction enzyme used, the chances are rather good that the gene of interest contains more than one restriction site recognized by that enzyme. If this is the case, and if the digestion is allowed to go to completion, the gene of interest is fragmented—that is, it is not contained in any one clone in the library. To avoid this usually undesirable result, a partial digestion is performed in which either the amount or the time of action of the enzyme is limited. This results in cleavage occurring at only a fraction of the restriction sites on any one DNA molecule, thus producing fragments of about 20 kb. Enzymes that cut very frequently (that is, those that recognize 4 bp sequences) are generally used for this purpose so that the result is an almost random collection of fragments. This ensures a high degree of probability that the gene of interest is contained, intact, in some fragment.

2. **cDNA libraries:** If a protein-coding gene of interest is expressed at a high level in a particular tissue, it is likely that the messenger RNA (mRNA) transcribed from that gene is also present at high concentrations in the cell. For example, reticulocyte mRNA is composed largely of molecules encoding the α-globin and β-globin chains of hemoglobin. This mRNA can be used as a template to make a complementary DNA (cDNA) molecule using the enzyme *reverse transcriptase* (Figure 33.7). [Note: mRNA is isolated from transfer RNA and ribosomal RNA by the presence of its polyA tail.] The resulting cDNA is thus a double-stranded copy of mRNA. cDNA can be amplified by cloning or by the polymerase chain reaction. It can be used as a probe to locate the gene that coded for the original mRNA (or fragments of the gene) in mixtures containing many unrelated DNA fragments. If the mRNA used as a template is a mixture of many different size species, the resulting cDNA is heterogeneous. These mixtures can be cloned to form a cDNA library. Because cDNA has no intervening sequences, it can be cloned into an expression vector for the synthesis of eukaryotic proteins by bacteria (Figure 33.8). These special plasmids contain a bacterial promoter for transcription of the

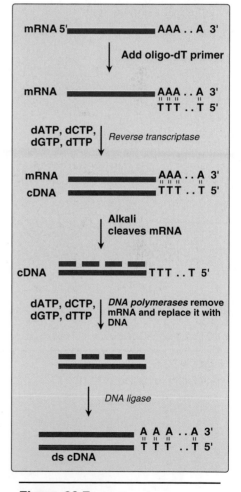

Figure 33.7
Synthesis of cDNA from mRNA using *reverse transcriptase*. Additional steps (not shown) are required to clone the cDNA.

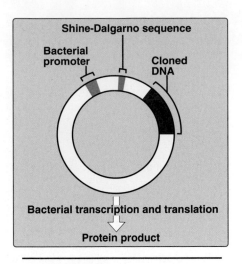

Figure 33.8
An expression vector.

cDNA, and a Shine-Dalgarno sequence (see p. 439) that allows the bacterial ribosome to initiate translation of the resulting mRNA molecule. [Note: Therapeutic human insulin is made in bacteria through this technology; however, the extensive co- and post-translational modifications (see p. 443) required for most other human proteins necessitates the use of eukaryotic hosts.]

C. Sequencing of cloned DNA fragments

The base sequence of DNA fragments that have been cloned can be determined. The original procedure for this purpose was the Sanger dideoxy method illustrated in Figure 33.9. The ssDNA to be sequenced is used as the template for DNA synthesis by *DNA polymerase*. A radiolabeled primer complementary to the 3'-end of the target DNA is added, along with the four deoxyribonucleoside triphosphates (dNTP). The sample is divided into four reaction tubes, and a small amount of one of the four dideoxyribonucleoside triphosphates (ddNTP) is added to each tube. Because it contains no 3'-hydroxyl group, incorporation of a ddNMP terminates elongation at that point. The products of this reaction, then, consist of a mixture of DNA strands of different lengths, each terminating at a specific base. Separation of the various DNA products by size using polyacrylamide gel electrophoresis, followed by autoradiography, yields a pattern of bands from which the DNA base sequence can be read. [Note: The shorter the fragment, the farther it travels on the gel, with the shortest fragment representing that which was made first, that is, the 5'-end.] The Human Genome Project used highly automated variations of this technique to determine the base sequence of the human genome.

IV. PROBES

Cleavage of large DNA molecules by restriction enzymes produces a bewildering array of fragments. How can the DNA sequence of interest be picked out of a mixture of thousands or even millions of irrelevant DNA fragments? The answer lies in the use of a probe—a short piece of ssDNA, labeled with a radioisotope, such as ^{32}P, or with a nonradioactive molecule, such as biotin. The sequence of a probe is complementary to a sequence in the DNA of interest, called the target DNA. Probes are used to identify which band on a gel or which clone in a library contains the target DNA, a process called screening.

A. Hybridization of a probe to DNA fragments

The utility of probes hinges on the phenomenon of hybridization (or annealing) in which a probe containing a complementary sequence binds a single-stranded sequence of a target DNA. ssDNA, produced by alkaline denaturation of dsDNA, is first bound to a solid support, such as a nitrocellulose membrane. The immobilized DNA strands are prevented from self-annealing, but are available for hybridization to an exogenous, radiolabeled, ssDNA probe. The extent of hybridization is measured by the retention of radioactivity on the membrane. Excess probe molecules that do not hybridize are removed by washing the filter.

B. Synthetic oligonucleotide probes

If the sequence of all or part of the target DNA is known, single-stranded oligonucleotide probes of 20–30 nucleotides can be synthesized that are complementary to a small region of the gene of interest. If the sequence of the gene is unknown, the amino acid sequence of the protein— the final gene product—may be used to construct a probe. Short, ssDNA sequences (15–30 nucleotides) are synthesized, using the genetic code as a guide. Because of the degeneracy of the genetic code, it is necessary to synthesize several oligonucleotides. [Note: Oligonucleotides can be used to detect single-base changes in the sequence to which they are complementary. In contrast, cDNA probes contain many thousands of bases, and their binding to a target DNA with a single-base change is unaffected.]

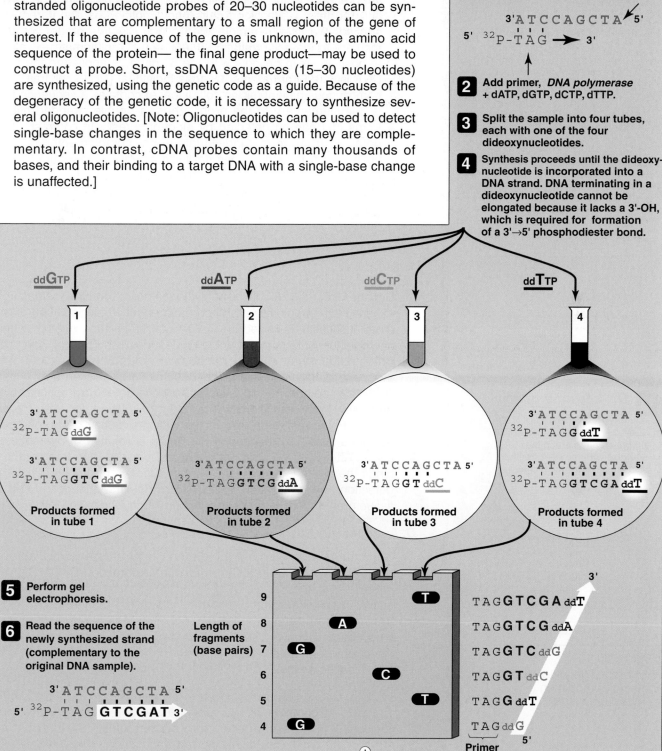

1 Single-stranded DNA of unknown sequence is used as a template.

2 Add primer, *DNA polymerase* + dATP, dGTP, dCTP, dTTP.

3 Split the sample into four tubes, each with one of the four dideoxynucleotides.

4 Synthesis proceeds until the dideoxynucleotide is incorporated into a DNA strand. DNA terminating in a dideoxynucleotide cannot be elongated because it lacks a 3'-OH, which is required for formation of a 3'→5' phosphodiester bond.

5 Perform gel electrophoresis.

6 Read the sequence of the newly synthesized strand (complementary to the original DNA sample).

Figure 33.9
DNA sequencing by the Sanger dideoxy method.

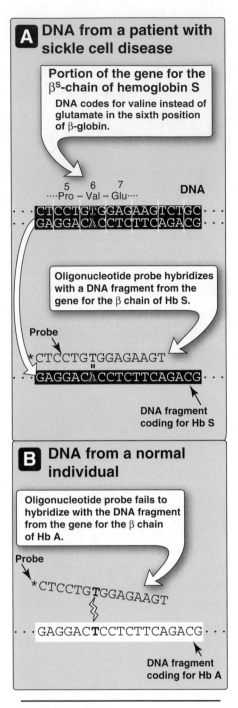

Figure 33.10
Allele-specific oligonucleotide probe detects hemoglobin (Hb) S allele. [Note: * indicates ^{32}P radiolabel.]

1. **Detecting the β^S-globin mutation:** Figure 33.10 shows how an allele-specific oligonucleotide (ASO) probe can be used to detect the presence of the sickle cell mutation in the β-globin gene. DNA, isolated from white blood cells and amplified, is denatured and applied to a filter. A radiolabeled oligonucleotide probe, complementary to the point mutation (GAG → GTG, glutamate → valine) at position six in patients with the β^S gene, is applied to the filter. DNA isolated from a heterozygous individual (sickle cell trait) or a homozygous patient (sickle cell disease) contains a sequence that is complementary to the probe; thus, a double-stranded hybrid forms that can be detected by electrophoresis. In contrast, DNA obtained from normal individuals is not complementary at this positon and, therefore, does not form a hybrid (see Figure 33.10). Use of a pair of such ASO probes (one specific for the normal allele and one specific for the mutant allele) allows all three possible genotypes—homozygous normal, heterozygous, and homozygous mutant (Figure 33.11)—to be distinguished. [Note: ASO probes are useful only if the mutation and its location are known.]

C. Biotinylated probes

Because the disposal of radioactive waste is becoming increasingly expensive, nonradioactive probes have been developed. One of the most successful is based on the vitamin biotin (see p. 381), which can be chemically coupled to the nucleotides used to synthesize the probe. Biotin was chosen because it binds very tenaciously to avidin—a readily available protein contained in chicken egg whites. Avidin can be attached to a fluorescent dye detectable optically with great sensitivity. Thus, a DNA fragment (displayed, for example, by gel electrophoresis) that hybridizes with the biotinylated probe can be made visible by immersing the gel in a solution of dye-coupled avidin. After washing away the excess avidin, the DNA fragment that binds the probe is fluorescent. [Note: Fluorescent probes can allow detection and localization of DNA (or mRNA) sequences in cell or tissue preparations, a process called in situ hybridization.]

D. Antibodies

Sometimes no amino acid sequence information is available to guide the synthesis of a probe for direct detection of the DNA of interest. In this case, a gene can be identified indirectly by cloning cDNA in an expression vector that allows the cloned cDNA to be transcribed and translated. A labeled antibody is used to identify which bacterial colony produces the protein and, therefore, contains the cDNA of interest. [Note: A library created using expression vectors is called an expression library.]

> Recombinant DNA technology has allowed the production, in nonhuman systems, of human enzymes that have been modified for appropriate targeting to lysosomes. Such recombinant enzyme replacement therapy (ERT) is used in the treatment of lysosomal storage diseases such as Pompe, Gaucher, and Hurler.

V. SOUTHERN BLOTTING

Southern blotting is a technique that can detect mutations in DNA. It combines the use of restriction enzymes, electrophoresis, and DNA probes.

A. Experimental procedure

This method, named after its inventor, Edward Southern, involves the following steps (Figure 33.12). First, DNA is extracted from cells, for example, a patient's leukocytes. Second, the DNA is cleaved into many fragments using a restriction enzyme. Third, the resulting fragments are separated on the basis of size by electrophoresis. [Note: As the large fragments move more slowly than the smaller ones, the lengths of the fragments, usually expressed as the number of base pairs, can be calculated from comparison of the position of the band relative to standard fragments of known size.] The DNA fragments in the gel are denatured and transferred (blotted) to a nitrocellulose membrane for analysis. If the original DNA represents the individual's entire genome, the enzymic digest contains a million or more fragments. The gene of interest is on only one (or a few if the gene itself was fragmented) of these pieces of DNA. If all the DNA segments were visualized by a nonspecific technique, they would appear as an unresolved blur of overlapping bands. To avoid this, the last step in Southern blotting uses a probe to identify the DNA fragments of interest. The patterns observed on Southern blot analysis depend both on the specific *restriction endonuclease* and on the probe used to visualize the restriction fragments. [Note: Variants of the Southern blot have been facetiously named "Northern" (electrophoresis of mRNA followed by hybridization with a specific probe), and "Western" (electrophoresis of protein followed by detection with an antibody directed against the protein of interest), neither of which relates to anyone's name or to points of the compass.]

B. Detection of mutations

Southern blotting can detect DNA mutations such as the insertion or deletion of nucleotides. It can also detect point mutations (replacement of one nucleotide by another, see p. 433) that cause the loss or gain of restriction enzyme cleavage sites. Such mutations cause the pattern of bands to differ from those seen with a normal gene. Longer fragments are generated if a restriction site is lost. For example, in Figure 33.12, Person 2 lacks a restriction site present in Person 1. Alternatively, the point mutation may create a new cleavage site with the production of shorter fragments. [Note: Most sequence differences at restriction sites represent normal variations present in the DNA.]

VI. RESTRICTION FRAGMENT LENGTH POLYMORPHISM

Genome variations are differences in the sequence of DNA among individuals. It has been estimated that the genomes of nonrelated people differ at about one in 1,200 DNA bases, or about 0.1% of the genome. These genome variations include both mutations and polymorphisms. A mutation refers to an infrequent, but potentially harmful, genome varia-

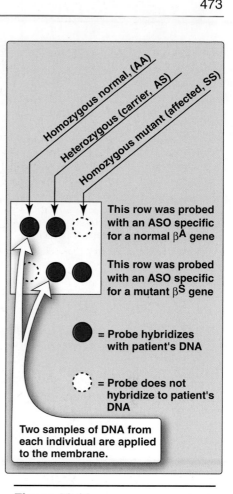

Figure 33.11
Allele-specific oligonucleotide (ASO) probes used to detect the sickle cell mutation and differentiate between sickle cell trait and disease.

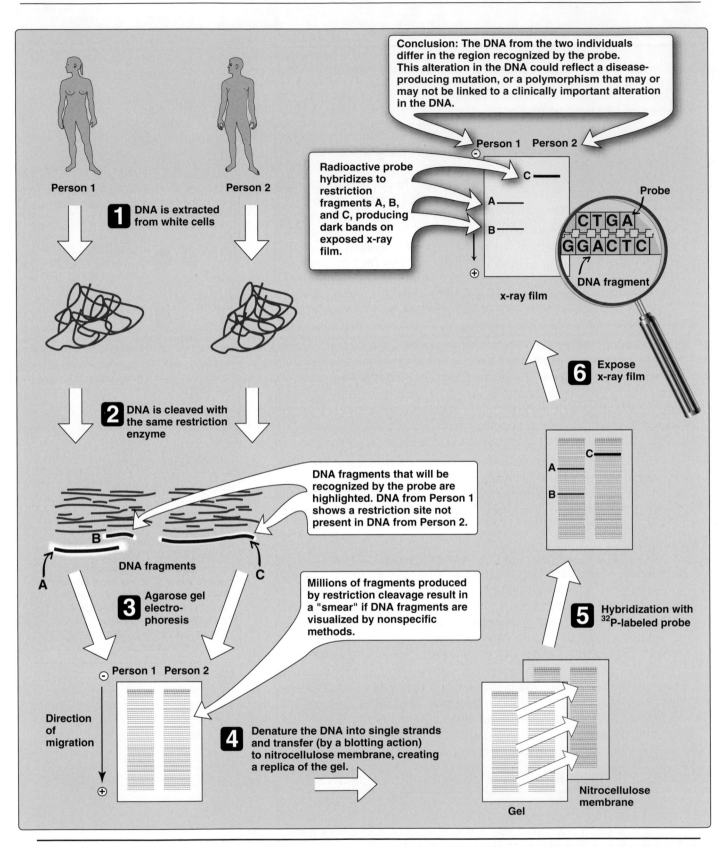

Figure 33.12
Southern blotting procedure.

tion that is associated with a specific human disease. In contrast, a polymorphism is a clinically harmless DNA variation that does not affect the phenotype. It is traditionally defined as a sequence variation at a given locus (allele) in more than 1% of a population. Polymorphisms primarily occur in regions of the genome that do not encode proteins, that is, in introns and intergenic regions. [Note: Less than 2% of the human genome actually encodes proteins.] A restriction fragment length polymorphism (RFLP) is a genetic variant that can be observed by cleaving the DNA into fragments (restriction fragments) with a restriction enzyme. The length of the restriction fragments is altered if the genetic variant alters the DNA so as to create or abolish a site of *restriction endonuclease* cleavage (a restriction site). RFLP can be used to detect human genetic variations, for example, in prospective parents or in fetal tissue.

A. DNA variations resulting in RFLP

Two types of DNA variation commonly result in RFLP: single-base changes in the nucleotide sequence, and tandem repeats of DNA sequences.

1. **Single base changes in DNA:** About 90% of human genome variation comes in the form of single-nucleotide polymorphisms, (SNPs, pronounced "snips"), that is, variations that involve just one base (Figure 33.13). The substitution of one nucleotide at a restriction site can render the site unrecognizable by a particular *restriction endonuclease*. A new restriction site can also be created by the same mechanism. In either case, cleavage with an *endonuclease* results in fragments of lengths differing from the normal, which can be detected by DNA hybridization (see Figure 33.12). [Note: The altered restriction site can be either at the site of a disease-causing mutation (rare) or at a site some distance from the mutation, see p. 477.]

2. **Tandem repeats:** Alternatively, polymorphism in chromosomal DNA can arise from the presence of a variable number of tandem repeats (VNTR, see Figure 33.14). These are short sequences of DNA at scattered locations in the genome, repeated in tandem (one after another). The number of these repeat units varies from person to person, but is unique for any given individual and, therefore, serves as a molecular fingerprint. Cleavage by restriction enzymes yields fragments that vary in length depending on how many repeated segments are contained in the fragment. Variation in the number of tandem repeats can lead to polymorphisms (Figure 33.14). Many different VNTR loci have been identified, and are extremely useful for DNA fingerprint analysis, such as in forensic and paternity identity cases. It is important to emphasize that these polymorphisms, whether SNP or VNTR, are simply markers, which, in most cases, have no known effect on the structure, function, or rate of production of any particular protein. [Note: Microsatellites are a type of VNTR.]

B. Tracing chromosomes from parent to offspring

If the DNA of an individual has gained a restriction site by base substitution, then enzymic cleavage yields at least one additional fragment. Conversely, if a mutation results in loss of a restriction site,

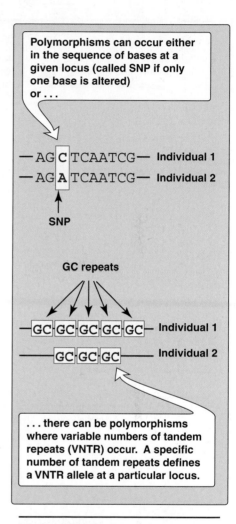

Figure 33.13
Common forms of genetic polymorphism. SNP = single-nucleotide polymorphism.

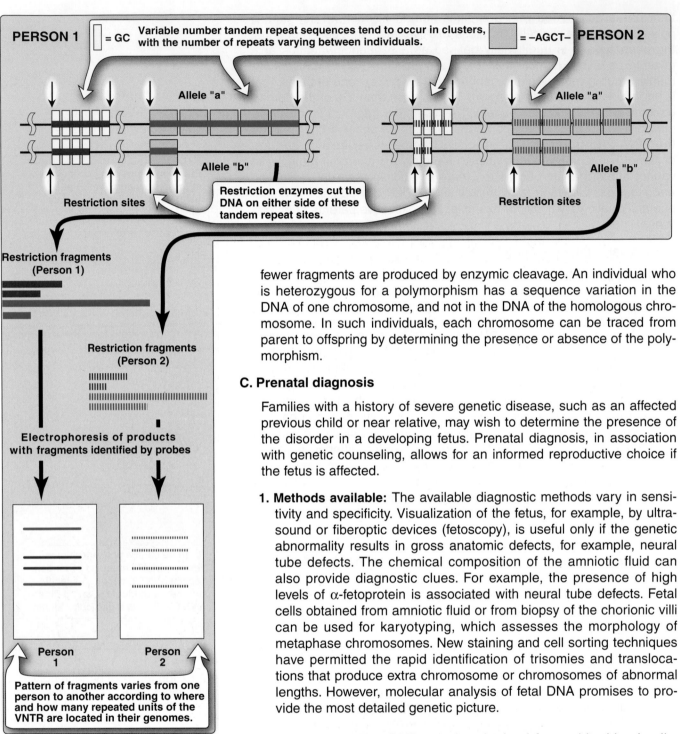

Figure 33.14
Restriction fragment length polymorphism (RFLP) of variable number tandem repeats (VNTR). For each person, a pair of homologous chromosomes is shown.

fewer fragments are produced by enzymic cleavage. An individual who is heterozygous for a polymorphism has a sequence variation in the DNA of one chromosome, and not in the DNA of the homologous chromosome. In such individuals, each chromosome can be traced from parent to offspring by determining the presence or absence of the polymorphism.

C. Prenatal diagnosis

Families with a history of severe genetic disease, such as an affected previous child or near relative, may wish to determine the presence of the disorder in a developing fetus. Prenatal diagnosis, in association with genetic counseling, allows for an informed reproductive choice if the fetus is affected.

1. **Methods available:** The available diagnostic methods vary in sensitivity and specificity. Visualization of the fetus, for example, by ultrasound or fiberoptic devices (fetoscopy), is useful only if the genetic abnormality results in gross anatomic defects, for example, neural tube defects. The chemical composition of the amniotic fluid can also provide diagnostic clues. For example, the presence of high levels of α-fetoprotein is associated with neural tube defects. Fetal cells obtained from amniotic fluid or from biopsy of the chorionic villi can be used for karyotyping, which assesses the morphology of metaphase chromosomes. New staining and cell sorting techniques have permitted the rapid identification of trisomies and translocations that produce extra chromosome or chromosomes of abnormal lengths. However, molecular analysis of fetal DNA promises to provide the most detailed genetic picture.

2. **Sources of DNA:** DNA may be obtained from white blood cells, amniotic fluid, or chorionic villi (Figure 33.15). For amniotic fluid, in the past, it was necessary to culture the cells in order to have sufficient DNA for analysis. This took 2–3 weeks to grow a sufficient number of cells. The development of the polymerase chain reaction (see below) has dramatically shortened the time needed for a DNA analysis.

3. **Direct diagnosis of sickle cell anemia using RFLP:** The genetic disorders of hemoglobin are the most common genetic diseases in humans. In the case of sickle cell anemia (Figure 33.16), the mutation that gives rise to the disease is actually one and the same as the mutation that gives rise to the polymorphism. Direct detection by RFLP of diseases that result from point mutations is, however, limited to only a few genetic diseases.

a. **Early efforts to diagnose sickle cell anemia:** Prenatal diagnosis of hemoglobinopathies has in the past involved the determination of the amount and kinds of hemoglobin (Hb) synthesized in red cells obtained from fetal blood. For example, the presence of Hb S in hemolysates indicated sickle cell anemia. However, the invasive procedures to obtain fetal blood have a high mortality rate (approximately 5%), and diagnosis cannot be carried out until late in the second trimester of pregnancy when Hb S begins to be produced.

b. **RFLP analysis:** Sickle cell anemia is an example of a genetic disease caused by a point mutation (see p. 35). The sequence altered by the mutation abolishes the recognition site of the *restriction endonuclease Mst*II that recognizes the nucleotide sequence CCTNAGG (where N is any nucleotide, see Figure 33.16). Thus, the A-to-T mutation within a codon of the β^S-globin gene eliminates a cleavage site for the enzyme. Normal DNA digested with *Mst*II yields a 1.15-kb fragment, whereas a 1.35-kb fragment is generated from the β^S gene as a result of the loss of one *Mst*II cleavage site. Diagnostic techniques for analyzing fetal DNA (from amniotic cells or chorionic villus sampling), rather than fetal blood, have proved valuable because they provide safe, early detection of sickle cell anemia, as well as other genetic diseases. [Note: Genetic disorders caused by the insertion or deletion of nucleotides between two restriction sites, rather than by the creation or loss of cleavage sites, will also display RFLP.]

4. **Indirect, prenatal diagnosis of phenylketonuria using RFLP:** The gene for *phenylalanine hydroxylase* (*PAH*), deficient in phenylketonuria (PKU, see p. 270), is located on chromosome 12. It spans about 90 kb of genomic DNA, and contains 13 exons separated by introns (Figure 33.17; see p. 426 for a description of exons and introns). Mutations in *PAH* usually do not directly affect any *restriction endonuclease* recognition site. To establish a diagnostic protocol for this disease, one has to analyze DNA of family members of the affected individual. The goal is to identify genetic markers (RFLP) that are tightly linked to the disease trait. Once these markers are identified, RFLP analysis can be used to carry out prenatal diagnosis.

a. **Identification of the gene:** One can determine the presence of the mutant gene by identifying the polymorphism marker if two conditions are satisfied. First, if the polymorphism is closely linked to a disease-producing mutation, the defective gene can be traced by detection of the RFLP. For example, if one exam-

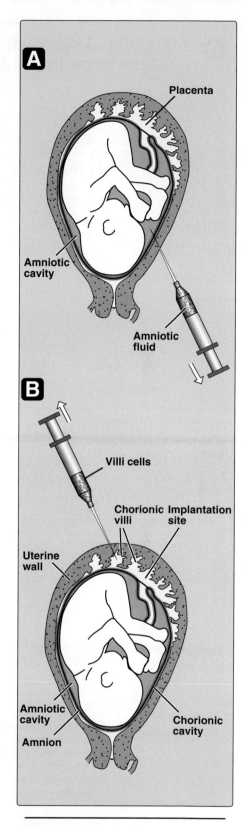

Figure 33.15
Sampling of fetal cells. A. Amniotic fluid. B. Chorionic villus.

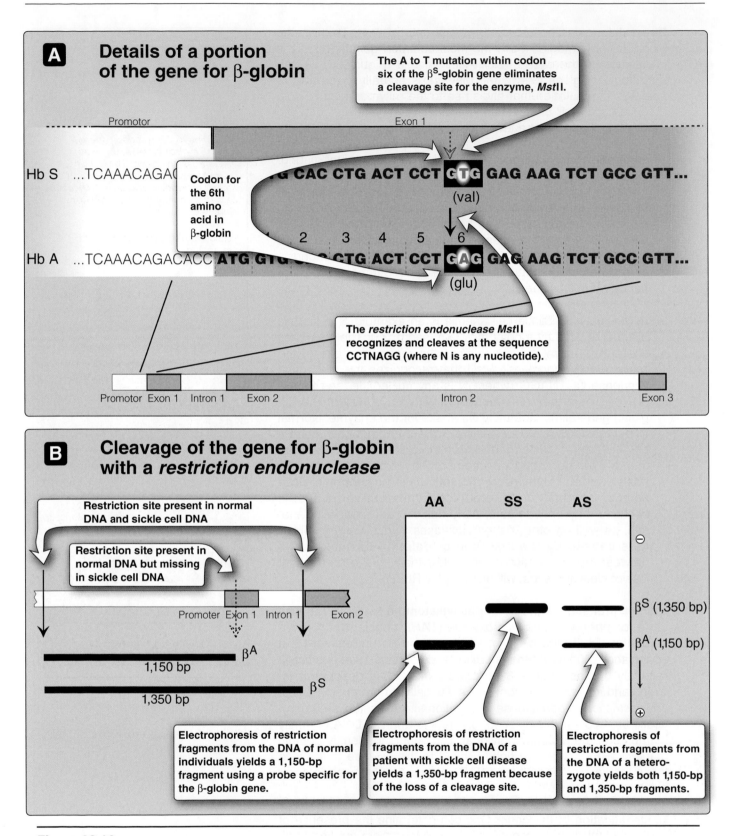

Figure 33.16
Detection of β^S-globin mutation. bp = base pair; Hb = hemoglobin

ines, by restriction enzyme cleavage and Southern blotting, the DNA from a family carrying a disease-producing gene, it is sometimes possible to find an RFLP that is consistently associated with that gene (that is, they show close linkage and are coinherited). It is then possible to trace the inheritance of the disease-producing DNA within a family without knowledge of the nature of the genetic defect or its precise location in the genome. [Note: The polymorphism may be known from the study of other families with the disorder, or may be discovered to be unique in the family under investigation.] Second, for autosomal recessive disorders, the presence of an affected individual in the family would aid in the diagnosis. This individual would have the mutation present on both chromosomes, allowing identification of the RFLP associated with the genetic disorder.

b. **RFLP analysis:** The presence of abnormal genes for *PAH* can be shown using DNA polymorphisms as markers to distinguish between normal and mutant genes. For example, Figure 33.18 shows a typical pattern obtained when DNA from the white blood cells of a family is cleaved with an appropriate restriction enzyme and subjected to electrophoresis. The vertical arrows represent the cleavage sites for the restriction enzyme used. The presence of a polymorphic site (see p. 473 for a discussion of polymorphisms) creates fragment "b" in the autoradiogram (after hybridization with a labeled *PAH*-cDNA probe), whereas the absence of this site yields only fragment "a." Note that Subject II-2 demonstrates that the polymorphism, as shown by the presence of fragment "b," is associated with the mutant gene. Therefore, in this particular family, the appearance of fragment "b" corresponds to the presence of a polymorphic site that tags the abnormal gene for *PAH*. The absence of fragment "b" corresponds to having only the normal gene. In Figure 33.18, examination of fetal DNA shows that the fetus inherited two abnormal genes from its parents and, therefore, has PKU.

c. **Value of screening:** DNA-based screening is useful not only in determining if an unborn fetus is affected, but also in detecting carriers of the mutated gene. PKU, like many inborn errors of amino acid metabolism, is inherited as an autosomal recessive trait. Identification of heterozygotes can aid in future family planning.

VII. POLYMERASE CHAIN REACTION

The polymerase chain reaction (PCR) is a test tube method for amplifying a selected DNA sequence that does not rely on the biologic cloning method described on p. 467. PCR permits the synthesis of millions of copies of a specific nucleotide sequence in a few hours. It can amplify the sequence, even when the targeted sequence makes up less than one part in a million of the total initial sample. The method can be used to amplify DNA sequences from any source—bacterial, viral, plant, or animal. The steps in PCR are summarized in Figures 33.19 and 33.20.

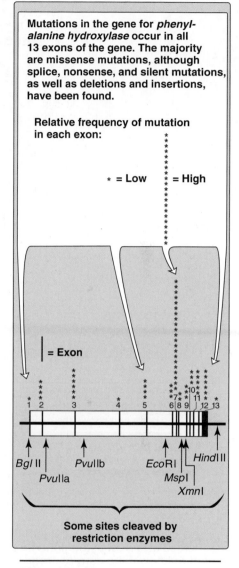

Mutations in the gene for *phenylalanine hydroxylase* occur in all 13 exons of the gene. The majority are missense mutations, although splice, nonsense, and silent mutations, as well as deletions and insertions, have been found.

Relative frequency of mutation in each exon:

* = Low   = High

= Exon

Bgl II   *Pvu*IIb   *Eco*RI   *Hind*III
*Pvu*IIa   *Msp*I
                              *Xmn*I

Some sites cleaved by restriction enzymes

Figure 33.17
The gene for *phenylalanine hydroxylase* showing 13 exons, restriction sites, and some of the mutations resulting in phenylketonuria.

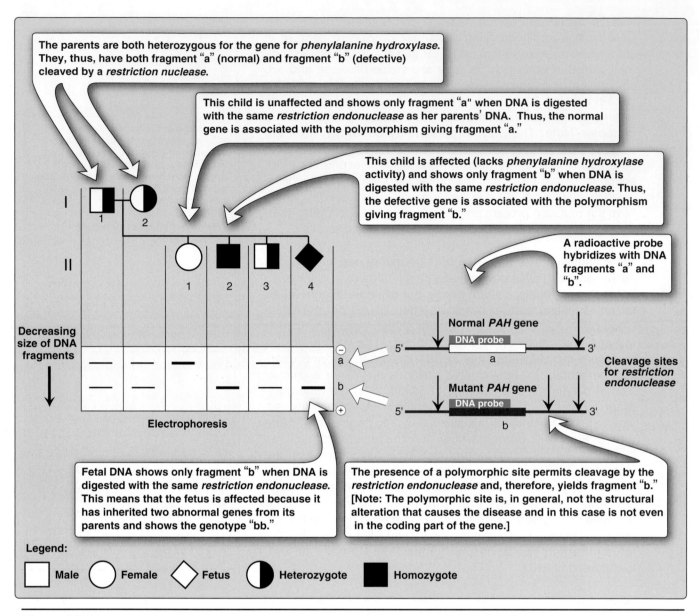

Figure 33.18
Analysis of restriction fragment length polymorphism in a family with a child affected by phenylketonuria. The molecular defect in the gene for *phenylalanine hydroxylase* (*PAH*) in the family is not known. The family wanted to know if the current pregnancy would be affected by phenylketonuria.

A. Steps of a PCR

PCR uses *DNA polymerase* to repetitively amplify targeted portions of DNA. Each cycle of amplification doubles the amount of DNA in the sample, leading to an exponential increase in DNA with repeated cycles of amplification. The amplified DNA sequence can then be analyzed by gel electrophoresis, Southern blotting, or direct sequence determination.

1. **Primer construction:** It is not necessary to know the nucleotide sequence of the target DNA in the PCR method. However, it is necessary to know the nucleotide sequence of short segments on

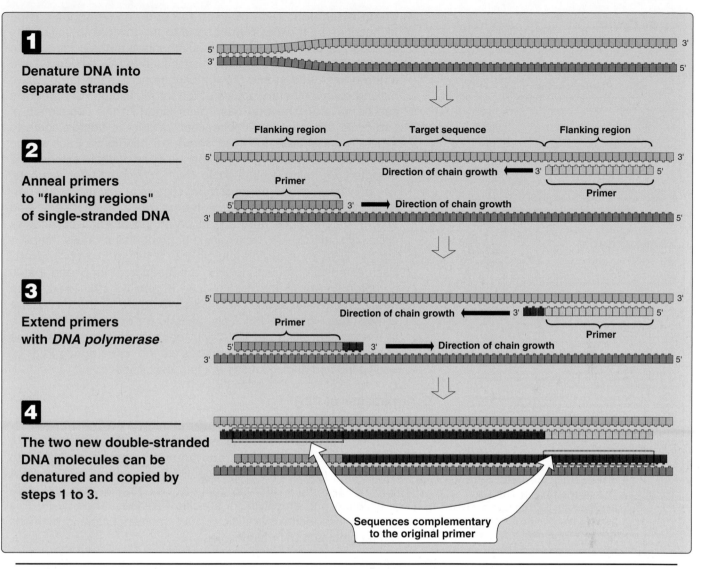

Figure 33.19
Steps in one cycle of the polymerase chain reaction.

each side of the target DNA. These stretches, called flanking sequences, bracket the DNA sequence of interest. The nucleotide sequences of the flanking regions are used to construct two, single-stranded oligonucleotides, usually 20–35 nucleotides long, which are complementary to the respective flanking sequences. The 3'-hydroxyl end of each oligonucleotide points toward the target sequence (see Figure 33.19). These synthetic oligonucleotides function as primers in PCR reactions.

2. **Denature the DNA:** The DNA to be amplified is heated to separate the double-stranded target DNA into single strands.

3. **Annealing of primers to ssDNA:** The separated strands are cooled and allowed to anneal to the two primers (one for each strand).

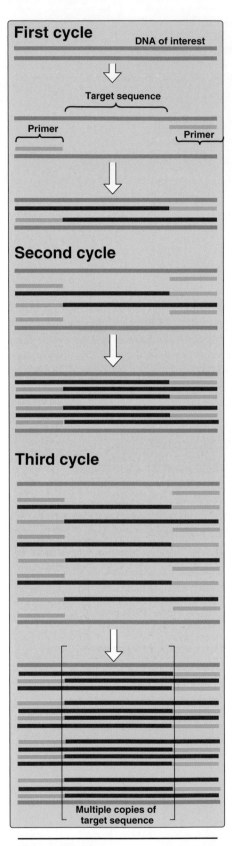

Figure 33.20
Multiple cycles of polymerase chain reaction.

4. **Chain extension:** *DNA polymerase* and deoxyribonucleoside triphosphates (in excess) are added to the mixture to initiate the synthesis of two new strands complementary to the original DNA strands. *DNA polymerase* adds nucleotides to the 3'-hydroxyl end of the primer, and strand growth extends across the target DNA, making complementary copies of the target. [Note: PCR products can be several thousand base pairs long.] At the completion of one cycle of replication, the reaction mixture is heated again to separate the strands (of which there are now four). Each strand binds a complementary primer, and the cycle of chain extension is repeated. By using a heat-stable *DNA polymerase* (for example, *Taq polymerase* from the bacterium, <u>Thermus</u> <u>aquaticus</u> that normally lives at high temperatures), the *polymerase* is not denatured and, therefore, does not have to be added at each successive cycle. Typically 20–30 cycles are run during this process, amplifying the DNA by a million-fold (2^{20}) to a billion-fold (2^{30}). [Note: Each extension product includes a sequence at its 5'-end that is complementary to the primer (see Figure 33.19). Thus, each newly synthesized strand can act as a template for the successive cycles (see Figure 33.20). This leads to an exponential increase in the amount of target DNA with each cycle hence the name "polymerase chain reaction."] Probes can be made during PCR by adding labeled nucleotides to the last few cycles.

B. Advantages of PCR

The major advantages of PCR over cloning as a mechanism for amplifying a specific DNA sequence are sensitivity and speed. DNA sequences present in only trace amounts can be amplified to become the predominant sequence. PCR is so sensitive that DNA sequences present in an individual cell can be amplified and studied. Isolating and amplifying a specific DNA sequence by PCR is faster and less technically difficult than traditional cloning methods using recombinant DNA techniques.

C. Applications

PCR has become a very common tool for a large number of applications. These include:

1. **Comparison of a normal cloned gene with an uncloned mutant form of the gene:** PCR allows the synthesis of mutant DNA in sufficient quantities for a sequencing protocol without laboriously cloning the altered DNA.

2. **Detection of low-abundance nucleic acid sequences:** For example, viruses that have a long latency period, such as human immunodeficiency virus (HIV), are difficult to detect at the early stage of infection using conventional methods. PCR offers a rapid and sensitive method for detecting viral DNA sequences even when only a small proportion of cells is harboring the virus.

3. **Forensic analysis of DNA samples:** DNA fingerprinting by means of PCR has revolutionized the analysis of evidence from crime scenes. DNA isolated from a single human hair, a tiny spot of

blood, or a sample of semen is sufficient to determine whether the sample comes from a specific individual. The DNA markers analyzed for such fingerprinting are most commonly short tandem repeat polymorphisms. These are very similar to the VNTRs described previously (see p. 475), but are smaller in size. [Note: Verification of paternity uses the same techniques.]

4. **Prenatal diagnosis and carrier detection of cystic fibrosis:** Cystic fibrosis is an autosomal recessive genetic disease resulting from mutations in the gene for the cystic fibrosis transmembrane conductance regulator (CFTR) protein. The most common mutation is a three-base deletion that results in the loss of a phenylalanine residue from the CFTR protein (see p. 434). Because the mutant allele is three bases shorter than the normal allele, it is possible to distinguish them from each other by the size of the PCR products obtained by amplifying that portion of the DNA. Figure 33.21 illustrates how the results of such a PCR test can distinguish between homozygous normal, heterozygous (carriers), and homozygous mutant (affected) individuals.

> PCR can generate 100 billion identical copies of a specific DNA sequence in an afternoon, using a highly automated system.

VIII. ANALYSIS OF GENE EXPRESSION

The tools of biotechnology not only allow the study of gene structure, but also provide ways of analyzing the products of gene expression— mRNA and proteins.

A. Determination of mRNA levels

Messenger RNA levels are usually determined by the hybridization of labeled probes to either mRNA itself or to cDNA produced from mRNA. [Note: Amplification of cDNA made from mRNA by retroviral *reverse transcriptase* (*RT*) is referred to as RT-PCR.]

1. **Northern blots:** Northern blots are very similar to Southern blots (see Figure 33.12, p. 474), except that the original sample contains a mixture of mRNA molecules that are separated by electrophoresis, then transferred to a membrane and hybridized to a radiolabeled probe. The bands obtained by autoradiography give a measure of the amount and size of particular mRNA molecules in the sample.

2. **Microarrays:** DNA microarrays contain thousands of immobilized DNA sequences organized in an area no larger than a microscope slide. These microarrays are used to analyze a sample for the presence of gene variations or mutations (genotyping), or to determine the patterns of mRNA production (gene expression analysis), analyzing thousands of genes at the same time. For genotyping analysis, the cellular sample is genomic DNA. For expression analysis, the population of mRNA molecules from a

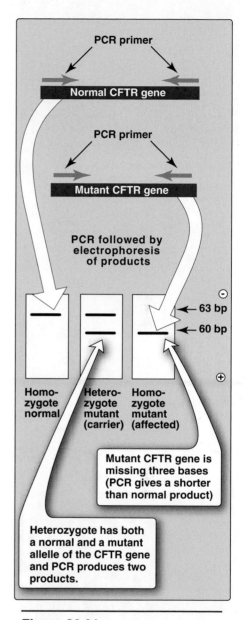

Figure 33.21
Genetic testing for cystic fibrosis using PCR. CFTR = cystic fibrosis transmembrane conductance regulator.

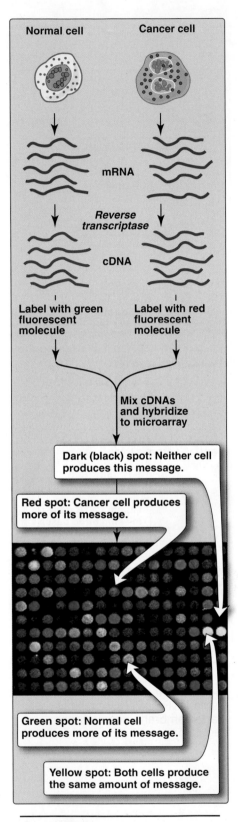

Figure 33.22
Microarray analysis of gene
expression.

particular cell type is converted to cDNA and labeled with a fluorescent tag (Figure 33.22). This mixture is then exposed to a gene chip, which is a glass slide or membrane containing thousands of tiny spots of DNA, each corresponding to a different gene. The amount of fluorescence bound to each spot is a measure of the amount of that particular mRNA in the sample. DNA microarrays are often used to determine the differing patterns of gene expression in two different types of cell—for example, normal and cancer cells (see Figure 33.22). Physicians hope to one day be able to tailor treatment regimens to each cancer patient, based on the specific microarray expression patterns exhibited by that patient's individual tumor.

B. Analysis of proteins

The kinds and amounts of proteins in cells do not always directly correspond to the amounts of mRNA present. Some mRNAs are translated more efficiently than others, and some proteins undergo posttranslational modifications by adding sugars or lipids, or both. When investigating one, or a limited number of gene products, it is convenient to use labeled antibodies to detect and quantify specific proteins. However, when analyzing the abundance and interactions of large numbers of cellular proteins (called proteomics, see below), automated methods employing two-dimensional gel electrophoresis, mass spectrometry, multidimensional liquid chromatography, and bioinformatics are employed.

1. **Enzyme-linked immunosorbent assays (ELISA):** These assays are performed in the wells of a plastic microtiter dish. The antigen (protein) is bound to the plastic of the dish. The probe used consists of an antibody specific for the particular protein to be measured. The antibody is covalently bound to an enzyme, which will produce a colored product when exposed to its substrate. The amount of color produced can be used to determine the amount of protein (or antibody) in the sample to be tested.

2. **Western blots:** Western blots (also called immunoblots) are similar to Southern blots, except that protein molecules in the sample are separated by electrophoresis and blotted (transferred) to a membrane. The probe is a labeled antibody, which produces a band at the location of its antigen.

3. **Detecting exposure to HIV:** ELISA and Western blots are commonly used to detect exposure to HIV by measuring the amount of anti-HIV antibodies present in a patient's blood sample. ELISAs are used as the primary screening tool, because they are very sensitive. These assays sometimes give false positives, however, so Western blots, which are more specific, are often used as a confirmatory test (Figure 33.23). [Note: ELISA and Western blots can only detect HIV exposure after anti-HIV antibodies appear in the bloodstream. PCR-based testing for HIV is more useful in the first few months after exposure.]

4. Proteomics: The study of all proteins expressed by a genome, including their relative abundance, distribution, posttranslational modifications, functions, and interactions with other macromolecules, is known as proteomics. The 20,000 to 30,000 protein-coding genes of the human genome translate into over 100,000 proteins when posttranscriptional and posttranslational modifications are considered. Although a genome remains unchanged, the amounts and types of proteins in any particular cell change dramatically as genes are turned on and off. Proteomics offers the potential of identifying new disease markers and drug targets. Figure 33.24 compares some of the analytic techniques discussed in this chapter.

IX. GENE THERAPY

The goal of gene therapy is to insert the normal, cloned DNA for a gene into the somatic cells of a patient who has a defect in that gene as a result of some disease-causing mutation. The DNA must become permanently integrated into the patient's chromosomes in such a way as to be properly expressed to produce the correct protein. For example, patients with severe combined immunodeficiency disease (SCID) have an immune deficiency as a result of mutations in either the gene for *adenosine deaminase* (see p. 301) or a gene coding for an interleukin receptor subunit (X-linked severe combined immunodeficiency, or SCID-X1). Patients with both kinds of SCID have been successfully treated by incorporating functional copies of the appropriate gene into their cells (Figure 33.25). [Note: This is often called "gene replacement therapy."] Although gene therapy is an attractive therapeutic strategy for individuals with inherited diseases, the method is not without risks. For example, retrovirus-mediated gene transfer was able to correct SCID-X1 in nine of ten patients. However, leukemias developed in several of the patients, presumably because of activation of a hematopoietic oncogene. Clearly, gene therapy is a work in progress.

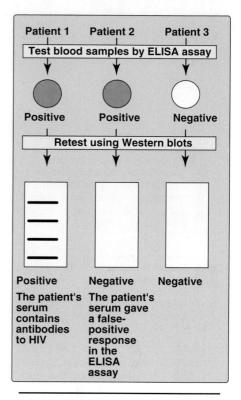

Figure 33.23
Testing for HIV exposure by enzyme-linked immunosorbent assays (ELISA) and Western blots.

TECHNIQUE	SAMPLE ANALYZED	GEL USED	PURPOSE
Southern blot	DNA	Yes	Detects DNA changes
Northern blot	RNA	Yes	Measures mRNA amounts and sizes
Western blot	Protein	Yes	Measures protein amounts
ASO	DNA	No	Detects DNA mutations
Microarray	cDNA or genomic DNA	No	Measures many mRNA levels at once; detects genomic changes
ELISA	Proteins or antibodies	No	Detects proteins (antigens) or antibodies; detects genomic changes
Proteomics	Proteins	Yes	Measures abundance, distribution, posttranslational modifications, functions, and interactions of cellular proteins

Figure 33.24
Techniques used to analyze DNA, RNA, and proteins. ASO = allele-specific oligonucleotides. ELISA = enzyme-linked immunosorbent assay.

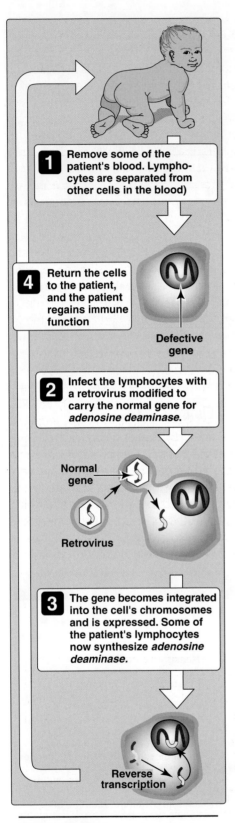

Figure 33.25
Gene therapy for a patient with severe combined immuno-deficiency caused by *adenosine deaminase* deficiency.

X. TRANSGENIC ANIMALS

Transgenic animals can be produced by injecting a cloned gene into the fertilized egg. If the gene becomes successfully integrated into a chromosome, it will be present in the germline of the resulting animal, and can be passed along from generation to generation. A giant mouse called "Supermouse" was produced in this way by injecting the gene for rat growth hormone into a fertilized mouse egg. In a similar way, transgenic goats and cows can now be designed that produce human proteins, such as blood clotting factors, in their milk. Sometimes, rather than introducing a functional gene into a mouse, a nonfunctional version is inserted. Such genetically engineered animals can be used to produce a colony of "knockout mice" that lack the product of the affected gene. Such animals can then serve as models for the study of a corresponding human disease. [Note: Knock-in mice result if the inserted gene expresses a mutated product or under (over)-expresses a product.]

XI. CHAPTER SUMMARY

Restriction endonucleases are bacterial enzymes that cleave double-stranded DNA into smaller fragments. Each enzyme cleaves dsDNA at a specific four to eight-base-long nucleotide sequence, producing DNA segments called **restriction fragments**. The sequences that are recognized are **palindromic**. These enzymes form either **staggered cuts (sticky ends)** or **blunt-end cuts** on the DNA. A DNA sequence that is recognized by a restriction enzyme is called a **restriction site**. **Bacterial DNA ligases** can anneal two DNA fragments from different sources if they have been cut by the same restriction endonuclease. This hybrid combination of two fragments is called a **recombinant DNA molecule**. Introduction of a foreign DNA molecule into a replicating cell permits the **amplification** (production of many copies) of the DNA—a process called **cloning**. A **vector** is a molecule of DNA to which the fragment of DNA to be cloned is attached. Vectors must be capable of **autonomous replication** within the host cell, and must contain at least one specific nucleotide sequence recognized by a restriction endonuclease. It must also carry at least one gene that confers the ability to select for the vector, such as an **antibiotic resistance gene**. Prokaryotic organisms normally contain small, circular, extrachromosomal DNA molecules called **plasmids** that can serve as **vectors**. They can be readily isolated from the bacterium, joined with the DNA of interest, and reintroduced into the bacterium which will replicate, thus making multiple copies of the **hybrid plasmid**. A **DNA library** is a collection of cloned restriction fragments of the DNA of an organism. **A genomic library** is a collection of fragments of double-stranded DNA obtained by digestion of the total DNA of the organism with a restriction endonuclease and subsequent ligation to an appropriate vector. It ideally contains a copy of every DNA nucleotide sequence in the genome. In contrast, **complementary DNA (cDNA) libraries** contain only those DNA sequences that are complementary to messenger RNA (mRNA) molecules present in a cell, and differ from one cell type to another. Because cDNA has no intervening sequences, it can be cloned into an **expression vector** for the synthesis of eukaryotic proteins by bacteria. Cloned, then purified, fragments of DNA can be sequenced, for example, using the **Sanger dideoxy method**. A **probe** is a small, single-stranded piece of DNA (usually labeled with a radioisotope, such as ^{32}P, or another recognizable compound, such as biotin) which has a nucleotide sequence complementary to the DNA molecule of interest (**target DNA**). Probes can be used to identify which clone of a library or which band on a gel contains the target DNA. **Southern blotting** is a technique that can be used to detect specific sequences present in DNA. The DNA is cleaved using a **restriction endonuclease**, and the pieces are separated by **gel electrophoresis** and are denatured and transferred (blotted) to a **nitrocellulose membrane** for analysis. The fragment of interest is detected using a **probe**. The human genome contains many thousands of polymorphisms (DNA sequence variations at a given locus) that do not affect the phenotype of the individual. Polymorphisms can arise from single base changes and from tandem repeats. A polymorphism can serve as a genetic marker that can be followed through families. A restriction fragment length polymorphism is a genetic variant that can be observed by cleaving the DNA into restriction fragments using a restriction enzyme. A base substitution in one or more nucleotides at a restriction site can render the site unrecognizable by a particular restriction endonuclease. A new restriction site also can be created by the same mechanism. In either case, cleavage with the endonuclease results in fragments of lengths differing from the normal that can be detected by DNA hybridization. This technique can be used to diagnose genetic diseases early in the gestation of a fetus. The **polymerase chain reaction (PCR)**, a test tube method for **amplifying** a selected DNA sequence, does not rely on the biologic cloning method. PCR permits the synthesis of millions of copies of a specific nucleotide sequence in a few hours. It can amplify the sequence, even when the targeted sequence makes up less than one part in a million of the total initial sample. The method can be used to amplify DNA sequences from any source. **Applications of the PCR technique** include: 1) efficient comparison of a normal cloned gene with an uncloned mutant form of the gene, 2) detection of low-abundance nucleic acid sequences, 3) forensic analysis of DNA samples, and 4) prenatal diagnosis and carrier detection, for example, of cystic fibrosis. The **products of gene expression** (mRNA and proteins) can be measured by techniques such as the following: **Northern blots** are very similar to Southern blots except that the original sample contains a mixture of **mRNA** molecules that are separated by electrophoresis, then hybridized to a radiolabeled probe. **Microarrays** are used to determine the differing patterns of gene expression in two different types of cells—for example, normal and cancer cells. **Enzyme-linked immunosorbent assays** and **Western blots (immunoblots)** are used to detect specific proteins. The goal of **gene therapy** is the insertion of a normal gene to replace a defective gene. Insertion of a foreign gene into an animal creates a **transgenic animal** that can produce therapeutic proteins or serve as a model for human diseases.

Study Questions

Choose the ONE correct answer.

33.1 *Hind*III is a restriction endonuclease commonly used to cut human DNA into pieces before inserting it into a plasmid. Which of the following is most likely to be the recognition sequence for this enzyme?

    A. AAGGAA.

    B. AAGAAG.

    C. AAGTTC.

    D. AAGCTT.

    E. AAGAGA.

Correct answer = D. The vast majority of restriction endonucleases recognize palindromes, and AAGCTT is the only palindrome among the choices. Because the sequence of only one DNA strand is given, one must determine the base sequence of the complementary strand. To be a palindrome, both strands must have the same sequence when read in the 5'→3' direction. Thus, the complement of 5'-AAGCTT-3' is also 5'-AAGCTT-3'.

33.2 An Ashkenazi Jewish couple brings their 6-month-old son to you for evaluation of listlessness, poor head control, and a fixed gaze. You determine that he has Tay-Sachs disease, an autosomal recessive disorder. The couple also has a daughter. The diagram below shows this family's pedigree, along with Southern blots of an RFLP very closely linked to the hexosaminidase A gene, which is defective in Tay-Sachs. Which of the statements below is most accurate with respect to the daughter?

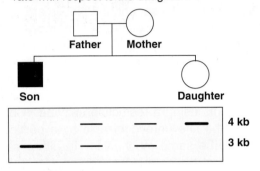

A. She has a 25% chance of having Tay-Sachs disease.

B. She has a 50% chance of having Tay-Sachs disease.

C. She has Tay-Sachs disease.

D. She is a carrier for Tay-Sachs disease.

E. She is homozygous normal.

Correct answer = E. Both the father and mother must be carriers for this disease. The son must have inherited a mutant allele from each parent. Because he shows only the 3-kb band on the Southern blot, the mutant allele for this disease must be linked to the 3-kb band for both parents. The normal allele must be linked to the 4-kb band in both parents. Because the daughter inherited the 4-kb band from both parents, she must be homozygous normal for the hexosaminidase A gene.

33.3 A physician would like to determine the global patterns of gene expression in two different types of tumor cells in order to develop the most appropriate form of chemotherapy for each patient. Which of the following techniques would be most appropriate for this purpose?

A. Southern blot.

B. Northern blot.

C. Western blot.

D. ELISA.

E. Microarray.

Correct answer = E. Microarray analysis allows the determination of mRNA production (thus, gene expression) from thousands of genes at once. A Northern blot only measures mRNA production from one gene at a time. Western blots and ELISA measure protein production (also gene expression), but only from one gene at a time. Southern blots are used to analyze DNA, not gene expression.

33.4 A 2-week-old infant is diagnosed with a urea cycle defect. Enzymic analysis showed no activity for ornithine transcarbamoylase (OTC). Molecular analysis revealed that the mRNA product of the gene for OTC was identical to that of a control. Which of the techniques listed below was most likely used to analyze the size and amount of the mRNA?

A. Dideoxy chain termination.

B. Northern blot.

C. Polymerase chain reaction.

D. Southern blot

E. Western blot

Correct answer = B. Northern blot allows analysis of the mRNA present (expressed) in a particular cell or tissue. Southern blot is used for DNA analysis, whereas Western blot is used for protein analysis. Dideoxy chain termination is used to sequence DNA. Polymerase chain reaction (PCR) is used to generate multiple, identical copies of a DNA sequence in vitro.

Index

25-Hydroxycholecalciferol 1-hydroxylase, 386
  regulation of, 386–388
5-Hydroxy-6,8,11,14 eicosatetraenoic acid (5-
  HPETE), 214, 215f
α-Hydroxylase, 195
11-β-Hydroxylase deficiency, 238f
17-α-Hydroxylase deficiency, 238f
21-α-Hydroxylase deficiency, 238f
Hydroxylation
  in collagen, 45, 45f, 46f, 47
  of proteins, 444, 444f
Hydroxylysine, in collagen, 45, 45f, 46f, 47
Hydroxymethylbilane, 279, 279f
Hydroxymethylbilane synthase, 281f
3-Hydroxy-3-methylglutaryl CoA (HMG CoA),
  220, 220f
*3-Hydroxy-3-methylglutaryl CoA (HMG CoA)
  reductase,* 220–221, 232
  gene expression of, sterol-dependent,
    222–223, 223f
  inhibition of, 232
  phosphorylation and dephosphorylation of,
    223, 223f
  regulation of, 222–224, 223f
*3-Hydroxy-3-methylglutaryl CoA (HMG CoA)
  synthase*
  in cholesterol synthesis, 220, 220f
  in ketone body synthesis, 196, 196f
*Hydroxymethylglutaryl CoA reductase (HMG
  CoA reductase),* 61
Hydroxyproline
  in collagen, 45, 45f, 46f, 47
  in elastin, 49
3-β-Hydroxysteroid dehydrogenase
  deficiency, 238f
5-Hydroxytryptamine. *See* Serotonin
5-Hydroxytryptophan, 287, 287f
Hydroxyurea, 36, 298
hyperammonemia, 257–258, 258f
  acquired, 258
  hereditary, 258
Hyperbilirubinemia, 284, 284f
Hypercalcemia, vitamin D and, 389
Hypercholesterolemia, 224, 226
Hyperglycemia
  in diabetes mellitus
    type 1, 338–339, 339
    type 2, 344
  glucose phosphorylation in, 98
  sorbitol and, 140
Hyperlipidemia/hyperlipoproteinemia
  niacin for, 380
  type I, 178, 229
  type II, 232
  type IIb, 380
  type III, familial, 231
Hyperoxaluria, primary Type 1, 253
Hyperphosphatemia, 389
Hypertension
  diabetes mellitus and, 346
  obesity and, 354f
  treatment of, 239
Hypertriacylglycerolemia, 229
  in diabetes mellitus
    type 1, 339–340
    in type 2, 344
Hyperuricemia, 296, 299
Hypervitaminosis A, 385–386
Hypocalcemia, 388, 389
Hypochlorous acid (HOCl), 150
Hypoglycemia, **314–318,** 319f
  alcohol-induced, 317–318, 317f
  brain damage in, 327
  characteristics of, 314

concept map, 319f
fasting, 317
glucagon and, 315, 315f, 316
glucoregulatory systems in, 315f, 316
insulin-induced, 316, 316f
postprandial, 316
symptoms of, 314–315
  adrenergic, 314
  neuroglycopenic, 314
in type 1 diabetes, 340–341, 341f
types of, 316–318
Hypoglycemia unawareness, 341
Hypoglycemic agents, for diabetes mellitus
  type 2, 344
Hypoparathyroidism, 389
Hypopigmentation, in PKU, 271
Hypoprothrombinemia, 390
Hypoxanthine, 299
*Hypoxanthine-guanine
  phosphoribosyltransferase (HGPRT),*
  296, 296f, 301
Hypoxia, 2,3-bisphosphoglycerate in, 32, 32f

I

I-cell disease, 169
Icterus. *See* Jaundice
Iduronate sulfatase deficiency, 164f
L-Iduronic acid
  in glycosaminoglycans, 157, 157f, 161
  synthesis of, 161
α-L-Iduronidase deficiency, 164f
Immunoblots, 484, 485f
Immunodeficiency syndromes. *See also*
  Human immunodeficiency virus
  (HIV); Severe combined
  immunodeficiency disease (SCID)
  DNA repair defects and, 413
Immunoglobulin G (IgG), 165
Immunoglobulins, production of, 461, 461f
IMP. *See* Inosine monophosphate
Inborn errors of metabolism, 270–274
Incretins, 310
Indomethacin, 214, 301
Infarction, in sickle cell disease, 36, 37f
Inflammatory processes, in gout, 299
Influenza, nutrition and, 361f
Initiation codons, 438f, 439
Initiator tRNA, 438f, 439
Inner membrane particles, 74
iNOS, 151
Inosine, for boosting 2,3-BPG levels in blood,
  32
Inosine monophosphate dehydrogenase, 295f
Inosine monophosphate (IMP)
  conversion to AMP and GMP, 295–296,
    295f
  as parent purine nucleotide, 293
  in purine synthesis, 293–296, 294f
  synthesis of, 293
Inositol 1,4,5-triphosphate (IP₃), in signal
  transmission, 205–206, 205f
Inositol triphosphate (ITP), in intracellular
  signaling, 205, 205f
Insig protein, 223
In situ hybridization, 472
Insulin, **307–313,** 353
  in absorptive/fed state, 328f
  in *acetyl CoA carboxylase* regulation, 184,
    184f
  anabolic effects of, 308
  carbohydrate metabolism and, 311
  concept map, 319f
  deficiency of
    absolute, in type 1 diabetes mellitus,

    336, 336f
    relative, in type 2 diabetes mellitus,
      341
  degradation of, 308
  epinephrine and, 310, 310f, 319f
  exogenous. *See* Insulin therapy
  fructose 2,6-bisphosphate and, 100, 100f
  glucagon opposing action of, 314, 319f
  glucagon secretion and, 309, 313
  glucokinase and, 310, 313
  glycerol phosphate synthesis and, 189
  glycogen degradation and, 133
  glycolysis and, 105, 105f
  in *HMG CoA reductase* regulation, 223
  hormone-sensitive lipase and, 190
  in hypoglycemia, 314–318, 315f
  hypoglycemia and
    alcohol consumption and, 318
  in integration of metabolism, 307
  lipid metabolism and, 311
  mechanism of action, 311–313, 311f
  membrane effects of, 312, 312f
  metabolic effects of, 311
  phosphofructokinase and, 313
  protein synthesis and, 311
  secretion of
    amino acids and, 310
    by β cells, 310, 310f
    coordination with glucagon secretion
      and, 309, 314
    gastrointestinal hormones and, 310
    glucose levels and, 310, 310f
    inhibition of, 310
    during onset of type 1 diabetes
      mellitus, 338, 338f
    regulation of, 309–310, 310f, 313
    stimulation of, 309–310
  in signal transduction, 311f, 312
  structure of, 308, 308f
  synthesis of, 308, 308f
  time course of actions, 313
  triacylglycerol degradation and, 189, 190f
Insulinase, 308
Insulin-dependent glucose transport (GLUT-4)
  proteins, 331
Insulin-induced hypoglycemia, 316, 316f
Insulin receptor, 311–312, 311f
Insulin receptor substrate (IRS) proteins, 311f,
  312
Insulin resistance
  causes of, 343
  obesity and, 342
  in type 2 diabetes mellitus, 342–343, 343f
Insulin resistance syndrome, 353
Insulin-sensitive glucose transporters (GLUT-
  4), 312
Insulin therapy
  hypoglycemia induced by, 316, 316f,
    340–341, 340f
  for type 1 diabetes mellitus, 340, 340f
    standard *vs.* intensive, 340, 340f
  for type 2 diabetes mellitus, 344
Insulitis, 338
Intercellular communication, 94, 94f
Intermediate-density lipoproteins (IDLs), 231
International Union of Biochemistry and
  Molecular Biology (IUBMB), enzyme
  nomenclature of, 53, 53f
Intestinal mucosal cells
  chylomicron assembly in, 177f, 228, 229f
  enzymes synthesized by, carbohydrate
    digestion by, 86–87, 87f
  lipid absorption by, 176, 177f
  lipid secretion by, 177f, 178

Figure Sources

Figure 2.12: Modified from Garrett, R. H. and Grisham, C. M. *Biochemistry.* Saunders College Publishing, 1995. Figure 6.36, p. 193.

Figure 2.13 (panel C, top): Abdulla, S. Basic mechanisms of protein folding disease. Nature Publishing Group.

Figure 3.1A: Illustration: Irving Geis. Rights owned by Howard Hughes Medical Institute. Not to be used without permission

Figure 3.20: Photo curtesy of Photodyne Incorporated, Hartland, WI.

Figure 3.21: Corbis

Figure 4.3: Electron micrograph of collagen: Natural Toxin Research Center. Texas A&M University-Kingsville. Collagen molecule modified from Mathews, C. K., van Holde, K. E. and Ahern, K. G. Biochemistry. 3rd Ed., Addison Wesley Longman, Inc. 2000. Figure 6.13, p.175.

Figure 4.4: modified from Yurchenco, P. D., Birk, D. E., and Mecham, R. P., eds. (1994) Extracellular Matrix Assembly and Structure, Academic Press, San Diego, California

Figure 4.8: Kronauer and Buhler, Images in Clinical Medicine, The New England Journal of Medicine, June 15, 1995 , Vol. 332, No. 24, p.1611.

Figure 4.10: Photo from Web site Derma.de

Figure 4.11: Jorde, L. B., Carey, J. C.,

Bamshad, M. J. and White, R. L. Medical Genetics, 2nd Ed.
http://medgen.genetics.utah.edu/index.htm

Question 4.3: from Berge LN, Marton V, Tranebjaerg L, Kearney MS, Kiserud T, Oian P. Prenatal diagnosis of osteogenesis imperfecta. Acta Obstetricia et Gynecologica Scandinavica. 74(4):321-3, 1995 Apr.

Figure 13.11: The Crookston Collection, University of Toronto.

Figure 17.13: Urbana Atlas of Pathology, University of Illinois College of Medicine at urbana-champaign. Image number 26.

Figure 17.19: Interactive Case Study Companion to Robbins Pathologic Basis of Disease.

Figure 18.12: Custom Medical Stock Photo.

Figure 20.20: Success in MRCO phth. http://www.mrcophth.com/iriscases/albinism.html

Figure 20.22 (top): Rubin, E. and Farber, J. L. Pathology (2nd edition). J. B. Lippincott. 194.Figure 6-30, p. 244.

Figure 20.22 (bottom): Gilbert-Barness, E. and Barness L. *Metabolic Disease.* Eaton Publishing, 2000. Figure 15, p.42.

Figure 21.6: Rich, M. W. Porphyria cutanea tarda, Postgraduate Medicine, 105: 208-214 (1999).

Figure 21.5: Department of Dermatlogy, University of Pittsburgh.
http://www.upmc.edu/dermatology/MedStudentInfo/introLecture/enlarged/vespct.htm.

Figure 21.10: Custom Medical Stock Photo, Inc.

Figure 21.13: Phototake.

Figure 22.16: Wuthrich, D. A., and Lebowitz. Tophaceous gout. Images in clinical Medicine. N Engl J Med, 332:646, 1995.

Figure 22.17: WebMD Inc.
http://www.samed.com/sam/forms/index.htm

Figure 22.18 : Corbis.

Figure 23.2: Childs, G.
http://www.cytochemistry.net/.

Figure 24.4: Phototake.

Figure 26.6: Corbis.

Figure 27.20: Joseph E. Armstrong Illinois State University.

Figure 28.4: Matthews, J. H. Queen's University Department of Medicine, Division of Hematology/Oncology, Kingston, Canada.

Figure 29.7: Nolan, J., Department of Biochemistry, Tulane University, New Orleans, LA.

Figure 23.13: Modified from Cryer, P. E., Fisher, J. N. and Shamoon, H. Hypoglycemia. Diabetes Care 17:734-753, 1994.